USER-CENTERED ASSESSMENT DESIGN

With my sincere thanks for
excellent care –
Madhabi Chatterji

User-Centered Assessment Design

An Integrated Methodology for Diverse Populations

Madhabi Chatterji

THE GUILFORD PRESS
New York London

A Division of Guilford Publications, Inc.
www.guilford.com

Printed in the United States of America

This book is printed on acid-free paper.

Last digit is print number: 9 8 7 6 5 4 3 2 1

Library of Congress Cataloging-in-Publication Data

Names: Chatterji, Madhabi, author.
Title: User-centered assessment design : an integrated methodology for diverse populations / Madhabi Chatterji.
Description: New York : The Guilford Press, [2025] | Includes bibliographical references and index. |
Identifiers: LCCN 2024013762 | ISBN 9781462555482 (cloth)
Subjects: LCSH: Educational tests and measurements—Methodology. | Evaluation.
Classification: LCC LB3051 .C455 2025 | DDC 371.26/2—dc23/eng/20240522
LC record available at *https://lccn.loc.gov/2024013762*

For my collaborators, mentees, advisees, and students—
past, present, and future—with gratitude

Preface

This book emerged from my 21-plus years of teaching experiences with graduate-level and professional audiences from multidisciplinary areas at Teachers College, Columbia University, in New York. To begin, I offer a quick glimpse into the essence of this book, what it will and will *not* provide, for whom it is intended, and its organization. I end with some necessary and grateful acknowledgments.

Why a New Assessment Book?

Why another assessment book and, specifically, a book on designing assessments? No doubt, there are numerous "off-the-shelf" assessment instruments available today for those interested, especially on the internet. In my graduate-level courses at Columbia, however, I routinely encountered participants from different disciplinary areas who were drawn to assessment with very particular instrumentation interests and problems in mind. Broadly from the social and behavioral sciences, these individuals were in a variety of professional roles in education, psychology, medicine, and the health fields. While most were still under training to become researchers or practitioners in their respective fields, many were already practicing professionals. Once enrolled, they almost always sought to strengthen their formal knowledge in measurement and evaluation methods in general, and in translating that knowledge to fulfill their immediate professional needs. For readers and adopters of this book who identify with this audience, I hope that this work provides useful solutions to their problems, while bolstering their background knowledge and technical skills in the desired directions.

What This Book Is About

True to its title, this book is in equal parts about *assessment design* and *assessment use*. In contrast to other textbooks on measurement–assessment topics for the above audiences, its point of departure lies in the incorporation of *user-centered design* principles throughout, founded on a realist view of science and informed by a socioecological perspective (more on this in Chapter 1). Fundamentally, this means that the book treats the theoretical and methodological considerations pertinent to designing instruments with the help of an integrative Process Model for Assessment Design, Validation, and Use®. This model is guided by what is likely to be most important to the primary users of assessment tools. In the book, I introduce a two-part concept of *utility* as a quality criterion for assessment instruments; utility comprises the dual notions of *usefulness* and *usability* of the tools for its primary users.

The subtitle of the book also includes the words "diverse populations." I have tried to situate the assessment design concepts, theory, and methods in a variety of disciplines and diverse application contexts. That is, the illustrative cases and examples assume that the instrument design projects of interest to readers and potential adopters could be from different fields of research or professional practice within the broad realm of the social and behavioral sciences. The instruments could be designed for socially and demographically diverse populations in local, national, or global settings.

Starting with the first chapter, the book introduces and elucidates in the chapters that follow the recommended user-centered approach to assessment design. It presents an argument for the approach with theoretical discussions, case studies, and applied instrumentation projects guided by the Process Model. The citations of my own and my students'/colleagues' works are presented as real-life applications of the Process Model by active researchers and professionals. In some cases, these are intended to demonstrate specific steps of the methodology. I hope these project descriptions add credence to the model and the book's recommendations.

What This Book Is Not

Beyond an occasional or a brief mention, this book does not provide in-depth treatments of any specialized or advanced methodological topics in measurement, psychometrics, or statistics (e.g., scaling methods, test equating, item response theory, generalizability theory, missing data treatments). Nevertheless, the book gives attention to the theoretical and historical foundations of selected measurement topics as relevant to applied aspects of assessment design and validation. To the extent possible, I have kept the discussions direct and practical, without diluting or avoiding any technical subject matter pertinent to sound assessment practices in a general sense. If some technical discussions or topics appear dense from time to time, the concepts and ideas are revisited with new applications and examples throughout, with added elaborations to facilitate readability and accessibility for nontechnical audiences outside measurement.

I hope readers will benefit from the large number of international and cross-disciplinary works cited throughout the book, as appropriate, including some historical and current literature sources on testing and measurement topics. A good deal of the early history of the testing field took place in the United States, where the field continues to evolve and influence global assessment practices (see Chapter 2). Should the older historical citations appear outdated to some, those are the seminal writings that could not be omitted here. Most are widely acknowledged as having stood the test of time and continue to influence thinking and practices in assessment and evaluation today. The United States is also where I myself have been immersed in measurement–evaluation for the past 35 years. In preparing this work, I have tried to draw on this firsthand learning and base of experience as a researcher, scholar, and professional in as honest a manner as possible.

Audience for This Book

The primary audience for the book, as suggested, includes graduate students, researchers, or professionals-in-training in various social science disciplines and related applied fields, including but not limited to education, psychology, social work, nursing, business, counseling, medicine/medical education, and other health professions. A second audience for this book consists of active consultants or consultants-in-training in the assessment and evaluation fields. This latter group typically includes individuals who are interested in providing technical consultation in measurement and evaluation methods to researchers, practitioners, and policymakers in other fields, and may include doctoral-level students in measurement–evaluation degree programs in education or psychology.

Organization of This Book

As the table of contents shows, the book is organized in three main sections. Section I (Chapters 1–3) deals with the foundations; Section II (Chapters 4–7) focuses on design; Section III (Chapters 9–12) is dedicated to validation and use. Chapter 8 is a supplementary chapter on basic statistics; this material is excerpted with adaptations from my earlier book (Chatterji, 2003).

To orient readers, each chapter begins with a brief overview and chapter objectives and ends with a chapter summary. Technical or new terminology is highlighted in bold font and defined in nearby text; definitions for those same terms again appear in the end-of-book Glossary. Intermittently, readers will find "Quick Recaps" and "Reflection Breaks" tied to chapter objectives for facilitating individual thinking or group discussions.

Suggestions: How to Use This Book

The book may be used as a textbook for graduate- and more advanced-level coursework in research methodology focused on instrument design and validation, *or* as a reference guide on instrument design for practicing researchers and professionals in the fields identified. Individual chapters are self-contained and could be used selectively for delivering short courses and workshops for professional development purposes. The material is adaptable for either online or more traditional in-class delivery.

The book is built in large part from my own lecture notes, collections of readings, and sections of my first book. These materials have undergone considerable changes over time—and this book reflects that evolution. Originally, the materials were designed to teach two 15-week semester-long courses in a sequence for graduate and doctoral degree programs in education, health, and psychology at Teachers College, Columbia University. In most of these programs, students were required to conduct research for their theses or dissertations, or prepare research papers for publication and grant applications, often necessitating some formal instrumentation effort. In this sequence, the first course was dedicated to instrument design and the second to conducting validation research. For those interested in adopting this delivery format, the corresponding chapters in the present book are Chapter 1–3, 4–7 (Course 1: Foundations and Design); Chapters 1–3, 8–12 (Course 2: Foundations, Validation, and Use).

MADHABI CHATTERJI

Acknowledgments

Books such as this tend to be arduous and long-term undertakings, even in the best of circumstances. This particular effort has taken me a good 7–8 years of thinking and rethinking, writing, and rewriting, interrupted by a 3-year pandemic and the vagaries of life and living. I persisted for one simple reason: I was offered the chance to do this work. Indeed, I am deeply and sincerely grateful to C. Deborah Laughton and everyone involved at The Guilford Press for their kindnesses. I consider myself fortunate to have had a publisher who placed her faith in my ability to deliver, supporting me with enormous patience, understanding, and encouragement despite the many unforeseen twists and turns. Thank you, CDeb!

I must thank the peer reviewers of early versions of the chapters (invited by the publisher) for their thoughtful, expert feedback and time: Robyn Thomas Pitts, College of Education, University of Denver; Matthew K. Burns, Special Education, University of Missouri–Columbia; Howard Everson, past Vice President of Research for the College Board; Paul Yovanoff, Department of Educational Psychology, Southern Methodist University; Scott L. Decker, Department of Psychology, University of South Carolina; and Beverly Fitzpatrick, School of Pharmacy and School of Education, Memorial University of Newfoundland. Critical as a few reviews were initially, I found them useful and took each one seriously. My own reviews—at points when I picked up the task of revising the material—were often harsher, leading me to continue the rethinking and reorganization efforts. I hope that learning is evident in the final product.

I am equally grateful to each and every one of my students, advisees, mentees, colleagues, and collaborators who enrolled in my courses or reached out to me for assistance with their respective assessment projects. It is for this reason alone that this effort became a labor of love that I just could not relinquish; several of their works are cited with my sincere thanks. Acknowledgments are especially due to Dr. Meiko Lin, Dr. Nancy Koh, Ms. Jooyoung Jeon, Dr. Xiaoxue Du, Ms. Dalveer Kaur, and other graduate research assistants at the Assessment and Evaluation Research Initiative who gave useful feedback or supported me with this work at Teachers College (TC); Dr. Peter Wyer, Dr. Mark Graham, Dr. John Encandela, Zoon Naqvi, Dr. Allison Lee, Dr. Maya Hastie, Dr. Hosam Arqiq, Dr. Amanda Sarafian, and other students, collaborators, and mentees from the Columbia University Medical Center and School of Dentistry; Dr. Jane Bogart, Dr. Bobby J. Belarmino, and others who enrolled in my courses from outside institutions and agreed to share their instrument design efforts as illustrations; my TC faculty colleagues, especially Professor Edmund W. Gordon, Professor John P. Allegrante, Professor Victoria Marsick, and many others who sent their students regularly to my classes over the years; and finally, Professor Eleanor Armour-Thomas (Queens College, CUNY) and Dr. Susan Lyons (Women in Measurement, Inc.), who read and reacted thoughtfully to an early draft of my first chapter that set the stage for the latest iteration of the book.

Lastly, I express my gratitude to the leadership at TC, especially Dr. Katie Embree, and to the Program of Social and Organizational Psychology for providing much-needed administrative support following my retirement, enabling me to bring this book to closure. And I must end this by acknowledging my closest family members, whose love, support, and encouragement boosted me through the most difficult periods in my finishing the project. Ruma, Raka, Alok, Kent, Kavi, Neel, Naveen, and Aura—thank you! I dedicate this effort humbly to all of you.

Madhabi Chatterji

Contents

SECTION I. FOUNDATIONS

SECTION I

FOUNDATIONS

CHAPTER 1

Foundational Concepts in Assessment Design

1.1 Chapter Overview

1.1.1 Introduction

The first chapter introduces selected foundational concepts in measurement alongside the basic elements of the assessment design process. To do so, it first describes three concrete instruments of different modalities, presents the theoretical foundations of a user-centered Process Model for Assessment Design, Validation, and Use®, and reviews the typical ways in which assessments are applied in a range of scientific and professional pursuits. As a preamble to the rest of the book, the first chapter argues for "user-centeredness" when designing tests and assessments. A recent case is analyzed to demonstrate the unexpected and sometimes adverse consequences that could result from an oversight of the primary assessment users' contexts and information needs.

1.1.2 Chapter Objectives

After reading this first chapter and completing the accompanying exercises, the reader should be able to:

1. Define the concept of *assessment*, distinguishing it from measurement, testing, and evaluation, including program evaluation and evaluation research.
2. Recognize the qualitative and quantitative components of the assessment design process.
3. Describe the five features of useful assessments, the principal elements of user-centered assessment design, and the four "portals" of the design process.
4. Describe the philosophical foundations of assessment as a science and field of practice, and its role in a range of scientific and professional human endeavors.
5. Define the quality criteria of validity, reliability, and utility, and unified validation as a part of a user-centered approach to developing high-caliber assessment tools and construct measures.
6. Present an argument for a principled, user-centered approach to assessment design or selection in a variety of user contexts.

1.2 Assessment: Old and Emerging Traditions, a Starting Definition, and Some Distinctions

> There is a distinct tradition in the literature on social science research methods that advocates convergent methodology . . . [the] conception that qualitative and quantitative methods should be viewed as complementary. . . .
>
> —TODD D. JICK (1979, p. 602)

From time immemorial, human beings have devised tests and assessment instruments to measure various characteristics of individuals, entities, or phenomena in the natural, physical, and social world. This book is concerned with the formalized methods, models, and procedures for doing so. Taking the point of view of the human users of the tools, the central question that the book asks is: How could we—as the interested assessment designers, researchers, or practitioners—build or select instruments that are best equipped to serve the interests of the projected human users, taking into account *their* situations, information needs, capacities, and limitations?

We begin by reviewing two quotes. The first, given at the top of this section, speaks to the advantages of combining qualitative and quantitative methods when engaging in social and behavioral inquiry, taken generally. That quote aligns in principle with another historical quote that helped open many a theoretical discussion tailored to measurement and instrumentation topics. The second quote is from Edward L. Thorndike, who once said, "Whatever exists at all exists in some amount. To know it thoroughly involves knowing its *quantity* as well as its *quality*" (E. L. Thorndike, 1918, p. 16; see also Crocker & Algina, 2006, p. 3, emphasis added). Indeed, effective approaches to assessment design require that we begin with deep qualitative understandings of the characteristics we wish to measure. We must then be able to translate those understandings into more succinct, quantified forms of information that facilitate specific kinds of human activity.

Thorndike's work, among that of many others, marked the beginnings of an early-20th-century tradition in testing and measurement that was prevalent in the fields of psychology and education. That tradition spread rapidly to the social and behavioral sciences at large, influencing test design and assessment practices in a vast number of other academic fields and applied professions. Today, tests and assessments are ubiquitous in multidisciplinary areas, both in the United States and overseas. This book stands on a good deal of that foundational knowledge, a tradition that relies predominantly on quantitative methods and psychometric models of research. At the same time, it will call for placing *human users* at the center of the assessment design and use processes (Giacomin, 2014; Norman, 2013), drawing on an equal plane from traditions of qualitative research with *its* methods, tools, and participatory approaches to social inquiry. There is a definitive tradition in social science research advocating for convergent methodology that this book will espouse.

We begin with that reminder, grounded in the philosophy of empirical science from a **social realist** perspective (Carter & New, 2004; see also Creswell & Creswell, 2023). When designing assessment instruments, we will consider both the **qualitative** and **quantitative** properties of characteristics we seek to measure in a convergent, conjoint, and complementary manner, keeping the information needs of prospective human users of the tool at the forefront (Giacomin, 2014)

To grasp what this means, consider an everyday assessment exercise with weather-related events and conditions. Routinely, we make broad-based, qualitative observations about atmospheric characteristics like the daily temperature. We might characterize a day as "pleasant," "too hot," or "too cold" for a particular purpose, such as engaging in an outdoor activity. Concurrently, we might seek to verify those casual observations with quantitative measurements taken with a thermometer. On occasions when our qualitative and quantitative observations align, we are able to conclude more confidently that our general assessments about a given day's temperature are probably accurate. There is greater meaning in the convergent inference we draw from that informal data gathering, as well as more precision.

While the typical mercury or alcohol thermometer is a useful tool for everyday uses by amateurs, meteorologists concerned with more serious weather-forecasting tasks tend to rely on considerably more specialized instrumentation. Weather stations today are equipped with simultaneous sensors that continually measure and track changes on various indicators like atmospheric temperatures, air pressure, rainfall, and so on. However, here too, the same convergence principle applies. The tools that are able to translate the observed *qualitative* properties of the weather characteristics more accurately into precise, *quantitative* forms of data, function better for the purposes that the meteorologists value. The more meaningful and trustworthy the measurements, the smaller the margins of error in the mathematical models that the scientists employ to make weather predictions (Byers, 1994; Glickman, 2000). In this example, the main human users of the instruments are the meteorologists. Their chief concern is the meaningfulness of the data produced by the instruments on given weather characteristics and their usefulness for making predictions. The better-performing assessment instruments would yield more refined, higher-caliber measures that are also dependable.

In the same vein, the most useful instruments in the social and behavioral sciences, and related applied fields where we work, also generate refined quantitative measures of the particular characteristics that interest us, and in terms that meaningfully depict their innate qualitative properties. Instruments that perform this basic function well enable more accurate differentiations of things that are similar versus dissimilar, have more versus less of a characteristic, or are better than worse for serving a specific human need.

QUICK RECAP: During assessment design, we seek to map the qualitative properties of the characteristics we intend to measure with their quantitative representations in a meaningful way. A user-centered approach to assessment design ensures that the tools and information produced by them serve the purposes that human users consider important.

Reflection Break 1.1: Objectives 1, 2, and 4

- Explain why the *principle of convergence* matters in assessment design. Give an example of an assessment tool from your own experience and describe how this principle was applied.
- Based on this section, what is a *user-centered assessment design* approach?
- Think of a clinical mercury thermometer for taking human body temperatures at home. Who are the *primary users* of this instrument? Would you characterize that instrument as *user-centered*? Explain why or why not.

1.2.1 What Is Assessment?

Immediate next questions to arise are: What is *assessment*? Is the concept interchangeable with *measurement*, as the preceding discussion might have suggested? In what ways are assessment and measurement similar? How are they different?

To arrive at acceptable definitions of these two central concepts in assessment design, we must first recognize what the defining features are of a *useful assessment procedure*. For this, let us next turn to examples of three assessment instruments in contrasting modalities. Examine Assessment Cases 1–3 that follow in tandem with Figures 1.1–1.3, intended to introduce selected technical concepts and nomenclature. As we progress, this section will also refer to Tables 1.1 and 1.2, and Box 1.1 that follow.

1.2.1.1 Elements of a Useful Assessment Procedure

ASSESSMENT CASE 1—
A DIAGNOSTIC STUDENT ASSESSMENT

Figure 1.1 shows a multiple-choice test item designed for delivery on a computer-based platform. This assessment item, meant for diagnosing and supporting high school students' learning of science topics, is invented as an illustration from two sources (Thissen-Row, Hunt, & Minstrell, 2004; see the Science Knowledge Quiz at *pewresearch.org*). Other easily accessible online examples appear in the Duolingo assessments, designed for supporting language learning and testing simultaneously with immediate feedback screens (see *www.duolingo.com*). The specific item shown focuses on canonical forms of reasoning dealing with the topic of experimental study designs in a biology unit. A set of similar items presented in paper-and-pencil format would fit our common definitions of a classroom test or quiz. But this assessment is unique in several respects.

First, the item is intended for delivery via a technology-based interface and presented online. Second, the item is a part of a computer adaptive testing system focusing on a specific science topic. Although the colors are not evident in Figure 1.1, an attractive computer interface would likely draw and engage young, post–millennial era students, for most of whom technology is a way of life. On a computer adaptive test, the assessment's administration and task delivery are *adapted* to the respondent's level. Hence, unlike a typical paper-and-pencil test, not everyone who takes the test responds to the same, fixed set of items. The computerized system's built-in algorithm selects a new question based on the student's prior response history to a series of similar questions on given topics.

Item on a computer screen	READ THIS SCENARIO TO ANSWER THE QUESTION BELOW. A scientist is looking for a cure for his rice plants that are infected with a fungus in his neighborhood. He creates a new fungicide (a chemical mixture that is expected to kill the fungus) and conducts a study to see if the fungicide is effective. He puts 20 drops of the fungicide in all the infected plants each day. After two (2) weeks, he finds that all the plants are healed. QUESTION Which of the following changes to the scientist's study would be most helpful in concluding that the fungicide worked? a. Use 20 drops to all plants for one (1) week only. b. Put 20 drops in unhealthy plants for two (2) weeks and compare the results with healthy rice plants in the neighborhood. c. Compare the results with a second, random group of unhealthy plants that did not get the fungicide at all during the two (2) weeks. d. Compare the results with a second, random group of unhealthy plants that got 10 drops of the fungicide daily for two (2) weeks.
Feedback to those selecting Option b	The best and correct answer is option c. You are close if you chose b or d! EXPLANATION Better experiments would randomly assign the treatment to *one* of two or more equivalent groups, before comparing the results. Having a comparison group strengthens the experiment (option b). However, to make sure that all the unhealthy plants had an equal chance to heal *before* the experiment was begun, start with the original group of unhealthy plants and divide them randomly into two subgroups. Then, give one subgroup the "treatment" of 20 drops of fungicide. This will give you a more certain answer on the effectiveness of the fungicide. Adding 10 drops (option d) changes the treatment, making it an unequal comparison.

FIGURE 1.1. A diagnostic science assessment for high school students: Item with feedback screens.

Computer adaptive testing (CAT) methods, elements of which are incorporated in the original assessment from which the illustrative item is devised (Thissen-Row et al., 2004), have proliferated in education since access to computers and the internet has grown. Adaptive assessments offer only the minimal number of items necessary matched to a person's mathematically estimated ability level so as to obtain a reliable picture of their performance, given their starting point and response patterns to the other items. Because of the fewer questions, CAT systems tend to be more time-efficient than traditional tests presented in written, multiple-choice format (Gershon, 2005).

A third feature of this particular item, mentioned at the top, is that it is designed specifically for error-detection and diagnosis of learning status. The item is scored as either right or wrong (the correct answer is option c in Figure 1.1, as shown). However, because of the item's design, a student's choice of a particular *incorrect answer* could point to specific learning issues that create opportunities for corrective feedback, further teaching, and relearning. Although not shown, formative online tasks could be designed in both multiple-choice and short answer format.

The diagnostic feature—unique to Case 1—shows that the assessment item is designed for **formative assessment** purposes. Intentionally, the item provides feedback immediately to its **primary users**—in this case, the students and teachers. Its purpose is to provide learning-relevant information directly back to the students as they engage in the assessment exercise to further their learning, as well as to the teachers who might provide added instructional supports. Depending on a student's responses, the feedback could be an error-related communication pointing to misconceptions; elsewhere, the feedback could be a prompt that makes suggestions for taking the next steps. Together, the results of a series of similar assessment items would allow both students and teachers to make inferences about individual students' learning needs, pointing also to their progress toward mastering the goals of the unit.

Computerized items could be beneficial in other ways. Many software-based assessments today can track the consistency of question-to-question errors made by individual respondents, the time needed to enter answers, and the number of attempts necessary before the final answer is entered. Based on such stored information, systems are programmed to offer immediate feedback to students or teachers on the screens as they engage, as shown in Figure 1.1. The instantaneous feedback, either in verbal, nonverbal, or quantitative form, carries the potential for both learners and teachers to *use* the information productively for supporting teaching–learning activities more effectively. All such built-in properties of items are directly relevant to the intended uses of an assessment and its results for *formative* purposes.

To sum up, by definition, formative classroom assessments should be designed purposefully to yield information that informs learning or instruction, enabling modifications, adjustments, and improvements to both as instruction continues (see Johnson, Sondergeld, & Walton, 2019; Shepard, 2006; Wiliam & Thompson, 2007). In addition, open-ended, person-to-person verbal feedback that teachers or peers provide could be equally or more valuable for shaping classroom learning and the growth of students in given areas, according to some (Hattie & Timperley, 2007). In contrast, **summative assessments** in a similar classroom setting are intended for making final and summary judgments of overall student performance. Hence, by design, a summative assessment's items *need not* yield data detailing a student's learning difficulties along the way. Typically performed at the end of an instructional unit or the school year, teacher-made "final" exams for grade-awarding purposes are common examples of summative assessments used in schools. Implemented frequently in contexts well beyond the classroom, *formative* and *summative decision making* have their roots in evaluation theory (Rossi, Lipsey, & Henry, 2018; Scriven, 1991).

ASSESSMENT CASE 2—A TEACHER OBSERVATION TOOL

Now, turn to Figure 1.2, which shows a framework for assessing a teacher's capacities in creating a diagnostic

Performance indicators		Low rating (1)	Mid-level rating (2)	High rating (3)
1. **Subject Area Knowledge**	• Shows in-depth understanding of topics and skills.			
2. **Knowledge of Students**	• Shows awareness of prior knowledge levels, home/family backgrounds, and special learning needs of students.			
3. **Diagnostic Teaching Practices**	• Breaks down the unit into sequenced objectives suited to different levels of learners. • Embeds assessments throughout instruction to identify student needs. • Adapts and differentiates teaching strategies for different levels of learners. • Encourages students to reflect on errors on tests and their learning progress.			
4. **Diagnostic Assessment Practices**	• Analyzes student errors, strengths, and weaknesses with appropriate assessments. • Uses assessment results formatively to redesign strategies, give student feedback, and intervene where needed.			
5. **Affirmative Classroom Culture**	• Creates a positive classroom environment to support teaching, learning, and assessment.			

FIGURE 1.2. A teacher observation tool for diagnostic classrooms.

learning environment in classrooms. This instrument could serve as a complementary tool for educators who utilize diagnostic assessments for students like that in Figure 1.1. As evident, the teacher assessment is built around five broad, theoretical indicators of expected behaviors that together reflect a model of good diagnostic teaching. To the right, we see a suggested 3-point rating scale for categorizing the observed teacher behaviors from low to high. Note that the tool would require outside observers to be directly involved during its application. That is, other school professionals, peer teachers, or school leaders would need to observe, record, and rate teachers while they are in action in live classroom contexts. The tool may also be used by the teachers themselves for conducting self-assessments, or as a professional development guide.

What inferences would be possible from the performance ratings in Assessment Case 2? All the inferences must refer back to the developer's theory of good diagnostic teaching on which the five-indicator framework is built. High ratings on all five would signify the best level of teacher performance measurable on the tool, as given by the underlying theory. As in Assessment Case 1, the primary users of the tool could make various decisions from the results, ranging from formative to summative actions on the teachers who are observed.

For example, the tool could yield a profile of ratings on the individual indicators, revealing a teacher's strengths and weaknesses. Such data could be useful for formative feedback and actions to help teachers further develop and refine specific skills. Or, we could obtain a "total score" for individual teachers by adding the five assigned ratings for making summative judgments. The latter score would indicate the degree to which the observed behaviors reached a desired maximum level of performance against the five-indicator theoretical framework.

ASSESSMENT CASE 3— THE PATIENT HEALTH QUESTIONNAIRE (PHQ)

Finally, take a look at Figure 1.3, which takes us out of a teaching and learning realm and into a clinical practice and health care setting. This tool is a self-reported survey questionnaire. It is intended to serve as an initial patient screening tool at a first visit, similar to an *intake assessment* for mental health screenings (American Psychological Association, 2011; Cohen & Swerdlik, 2010; Cohen, Tobin, & Schneider, 2022).

The excerpted tool has two discernible parts: a section with a few dissimilar items on patient background characteristics; next, we see a cluster of related items that share a common rating scale. This item set (Items *a–m*) asks for a person's self-experienced discomforts on 13 preselected physical and physiological symptoms within a 4-week timeframe. Unlike Assessment Cases 1 and 2, the PHQ's assessment results are intended for making health-related inferences on patients. The primary users of the assessment results would likely be doctors or health care professionals interested in a quick screening of their patients' health needs. Decisions contingent on the PHQ's results could involve further diagnostic testing or medical consultations leading toward appropriate treatments and care. Determinations on the next steps often involve consultation with the patients themselves or patient families. Like students in a classroom, most adult patients themselves are among the primary users of such health information.

Notice that, similar to the items in Assessment Case 2, each survey item could be categorically checked or rated numerically. There is an increasing gradient on the 3-point response scale tied to Items *a–m*, suggesting perceived levels of severity on the listed symptoms that patients are asked to recall. The response scale for the items varies from the lowest point (Not bothered) to a midpoint leading up to the highest point (Bothered a lot). But, unlike the first two assessments, there is *no* correct answer to any of the PHQ items; nor is there a desirable "high" performance implicit in the instrument.

1.2.2 Five Common Features of "Useful" Assessments

Now, with Assessment Cases 1–3 in mind, let us identify the defining elements and properties of a *useful* assessment tool. While each tool has its distinctive properties, there is much in common across the three assessment instruments. We will arrive at a general, working definition of "assessment" by focusing on five common features that are recognizable in all three. As we proceed, this section will provide relevant background theory to

PATIENT HEALTH QUESTIONNAIRE (PHQ)

This questionnaire is an important part of providing you with the best health care possible. Your answers will help in understanding problems that you may have. Please answer every question to the best of your ability unless you are requested to skip over a question.

Name__________ Age____ Sex: ☐ Female ☐ Male Today's Date______

1. During the <u>last 4 weeks</u>, how much have you been bothered by any of the following problems?	Not bothered	Bothered a little	Bothered a lot
a. Stomach pain	☐	☐	☐
b. Back pain	☐	☐	☐
c. Pain in your arms, legs, or joints (knees, hips, etc.)	☐	☐	☐
d. Menstrual cramps or other problems with your periods	☐	☐	☐
e. Pain or problems during sexual intercourse	☐	☐	☐
f. Headaches	☐	☐	☐
g. Chest pain	☐	☐	☐
h. Dizziness	☐	☐	☐
i. Fainting spells	☐	☐	☐
j. Feeling your heart pound or race	☐	☐	☐
k. Shortness of breath	☐	☐	☐
l. Constipation, loose bowels, or diarrhea	☐	☐	☐
m. Nausea, gas, or indigestion	☐	☐	☐

FIGURE 1.3. Reprinted as in original in the public domain, developed by Drs. Robert L. Spitzer, Janet B. W. Williams, Kurt Kroenke, and colleagues, with an educational grant from Pfizer Inc. No permission required to reproduce, translate, display, or distribute.

introduce selected measurement concepts, referring to Tables 1.1 and 1.2 and Box 1.1 as we go.

- **Feature 1: Useful assessment instruments focus on measuring well-defined characteristics of the persons, objects, or entities that interest the primary users.** Human beings are defined by multiple attributes and characteristics. Regardless, useful assessment instruments home in on, and select only *one* or *a few* among those to measure, guided by the purposes of the assessment tool for its primary users. Characteristics of persons, groups, or entities that we measure are referred to as **constructs** in the educational and psychological literature. They are labeled elsewhere as **concepts**, **attributes**, **traits**, or **latent traits** (Babbie, 2020; Bandalos, 2018; Crocker & Algina, 2006; Price, 2018). Identifying the construct helps address the question dealing with *What?* we desire to measure with an assessment instrument or a multipart assessment system that we might design with a particular purpose in mind.

See Table 1.1. Common objects, such as chairs or tables and natural events like the weather, are also similarly defined by a number of different attributes. To design effective assessment instruments, however, we must select *one* or *a few* clearly defined characteristic(s) to measure. For instance, when devising thermometers best suited for weather-forecasting tasks, the scientists deliberately choose to focus only on measuring atmospheric temperatures (one characteristic). Similarly, in Case 1, we found a unitary focus on student learning tied to a single, well-defined curriculum unit on designing experiments in biology. For developing a student assessment useful for diagnostic and formative decision making in that science unit, the relevant construct has a boundary of knowledge and skills.

In Case 2, the assessment is similarly focused on measuring only *one coherent set* of skills pertinent to teachers' abilities to create diagnostic classroom learning environments. This singular skill set was considered necessary for teachers to operate effective diagnostic classrooms—no more, no less. A similar defining feature is evident in Case 3, where the instrument's focal point is Items *a–m*. As a set, these items are expected to yield a quick picture of a patient's general sense of well-being or malaise so as to inform the health-screening decisions desired by clinicians and medical doctors, the primary users. In all three cases, the unitary attribute(s) measured is called the *construct*.

In an early usage, Cronbach and Meehl (1955) defined the term construct as a hypothetical concept that cannot be observed directly but must be inferred indirectly from multiple referents that *are* observable. While some constructs—like the physical length of a table—may be directly observable and more easily measured, others pose assessment barriers when they are not visible to the naked eye. A student's learning levels and misconceptions in a science unit (Assessment Case 1), a teacher's skills and abilities to create diagnostic classroom environments (Assessment Case 2), or a patient's overall sense of well-being (Assessment Case 3) are all unobservable characteristics; hence, we must rely on *multiple, indirect indicators* for making inferences about the extent of their presence. The response data we get from the items are those indirect referents; collectively, the responses would allow inferences on the degree to which that underlying construct exists in different persons. Because the item responses are, at best, proxy signals for the hypothesized construct, we should always draw on some established theory or agreed upon knowledge bases to compile the items for an assessment tool.

While reliance on multiple indicators for measuring an unobservable construct is the general rule, there are occasional exceptions. Notice the patient background items in the PHQ in Figure 1.3. For relatively unambiguous background characteristics like age, assessment designers often rely on a single item rather than multiple item-referents. This is because these items aim to tap into "fact-based" constructs with socially accepted definitions that are in common usage. Fact-based items are not vulnerable to potential ambiguities in making interpretations. With a credible defense, the targeted information can be, and often is, obtainable with a single item.

Assessment Case 3 also illustrates that, when it is reasonable to do so for the purposes at hand, a single assessment tool could aim to measure *more than one* construct. The assessment designers here—given their medical knowledge—expected that inferences about a patient's health condition could be enhanced with added data on their age and sex. As such, a single instrument that gathers data concurrently on a number of substantively different yet useful constructs for decision-making purposes is justifiable. This approach is also more efficient and practical. To sum up, then, a first general feature of useful assessments is a specified focus on a single construct, or a number of constructs that together serve a clearly set forth purpose that the primary users value.

- **Feature 2: Useful assessment instruments are designed for well-defined populations and population units, and closely matched to their background profiles and settings.** A second principle that binds together all three cases in Figures 1.1–1.3 is that each assessment is intentionally designed for individuals of a clearly *bounded group*, all of whom share some similar background characteristics. Consistent with traditions of social science, the defined group of persons, objects, or entities on which we focus for assessment design purposes is the **population**; each member of that defined group is the **population unit** (Babbie, 2020). For most assessment instruments, the population units are individual persons—as in the students, teachers, or patients in Cases 1–3, respectively. Table 1.1 illustrates that in other instances, the population units could be objects, events, or organized groups, such as classrooms or communities. This aspect of a useful assessment procedure speaks to the question as to *Who?* is to be assessed, or *For whom?* an assessment instrument is to be designed, taking into consideration their sociocultural, ecological, and demographic backgrounds.

When developing an assessment tool, we need to specify who belongs in the population and where the population's limits lie. We must also ensure that all the population units share some common contextual characteristics. The diagnostic assessment system in Assessment Case 1, for example, is expected to function best for high school students in technology-supported science classrooms, preferably taught by teachers competent in creating diagnostic learning environments—a tightly defined group. Should these population-specific

TABLE 1.1. Analyzing Assessment Tools: Four Guiding Questions

Instrument (examples)	*What?* Construct	*Who?* Population	*Why?* Assessment purposes (inferences, uses)	*How?* Assessment operations (selected)
1. A computer-based diagnostic science assessment	Learner needs in science units	**Population:** High school students **Population Units:** Individual students	***Measure-based inferences:*** Student misconceptions and learning needs in science units ***Uses:*** Diagnosing students' learning needs, adjusting teaching–learning strategies	Multiple-choice items on a computer interface with immediate feedback
2. A diagnostic classroom observation tool	Diagnostic classroom skills	**Population:** Teachers **Population Units:** Individual teachers	***Measure-based inferences:*** Teachers' diagnostic skill levels ***Uses:*** Evaluating teacher performance	Performance observation tool with five indicators and a 3-point rating scale
3. The Patient Health Questionnaire (PHQ)	Well-being and general health status	**Population:** Adult patients in given communities **Population Units:** Individual patients	***Measure-based inferences:*** Patient health needs ***Uses:*** Health care screening	Self-report survey, items with 3-point rating scales
4. A thermometer	Atmospheric temperature	**Population:** Days in a given season **Population Units:** Individual days	***Measure-based inferences:*** Temperature in degrees Fahrenheit ***Uses:*** Applied research, weather-prediction models	An equal interval scale, with units in degrees Fahrenheit
5. A meter rule	Length Height Width	**Population:** Everyday household objects **Population Units:** Individual objects (chairs, tables, beds)	***Inferences:*** Dimensional inferences (How long? How wide?) ***Uses:*** Architectural decisions for homes	Ratio scales, units marked in millimeters, centimeters, and meters
6. Customer satisfaction surveys	Satisfaction levels	**Population:** Customers of a service entity **Population Units:** Groups of customers by region	***Measure-based inferences:*** Group satisfaction levels by region ***Uses:*** Improving services	Self-rated opinion survey, items dealing with service areas

parameters be violated for some students, they may not be able to respond as easily or freely as expected. For example, if the assessment is administered in settings where students are unfamiliar or uncomfortable with the technology platform, the results will likely be compromised and less useful for the desired learning-relevant inferences and decisions. Poorer students located in regions of high poverty—typically, also with higher proportions of ethnic minority or immigrant students in the United States—could be placed at such a disadvantage. With the PHQ, likewise, patients who face linguistic or other barriers in taking a survey in English could tilt the resulting inferences about their health status and the decisions made with the survey's scores. Alternatively, notice a possible issue with Items *d–e* in Case 3; the survey assumes that the respondents are all *adults*. Should preadolescents be surveyed mistakenly with the PHQ, there could be interpretive issues with missing item responses or erroneous answers in the data—especially, in the absence of a "Not applicable" response option. A long-documented issue for demographically different groups is the unequal levels of care that they tend to receive in U.S. health care systems (Laster Pirtle, 2020; Smedley et al., 2003). Population-specific intake instrumentation is a first step toward addressing the health needs of socially diverse patients.

A technical standard for designing high-quality assessments therefore, as given by the American Educational Research Association (AERA), American Psychological Association (APA), and National Council on Measurement in Education (NCME) (AERA, APA, & NCME, 2014), is attention to the population to be assessed. To maximize the meaningfulness and functionality of the assessment's results, the population must be specified in advance. Prospective test-takers and respondents must "fit" the parameters that assessment designers had in mind on these relevant background characteristics.

• **Feature 3: Useful assessments incorporate assessment operations in a disciplined manner to provide an** operational definition **of the construct(s) measured.** All assessment instruments are built with a set of procedures, collectively referred to as the **assessment operations** (AERA et al., 2014). These operations deal with the questions or items with which an assessment tool is constructed, and steps specifying how it should be administered, scored, the resulting information interpreted and put to use. Assessment operations address the question as to *How?* an assessment tool or system is constructed, as well as *How?* it should be applied, by design, in specified circumstances. To maximize the quality of the assessment's results for the purposes that users prioritize, the assessment procedures must be selected and deployed in a disciplined, integrative, and methodical manner. To be defensible, the operations must be grounded in some relevant and established body of knowledge and/or theory about the constructs.

Back to Assessment Case 1, what are some operations that the designer selected to build that assessment system? Collectively, the procedures include the items themselves, designed to test very specific content and thinking processes from the instructional unit; the multiple-choice item format allowing structured answers to be entered and objectively scored by the computer without any subjective involvement of teachers; the computer interface allowing students to navigate the platform autonomously and enter their responses; screens that offer instant quantitative or qualitative feedback to students; and finally, the CAT algorithm built into the system for selecting ability-adapted items for individual students. Other procedures, not shown, could include guidelines for teachers to implement the assessment system as designed—such as controlling for the conditions under which students take the assessment, the time limits permitted for each question, student assistance or accommodations allowed, and so on.

The operations must all be selected to aptly serve the planned uses of the assessment results in the overall user context. Essentially, this *assessment context* is defined by the constructs and the populations that the primary users wish to measure, and purposes that interest them. The purposes (see Feature 5) include the inferences and specific decisions that users intend to take with the assessment's results. As different assessments could have entirely different uses and user contexts, the assessment operations will have to be varied accordingly. In comparing Assessment Cases 1–3, we see three completely different instruments, with operations ranging from mixed diagnostic item formats to a behavior-based, performance assessment to a self-reported survey. Yet, respectively, each is reasonable and appropriate for the assessment's intended functions.

Note that when crafting the assessment operations, designers could opt for a more or less disciplined approach. Where errors are tolerable and relatively inconsequential, the assessment operations can be loosely conceptualized and the instrument informally assembled. In Assessment Cases 1–3, however, we find that the procedures are quite systematic, deliberate, and thoughtful, as opposed to sloppy, random, hasty, or arbitrary. Some level of discipline is almost always necessary for users to be able to trust the information produced by an assessment instrument.

Once a designer selects and formalizes the operations, the finished assessment tool provides an **operational definition** of the construct(s) measured. For each assessment, the structural parts collectively provide the operational definitions of the constructs that designers intended to measure.

Note here that there could be *more than one way* to operationally define a given construct. For example, we could devise a diagnostic classroom assessment for students without opting for a technology interface or a CAT system at all! Regardless, the operational choices we make should all be reasonable and theoretically defensible; and in every case, the resulting instrument would provide a unique operational definition of the targeted constructs. This operational definition should tie directly back to the preplanned inferences and uses that the main users consider important.

• **Feature 4: Useful assessments incorporate measurement scales as a part of the assessment operations.** A vital part of the overall assessment operations is devising the **measurement scale**. The measurement scale is generated directly from the numeric scoring procedures that the designer decides on and formalizes. This quantification step is called **scaling** (Brennan, 2006); when completed, the measurement scale is useful in revealing how a measured construct varies from person to person (or in the different units of the population), in numeric terms. The general term **variable** refers to a measured construct that takes on different values in different units of the population. This book refers to the numeric "scores" generated by the measurement scale of an instrument as the **construct measures** or, simply, the **measures**.

Although some instruments may incorporate items or tasks that invite open-ended responses, a numeric measurement scale is a necessary operational component of all instruments that yield quantified information. Review again how Assessment Cases 1–3 illustrate different ways by which the scaling step could be executed, depending on user needs.

- **Case 1:** The online assessment utilizes multiple-choice items. These are usually scored with correct responses coded as 1 and incorrect responses as 0. Summing the 1s would yield a total score; alternatively, a series of 0s and 1s tied to the tested concepts and skills could yield *error patterns* and *diagnostic profiles* for students.
- **Case 2:** The teacher-behavioral "indicators" are rated items on the teacher observation tool. The rating categories could be quantified with: High = 3, Mid-level = 2, and Low-level = 1. These could similarly yield a total score or a rating profile.
- **Case 3:** Here, we see items with more than one response format. The item data on sex could be coded categorically, for example, Male = 1 versus Female = 2. The rating categories of Items *a–m* could range from 1 to 3, yielding either rated item profiles or total scores for patients, as with Cases 1–2.

The scaling methods in Cases 1–3 are relatively straightforward and commonly applied; no matter, these illustrate different ways by which the designers undertook this operational step. In theory, we could intentionally create scales to generate the specific forms of data best suited for informing our desired inferences and decisions. So, if the designers and human users of an instrument specified a formative or a summative decision-making need, or some combination of both, the scaling step could be appropriately executed to best serve those separate purposes. When effectively operationalized, the scale should reveal the innate or natural variability of the characteristics we desire to measure as closely as possible.

In an often cited historical definition, the concept of **measurement** is defined as "the assignment of numbers to aspects of objects or events, according to one or another rule or convention" (Stevens, 1968, pp. 849–851; see also Stevens, 1946, 1951). This definition has appeared in many 20th- and 21st-century measurement textbooks in original or modified form (see Allen & Yen, 2002; Crocker & Algina, 2006; Nunnally & Bernstien, 1994; R. M. Thorndike, 1997) and, as may by now be obvious, equated with the *scaling operations* of assessment design. Alongside the above definition, Stevens (1946) offered a classification system identifying four major types of measurement scales.

Take a moment to read Table 1.2 that follows next. Stevens's taxonomy distinguished among four hierarchically arranged *levels of measurement*, corresponding to four scale types: **nominal**, **ordinal**, **interval**, and **ratio**. As shown, a categorical, binary-coded variable like sex measured with a single item on the PHQ is on a *nominal scale*; this is the lowest level of measurement in Stevens's classification. The next highest would be an *ordinal scale*, where the data are categorical but ordered from low to high; an example of an ordinal scale is the 3-point rating scale for each indicator of the teacher performance assessment. Possible total scores generated by several items on a diagnostic student assessment would yield what is treated generally as an *equal-interval scale*. Finally, the highest level of Stevens's scaling taxonomy is a *ratio scale*, where the units start from a true zero point and are equal-sized; a common yardstick used to measure height is an example of an instrument that is on a ratio scale.

There is some controversy associated with Stevens's taxonomy, mostly surrounding the mathematical properties and correct statistical treatments of numerals produced by each scale type (e.g., Lord, 1953; Stevens, 1946, 1968; more to follow in Chapter 8). Given that, what would be the best approach to take on the scaling aspect when we design assessments? This book will adopt Stevens's typology as a general guide. Note,

TABLE 1.2. Four Types of Measurement Scales

Scale type and definition	Applications
1. Nominal scale A categorical scale where the numeral serves as a name/code for mutually exclusive classes or groups. A zero, if used, carries no true arithmetic property or meaning.	*Nationality measured on a survey item* USA (code 0) Canada (code 1) Mexico (code 2) Other (code 3)
2. Ordinal scale A scale where the numerals indicate ordered categories, increasing in tandem with the underlying attribute. There is no true or meaningful zero and units are not necessarily equal-sized.	*Annual income levels rated on a survey item* 5. Very high ($100, 000 or more per year) 4. High ($60,000–99,999 per year) 3. Moderate ($40,000–59,999 per year) 2. Low ($20,000–39,999 per year) 1. Very low (Less than $20,000 per year)
3. Interval scale This linear scale starts at an "arbitrary" zero point followed by equal-sized units that correspond to equal increases in amounts of the attribute. Numbers on the scale can be meaningfully added and subtracted.	*A Centigrade thermometer for measuring temperature* The freezing point of water corresponds to the starting point on the Centigrade scale, set at 0. From that origin, units increase linearly in equal amounts. *Note:* The "true zero" for temperature is the absolute zero on the Kelvin scale at –273°C, but it is not marked on a Centigrade scale.
4. Ratio scale This is a linear scale with a true zero as the starting point and equal-sized units that correspond with equivalent changes in the attributes measured. The properties of numbers permit meaningful addition, subtraction, multiplication, and division.	*A yardstick for measuring length* Calibrated in feet and inches, the starting point is a true zero, the units are consistently equal-sized and increase on a number line as length changes.

BOX 1.1 Five Features of Useful Assessments

Feature 1: What is measured?

Constructs and Characteristics

- Useful assessments focus on measuring a single, well-defined construct, or a predefined number of constructs in the persons, groups, objects, or entities that interest the primary users.

Feature 2: Who is measured?

Populations and Population Units

- Useful assessments are designed for well-defined populations and population units, and matched to their key background characteristics.

Feature 3: How is it measured?

Assessment Operations

- Useful assessments incorporate a disciplined set of assessment operations that provide a so-called operational definition of the constructs measured.

Feature 4: How is it scaled?

Measurement Scales

- Useful assessments incorporate suitable measurement scales as a part of the assessment operations, yielding scaled construct measures.

Feature 5: Why is it measured?

Purposeful Assessment Tools and Measures

- Useful assessments are purposefully designed and user-centered, supporting the users' desired inferences and uses of the information produced.

however, that any given construct could be scaled in *more than one way*. Again, as assessment designers, we have the options to choose the assessment operations, including the scale type (or level of measurement) that would be most apposite for the particular inferences and uses that the human users prioritize for an instrument.

- **Feature 5: Useful assessments are purposefully designed and user-centered.** Finally, and critically for implementing the user-centered design approach that this book advocates, the two questions *Why assess?* and *Who are the primary users?* hold the key for designers to build assessments that function optimally in the desired application contexts, meeting user-specified needs. Assessment is fundamentally a utilitarian endeavor that is rarely (if ever) conducted in a purpose-free space. In Assessment Cases 1–3, we see that each assessment was built to obtain very specific but different kinds of information for particular groups of users—science teachers, students, and others concerned with student learning (Case 1); science teachers, school leaders, professional peers in professional development contexts for educators/teachers (Case 2); and doctors, clinicians, patients, and their families in health care settings (Case 3). Situated in their respective contexts, each instrument is meant to support different kinds of action-taking with the construct measures.

Under the broad umbrella of **assessment purposes**, two key concepts (referenced throughout) are now distinguished. What do the construct measures produced by an instrument mean? And what decisions or actions do the primary users have in mind for those construct measures?

- *Measure-based inferences.* The term *inferences* in assessment design refers to the interpretations and meanings that the test scores/construct measures will connote vis-à-vis the constructs being measured, as distributed in different members of the population.
- *Assessment uses.* The term *uses* in assessment design refers to the specific decisions and actions that the primary users of the tool plan to take with the test scores/construct measures in the contexts where the targeted population is situated.

Having a proactive answer to the *Why assess?* question is helpful for both designers and users. From the designers' perspective, it helps in creating or selecting instruments that function optimally in the desired assessment use and user contexts. From the users' standpoint, it helps in adopting, implementing, and using the assessments and construct measures in a manner consistent with the original intentions of the designers.

Whether, and how well, a given assessment tool actually serves its intended purposes in the assessment contexts identified is an open question. Indeed, it is a central quality control question that guides an evaluative inquiry process called **validation** (AERA et al., 2014). How do we know that the inferences that primary users desire from the construct measures are defensible and will support the actions they prioritize? What evidence tells us that the construct measures actually manifest in the ways we expect in the populations? All tests and assessments should be checked and validated. Before an instrument can be applied, both designers and user groups should be interested in the validation results.

1.2.3 A Formal Definition of Assessment

See Box 1.1 again, summarizing the guiding questions that will serve as the "portals" to the assessment design process that this book presents: *What? Who? Why? How?* Building on the five features of useful assessment instruments, we arrive at the following definition of the term **assessment**.

> *Assessment is a disciplined set of procedures that yields quantified information on given constructs in defined groups of persons, objects, events, or entities, revealing their innate qualitative properties meaningfully, and facilitating inferences that the primary users desire for making specific uses of the results.*

Based on this broad definition, the work of assessment design could focus on a wide variety of assessment instruments with different response modalities, such as:

- Structured-response tests built with multiple-choice, true–false, fill-in-the-blank, or similar selected choice item formats (e.g., Assessment Case 1)
- Constructed-response assessment tasks requiring open-ended responses in writing or other modalities like essay tests
- Questionnaires, survey-based, or interview-based instruments requiring self-report responses (e.g., Assessment Case 3)
- Behavior-based, product-based, portfolio-based, or other performance-based assessments (e.g., Assessment Case 2)
- Computer adaptive tests, technology-mediated assessments, and a variety of more complex assessment systems (e.g., Assessment Case 1)

Just the term *assessment* is sometimes used in shorthand to refer to tests, instruments, or tools intended for a given purpose. So, instead of saying, "This assessment is used for psychological purposes," one might simply say, "This is a psychological assessment."

QUICK RECAP: Useful assessments are characterized by five features: clearly defined constructs (*What is being assessed?*); clearly specified populations, population units, and settings (*Who is being assessed?*); clearly set forth assessment purposes, identifying the inferences and uses that the primary users value (*Why is it being assessed?*); systematically compiled assessment operations (*How is it assessed?*); and rule-guided, numeric scaling operations (*How is it scaled?*). Validation is a part of the design process. It is concerned with evaluating how well an instrument and the construct measures actually function in given user contexts and must be supported with evidence.

Reflection Break 1.2: Objectives 1 and 2

- Analyze an assessment tool with which you are familiar as follows (see Table 1.1):
  - *What* is measured? Indicate if the assessment aims to measure more than one construct.
  - *Who* is measured?
  - *Why* is it measured?
  - *How* is it measured?
  - Who is/are the *primary user(s)* of the tool?
  - What is/are the main *inferences* they desire from assessment's results?

- What are the *uses* that the users prioritize?
- Is the instrument "useful" based on the five criteria in Box 1.1, in your opinion?
- Define the term *operational definition* of a construct. What is the difference between an operational definition and a *conceptual definition* of a construct?
- Define the term *variable* with an example. Distinguish it from the term *construct*.
- From a measurement perspective, define the terms *scale* and *scaling operations*.
- Define and name the *four levels of measurement*. How do these levels relate to the work of designing instruments?
- Define the term *inference* as it applies to assessment design. Distinguish it from the term *assessment use*. Give an example of each.

1.3 Viewpoints on Assessment, Measurement, Testing, and Evaluation

1.3.1 Some Distinctions: Assessment, Measurement, and Testing

In many respects, the definition of *assessment* this book offers is consistent with a consensus-based definition offered in the most recent *Standards for Educational and Psychological Measurement* (Standards hereafter; AERA et al., 2014). Although written for guiding standardized and formal test development projects, the Standards serve as a helpful resource for all assessment development endeavors. The 2014 Standards define *assessment* as

> any systematic method for obtaining information, used to draw inferences about characteristics of people, objects or programs; [or] a systematic process to measure and evaluate the characteristics or performance of individuals, programs or other entities, for the purposes of drawing inferences. . . . (p. 216)

In educational assessment, historically, we find that the degree of objectivity in the administration and scoring procedures of an assessment tool serves as the criterion for distinguishing between *measurement* and *testing* on the one hand, and *assessment* on the other. A higher degree of standardization, objectivity, control, or structure in the assessment exercise is traditionally associated with testing or measurement. Less structure and greater involvement of human judgments in the scoring of items and tasks, as in an essay examination, are called assessment. For example, Stiggins (2002) referred to tools that involved human observers as *performance assessments*, while he called multiple-choice instruments *tests*. Because the latter included items with a preset right/wrong answer, they are viewed to be more objective (see also Hopkins, 1998, and many measurement textbooks in psychology and education).

Authors from clinical traditions in psychology also treat the concept of assessment quite differently from measurement and testing. Walsh and Betz (2001, p. 19), an old but still respected resource in psychological testing, defined a psychological test as an objective sample of human behavior gathered under controlled conditions. These authors equated **psychological testing** with measurement, which they considered as one of several means for obtaining objective data necessary for addressing the psychological needs of people. In contrast, they saw **psychological assessment** as a broad and general process for understanding and "helping people cope with problems" (pp. 19–20). In this view, psychological testing and measurement are interchangeable, and a means for gathering information from objective samples of client behaviors to help psychologists gain insights into their needs. Psychological assessment is closer to what we would refer to as evaluation, as defined in the next section.

Cohen and Swerdlik (2010, p. 3), speaking also from a psychologist's vantage point, similarly referred to the levels of subjectivity and professional judgment involved in the process as a basis for making distinctions. They referred to the use of objectively scored psychological tests as testing and measurement because these tools generate traditionally derived test scores under more controlled conditions. In contrast, they viewed individualized administrations of behavioral assessments by trained psychologists as assessment. In their view, the latter incorporates greater levels of subjective and evaluative judgments, and problem-solving skills of human examiners.

Today, perspectives on assessment are more consistent with the Standards and the definition this book offers. In a National Research Council report, Pellegrino, Chudowsky, and Glaser (2001, p. 20) focused on assessments used in education, for example. They defined the term as a "comprehensive set of means for eliciting evidence of student performance than the traditional paper and pencil test." Various kinds of assessments with different response modalities, structures, and item delivery formats would fall under this broad umbrella. Added, alternative opinions of the concept of assessment overlap with the closely related concept of evaluation, treated next.

1.3.2 Another Distinction: Assessment versus Evaluation

The related term—**evaluation**—needs to be distinguished from assessment to avoid confusions. We will make a distinction between the concepts of assessment and evaluation drawing on the literature in evaluation research and program evaluation (Fitzpatrick, Sanders, & Worthen, 2003; Mertens, 2020; Rossi et al., 2018; Yarborough, Caruthers, Shulha, & Hopson, 2011).

Like assessment, evaluation is also a process. But the evaluative process follows *after* assessment is completed. In an instructional context, for example, the operational procedures for generating a test with a score for a person of 5/10, would be labeled as *assessment*; however, the process of arriving at a Pass or Fail decision with that score, would be *evaluation*. Evaluation involves making decisions, applying value-based criteria and judgments with the assessment results; in our usage, it involves making *uses* of the assessment results.

Returning to Figure 1.1, we see that a teacher's judgment as to whether a student's error patterns call for reteaching in a different way is an example of evaluation. In contrast, all the operations leading up to producing the quantitative error scores would involve assessment. Any decisions teachers might make using the results of a similar diagnostic assessment would be called evaluation, as it is a judgment-based activity. This distinction suggests an ideal sequence in which the two activities should be carried out, with assessment coming first and evaluation next.

In most cases, the act of evaluation requires the integration of different kinds of data from various sources, including the results of multiple assessments. Along with the performance history and background information, student evaluations by teachers could be based on results from an array of classroom tests, anecdotal records, parent observations, student attitude surveys, and students' standardized test scores. Such practices are common in schools.

Program evaluation, or evaluation research, often involves making judgments regarding the merit or worth of entire organizations or organizational units, projects, programs, or other entities, using data gathered from multiple data sources, including assessments. In such cases, too, researchers and evaluators may similarly rely on the assessment-based information on relevant constructs and variables as an antecedent exercise. Then, the evaluations would follow, and could involve formative or summative decisions. Program evaluations that call for making consequential, value-based decisions should rely on practices that are guided by agreed-upon standards set by societies, organizations, professions, or fields of scholarly activity. Ethical guidelines for such practices, for instance, are posted online by the American Evaluation Association (AEA) (see AEA's Guiding Principles for Ethical Practices at *www.eval.org*).

Importantly, acts of evaluation involve **stakeholders**—these are individuals with vested interests in the outcomes of the assessments and associated evaluative actions that follow. For instance, the primary users of the assessments employed by schools are among the key stakeholders of educational programs. They include the students/test-takers and their families, teachers, test designers, and other persons linked to the students in classrooms, schools, and school district organizations.

Stakeholders may be directly involved in making the judgments with assessment results in given decision-making contexts, or not at all. In Assessment Case 1, a student, the student's family, concerned teachers and administrators would all be stakeholders in the evaluative process. But the student and family may not be directly engaged in setting criteria for making judgments on the student's learning needs, nor on the merits of a student's growth; these actions would likely be led by teachers and other school-based staff. Regardless, they are all stakeholders. Directly or indirectly, each group stands to benefit from the evaluative actions that may follow or suffer any possible negative consequences of the same.

The more formal term, **evaluation research** refers to systematic data-gathering efforts and research studies aimed at answering questions that stakeholders might raise regarding the worth and effectiveness of particular social service programs, policies, projects, or interventions. Most such programs are established to ameliorate acknowledged societal problems (Rossi et al., 2018). For instance, we witnessed extensive evaluative inquiry in the context of the recent COVID-19 pandemic (see, e.g., Lau et al., 2020). In all such evaluation studies, the administration of assessments (as we define the term) precedes the evaluative research activities. Judgments made with the results and actions taken by researchers, medical professionals, or regional policymakers—the stakeholders of research efforts on the pandemic—all fall under what we call evaluation here.

QUICK RECAP: *Assessment*, as defined in this book, includes the operations and procedures compiled systematically in the form of an instrument to measure given constructs in defined contexts of use. *Measurement* refers to the numeric scaling components of the assessment operations. *Evaluation* is a judgment-based activity that follows assessment activities; it could rely on data from various assessments and other sources. Evaluation always involves stakeholders.

Reflection Break 1.3: Objective 1

- Differentiate among the concepts below, with a concrete example of each in your own field:
  - Measurement
  - Assessment
  - Evaluation
  - Evaluation research
  - Program evaluation

  Do you find conflicting definitions of the above terms elsewhere? Explain where you stand with each concept.
- Classify the following as *assessment* versus *evaluation*. Explain your answers.
  - A psychologist administering a survey tool to obtain measures of a client's anxiety levels
  - A teacher awarding A, B, C, D, or F grades to students based on their results on semester exams
  - School leaders increasing the salaries of teachers based on student survey ratings
  - Managers in an industry using a numeric checklist to sort products by different levels of quality
  - Supervisors providing ratings of their workers' performance levels in different divisions of an organization

1.4 Role of Assessment in Scientific, Professional, and Practical Endeavors

Is assessment design a science or a practical craft? What role does assessment play in scientific endeavors? In what ways are these roles different to those we find in professional applications or everyday uses of assessments? Consider now the philosophical basis of assessment and where it might fit within the larger scope of human pursuits. This section will refer to Box 1.2 that follows.

1.4.1 Assessment in the Social Sciences and Applied Research Endeavors

1.4.1.1 Assessment in the Context of Scientific Inquiry—Different Philosophical Views

In the classical conception, the aim of science is to improve understandings of the world around us and to continually expand that base of formally produced knowledge in different academic and scientific disciplines. Assessment design, with measurement as a component of it, is central to the pursuit of science in various quantitative fields founded on this tradition. Here, a first building block in the practice of science *is* measurement, and to measure well, one needs to have the appropriate instrumentation in hand (Babbie, 2020; Beveridge, 1950; Robson, 2024; Robson & McCartan, 2016).

From this classical science perspective, the universe exists independent of the researcher. Methods and tools stemming from this tradition of inquiry hold that most phenomena can be observed, described, measured, and analyzed from an objective distance and in quantitative terms, without necessitating direct involvement of the scientists themselves. Given this view, instrumentation procedures seek to yield objective forms of data on constructs and variables that interest researchers in the natural and physical world. Scientists and researchers trained in this tradition believe that more precise communication is made possible with quantified measures (Hopkins, 1998; R. M. Thorndike, 1997).

There are three basic types of activity that interest social and behavioral researchers who subscribe to the philosophy of science in the classical sense, referred to as the positivistic or postpositivistic philosophy of science (Babbie, 2020):

- Observation and description of phenomena in terms of relevant constructs and variables
- Discovery of causes, patterns, order, and regularities in their interrelationships
- Generation of principles, laws, and theories based on those empirical observations

The positivist belief system on the nature of reality, and how best to study it, is rooted in the natural and physical sciences (e.g., physics).

The difficulty in transferring classical methods of science to assessment and measurement in the social sciences lies in the fact that researchers are themselves a part of the social world, aspects of which they wish to observe, measure, and study. In the minds of some scholars, this conflict poses barriers to applying positivistic principles in a purist sense to social science (Babbie, 2015; Robson, 2024).

In contrast to the positivistic view, qualitative traditions of social research—which originated in fields like anthropology and sociology—are built on an opposing, constructivist, and phenomenological philosophy on the nature of social reality (Creswell & Creswell, 2023; Robson & McCartan, 2016). Here, the ontological status of social phenomena is viewed as dependent on the subjective experiences of researchers themselves. Knowledge of the social reality is gained through their direct immersion and experiential learnings, called the *lived experiences* of researchers. Researchers who subscribe to this second philosophy serve as instruments themselves, constructing meanings about processes, people, objects, social structures, and their interrelationships by immersion within the entities in their natural settings. They rely on emergent designs and non-numeric forms of data gathered via open-ended observation notes, interviews, narratives, and other text-based, audio, pictorial, or graphic methods for documentation of observations (Creswell & Creswell, 2023; Robson, 2024).

There is a "blind spot" when embracing a purely qualitative tradition of research for assessment in the social sciences as well. The difficulty lies in the exclusion of any form of objective inquiry altogether, even for social phenomena with preexisting structures and processes that precede any inquiry by researchers. Most social entities, aspects of which we wish to assess, measure, or study, are already there (preexisting characteristics of individuals, groups, schools, hospitals, governmental organizations, legal systems, or communities). These are available for objective and independent examinations after the fact. Furthermore, the constructivist tradition also eliminates the possibility that there could be lawful regularities and patterns in how persons, social structures, or systems behave that can *also* be studied systematically in quantitative terms, generating viable new theories.

A more modern view of the social and behavioral sciences stems from *social realism*. This worldview creates a space for empirical methods of assessment and measurement, tying together the philosophical lenses from quantitative and qualitative traditions of inquiry pragmatically. The complementary and convergent reliance on both qualitative and quantitative information mentioned in the opening section is undergirded in the social realist theory of science (Carter & New, 2004; Pawson, 1989; Pawson & Tilley, 1997). A basic principle from social realism is *naturalism*, the view that aspects of the social world can be studied in essentially the same ways as aspects of nature and the natural world. This is because a vast number of social structures (e.g., governments, schools, corporations, legal systems, societies) exist well before researchers or observers do. What might change, or be advantageous, if we aspire to design assessments or create useful construct measures adopting a social realist perspective of science?

The methodological options and possibilities broaden. Deeper forms of qualitative inquiry into the nature of new or unknown constructs could shed greater light on their properties. This step could either precede or be conducted in tandem with quantitative inquiry into the best ways to scale the construct. For example, think of *COVID-19 disease severity* as a novel construct that emerged in the context of the recent pandemic. Researchers could first engage in descriptive, qualitative inquiry into the symptomatology and experiences of a few patient cases. Given that learning, they could then identify the most appropriate item formats, response structures, and scaling methods to map the observed differences in disease severity in quantitative terms. A dual and reciprocal approach would enable the choice of the most apt assessment operations and scaling methodologies, strengthening connections between the construct and the data produced by an assessment tool.

This method is more or less what S. S. Stevens attempted when developing measurement scales for psychoacoustics constructs, labeling it the *schemapiric* approach (Stevens, 1968, pp. 849–851). Stevens was an experimental psychologist whose research interests were in human-perceived loudness of sounds. Through laboratory-based research on how well human subjects could discern and map a series of increasingly louder sounds on a number line, he tried to unify his *qualitative* observations onto *quantitative* scale continua. One study examined the degree to which humans could hear deliberately produced sounds and match these with hand sensations of vibrating objects at corresponding levels of intensity. His interest was in creating a scale to measure human perceptions with equidistant linear units similar to those on a decibel scale used in audio instrumentation. Several experiments along these lines led to his proposal for the taxonomy with four levels of measurement shown in Table 1.2. One of Stevens's discoveries was that human perceptions of sounds tended to be *ordinal* by nature, not precise enough to be scaled on an equal interval or a ratio scale (Stevens, 1946, 1968).

Another advantage afforded by a social realist approach to assessment design is that it enables greater contextualization and "user-centeredness" of the processes involved in the design, validation, and use phases. Once assessment designers are able to recognize the existing social structures within which the major users and stakeholders operate, they can obtain better understandings of their interests, values, agendas, limitations, and societal roles. These user-specific factors could drive how assessments are designed and eventually used in both basic and applied forms of research.

1.4.2 Assessments in Practice, Policy, and Everyday Applications

The need for instrumentation is not exclusive to conducting research in the social and behavioral sciences. Indeed, from a chef's measurement of ingredients for a recipe, to the careful physical examinations by physicians when screening patient needs (Assessment Case 3), to a teacher's use of classroom assessments for instructional purposes (Assessment Case 1), the need for suitable instrumentation is ever present today, no matter the profession. Box 1.2 provides illustrative scenarios depicting instrumentation needs for a variety of assessment users in different fields of professional practice and policy contexts.

Unlike scientists and researchers who typically prefer to design their own instruments, most practitioners, organizational leaders, and policymakers tend to rely on instruments *designed by others*. Some of these could be commercial products like a standardized test; others may be designed and published by other researchers or practitioners in given professional fields (e.g., Assessment Case 3). A major requirement for prospective users is, therefore, *selection* of appropriate assessments for their own particularized contexts.

See Scenario 5 for an example describing an elder care context. Hearing loss in older people is a common health issue, usually confirmed with specialized instrumentation in audiology with advanced technologies. As these formal assessments are costly and need trained health care professionals, a more feasible initial step is an evaluation with data obtained from an easy-to-apply self-report tool that permits a quick screening of elderly persons (like the PHQ). The Hearing Handicap Inventory (Newman, Weinstein, Jacobson, & Hug, 1990), for example, is a survey developed by audiologists and hearing experts in medicine for such a purpose. In Scenario 5, the users would include the survey respondents (elderly patients), as well as the clinical and caregiving practitioners who adopt the assessment tool.

Survey-based assessments, we should note, measure *perceived* levels of hearing loss and associated barriers in day-to-day living as reported by the patients. Although these results might correlate to some degree with audiometric data, the two methods will not yield exactly the same information. For consequential decisions on elderly patients, therefore, the construct measures from surveys must be validated and proven to function adequately for the actions that adopters of the tool desire. Some uses may even demand higher or different validation requirements. On this issue, the literature differentiates between "high-stakes" versus

BOX 1.2 Five Scenarios: How Practitioners and Professionals in Different Fields Use Assessments

Scenario 1

How could we hire teachers with the highest levels of reform-readiness and learning agility as we implement innovations in our schools?

A team of school leaders needs an instrument to help recruit classroom teachers most likely to adapt to curricular innovations energetically and enthusiastically. They believe that teachers differ in their attitudes toward reforms and in their mental agility to learn new things.

Scenario 2

Can emotional intelligence, *a construct known to correlate with leadership characteristics in some organizations, be nurtured in workers with the potential to become leaders in ours?*

A global corporate organization wants to identify and develop leaders from its own employee pool that includes multilingual and culturally diverse employees. Their psychologist is, therefore, designing a new instrument to measure emotional intelligence levels matched to their work backgrounds.

Scenario 3

Are postsurgery patients recovering as expected? Are they sufficiently compliant with postsurgical treatments prescribed by their doctors after they leave the hospital?

A clinical team at a hospital is interested in locating a psychological tool to monitor patients' treatment-compliance attitudes and postsurgical behaviors.

Scenario 4

Which college entrance test will give us balanced and fair information on a student applicant's potential for future success, when combined with their high school records and materials in their application portfolios?

Decision makers at the admissions office of an undergraduate liberal arts college need a standardized college entrance test that they can add to applicant portfolios to help identify the most promising candidates fairly and equitably.

Scenario 5

Is there an inexpensive and easy-to-use tool to identify elderly community members suffering from early signs of hearing loss?

Professionals at an elder care center need a suitable instrument to screen for beginning signs of hearing loss in their community members. How well elders are able to hear very soft sounds and cope with day-to-day frustrations with hearing issues, point to needs for further testing and medical attention.

"low-stakes" assessment uses (Hafferty, O'Brien, & Tilburt, 2020).

On every occasion when we use the results of tests and assessments, there is a consequence (Messick, 1989). Most designers and users intend assessment uses to have a *positive impact* for those assessed and others concerned. For example, the use of a hearing handicap survey is expected to benefit the elderly with early detection of issues and timely medical care. A **high-stakes assessment** refers to instances where the actions based on the assessment's results could also have unexpected, and sometimes, harmful effects for the individuals assessed and other stakeholders (e.g., an improper or mistaken diagnosis with treatments that have bad side effects for patients). In some instances, these effects could be irreversible and long-lasting. Conversely, with a **low-stakes assessment**, any unexpected or undesirable impacts are considered to be minor, temporary, or relatively inconsequential for the respondents/test-takers and other stakeholders; furthermore, possible mistakes are deemed easily reversible. Most uses of assessment instruments fall somewhere in the range from carrying very high to very low stakes for primary users.

For all high-stakes assessment scenarios, appropriate assessment selection, and accurate interpretation and uses of the results, are essential requirements. Credible evidence from validation activities assuring that the measures meet quality standards for the intended uses is equally important. The next section addresses the major quality criteria that we would typically employ for most tests and assessments.

QUICK RECAP: This book adopts the social realist perspective in science, combining quantitative and qualitative methods to address assessment design problems. Assessments could be designed "from scratch" or adopted from elsewhere for serving an array of purposes in basic science, applied research, professional practice, and/or policy settings. Information from assessments could be useful for making high- or low-stakes decisions that users and stakeholders value. *High-stakes* assessments should be designed and validated more rigorously.

Reflection Break 1.4: Objectives 2–4

- In any field of your choice, locate examples of assessment instruments typically employed for (1) basic science, (2) applied research, (3) practice-based professional decision making, and (4) policy-related decisions. Identify the *inferences* and *uses* of the construct measures in each.
- Contrast the *classical* perspective in social science inquiry, with the *constructivist* and *social realist* views. Which one do you lean toward? Explain.
- See Scenario 5 in Box 1.2. Suppose the staff selected the Hearing Handicap Inventory to identify how many elderly members showed signs of *severe hearing loss* so as to recommend medical follow-ups. In this scenario, what would be an *inference* using the assessment's results? What is the *use* of the results?
- Review Assessment Cases 1–3. Which, in your view, depicts a higher-stakes use? Explain.
- Define these concepts, with examples from your own experience: (1) *formative assessment uses*, (2) *summative assessment uses*, (3) *high-stakes assessment uses*, (4) *low-stakes assessment uses*.

1.5 Evaluating the Quality of Assessments and Construct Measures: Validity, Reliability, and Utility

Every assessment instrument we build or select, and the assessment results it produces, will be limited in one way or another. There is no such thing as perfect or error-free measurement! Validation, therefore, is a necessary part of the assessment design or selection process. A modern (and dominant) view of validation is that we gather and evaluate a body of evidence in a *unified* manner, situated in the contexts where the assessment's results will be interpreted and used (AERA et al., 1999, 2014; Cronbach & Meehl, 1955). This collective body of evidence should shed light on the overall **construct validity** of the measures in those contexts. The exact kinds of evidence we gather, and how much of it may be necessary, would depend on the particular assessment use scenario. As we saw, for high-stakes uses of the assessment's results, the threshold should be set higher for the evidence gathered. The major criteria for evaluating the quality of instruments and construct measures are validity, reliability, and utility. These concepts are now defined and summarized in Box 1.3.

1.5.1 Validity

In psychometric terms, **validity** refers to the extent to which **systematic variance** in the measures is attributable to the construct(s) we intended to measure, ruling out all other outside factors (AERA et al., 2014; Stanley, 1971). When external factors interfere systematically, they cloud the meaning of the assessment results to different degrees, diminishing validity levels. We then have what is called **construct-irrelevant variance** in the measures. To investigate validity, we ask: How meaningful and accurate are the measures in depicting the "true" nature of the constructs, as dis-

BOX 1.3 Quality Criteria for Assessments and Construct Measures

Validity

- The meaningfulness and accuracy levels of the measures in depicting the "true" nature and variability of the constructs in the population units of interest to primary users
- The extent to which the systematic variance in the measures is attributable to the constructs measured, ruling out outside factors

Reliability

- The consistency and replicability of the measures under different conditions in the population units
- The extent to which the construct measures are free from random or unknown disturbances

Utility

- *Usefulness:* The benefits and expected positive consequences of using the assessment tool and the construct measures by primary users in the desired application contexts
- *Usability:* The practicality, ease of use, transparency, accessibility, and suitability of the assessment tool and the construct measures for the primary users

tributed in the population units? Essentially, validity deals with the *What is assessed?* question. A corollary question from the *Why assess?* perspective is: Are the measure-based inferences and the uses that the primary users desire supported with credible evidence?

For an example of how validity is affected, consider Assessment Case 1 again (Figure 1.1). Suppose that, without the intention of the designers, a subset of science items also required sophisticated levels of reading vocabulary. Students who lacked the required vocabulary would likely provide wrong answers due to their reading comprehension difficulties, rather than their science knowledge/skills. Or the vocabulary in the test items would serve as a *systematic source of error* in their response data, lowering the validity levels of any inferences we make about students' learning difficulties in the science unit. Chapter 3 discusses external factors known to lower validity levels of standardized test scores, in particular subgroups of examinees or respondents, such as their background differences in language, race, gender, or social class.

In other circumstances, validity levels are affected due to misinterpretations or misuses of the assessment results for purposes that were unintended by the original designers. In Case 1, we see an assessment intended for making formative, diagnostic decisions while teaching and learning is still continuing. If a teacher misuses the results by assigning a summative pass/fail grade prematurely to a student, it may lead to an invalid inference about what the student could have eventually learned. When instruments designed for a given purpose, population, or user context are applied in a disparate or novel context without attention to the limitations, issues of validity arise (Chatterji, 2013a, 2013b, 2019).

Appropriate kinds of evidence, gathered and evaluated carefully in context, provide insights into the validity levels of the construct measures. Chapters 10 and 11 detail the major evidence clusters that assessment designers and users could seek out, depending on the user contexts, including five broad classes of validity evidence that the Standards identify (AERA et al., 2014, pp. 13–21).

1.5.2 Reliability

Reliability refers to the consistency and replicability of construct measures. Whereas validity is associated with the notion of systematic errors of measurement, the concept of reliability is built on the premise that we will always encounter some amount of **random measurement error** in the results (AERA et al., 2014; Stanley, 1971). As random errors lead to inconsistent measures, they are treated as unwanted "noise" in the assessment results. Empirical reliability investigations attempt to estimate the amounts of **variance** in the test scores/measures that is due to random errors. Different techniques are available for this purpose.

Although typically, random errors will lead to unpredictable variations in the measures, many can be anticipated and controlled as a part of the assessment design process. For example, we could address:

- Random fluctuations in the mindsets or behaviors of respondents during the assessment process by controlling the environment where assessments are administered
- Idiosyncratic examiner or observer behaviors by giving orientation, training, and structured guidance to these persons (see Assessment Case 2)
- Random errors introduced through ambiguous, vague, or unclear assessment procedures, items, or directions through careful construction, reviews, and revisions
- Random errors that arise from sudden environmental disruptions by setting up constraints in the assessment environment
- Random errors introduced by selecting too few items, or too small a number of behaviors to observe as a part of the assessment—called behavioral sampling errors—by pilot-testing assessments of different lengths

More on reliability theory, types of reliability coefficients, and various estimation and evidence-gathering methods follows in Chapters 10 and 11.

1.5.3 Utility

Finally, **utility** is a major quality criterion for construct measures and instruments overall, and central to a **user-centered assessment design** approach. Utility has two aspects that must cohere in assessment design and use practices.

- **Usefulness:** Usefulness refers to the benefits and expected positive consequences of using an assessment tool and construct measures for the respondents and primary users, keeping in mind their information needs, situations, capacities, and limitations, ruling out any unintended consequences.
- **Usability:** Usability refers to the degree to which the instruments and measures are easy to apply/practical, accessible, transparent, and suitable for use by the respondents and primary users.

When applying utility concepts, we should note that the "primary users" include the test-takers or respondents themselves, along with the designers, adopters, and other stakeholders who may rely on an assessment's results for making decisions.

Of the three quality criteria, utility affects the assessment users most directly. For example, high material costs, implementation demands of an overly complex instrument or assessment system, taxing administration conditions, dependence on specialized human resources, excessive technical complexity, and inaccessibility of the reports/results—sometimes called "black box" assessment reports—are all utility issues. The last could lead to invalidity levels due to increased likelihood of misinterpretation and misuse of results.

Thoughtful actions during the design process could address several utility issues. Studies investigating utility help evaluate issues of the usefulness, usability, and desired impacts of the measures on primary users and stakeholders. Examining any potential adverse consequences for actors/groups should be a key component of such investigations. Types of evidence that could be gathered, and methods for examining usability and usefulness issues, follow in Chapters 10 and 11.

QUICK RECAP: Guided by the assessment context, we should gather and evaluate evidence of validity, reliability, and utility of the construct measures in a unified manner. Each quality criterion is defined differently and calls for different questions and methods of evidence gathering during validation. Overall, *construct validity* refers to the combined body of evidence on validity, reliability, and utility of the measures in given user contexts.

Reflection Break 1.5: Objectives 3 and 4

- Define the concepts of *validity*, *reliability*, and *utility* and distinguish these from *construct validity* as a whole.
- How are *validity* and *reliability* (1) similar and (2) different? (3) How is *utility* different from both?
- What does validation in a "unified manner" mean? Explain with an example. Do you agree with taking this approach?

- What does "validity in the context of test use" mean? Explain with an example.
- Do you agree that many widely used tests and commercially distributed assessments are "black boxes" for their primary users? Explain with examples.

1.6 Integrating Assessment Design, Validation, and Use: A User-Centered Process Model

To end the first chapter, this section now integrates the foundational concepts presented thus far, with the main components of a user-centered assessment design framework. See Figure 1.4 on page 28 for the Process Model of Assessment Design, Validation, and Use®. The *What?*, *Who?*, *Why?*, and *How?* questions are now situated within that framework as the main portals of the assessment design process. To reiterate the arguments for the framework, this section first begins with a case study of high-stakes test use in a visible public policy arena—immigration and naturalization in the United States (Box 1.4)—and provides the theoretical foundations of the Process Model. Refer again to Boxes 1.1–1.3 as we proceed.

1.6.1 A High-Stakes Assessment Scenario: Testing for Immigration and Naturalization

1.6.1.1 Identifying High-Stakes Assessment Cases

Reconsidering Assessment Cases 1–3 briefly, we find that the implicit benefits of the assessment uses were evident in each. Namely, these were to improve diagnostic teaching and learning processes in classrooms, and health care screening in clinics and hospitals. All three may be cast as relatively low-stakes assessment uses. Errors or issues that arise could be corrected along the way; possible negative impacts would likely be short-term and alterable.

In contrast, review Box 1.4, which illustrates a case where well-intentioned assessment reforms in the immigration and naturalization sector went temporarily amiss. Testing-for-citizenship is a socially and politi-

BOX 1.4 High-Stakes Case Study in Testing for Immigration and Naturalization

Is a new mandatory test for naturalization intended to exclude some individuals or groups from entering the country?

The U.S. Immigration and Naturalization Services requires that all applicants for citizenship pass a civics test before they become American citizens. The test is completed in the final stages of the citizenship acquisition process. The passing score is kept low to allow a high pass rate at this final point of a usually lengthy process.

In December 2020, the federal government launched a revamped civics test. Compared to the earlier version that had been in use from 2008, the new test was longer, more rigorously designed, and found to be more difficult for test-takers.

Protests rose against the new version of the citizenship test almost immediately after its release. At first, the concerns came from immigrant advocacy groups, next from lawyers and human rights experts, and finally, from political groups. Enforcement of the new test just prior to a national election was viewed as "a last-ditch effort . . . to prevent immigrants from gaining the benefits of U.S. citizenship, including the ability to vote."

The pool of test-takers applying for citizenship in 2020 had grown more diverse. Applicants included educated individuals who were unschooled in the English language (the language of the test), relatively less educated minors or aged family members who were entering as dependents of recent immigrants, and refugees from regions of the world affected by political turmoil, war, or natural disasters. Some were indigent with very low literacy levels, even in their native language.

In February 2021, the Biden administration discarded the new civics test, reverting back to the 2008 version for immigrants to avoid "unnecessary barriers to naturalization."

Source: Adapted from Romero (2021), www.kqed.org/news/11849159/new-citizenship-test-is-longer-and-could-deter-immigrvants-from-applying-advocates-say.

cally charged topic in the best of circumstances. In this particular case, the test was meant originally to impact society positively. We find two primary user groups: the test-takers themselves, who are the aspiring immigrant-citizen applicants; and the federal government authorities, which adopted the new civics test as a step in the usually long and demanding process of the applicants' acquiring citizenship. A major stakeholder group is the American public and citizenry at large. Keeping validity, reliability, utility needs uppermost as we review the case, could a user-centered assessment design approach have prevented the anti-testing protests and public fears?

1.6.1.2 Analyzing the Naturalization Case

In testing-for-citizenship contexts (Box 1.4), the anticipated consequences of implementing a new, seemingly more rigorous test could be manifold. The positive consequences, consistent with the presumptive motivations of the implementers of the new civics test, are to ensure that naturalized citizens are able to participate more effectively in the American democracy and related societal functions. Other impacts, however, could be viewed as potentially negative and long-lasting, even if unintended. Consider the following possibilities:

- *Perceptions of unfair or biased testing outcomes.* If groups or individuals from particular regions of the world found the new test too difficult, there could be a public perception of bias. Beliefs could spread that the decision-making process is systematically limiting entry to some, while favoring others.
- *Validity issues due to a lack of culturally or ecologically responsive testing.* For applicants who lacked the presumed levels of prior education from their home countries, or had an unanticipated language, age-related, religious, or cultural barrier that the test designers overlooked, there could be challenges in interpreting their test scores accurately.
- *Human rights issues.* As the public advocacy groups asking for equitable treatment pointed out, there could be possible violations of human and legal rights. When test-based actions delayed entry of some, for example, it could alter the composition of groups that were eligible to vote.
- *Possible changes of a country's demographic composition.* If potentially talented but more globally diverse applicants faced barriers during the testing process due to their background characteristics (but not civics knowledge), other validity issues could arise with related impacts on the nation's population, such as limited numbers of people who could contribute productively to society.

The list could be continued. Happily, and quickly in this case, federal policy actions under a new administration preempted further complications.

1.6.1.3 Advantages of User-Centeredness

For stakeholders in this case, adopting a more user-centered approach may have obviated some of the observed issues and unexpected consequences. With more deliberate attention to the *Who?* question, the test design and validation efforts could have been performed with more current applicant groups, accounting for the changing demographics of test-takers. A comparability study of the properties of test scores from the old versus the new version of the civics test could have informed decisions on whether replacing one test with the other is reasonable. This is a type of correlational evidence of validity called **concurrent validity** (more in Chapters 10 and 11). Attention to the turbulent global and internal political conditions could have helped define more accurately the contexts of test use and primary users of the test-based information. Greater openness and involvement of key stakeholders in the essential phases of test design might have reduced the climate of distrust—such as among recent immigrants and human rights advocacy groups.

1.6.2 A User-Centered Process Model

The user-centered framework in Figure 1.4 recommends a cyclic and iterative process involving five activity phases during *assessment design*, *validation*, and/or *use* as follows:

- **Phase I:** Specifying the context(s) of assessment use. The constructs; populations (population

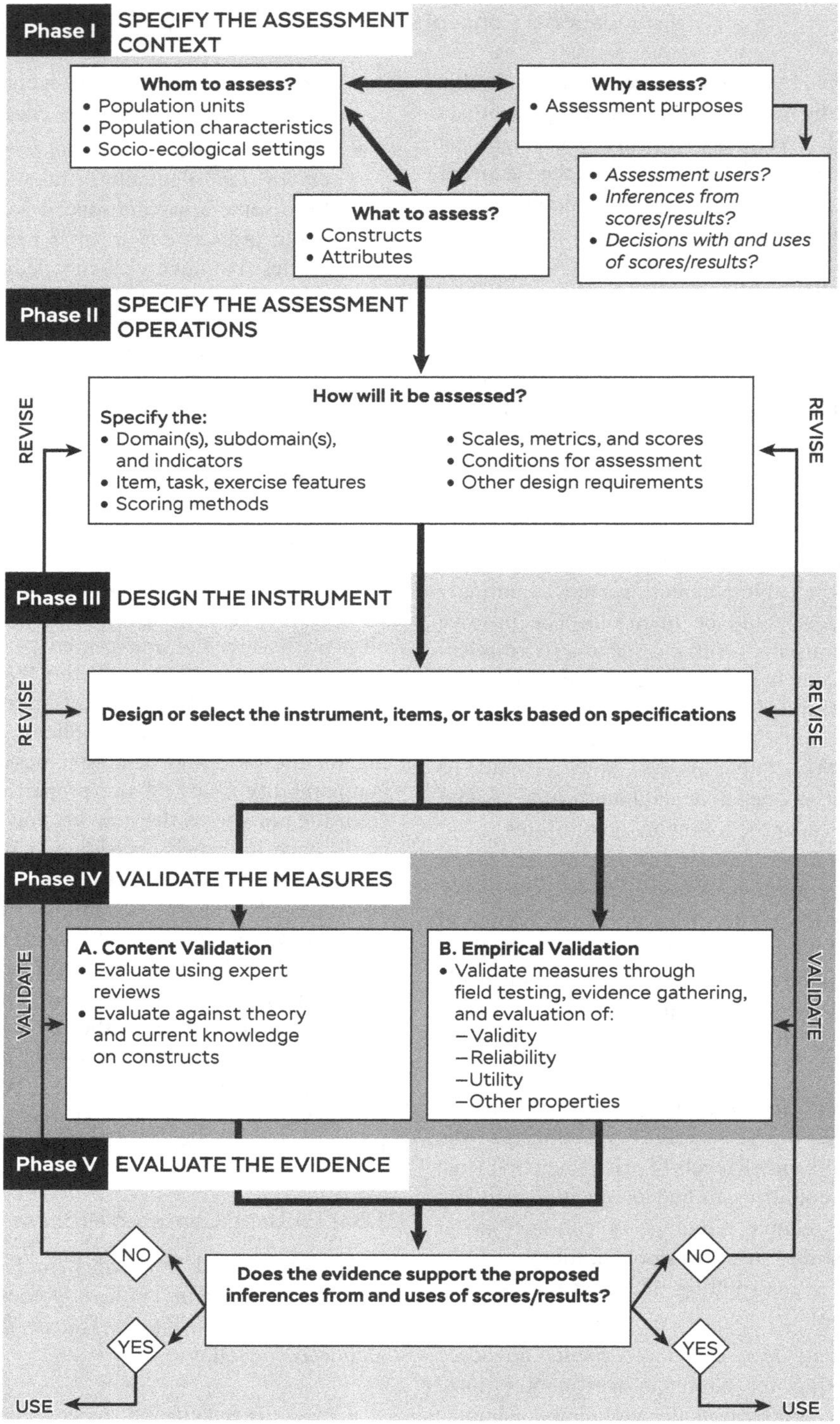

FIGURE 1.4. A user-centered Process Model for Assessment Design, Validation, and Use.

units, characteristics, and settings); and assessment purposes (primary users, measure-based inferences, and uses) are first clarified.

- **Phase II:** Specifying the assessment operations needed to build or select the instrument matched to the context parameters.
- **Phase III:** Building the assessment guided by the design specifications in Phases I and II.
- **Phase IV:** Validating the instrument and construct measure(s) in context.
- **Phase V:** Gathering and evaluating the evidence in a unified manner in context.
- **Iterate as needed:** Iterating the process of designing, validating, refining, and revising the instrument and its parts until optimally functioning measures are obtained for the specified inferences, uses, and user contexts.

1.6.2.1 The Portals of Assessment Design or Selection

In the Process Model, the four questions in Box 1.1 are viewed as the doorways or "portals" through which we engage in the assessment design or selection process. In a best-case scenario, the *What?*, *Who?*, and *Why?* questions are clarified upfront. This information then guides the entire assessment design or selection process that follows. Phase I is also critical in informing the validation and evidence evaluation phases (Phases IV and V). The model is a general framework for user-centered assessment design, where the instrument, construct measures, and any ancillary materials, reports, or data produced for users are all viewed as purposefully designed "products."

The *How?* question appears twice, in Phases II and III of the Process Model. In its first appearance, it helps designers lay out a blueprint for designing the assessment tool. This is the practice of setting forth the assessment design specifications to fit the user context. On the second occasion, it aids in constructing, assembling, or compiling the different parts of the assessment instrument or system guided by that blueprint. The blueprints for designing tests and assessments are also called **assessment (or test) design specifications**. The parameters in the assessment design blueprints (Phase II) should aim to produce optimally functioning measures for the specified user contexts (Phase I).

1.6.2.2 Validation as a Component of the Design Process

Validation occurs in Phase IV. Depending on the stakes involved, this phase could be a brief and informal process, or more involved evaluative studies focusing on specific validity, reliability, and utility questions. So as to avoid inevitable "cracks" in the assessment design or selection processes, the validation phase is almost always necessary.

1.6.2.3 Realist and Pragmatist Philosophy of Science

A variety of techniques and tools of inquiry could be employed within the user-centered framework for design and validation. Founded on a realist philosophy of science, the Process Model is use- and user-driven, but broad and eclectic in its methodological and theoretical orientations. It does not lean toward any particular psychometric traditions, methodological approach, or theories in measurement or social research methods. Guided by the instrument use contexts, it is open to methods under classical test theory, item response theory, or other theoretical, statistical, or mathematical models of assessment design, and to qualitative and quantitative research methods.

1.6.2.4 Iterative Cycles toward Optimally Functioning Measures

The iterative validation and redesign processes are *not* unending. To decide whether an assessment instrument and its measures are ready for use, the Process Model calls for evidence gathering and evaluation procedures appropriate for prespecified application contexts. Phase V's results are carefully considered against the contextual parameters set forth in Phase I. Studies continue until the instruments and measures function optimally in the specified user context; no further iterations are necessary. In high-stakes contexts, appropriate degrees of stakeholder involvement and deliberation are desirable to end the evidence evaluation phase.

1.6.2.5 Generalizable Process

Different academic disciplines, professions, or policy arenas are known to have specific interests in particular types of instrumentation. Inferential needs and uses for the assessment results are discipline-centric. Regardless, the five features that define useful assessments (Box 1.1) and the five phases of the Process Model (Figure 1.4) would apply across these different disciplinary and professional settings. The approach also assumes that instruments will be employed with diverse and global populations.

1.6.3 Theoretical Foundations of the Process Model

> Good design . . . is a lot harder to notice than poor design, in part because good designs fit our needs so well that the design is invisible. Bad design, on the other hand, screams out its inadequacies. . . .
>
> —Don Norman (2013, p. xi)

The Process Model draws from the measurement literature on validity theory tied to test uses and unified construct validation as a form of evaluative inquiry. It stands in large measure on the theory of user-centered design taken from the fields of engineering and technology, as well as from evaluation theory on utilization-focused evaluation, product evaluation, and, specifically, the *program evaluation standards* on utility, cultural responsiveness, and contexts of evaluation use (Yarborough et al., 2011). A brief discussion of this foundational literature follows.

1.6.3.1 Foundations in User-Centered Product Design

Several design theorists in the fields of architecture, engineering, technology, and software development think of sound product design as one where the "function" (use) of a product to be developed is given precedence over its "form" (physical features and structure). A major guiding principle in this literature is prioritizing the needs of product users and the quality of user experience.

When designing "everyday things," the user is at the crux of the design process (Norman, 1986, 2013). In human-centered design, the focus at all stages of a product design process is the human users' interests, capacities, needs, and limitations (Giacomin, 2014, pp. 1–2). Feedback from potential users is sought throughout to shape the product design processes. A user-centered design philosophy is commonly applied for software development, and for engineering solutions in technology and health care systems (Lowdermilk, 2013).

The conception and development of the Process Model were influenced by the notions of both user-centered design and *human-centered design* (Giacomin, 2014; Norman, 2013; Still & Crane, 2017). Rather than forcing end users to change behaviors to use a product appropriately (here, a test, assessment, and ancillary materials), the product would be designed to maximize its intuitive utility and meaningfulness for users. Hence, the product development lifecycle is stakeholder-oriented, iterative, and involves cycles of product testing, data gathering, and evaluation until the products have desired levels of quality for the user-intended functions. Evidence of an assessment's *usefulness*, and specifically, *usability*, is of prime importance in informing this approach to assessment design (see definitions in Box 1.3; Figure 1.4).

1.6.3.2 Foundations in Utilization-Focused Evaluation

Another major set of foundational ideas come from utilization-focused evaluation (UFE; Patton & Campbell-Patton, 2022). Originally, UFE was conceived as an approach to conducting *program evaluations* guided by the usefulness of the evaluative processes and outcomes for the intended users. From this viewpoint, evaluations should be planned and conducted in ways that enhance the likely utilization of the findings and the overall evaluation process. UFE aims to better inform the decisions by primary users, while improving the performance of the overall entity that is being evaluated.

Applicable to program, process, or product evaluations, Patton and Campbell-Patton's (2022) ideas on UFE offered two essential elements that were incorporated in the Process Model. First, UFE requires that the *primary intended users* be clearly identified when the design process begins. In assessment design practice, this is a simple but potentially outcome-altering step. It is very different from starting with an abstract or general notion of who the users might eventually be, and identifying in vague terms the uses that they would likely prioritize (the typical case today).

Second, UFE emphasizes that *users must be en-*

gaged in the design process from the beginning to the end, even guiding the process at times, if needed. Likewise, the Process Model is built on the premise that involving relevant groups of potential users (see Phase I) would maximize utility levels of assessments, also positively impacting validity and reliability of the measures, no matter the forms in which the assessment's results may be produced (see Phases IV and V).

Several aspects of the product evaluation literature (Scriven, 1991) and the program evaluation standards emphasizing contextual and cultural responsiveness (Yarbrough et al., 2011) underpin the principles that guided the Process Model. The notions of utility as a quality criterion, as well as responsiveness to socio-ecological diversity of the populations and population units during assessment design, stem from this literature base. Viewed from an improvement science perspective (LeMahieu, Bryk, Grunow, & Gomez, 2017), the iterative product testing and evaluation phases in the Process Model depict parallels with the continuous quality improvement cycles described in that literature. Again, in formal or large-scale test design applications, the assessment "products" could be complex and multilayered. For example, the items and tasks, the instrument; directions and scoring protocols; guides, manuals, reporting materials for users; and the scales and derived scores—all could be viewed as products.

1.6.3.3 Foundations in Validity Theory

Several theoretical perspectives on validity related to test uses, and validation as a form of evaluative inquiry, informed the Process Model as well. These ideas go back several decades, with many now incorporated in the 2014 Standards (AERA et al., 2014; Cronbach, 1971, 1988; Ebel, 1961; Kane, 2006; Messick, 1989; Shepard, 2013). These selected perspectives align closely with the notions on investigating the construct validity of measures and an overall instrument holistically tied to given contexts of use (Phases I, IV, and V).

Lee Cronbach (1971, pp. 451–455) asserted that validation research calls for "an integration of multiple kinds of evidence . . . and varieties of investigations . . . [that] must be a comprehensive, integrated evaluation of the test. . . ." Speaking about educational and psychological tests at the time, he recognized that test uses are frequently situation-bound, endorsing appropriate kinds of evidence for given circumstances of test use. In his view, evidence gathering to establish validity should be guided by logically framed arguments and hypotheses about what the test scores are supposed to mean in given contexts. He pointed out that while all tests and assessments may generate test scores, they all aim to measure some underlying constructs. Hence, it is the *interpretations* of those test scores vis-à-vis the targeted constructs that must be the focus of validation efforts, not the test. What matters is the overall construct validity of the assessment results for the intended uses.

Adding to this perspective, Samuel J. Messick (1989) defined validity explicitly in terms of the inferences and actions associated with assessment results. In his words, validity is also "an integrated evaluative judgment of the degree to which empirical evidence and theoretical rationales support the *adequacy* and *appropriateness of inferences* and *actions* based on test scores and other forms of assessment (p. 13, original emphasis). By identifying the "inferential" and "action" dimensions separately, Messick emphasized that validity evidence we gather must speak to both of these aspects of the assessment use context. Furthermore, he pointed out that scores from assessments and tests simply cannot be assumed to be valid once an instrument is designed—every new use of the tool must be validated, along with any new score-based inferences. Importantly, Messick recognized explicitly that test uses always have consequences for users and stakeholders that should be subjected to careful study.

Subsequently, Kane (2006) provided an argument-based framework for validation. His approach recommends that we gather the requisite evidence to validate any theoretical claims underpinning the construct measures. In addition, he posited that every action or decision stemming from those score-based interpretations should also be validated in an interconnected chain.

The Process Model draws on all of these perspectives and others cited previously by stressing the interlinkages among the activity cycles of Phases I–V. A lack of connectivity of Phase I with Phases IV and V, for instance, could shortchange the evidence we gather on validity, reliability, and utility. The testing-for-citizenship case shows that, in a rapidly changing setting, the results of a well-designed and well-intentioned assessment may become vulnerable to misinterpretations or misuse (see also AERA et al., 2014).

1.6.3.4 Equitable Assessment Practices with the Process Model

Today, we find ever-expanding testing programs in numerous sectors of society with increasingly diverse and international populations. Over and over, the results uncover persistent gaps between ethnic minority and majority groups, males and females, or the "haves" versus "have-nots." According to some, actions based on test results have led to documentable disparities and inequities in educational, professional, and life opportunities, opening doors to some while blocking others (see Mendoza-Denton, 2014; Organisation for Economic Co-operation and Development, 2010; Reynolds & Suzuki, 2012; see also Arbuthnot, 2020; Ortiz, 2016). These forms of assessment-based problems are characterized as institutionalized, structural, and systemic. The issues are not restricted just to the United States, but in societies with diverse demographics worldwide.

This book stands on the premise that the observed test-based societal issues and inequalities are fundamentally preventable and, sometimes, attributable to problematic assessment practices that can be turned around. The Process Model, updated since the original version (Chatterji, 2003), is intended to offer solutions toward these ends.

1.6.3.5 Comparisons with Other Models of Assessment Design

Chapter 12 will compare and contrast the user-centered framework of the Process Model, against other predominant approaches to assessment development found in the measurement and social sciences literature. It will also compare the essential elements of the Process Model against recommendations given in the 2014 Standards.

1.6.3.6 Applications of the Process Model

The Process Model has been applied in numerous moderate-sized and larger-scale assessment design projects for over two decades. The projects are referenced where appropriate, and selected projects led by multidisciplinary researchers and professionals (including this author) are described and presented as case studies (Chapters 5–7 and 12). Variously, the projects focused on instrument design for accreditation and evaluation of graduate medical education programs, anesthesia education research, community health-worker testing programs, education reform projects in grades K–12 systems, and a national curriculum design project for workforce development in health information technology.

QUICK RECAP: Founded on a broad literature base from the measurement, evaluation, technology and product design fields, the Process Model starts with the *What?*, *Who?*, *Why?*, and *How?* questions. Given predesignated users and contexts of use, it outlines a cyclic and integrative methodology for optimizing the quality of instruments and construct measures. Validation is a part of the design process in this framework.

Reflection Break 1.6: Objectives 5 and 6

- Define the concept of *user-centered assessment design*. What are its advantages? Disadvantages?
- Review the Process Model in Figure 1.4 and compare it to a different assessment design approach you may have seen elsewhere. What advantages or disadvantages did the other model afford over the Process Model?
- Weigh the pros and cons of a user-centered approach to designing a high-stakes assessment in your field (as opposed to an alternative method).
- Make a theoretical and practical argument to support the Process Model.

1.7 Summary

A test or assessment instrument is about as "everyday" a thing as we can get today; however, deliberate attention to the *assessment contexts*, *uses*, and *users* during the design process is still a rare practice. To date, the author found just one published instance of "user-centered design" mentioned in the professional literature on educational test development (Nichols, Mittelholtz, Adams, & van Deusen, 2008); added references to human-centered design are just entering the assessment literature as of this writing. This is an encouraging trend.

Chapter 1 presented a theoretical and case-based argument for user-centered assessment design, elaborating on several foundational concepts and presenting a five-phase Process Model. Several theoretical measurement concepts were defined and introduced. The term *assessment* was distinguished from the concepts of measurement, evaluation, evaluation research, and program evaluation.

Philosophically, the chapter highlighted a social realist perspective on science as applied to assessment design and measurement problems. From this viewpoint, we could draw on a range of quantitative and qualitative methodologies pragmatically during the instrument design and validation processes. Instrument design efforts using the Process Model could focus on tests, surveys, observation protocols, and a variety of performance assessment devices, including more complex assessment systems and standardized tests. Updated in Figure 1.4, the Process Model treats the assessment design, selection, validation, and use processes as integrated and interdependent activities.

CHAPTER 2

Why Assess?

Measure-Based Inferences, Uses, Users, and Consequences

2.1 Chapter Overview

2.1.1 Introduction

The central concern of Chapter 2 is to examine the role that *assessment uses* play in the overall design process and what that implies for both assessment developers and the primary users of an assessment instrument and its results. A related concern has to do with *assessment misuses* and the repercussions of misinterpreted results, or inappropriately used assessments, on the respondents and all concerned stakeholders.

See Figure 2.1. It excerpts the *Why assess?* boxes in the Process Model for Assessment Design, Validation, and Use®. Chapter 2 connects with the rest of the book, and more specifically, with the Process Model through the *Why?* portal of assessment design, interlinked tightly with the *What?* and *Who?* portals in Phase 1. This chapter elaborates on two foundational ideas introduced in the first chapter, namely, the importance of specifying the (1) larger assessment user context and (2) the assessment purposes within that context, to begin the instrument design, selection, or use processes.

2.1.2 Chapter Objectives

After reading the second chapter and completing the accompanying exercises, the reader should be able to:

1. Trace the major historical and modern drivers of assessment uses in different fields.
2. Given assessment scenarios from different fields, identify the assessment purposes, measure-based inferences, and specific uses that the primary users desire, within the larger user context.
3. Evaluate the implications for appropriate interpretations and uses of the assessment results in given contexts, with attention to validity, utility, and anticipated consequences of specific uses.
4. Brainstorm the instrument design and validation implications guided by given assessment user contexts.
5. Classify the major "user paths" where tests and assessments are employed today in the social and behavioral sciences and related fields.
6. Identify the relevance of "user-centered" design principles and the Process Model for improving *assessment uses*.

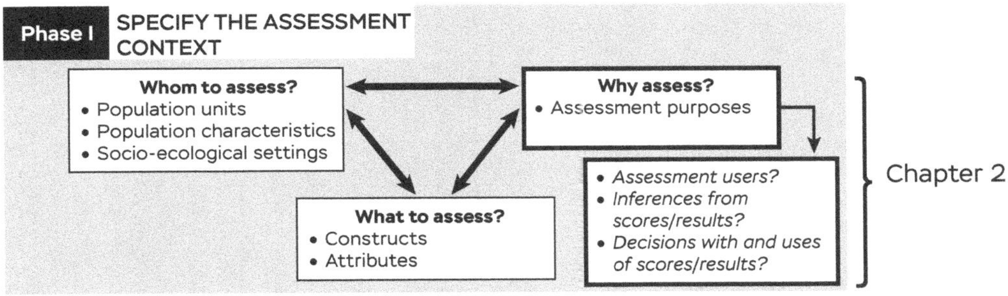

FIGURE 2.1. Connecting Chapter 2 to the Process Model and the rest of the book.

2.2 Back to the Future: Early Drivers, Milestones, and Consequences of Assessment Use

The same test may be used for several different purposes, and its validity may be high for one, moderate for another, and low for a third. The essential question . . . is how well the test does the job it is employed to do.

—EDWARD E. CURETON (1951, p. 621)

2.2.1 Historical Trend Lines and Patterns of Assessment Use

Should the intended uses for an instrument drive the assessment design and selection processes? Or should it be the other way around, with assessments designed or selected first, giving less importance to how and where the tool or the results may be used in specific ways? By describing the Process Model as "user-centered," this author's position on this question should be obvious. A look back at the history of testing and assessment practices, however, yields other answers.

Recall the early studies on measuring and scaling of psychoacoustic constructs from Chapter 1 (Stevens, 1946, 1968). From those origins in the then emergent field of experimental psychology, testing and assessment practices became widespread in psychology writ large, branching out and spreading rapidly to the social and behavioral sciences and several fields of professional practice. Notable among these were mental health, medicine, and health care; education, including higher and professional education; business and the workplace; social work, clinical and counseling psychology; and a number of public policy sectors, such as immigration and naturalization (recall the case in Chapter 1).

To view selected historical trends in assessment and testing, examine Figure 2.2 next. These charts were created using the search period 1900–2010 with Google's *ngram* viewer, an online tool that identifies how often terms such as *testing* or *psychological assessment* appear in books housed in the Google archives. Recorded in the top graph, we find a chart marking the birth of "testing" as a general field—a line that rises steadily from the 1900s and holds strong through 2000, with a visible dip later. The bottom graph depicts corresponding trends in specialized branches where tests and assessments came to be used widely. The lines begin, ascend, plateau, or dip, suggesting different historical patterns for each. (Readers might try using the *ngram* viewer for specific branches, e.g., clinical assessment for the period up to 2021.)

We might perhaps question the reliability of the *ngram* as a historical tracing tool, recognizing that the data are possibly skewed toward books written in the English language in the United States and the West. However, a series of historical accounts corroborate the general trends suggested in Figure 2.2. The world, in fact, witnessed an exponential growth in testing and assessment over those years, with applications spreading to multiple fields globally. Some writers trace the earliest examples of formal examinations to China; developments thereafter were documented in the United States, United Kingdom, Europe, and elsewhere on a

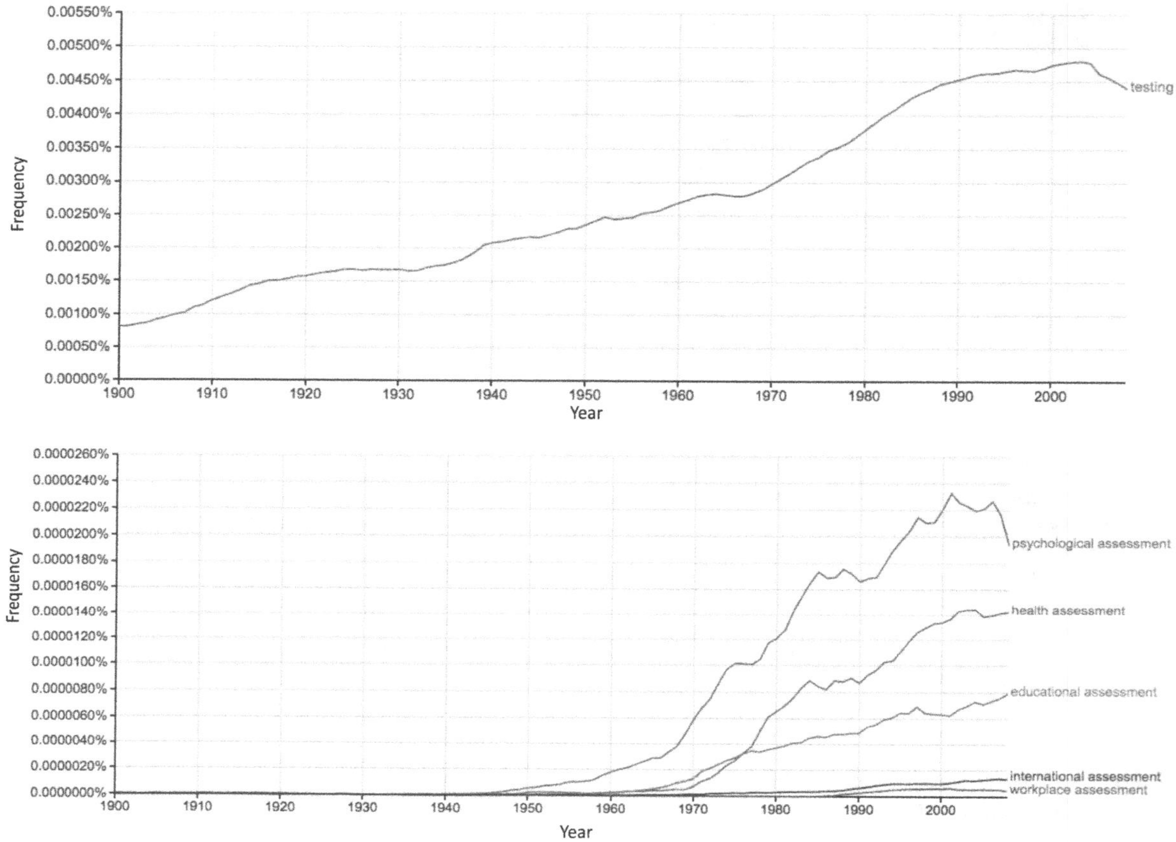

FIGURE 2.2. Google's ngram viewer charts: Trend lines in *testing* and *assessment* in different fields for 1900–2010.

much larger scale (Cohen et al., 2022; Du Bois, 1970; Ryan & Cousins, 2009; R. M. Thorndike, 1997; Ward, Stoker, & Murray-Ward, 1996).

Psychological assessments—the earliest trend line to arise in the bottom panel of Figure 2.2—were dominant at first. The line peaks to the highest point and is sustained for a long period until a drop-off begins to register in recent years. A question arises: *Why?* Through 2000, however, that same line stands as the most prominent. The lines in health and education assessments follow as the next most dominant, with the international assessment and workplace assessment lines relatively less so.

In step with the story suggested in Figure 2.2, the number and availability of new tests and assessment instruments expanded voluminously, many catalogued and critically reviewed in publications like *Tests in Print* and the Buros Center's *Mental Measurements Yearbook* (see, e.g., Spies & Plake, 2003). A testing industry developed, with nonprofit and commercial test development organizations gaining in stature and reach. Internationally, different governmental entities and institutions developed testing and assessment programs guided by their own missions. The observed expansion in individualized, small- and large-group testing and assessment practices was accompanied with significant theoretical developments in a formalized academic discipline, *measurement* (see, e.g., Cronbach, Gleser, Nanda, & Rajaratnam, 1972; Gulliksen, 1950; Lord, 2009; E. L. Thorndike, 1918; Wright & Stone, 1979).

2.2.2 Drivers of the Earliest Assessment Uses

What did the earliest assessment tools look like, why were they designed, and whose interests did they serve? What were the social, organizational, or larger contextual factors that drove those assessment uses? What were their intended impacts on the individuals assessed, or organizations and societies where the instruments appeared? With these questions as a general guide, we will now look briefly at *selected milestones* in assessment use. Table 2.1 summarizes the range of assessment purposes evident in these historical instances. Consistent with segments highlighted in Figure 2.1, Table 2.1 identifies the *primary users*, *measure-based inferences*, and *specific uses* of assessment results that the major actors appeared to value.

2.2.2.1 Science and Discovery—Scaling of Human Attributes and the Study of Individual Differences

The study of psychology as an experimental science began in early-19th-century Germany, where scientists worked in so-called perceptual laboratories that led the way toward the scaling of human perceptions (see Stevens, 1946, in Chapter 1; Wundt, 1948). Disciples of the Wundt (1948) tradition pursued **scale construction** as a purely scientific activity. Subsequently, experimental psychologists in Germany, Great Britain, France, and the United States initiated distinctive traditions in scaling methods, working in the broader area of psychophysics and moving psychology away from the field of philosophy where it originated. Many of the same psychologists also pursued the study of **individual differences** on measured human characteristics driven by interests in understanding variabilities in human intelligence, mental abilities, attitudes, and perceptions.

Two fairly clear-cut theoretical "scaling camps" emerged from these early efforts in measurement. One endorsed scaling by ordering of test items on a linear scale, with the objective of building unidimensional scales. This trend evolved into scale construction methods attempting to order both the items and persons conjointly on a straight-line continuum, based, respectively, on differences in difficulty or ability levels (Guttman, 1941; Thurstone & Chave, 1929). Another trend disregarded the item order altogether and sought to "scale people" only on construct continua based on the observed differences in their "total scores" on the measured attribute (Crocker & Algina, 2006; see Likert, 1932, for the original). Interestingly, elements of these scaling approaches stood the test of time, and we encounter applications with variations of the originals in Chapters 5–9.

2.2.2.2 Measurement of Human Intelligence as an "Educable" Construct

The arrival of the Binet–Simon Intelligence Scale in 1905 marked a new beginning of sorts. Unlike the scientifically motivated research on scaling techniques and individual differences, the outcomes of the Binet scale were meant to inform applied decisions regarding where cognitively impaired children should be placed educationally (Crocker & Algina, 2006).

Binet's work was distinctive in an important way. While many of his contemporaries viewed **human intelligence** as a genetically predetermined and fixed trait, Binet believed in the "educability" of children's intelligence (Binet, 1909). That is, he expected that intelligence could be developed and could change and evolve in children with appropriate educational interventions—even when they were mentally challenged. To tackle the need for tracking and interpreting those changes, he designed an individually administered test with developmentally ordered tasks. Binet's instrument was one of the earliest **developmental assessments** of intelligence. It was designed for measuring children's "mental age" during the ages of 3–13, yielding scores that were interpreted against multi-age **norms tables** that he was among the first to develop.

In the United States, the original Binet scale became the precursor to the subsequent Stanford–Binet Intelligence Scale (S-B) to follow. While the modern S-B test is also an individualized, developmental assessment designed for multi-age populations, it is applied with both children, youth and older adults today. The S-B is administered by trained psychologists nowadays. Grouped under **assessments for screening, diagnosis, and placement** in this book, it is used mainly with "special needs populations." In American public education settings, for instance, the modern S-B test's results are used regularly for identifying giftedness, cognitive impairments, or disabilities in children and youth from grades K–12, guided by somewhat differ-

TABLE 2.1. Historical Drivers of Assessment Uses

Assessment purposes	Historical markers	Primary users	Historical uses and measure-based inferences
Research and scientific discovery	Emergence of psychology as a field of social science	Scientists and researchers in psychology	***Specific uses:*** Generating new knowledge on scaling methods and measurement of human attributes ***Measure-based inferences:*** Individual differences on selected psychological constructs
Educability assessments	Development of the Binet–Simon Intelligence Scale	Researchers/assessment designers, educators, tested children and families	***Specific uses:*** Educational placements of mentally impaired children ***Measure-based inferences:*** Intellectual developmental status
Selecting the "most able-minded" for societal roles	Intelligence testing in the U.S. military and government institutions	Researchers, assessment designers, government institutions, societal leaders, tested individuals and families	***Specific uses:*** Identifying the most able-minded for various societal roles and functions ***Measure-based inferences:*** Mental ability levels
Workplace recruitment and selection	Civil service examinations in the Chinese empire *c.* 1000 B.C.E. Group intelligence testing in the U.S. Army	Researchers, assessment designers, government institutions, societal leaders, tested individuals and families	***Specific uses:*** Identifying the most able-minded for specific job placements ***Measure-based inferences:*** Mental ability levels
School evaluation and accountability	Scientific management movement in U.S. schools with Rice's "common" tests	Test developers, researchers, "scientific managers" of schools, and school-based and societal stakeholders	***Specific uses:*** Mainly summative decisions focused on student and school performance ***Measure-based inferences:*** Quality of schools; students' mastery of the curriculum
Classroom assessments of students	Progressive education movement Tyler's objectives-based tests for educational evaluation	Teachers, test developers, researchers, public school educators, tested students, families, and the general public	***Specific uses:*** Formative and summative decisions to improve classroom instruction and student learning ***Measure-based inferences:*** Instructional quality; students' mastery of the curriculum

ent assessment purposes from the original (Roid, 2003; Walsh & Betz, 2001).

2.2.2.3 Spread of Intelligence Testing Practices in the United States

The interest in individual differences in human intellect engendered pervasive intelligence-testing practices during the years that followed. Unlike Binet's "educable" perspective of the construct, mental testing in the United States became associated with the firm belief that individual intelligence levels were not only inherited attributes but also permanently fixed at birth—a now outdated notion. What followed were serious social policy actions with long-lasting, and sometimes, adverse consequences for particular individuals and social groups (Gould, 1996).

The name of Henry Herbert Goddard (1866–1957), in particular, is associated with the promotion of intelligence-testing practices in the United States. Goddard was responsible for translating the original 1905 Binet test from French to English and using it for the first time with institutionalized children and youth in New Jersey who were mentally disabled. The practice spread rapidly to military, hospital, public school, and immigration settings (Benjamin, 2009).

Ideologically, Goddard subscribed to a now-discredited movement known as **eugenics**. The collective eugenics mindset held that society should keep so-called feebleminded individuals (identified on the basis of intelligence test scores) from having children—either through institutional isolation or sexual sterilization. At the time, African American descendants of slaves and recent immigrants were among the poorest in American society. They tended to perform poorly on intelligence tests of the period, especially compared to the norm groups comprising the dominant sociocultural segments of American society. Believers often attributed poverty to be a direct result of the measured mental capacities of individuals, disregarding the limitations of the assessments, or the possibility that it could be the other way around! Inaccurate test scores are often affected by the socioeconomic, cultural, linguistic, and poverty-related backgrounds of the tested individuals (Gould, 1996; more in Chapter 3).

Exacerbated by a sweeping and blind faith in psychological tests as sources of objective and scientifically trusted data, these intelligence-testing practices led to a pattern of serious misuses of the tests' results, on occasion, coupled with legislated segregation of some groups from given societal roles and functions. Over the long term, these actions harmed particular racial, immigrant, and minority groups significantly (Lombardo, 2011). Most psychologists today describe the eugenics movement and associated intelligence-testing practices as "a dark chapter in American history" (Benjamin, 2009, p. 20).

Decried in retrospect (Gould, 1996), what caused the large-scale social abuses stemming from misuses of intelligence test results? Five misguided ideas embraced by politically powerful voices lay at the bottom of these early-20th-century assessment practices that had negative societal consequences. These were as follows:

1. Human mental capacities are inherited and unalterable traits.
2. Tests and assessment instruments—once designed with "scientific methods"—are infallible tools that measure human attributes and abilities with little or no errors.
3. Assessment instruments (like Binet's original test), once designed, could be moved and applied indiscriminately elsewhere, regardless of the major differences in assessment user contexts. Shifts in the assessment purposes, regions, or population characteristics do not matter.
4. Test-based practices to sort, select, and offer better opportunities in education, work, or other aspects of life to some groups versus others would actually benefit society in the long run.
5. The use of intelligence tests could help engineer and create a socially superior race of people, a belief consistent with the eugenics movement.

In retrospect, one finds a lack of adequate public questioning or a collective social conscience about intelligence-testing practices of that period. Intelligence test developers, and advocates of these tests and test-based actions, also seemingly abdicated their responsibilities in examining the technical properties thoroughly, and conveying the limitations of those early measuring instruments to public users of the tests. That the economically disadvantaged, disabled, or perhaps those simply born into difficult circumstances performed poorly on the tests, did not alter societal perspectives.

2.2.2.4 Early High-Stakes Assessments in the Workplace—China

The emergence of workplace recruitment assessments is attributed to China, dating as far back as 1000–2000 B.C.E. (Du Bois, 1970; R. M. Thorndike, 1990). The Chinese conducted very high-stakes examinations for appointing civil service officers. Other than documentation of the various types of performance assessment tasks that they employed (more on this in Chapter 6), there is little information on the broader social contexts of this highly competitive examination system. The singular priority of the Chinese emperors, it seems, was to select, recruit, and promote only the most able public officials to top-level ministerial positions (Ward et al., 1996).

As with early intelligence testing in the United States, these ancient testing practices in China were consequential in societal terms. With high-stakes recruitment actions linked to workplace testing, both positive and negative consequences could ensue. If the emperors were able to hire well, the implicit positive outcomes—such as good governance practices—would follow for Chinese society. With evidence to support the latter, the essential reasoning underlying the highly competitive examinations would be validated. At the same time, several possible unintended (and negative) consequences could befall the unsuccessful candidates, who could suffer the social stigma of being "failures," lose subsequent job opportunities, or face other barriers in life. Furthermore, if the unselected candidates were found to belong consistently to particular minority groups, social discrimination against these individuals may be viewed as another negative consequence in today's world.

2.2.2.5 Early High-Stakes Workplace Assessments in the United States

Like the examinations in China, the Army Alpha and Army Beta intelligence tests are among the earliest examples of **assessments for job selection and recruitment** purposes in the United States. The armed services employed the tests to recruit soldiers during World War I (*c.* 1910–1917). Albeit applied in this particularized setting at first, the Army Alpha/Beta testing programs exemplify another high-stakes application of early intelligence tests in the American workplace.

Unlike the Binet scale that was individually administered, the Alpha/Beta instruments were a part of a *group testing* program. As a method, large group testing quickly became a popular practice as it is far more efficient than administering assessments individually. In addition, the group tests were among the first examples of **standardized tests**. *Standardization* here implies that common instruments were administered to all the test-takers and scored under the same controlled conditions. Furthermore, the scores were **norm-referenced** to improve comparative score interpretations among test-takers. When test scores are norm-referenced, a person's performance level is determined not so much by the measured level of knowledge mastery but the score's ranked placement, as compared with a defined group of similar test-takers (see the further discussion in Chapter 9). As characteristic of this period, users of the Army Alpha/Beta assessments labeled individuals with poor results as "feebleminded" (Benjamin, 2009, p. 20). Despite controversial evidence suggesting several empirically found limitations of the Alpha/Beta, the tests continued to be applied widely (Atwell, 1937).

2.2.2.6 Early "Common" Tests to Evaluate U.S. Schools

The name of Joseph Mayer Rice is associated with the history of two movements that persist today: standardized educational testing and research conducted in U.S. public schools relying predominantly on student test scores as indicators of school performance (Johanningmeier & Richardson, 2008; Tyack, 1974). Rice's 1890s studies provide the rudiments of what evolved into large-scale student testing practices in schools for *educational evaluation* and *public accountability* purposes. Furthermore, Rice (1893, 1898, 1913) designed the first "common" spelling and arithmetic tests that could be administered simultaneously at multiple schools.

Historians characterize Rice, who was a pediatrician by avocation, as a muckraking journalist (Tyack, 1974). An early empiricist, Rice raised unsettling questions about the quality of public schools in the 1880s, disseminating his views through the popular press. In his initial investigations, Rice visited the schools in person, recording descriptions of classroom teaching and school activities qualitatively, based on his direct observations. Appalled by the conditions he saw, he persisted by administering his self-devised tests of spelling and arithmetic to large groups of students in several grades (Tyack, 1974). His publicly released test results depicted schools of the period unfavorably. Much like accountability-driven educational testing today, a primary purpose of Rice's testing efforts was to evaluate how the *schools* were doing based on how well their *students* performed on the tests (Kliebard, 1992, 2004). Rice's implicit intent was to jolt the schools into improving their teaching practices and student performance. All of the above caused his name to become inextricably associated with the *scientific management* movement of 19th-century American education. In fact, Rice's studies were the harbinger for test-based models of school accountability that followed.

2.2.2.7 Assessments of the "Progressives" in U.S. Education

Contemporaneous with origins of the *common test* and the scientific management movement, we find an almost opposing assessment movement under the rubric of **progressive education** (Cremin, 1961). In general, progressives viewed education as a pragmatic means for serving larger societal goals, such as bringing about social reform, community building, and developing social responsibility and democratic ideals in pupils. John Dewey, who is remembered as a leading and influential scholar-advocate of this pedagogical movement, emphasized the progressive principles of *learning by doing* in his notable works (Dewey, 1897, 1902).

The progressives' teaching and learning ideals were typified with student-developed projects and products. These assessment exercises sought to build students' problem-solving, creative, and critical thinking skills. Important outcomes of the Eight-Year Study—an experimental project conducted between 1930 to 1942 in multiple schools by the Progressive Education Association—included the development of more "sophisticated" tests and alternative forms of student assessment beyond paper-and-pencil tests (Aikin, 1942; Smith & Tyler, 1942).

2.2.2.8 Origins of Objectives-Based Tests in Education

The name of Ralph Tyler (1949) is widely recognized for pioneering the most influential ideas in curriculum development and achievement test design guided by educational objectives. Tyler proposed a model of **objectives-based evaluation** to examine the effectiveness of classroom instruction and education programs more generally (Fitzpatrick, Sanders, & Worthen, 2003). He introduced the straightforward, but then novel, idea that *both* instruction and assessment should be fashioned around a common framework of **educational objectives**. Designed in alignment with objectives, Tyler (1949, 1951) believed that the results of educational tests would have greater utility for improving instruction, as well as raising the achievement outcomes for students, classrooms, and schools in a multitude of ways. He identified the following specific types of uses of the information obtained from objective-based educational tests (see Tyler, 1951, pp. 65–80).

1. **Providing instructional guidance to students:** These were potentially formative decisions that could be made by teachers as instruction continued, focusing on individual students or at the classroom level.
2. **Evaluating pupil performance:** These could be summative decisions that teachers made once instruction was completed, typically at the individual student level.
3. **Organizing learning experiences:** These were the formative actions that teachers could take to help design, organize, and/or deliver instruction at the classroom level.
4. **Appraising the effectiveness of classroom instruction:** These summative decisions could be made by administrators, leaders, and staff at the school or district levels, sometimes also involving teachers at the classroom levels.
5. **Making instructional and administrative improvements to education programs:** These formative decisions could be made by school leaders, teachers, and other staff at the classroom, school, and/or district levels to support quality improvements in education systems.

Notice the *levels of decision making* within school organizations that Tyler had in mind. Note also the wide range of possible uses of data from objective-based student tests for educators, including both formative and summative actions. For example, performed with aggregated test data gathered from large groups of students, uses 4 and 5 above could be applied to multiple levels of decision making in a large school organization—classrooms, schools, and school districts. Notice finally that the *inferences* to be drawn from the students' test results would change significantly as the levels of decision making changed. At the student level, the results of objectives-based tests would indicate their *individual* level of achievement or mastery of the curriculum taught. At the organizational level (classroom, school, or district), the *grouped* test scores would signify the quality of teaching or the effectiveness of schooling processes overall.

Tyler's (1949) trendsetting ideas on objectives-based test design also introduced a key distinction between *learning experiences* (the activities organized by teachers to teach) and the desired *learning outcomes* (performance expectations for students at the end of instruction). To guide education and attain the expected learning outcomes for students, Tyler (1949) prescribed that teachers state the instructional objectives beforehand.

Educational test development entities still apply the essentials of Tyler's approach (see, e.g., Lane, Raymond, Haladyna, & Downing, 2016; Schmeiser & Welch, 2006). This body of work was significantly bolstered by the influential works of Benjamin Bloom and colleagues (1956), Robert Gagné (1965), and others that followed who crafted taxonomies of learning levels (e.g., Bloom's **Taxonomy of Educational Objectives**) to guide the design of educational curricula, instructional strategies, and assessments (more in Chapters 5–7).

QUICK RECAP: Organically generated interests of individuals, groups, or society as a whole gave rise to multiple uses of tests and assessments for different strands of decision making. The historical drivers are summarized in Table 2.1. Although each historical instance began discretely, cases show where assessments were transplanted into new regional contexts, with little or no changes to the test itself (e.g., Binet–Simon's test). The historical inferences and specific uses of a given assessment's results include both formative and summative action taking, sometimes intended for different organizational or societal levels and with different population units. Some past uses of test-based data had egregious societal consequences with little attention to a test's limitations; others show that there could be both positive (usually intended) and negative (usually unintended) consequences of testing on test-takers and societal stakeholders.

Reflection Break 2.1: Objectives 1–3

- In which historical case(s), did the projected *use* appear to drive the assessment design process, dictating how the assessment tool was created? In which of the cases was the assessment *already designed* (in large part) before a new application of the test was found? Explain which approach you'd prefer and why.
- Choose a historical case of assessment use *in your own field.* Identify the larger assessment purpose, the primary users, and measure-based inferences and specific uses that the primary users valued. See Table 2.1 for a guide.
- Do you agree that every assessment use always has a consequence? Distinguish between a *positive consequence* and an *adverse consequence* of a testing scenario. Explain your answers.
- What were the population units or *level of decision making* that the following assessment designers/users valued? Explain your answers. (Choose between individuals, groups, organizations like classrooms or schools, society as a whole, or more than one.)
  - J. M. Rice with his common spelling test
  - Ralph Tyler with objective-based educational tests
  - Army Alpha/Beta intelligence tests
  - Alfred Binet with his educable intelligence scale
  - Chinese emperors with their ancient personnel recruitment tests

2.3 Modern Drivers and Consequences of Assessment Uses in Education

[In] truth, testing is like an iceberg. The part that shows as change is the one-ninth of the berg that is above the water level, and the part that remains the same is the vast underwater bulk.
—ROBERT L. THORNDIKE (1971, p. 3)

How much and what specifically changed in terms of assessment uses as testing and measurement burgeoned in the manner shown in Figure 2.2? This section examines modern assessment uses in education first, followed by a combined discussion of assessment uses found in psychology, health, business, and other fields in the next section. We begin the modern era in the 1960s and 1970s.

2.3.1 Modern Assessment Uses in Grades K–12 Education: The Ups and Downs

2.3.1.1 The Minimum Competency Testing Era

The testing era through the 1970s emphasized the mastery of basic skills and **minimum competency testing** (Jaeger & Tittle, 1980). This era led R. L. Thorndike (1971), cited above, to also observe that there were two undesirable effects of educational test uses: "One [issue] . . . is that there is too much testing and too much weight is given to it. The other is that objective tests . . . tend to pervert the learning process, either because they are poorly constructed or because they inherently measure limited and trivial learning outcomes" (p. 101). See Table 2.2, top panel, as we proceed.

Ralph Tyler's (1949) ideas on curriculum and assessment design became operationalized extensively in education in the form of **objective-type tests**. By and large, whether for pedagogical or educational evaluation and accountability purposes, multiple-choice tests dominated the scene. These test items measured cognitive abilities at the lowest levels, such as rote memorization and recall of basic facts. Efficiency and utility overruled other quality concerns for the assessments. Tyler had been a lead researcher in the Eight-Year Study that included innovative assessments endorsed by progressive educators (Smith & Tyler, 1942). Hence, he may not have anticipated or advocated for the testing trends that followed in the 1970s.

Ideas from behavioral psychology influenced the test design methods of the *minimum competency* era (see Holland & Skinner, 1961, for a treatise on behaviorism). Consistent with the understanding that animal learning occurs via stimulus–response chains, these tests tended to focus on measurement of discrete and often decontextualized elements of knowledge and skill extracted from broader curricula. An excessive reliance on highly **structured-response test** items led to a focus on the easy-to-measure curricular objectives. Regardless of their suitability for the underlying constructs or curricular areas tested, **multiple-choice tests** were adopted by a vast and growing testing industry, as well as by publishers of textbooks and teachers' guides.

2.3.1.2 Toward "Constructivist" Assessments in Education

See Table 2.2, focusing first on its middle and bottom panels. From the 1980s onward, a shift began to occur (Glaser, 1984; Greeno, Moore, & Smith, 1993; Pellegrino et al., 2001, 2014; Shepard, 2000; Sternberg, 2003). New knowledge from cognitive psychology and the neurosciences brought about revised understandings of how human learning occurs, with implications for altered educational practices. There was soon enough organized knowledge pointing to important changes that were necessary in assessment design approaches. Concomitantly, there were public and federal government calls to raise academic standards in education with challenging "content standards" and "world-class" expectations of student performance.

The pushback movement against minimum competency testing reversed the assessment priorities, as shown in the bottom panels of Table 2.2. Curricular domains for instruction and assessment targeted more complex learning outcomes in the 1990s, adding constructed-response and performance assessments to the testing regimens in K–12 schools.

In educational assessments, a **domain** is a defined body of knowledge and skills tied to a subject area curriculum that students are expected to master. Several principles, grounded in the cognitive and learning sciences literature, prompted educators and educational researchers to recommend changes in how assessments were designed and used for educational purposes (Pellegrino et al., 2001). A few of these tenets are sum-

TABLE 2.2. Content Standards and Educational Objectives from Different Eras: Illustrations from Grades K–12

Period	Subject area	Grade level	Content standards and educational objectives
1970–1989 Minimum Competency Testing Era	Reading comprehension	11	*The student will paraphrase verbal information in everyday maps or signs.* ***Test type and items:*** Multiple-choice test items requiring reading of everyday signage
1990–2000 Standards-Based Reforms Era	Reading comprehension	10	*Student will use strategies to understand words and text, confirm predictions, and make inferences from what is read.* ***Test type and items:*** Passage-dependent complex interpretive tasks with multiple-choice and constructed-response items
2001–2020s No Child Left Behind Act of 2001, Common Core State Standards, and Every Student Succeeds Act of 2015	Mathematical reasoning and communication skills	PreK–grade 5	*The student solves everyday computation problems and explains the answers using mathematical reasoning.* ***Test type and items:*** Problem-solving tasks with multiple-choice and constructed-response test items

marized next; what they emphasized was that learning in given domains does not simply occur through the associative, stimulus–response chains popularized by behavioral psychologists (more on this in Chapter 5).

- Individuals *construct new meanings* of the world situated in social and cultural contexts. Most human abilities and skills are developed in this manner.
- New learning occurs by building upon *preexisting knowledge structures* in the human brain. Strengthening these prior connections brings about greater success with new tasks to be learned.
- Human learning and thought are facilitated by a skill set called *metacognition*, which involves the capacity to reflect on, self-monitor, and regulate one's own learning.
- Learning in any domain is influenced by a *learner's feelings*, as well as their attitudinal dispositions and personal-cultural identities. These "noncognitive" factors could either promote or impede learning in given domains.
- Deeper understandings of a domain, when acquired, tend to enable easier *transfer of knowledge* to new or different contexts *and* to other domains of learning.

2.3.1.3 Standards-Based Assessment Reforms

A series of **standards-based reform** initiatives followed in U.S. education, which continue as of this writing. A major federal policy driver was the publication of a labor department report titled *A Nation at Risk* (National Commission for Excellence in Education, 1983). Employee competence levels in workplaces were found to be wanting; the federal report called for higher standards and challenging assessments in education that could change that status quo.

Table 2.2 compares substantive differences in the wording, content, and cognitive demands of curriculum standards with three illustrative educational objectives from the 1970s, 1990s, and 2000s for grades K–12. Standards-based assessments in the new era were intended to match the increasing cognitive complexity of new learning goals and content standards that were endorsed at the federal government level. The emphasis in grades K–12 shifted to the teaching of "big ideas" of the curriculum, accompanied by the use of **alternative assessments** in different performance modalities. Calls for more **authentic assessments** began, incorporating problem-solving and thinking tasks that reflected real-life scenarios (Herman, Aschbacher, & Winters, 1992; Wiggins, 1989).

The passage of the No Child Left Behind (NCLB) Act of 2002 reiterated the earlier calls for world-class education standards. These initiatives were reinforced with new vigor with the Common Core State Standards reforms, reauthorized again with the Every Student Succeeds Act in 2015 (ESSA; U.S. Department of Education, 2015; see www.ed.gov/essa). Each set of these federally legislated reforms was accompanied with stringent student testing requirements for schools and school systems, where every pupil was tested and results publicly released—just as in the era of Joseph Mayer Rice.

The reforms also called for schools to eradicate **achievement gaps** observed in different tested subgroups of students. For example, clear test-based gaps were evident in reading and mathematics for students from high and low socioeconomic levels, males and females, different ethnic and racial groups, and those with and without diagnosed disabilities (Lee, 2002, 2006; National Assessment of Educational Progress [NAEP], 2015).

The implementation of the school reforms was monitored by state departments of education, with high-stakes, public accountability measures tied to students' test scores (National Research Council, 2013; Porter, McMaken, Hwang, & Yang, 2011; Wiggins, 2011). These actions, directly and often adversely, impacted teachers, leaders, and schools in various communities. Under the NCLB and ESSA laws, for example, Ravitch (2016) identified the following types of high-stakes actions based on the results of student testing:

- Schools and education systems that performed well were publicly recognized and rewarded.
- Schools that did not faced large funding cuts; corporate or private takeovers of school system operations; shifts in (or firing of) a school's leadership, teachers, and staff; publicized school rankings and school "report cards"; and merit pay to recognize better-performing schools, leaders, and teachers.

2.3.1.4 Consequences of High-Stakes Testing in U.S. Schools

Tied to the sanctions and rewards, the state tests designed for accountability purposes became the most dominant instruments used in schools. The consequences for individual schools, students, parents, and larger communities were manifold. One ill effect was *teaching-to-the-test*—or student drilling practices where the external state tests (or the content of the test items) heavily influenced classroom-level instruction carried out by teachers, competing with potentially richer curricula for supporting student learning and closing achievement gaps in an all-around manner (Shepard, 1989). Another issue was an *opt-out* movement that began in schools, where parents and families chose to *not* allow their children to participate at all in the state testing programs (Sireci, 2021).

In theory, classroom teachers have more opportunities to engage in formative uses of assessments to foster student learning (Black, Harrison, Lee, Marshall, & Wiliam, 2007; Black & Wiliam, 1998; Shepard, 2006). Much research showed, under ESSA and NCLB, that they focused instead on test drills in an effort to improve student performance on the external accountability tests. A net consequence was that learning opportunities appropriate for the neediest students were shortchanged, with achievement gaps persisting at the end of each school year (Lee, 2002; NAEP, 2015; see also the latest achievement gaps on the NAEP tests, as recorded after the COVID-19 pandemic, at *www.nationsreportcard.gov*). Consider now two case studies in Figure 2.3 and Box 2.1, presenting some well-documented consequences of high-stakes student testing in school evaluation and accountability contexts.

CASE STUDY 1—THE LAKE WOBEGON EFFECT OF THE 1990S

Teaching-to-the-test first became a "hot-button" issue in the 1980s due to a phenomenon called the Lake Wobegon effect (Figure 2.3; Cannell, 1988). Lake Wobegon, from the radio program conceived by the late Garrison Keillor, is a mythical place where "all the men are strong, all the women beautiful, and all the children above average." John Jacob Cannell (1988)—a physician and outsider to education—was able to show empirically that a vast majority of school districts and states were *all above average* on the norm-referenced achievement tests they adopted then, while performing *below average* on other quality indicators at the schools. This inconsistency raised serious questions.

Guided by local school evaluation and accountability needs at the time, the school districts had all adopted commercially designed, norm-referenced tests in reading and mathematics for their annual student testing programs. The tests were normed when designed several years before they were adopted and administered on a large scale in the school systems. Figure 2.3 shows how a Lake Wobegon effect could result from teaching only to the adopted test's items, or to the narrow set of curricular objectives covered by a test. Compared to students in the norm group who did not receive similar drilling and test item exposure, local student cohorts developed an advantage after repeated exposure to the annual tests. Figure 2.3 illustrates how distributions of test scores in a local school system could shift favorably rightward after a few years, as compared to the fixed distribution of a norm group.

The Lake Wobegon effect was first documented during a policy era of relatively *low-stakes testing* requirements, an unexpected consequence of testing for school evaluation purposes. In the 1990s, there were no federal government laws like the NCLB or ESSA requiring every-pupil testing, nor were there public rewards or punitive sanctions linked to the students' test results.

Researchers have since identified a combination of possible factors that could lead to spuriously high scores in schools on external tests. These include teaching-to-the-test practices, outdated norms for the adopted standardized tests, a lack of adequate test security (or too much item exposure), and some forms of widespread cheating documented to occur under high-stakes testing conditions (Phelps, 2017). Most educational experts discourage teaching-to-the-test, as it narrows what could otherwise be a broader, more comprehensive curriculum. Importantly, research shows that these inflated scores rarely reflect lasting forms of student learning. There is a greater consensus today that commercially developed tests should be renormed every 5–10 years to avoid a Lake Wobegon effect (AERA et al., 2014). More information on norming and norm-referenced tests follows in Chapters 3 and 9.

CASE STUDY 2—OPT-OUT MOVEMENTS UNDER ESSA TESTING

Now, take a look at Box 2.1, which presents a news story from the *Huffington Post*. When the reforms began, there was little public dispute that the goals of the Common Core and ESSA were worthwhile. However, due to uneven levels of reform implementation, inadequate distribution of resources, and too-early administrations of the high-stakes tests at schools, a feeling of public distrust grew around the state tests and test development entities. The tests were criticized as being too long, superficial, or overly narrow, and out of alignment with the then prevalent curriculum in public schools. Most school systems were still operating with

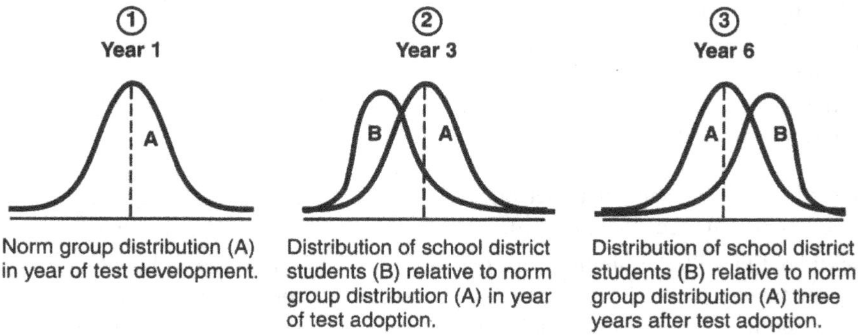

FIGURE 2.3. The Lake Wobegon effect in educational testing: A hypothetical illustration. Reprinted with permission from Chatterji (2003). Allyn & Bacon. © Madhabi Chatterji.

BOX 2.1 Opt-Out Movements in Grades K–12 Education

Consequences of High-Stakes Testing

An excerpt from a news article:

> New York State began 2016 Common Core aligned English-Language Arts testing on April 5. On Long Island, a major opt-out center, thousands of students refused to take the tests. Based on a survey that included 60% of Long Island school districts, *Newsday* estimated that 58,000 out of a potential 115,000 test-takers in third through eighth grade, a little more than half the eligible students, sat out the tests. In one district, Patchogue-Medford, over 70% of the students refused to take the tests. . . . Critics have dismissed the opt-out movement as limited to White parents who are over-protective of their kids. However at Westbury Middle School on Long Island, where 97% of the students are Black and Latino, half the students [will] opt-out of the tests this year, compared to only 2% in 2015.

Source: Reprinted from "Thousands Refuse Common Core Testing." *The Huffington Post.* www.huffingtonpost.com/alan-singer/thousands-refuse-common-c_b_9631956/html.

the previously legislated, NCLB-endorsed curricula! Largely excluded from a top-down process of reform implementation, educators and other stakeholders on the ground viewed the tests as blunt policy instruments to enforce the new ESSA reforms before schools were ready. The news on initially poor test results was often dramatically portrayed by politicians or the media, embarrassing school systems and local communities. A consequence was the widespread opt-out movement.

In one school district, according to a recent report by Sireci (2021), the parents and guardians of almost 90% of the students opted out of the federally mandated testing requirements for their children. The Massachusetts Teachers Association's website apparently included "A Parent's Guide to Opting Out of State Standardized Tests" with one section titled "What Else Can I Do to Support Less Testing, More Learning?"

A fundamental validity issue was the following: With ill-prepared schools, teachers, and students, what did the ESSA test results indicate about actual student learning, or the quality of schooling they had received? (Bennett, 2016; Chatterji, 2013a, 2014a, 2014b; Popham, 2014). To date, the evidence on measured levels of student achievement and transfer as a *positive consequence* of implementing standards-based reforms in schools under ESSA is limited or mixed. Achievement gaps between racial-ethnic and different socioeconomic groups persist on major external assessments, including the NAEP (2024).

2.3.1.5 International Large-Scale Assessment Studies in Education

In Figure 2.2, we saw *international assessment* emerging relatively recently on the historical timeline. International testing programs in K–12 education systems arrived in the 1960s, leading to **international large-scale assessment (ILSA)** studies comparing education systems of different nations. Several ILSA studies are now ongoing and a rapidly growing phenomenon in global research and policy contexts (Feuer, 2013; Ryan & Cousins, 2009).

For example, the Programme for International Student Assessment (PISA) is an ILSA program operated by the Organisation for Economic Co-operation and Development. Typically, the tests focus on mathematics, reading, and science domains. ILSA programs like the Trends in International Mathematics and Science Studies (TIMSS) also measure proficiency in subject areas like civics (see *https://nces.ed.gov/timss*).

In 2015, the PISA tests were administered in some 70 participating regions/nations, including both industrialized and developing countries. That number is growing, supported by different regional governments. In the typical case, participating regions and countries are ranked in *league tables* that compare averages on their student test scores. These country-level ranks have led to many myths, exaggerations, misunderstandings, and misuses of ILSA results in global, national, and public policy contexts. Debates on the ILSA tests are often exacerbated by attention from the media or local politicians. See Box 2.2.

The first ILSA program was established by the International Association for the Evaluation of Educational Achievement in 1958 under the auspices of the United Nations Educational, Scientific and Cultural Organization's Institute for Education. The goal then was to

BOX 2.2 Six Myths about Country Ranks in International Large-Scale Assessment Studies

1. ***Myth:*** The international average test score to which a country's average test score is compared for ranking purposes is the average for every student from every nation of the world.

   Reality: The international mean score is the mean of *participating* countries and regions in a given testing cycle. Schools and students of a given age or grade level are a sample selected from each participating country. The participating nations change in testing cycles.

2. ***Myth:*** If Japan is ranked higher than the United States on the mathematics test, we can generalize that result to conclude that every Japanese student performs better in math than every U.S. student in any year.

   Reality: The test scores in a given region can vary a great deal. Research shows that there is higher variability in test scores within countries than between countries in a typical testing cycle. Results from a given cycle can only be generalized to other years or regions after the sampling differences and other errors are taken into account.

3. ***Myth:*** The international average score from an international large-scale assessment (ILSA) study is a universal quality standard against which all schools and education systems in the world should be judged.

   Reality: The average test score for all the participating countries in a given ILSA cycle is not designed to serve as the "gold standard" for educational quality. As education policies, the curriculum, and local conditions can vary a great deal from country to country, school- and systemwide evaluations using ILSA data make better sense when contextualized data are collected in individual nations.

4. ***Myth:*** The ILSA rank for the United States among industrialized Western nations is an indicator of its economic standing and future economic prospects in the world.

   Reality: Research shows there is little or no relationship between ILSA test results and economic productivity indicators of nations. Nor is there a strong relationship between the development of human capital in the science, technology, engineering, and mathematics (STEM) fields and ILSA results for different nations.

5. ***Myth:*** The average scores on which the country ranks are based is sufficient information to initiate major reforms of the education system in a country.

   Reality: Leaders, educators, and regional stakeholders should be very cautious when interpreting the country ranks without accounting for regional factors, such as the history, politics, and governance of education systems, regional curriculum, the time of testing against the school calendars, and the participants in a testing cycle.

6. ***Myth:*** ILSA country ranks, taken at face value, are sound indicators of a nation's overall educational effectiveness and standing in the world.

   Reality: ILSA studies are based on survey research methods and similar to public opinion polls. By design, the results do not allow meaningful or fair intercountry comparisons. A country's average score should be interpreted only as a descriptor of student achievement status in the subject tested in a given year, accounting for sampling errors.

conduct research to compare educational systems in various nations as an intellectual exercise. The effort was led by researchers. Today, multiple such programs have mushroomed, guided instead by economic development goals, often tied closely to education program development with high-stakes accountability policies (Pizmony-Levy et al., 2014).

In Mexico, for example, Backhoff (2013, p. 245) reported how the results of the PISA and other student tests were touted in a documentary film titled *De panzazo*. Test scores were used to promote higher salaries for successful teachers, with dismissal of teachers when the results were deemed too low. Front-page newspaper headlines and editorials tend to directly interpret the high- or low-country ranks on the PISA as indicators of how a nation's overall education system or economy is performing. Both these inferences are largely unsupported with evidence of validity (Feuer, 2013; Rotberg, 2014). In the United States, politicians have similarly used PISA rankings to raise concerns about American education or to sponsor legislation to spur added reforms (see *https://blog.ed.gov/2013/12/duncan-calls-for-higher-standards-and-expectations*).

ILSA researchers and experts have tried to refute the most common, but often unwarranted inferences and uses of ILSA study results (Box 2.2; after Pizmony-Levy et al., 2014). Box 2.2 clarifies that each ILSA study, in reality, is conducted in periodic cycles. Each is a technically complex, survey-testing endeavor that generates large, multivariate datasets. Different ILSA reports yield useful information for certain purposes. Countries that participate tend to change from testing cycle to cycle. For example, in the 2012 TIMSS, only the state of Florida participated on behalf of the entire United States. Interpretations of country ranks, therefore, should be conducted in an informed and careful manner.

Appropriately interpreted and used, the *within-nation* ILSA reports could yield valuable information for improving local educational systems. Similarly, contextualized and appropriately analyzed ILSA data could permit some comparative interpretations of results for nations trying to model their own education systems against others with similar backgrounds, governments, economies, histories, and geographic profiles. For nations without the resources to mount and maintain their own large-scale educational testing programs, ILSA studies can yield helpful data for educational policymakers (Backhoff, 2013; Feuer, 2013; Laurie, 2013; Plisko, 2013; Wagemaker, 2013).

2.3.2 Assessment Uses in Higher Education

With a few exceptions, we see parallel types of assessment uses in higher and professional education contexts, as in PreK–12 systems. Programs and institutions in higher education tend to rely on data on multiple constructs and indicators of quality, measured at different levels of an organizational entity (Eaton, 2015). In a well-regarded book, Astin (2012) identified the main assessment uses in higher and professional education that hold up today, pointing to the widespread use of student tests and surveys. For example, student-level assessments are a routine component of coursework and instructional program delivery. Faculty and instructors often use **classroom assessments** for providing formative feedback and individualized mentoring or apprenticeship opportunities. Likewise, tests and assessments are used for assigning summative grades to signify student performance levels at the end of a course or degree program. For students involved, these different actions could carry either low or high stakes. Similarly, assessments for *professional certification* are common in training programs for specialized occupations, like teaching, medicine, and the health professions; this is a relatively high-stakes use that impacts individual candidates directly.

Assessments for program evaluation and accreditation purposes could be varied and performed at the student, program, and institutional levels in higher and professional education. The main user groups include students, instructors, administrators, and the oversight constituencies. *Accreditation* of programs and institutions by external certification agencies is a high-stakes evaluative activity involving site visits and extensive data reviews by recognized external associations and national credentialing bodies. Accreditations are typically conducted to certify degree-awarding programs and their supporting entities.

Three long-recognized issues with assessment uses in higher education are as follows (Astin, 2012):

- Instructor-implemented assessments are highly variable and subjective, along with grade-inflation issues that accompany a lowering of students' performance standards.

- Institutional and program evaluations tend to rely too much on subjective questionnaires and surveys.
- The assessment information gathered routinely has little or no collective benefit or value for students and stakeholders.
- College admissions tests are flawed, as these tools tend to favor Whites and socioeconomically wealthier students, leaving minority groups behind.

Testing for college entrance purposes, the last bullet, tends to be a controversial practice. For decades now in the United States, well-known standardized tests like the SAT and ACT are employed by many colleges for undergraduate admissions. At the graduate and professional levels, tests like the GRE and GMAT are used for the same reasons. To complicate matters, adopters often use the same tests for awarding scholarships and other recognitions to further select smaller numbers of candidates for potentially better opportunities; this second competitive use involves even higher-stakes decisions. As often rationalized by both test developers and adopters, such tools are designed to serve as common entrance examinations to be taken by applicants who may come from variable scholastic settings, whether in the nation or globally. Therefore, use of the tests offers everyone a comparable and fair performance platform prior to college entry.

To understand the controversy, let us consider the SAT in-depth as a case in point. Administered typically to high school students who aspire to a college-level education, the SAT provides verbal and math ability scores. The current version was completely redesigned by the test developers in 2016. Based on statistics posted by the National Center for Educational Statistics, the mean SAT score for all existing high school–level test-takers in the United States in 2017 was 1060 (SD of 195; see *www.nces.ed.gov*).

These SAT test scores, collected at the end of high school, are expected to predict students' future academic performance in college. Accordingly, the tests used for admission require evidence of **predictive validity**, showing that the test scores adequately and reliably predict student success on college-level performance measures. This evidence is usually gathered longitudinally with correlational statistics (AERA et al., 2014). To claim fairness in the college entrance decisions, the results should further show similar levels of predictive validity for *all* groups of test-takers, without favoring any gender-related, ethnic, or social group. Historically, however, when taken alone, SAT results have shown only modest to low levels of predictive validity, revealing instead some systematic performance differences between males versus females, and applicants belonging in ethnic majority and minority groups (Marini et al., 2019; Shaw & McKenzie, 2010).

Figure 2.4 presents illustrative gaps on the SAT as recently reported by the University of California system with 2018 and 2019 data. Note that this table suggests that all the applicants from the University of California system, regardless of racial-ethnic group, actually outperformed the typical U.S. applicant based on the national average score. But, as compared with the two highest-performing groups (Whites and Asians) within this particular university system, we see that there are distinct performance gaps in the other applicant groups. Following an internal review of these and other data trends, the University of California system decided to abandon use of the SAT as an undergraduate admissions measure (University of California).

Multipurposing of college entrance tests for performing research and evaluation of K–12 school systems is another problematic issue but also a common practice. Sometimes media reports draw the public's attention with alarmist headlines when SAT scores decline in an education system (see, e.g., "SAT Reading Scores Hit a Four-Decade Low" in the *Washington Post*, September 24, 2012). When decision-makers, education observers, and other stakeholders make direct causal inferences about the quality of a particular high school program or a school system on the basis of average SAT or ACT scores, it is often a *misinterpretation* of that data.

Validity issues arise because tests like the SAT are not designed for evaluating the quality of school programs or the effectiveness of specific teaching practices. The items on the test may have little or no match with the coursework and curriculum that students tend to receive. Hence, without added validation and locally gathered evidence to show that the SAT items actually

2018 (left) and 2019 (right)

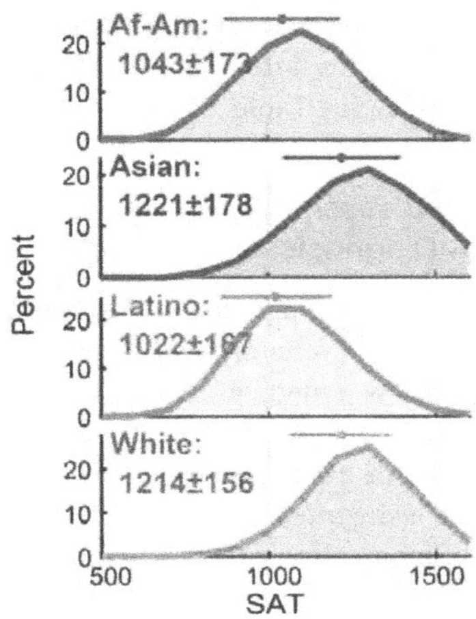

Race/Ethnicity	Mean SAT	Gap Vs. Asian
African-American	1166	190
Native American	**1259**	**97**
Asian	1356	0
Latino	1122	234
Pacific Islander	**1216**	**140**
White	1338	18
Unknown	**1356**	**0**

FIGURE 2.4. Illustrative data on college entrance examination scores: SAT gaps in scale score points for different ethnic groups against the highest-performing group (Asian). Reprinted with permission from University of California Academic Senate (2020), https://senate.universityofcalifornia.edu/_files/committees/sttf/sttf-report.pdf.

match the curriculum delivered, the test scores would have unknown levels of **content-based validity**. In addition, when students from wealthier households opt to take the SAT in larger numbers, there could be *selection biases* in the sample of test-takers at a school or school system. Well-to-do students frequently have greater educational advantages at home and are, therefore, better prepared for college entrance exams. Issues like greater chances to take more challenging coursework at schools located in wealthier neighborhoods could further cloud the inferences about effective schools, programs, and practices using data from college entrance tests.

QUICK RECAP: See Table 2.3. Modern purposes for tests and assessments in grades K–12 and higher education link back to the historical roots of testing, with some new uses emerging over time. Among these are large-scale, international assessments for national policy evaluations. Modern assessment purposes span seven areas, including both high- and low-stakes uses. As with historical instances, modern assessment users tend to use the same test for more than one purpose, sometimes without attention to the purposes of the original test or limitations of the measures. Use of the SAT as a curriculum-based outcome measure is an example. This can lead to serious validity issues, with adverse or unexpected consequences for some users and stakeholders.

Reflection Break 2.2: Objectives 1–4

- How is *teaching-to-the-test* in the Lake Wobegon case different from classroom teaching and assessment guided by a curriculum?
- Identify a *positive consequence* of high-stakes college admissions testing policies.
- Compare Rice's and Tyler's assessment uses in education to *modern uses* we find in K–12 education today (with which you are familiar). What are the (1) similarities and (2) differences with respect to constructs measured, inferences and uses valued, primary users, and levels of decision making?

- What would be a *low-stakes* and *appropriate use of ILSA* results in a country? Explain.
- List examples of modern assessment applications in *higher education* from your experience, where the users make both high-stakes and low-stakes decisions with results.
    - What is the expected *positive consequence* of each use?
    - What, if any, is a possible *negative consequence* of each use?
    - Who could be most affected by each action?
- Think of different levels of education systems: students, classrooms/courses, programs, institutions. Give examples of *formative* and *summative uses* of assessment results at each level, and the different *measure-based inferences* that users desire. Explain your answer.
- What is *multipurposing* an assessment? Why is it problematic from a validity standpoint? Give an example of a multipurposed assessment with which you are familiar.

2.4 Modern Drivers and Consequences of Assessment Uses in Psychology, Health, Business, and Other Fields

An edited series of books by McReynolds and colleagues (2012) provides a window into some major ways in which assessment instruments came to be employed in psychology and mental health areas, spreading to other applied professions. Looking back to Figure 2.2 with a focus on psychological assessment specifically, recall the observable drop in the trend line after 2010: What may have caused it?

Four broad trends in assessment use emerged outside education (McReynolds et al., 2012). These were (1) research and scientific activity, with new interests on correlational studies of human abilities, personality traits, and behaviors; (2) clinical screenings, diagnoses, and/or treatment of health disorders and diseases; (3) counseling and guidance of individuals for educational, life, or career planning, a novel direction: (4) specialized workplace applications in industrial, organizational and employment settings, offshoots of the old traditions in the United States and China; and (5) professional certification testing. As most of these categories have already been discussed at length, this section devotes attention to the second, third, and fourth uses. See Table 2.3.

2.4.1 Assessment Uses for Screening, Diagnosis, and Therapeutic Purposes

Screening and diagnosis of disabilities or health disorders are common clinical assessment uses that generally follow a medical model. Most such applications are individual assessments. The goal for clinically oriented health assessments is to provide treatments to address a diagnosed disease, disorder, or health care need. Technically, screening is the first step, followed by use of more rigorous assessments to make a final diagnosis of the condition (Cohen et al., 2022). Screening decisions carry lower stakes as these are changeable, less firm or long-lasting, and therefore less consequential for those examined. Diagnostic and placement decisions in treatment courses, on the other hand, can have serious long-term consequences. Three examples of diagnosed mental health conditions are, for instance, depression, attention deficit disorder (ADD), and schizophrenia. Personality disorders include, for example, paranoid personality disorder.

The design and properties of measures employed for each separate purpose, therefore, must meet appropriate standards of rigor with respect to validity, reliability, and utility. Specifically, diagnostic tools should meet demonstrably higher standards for *predictive validity* and *classification accuracy* rates so that the treatment placements are dependable, or within tolerable margins of error when individuals are placed for treatment.

Clinical screening and diagnostic applications of tests could also focus on identifying mild handicaps or learning disabilities of students in education systems (Shepard, 1989). The assessment purposes, here again, are for clinical screening, diagnosis, treatment placements, and/or delivery of interventions to students identified with special needs. A typical testing regimen to identify a student's speech impairment, for example, could involve an early screening followed by diagnostic assessments by speech therapists. The assessment tools, diagnostic categories and criteria are standardized and specific to the constructs.

To facilitate best practices, leading professional organizations have developed resources and practitioner guides on interpreting the data from given assessments correctly. One example is the *Diagnostic and Statistical Manual of Mental Disorders* (DSM) published by the American Psychiatric Association. This manual offers a common set of criteria for the classification of mental disorders using an array of mental health assessment tools. Among the primary users and stakeholders who rely on the DSM for guidance are clinicians, psychologists, researchers, psychiatric drug regulation agencies, health insurance companies, pharmaceutical companies, the legal system, as well as policymakers.

The *International Statistical Classification of Diseases and Related Health Problems* (ICD), produced by the World Health Organization, is another commonly used manual for guiding appropriate uses of assessments designed for the diagnosis of health-related disorders. The ICD is distinguished from the DSM in that it covers all health issues and conditions and is not restricted to mental health issues alone.

Regardless of the guidelines and resources, serious concerns often surround clinical uses of tests used for high-stakes diagnoses of health issues. Speaking in particular about DSM assessments and associated clinical criteria for classification of diseased conditions, Lane (2013) raised the following issues:

- The predictive validity and reliability of measures used for diagnostic purposes, and diagnostic categories, are sometimes scientifically suspect. The reliance on superficial symptoms of a disease or disorder based on still evolving scientific knowledge on a construct is a source of concern.
- The use of artificially set dividing lines between "normal" versus abnormal, unhealthy, or disabled categories of individuals is controversial.
- The possibility of **systematic measurement biases** inherent in items and instruments applied with different gender, ethnic, linguistic, or cultural groups is a major and perpetual concern.
- Finally, there are concerns that human distress conditions are often "medicalized" as abnormalities. (This issue arose in the 2010s with the diagnoses of mental illnesses in displaced refugees and vulnerable populations migrating from war-torn regions like Tunisia to refugee camps in Jordan.)

Critics of the DSM today include the National Institute of Mental Health (NIMH) in the United States, a group that no longer funds research using instruments associated with the criteria. According to Lane (2013), the NIMH rejected DSM criteria as an unscientific and subjective system for diagnosing mental illnesses and disorders. Recent versions, like the DSM-5-TR (American Psychiatric Association, 2022), follow a more holistic set of diagnostic criteria for identifying particular health conditions than prior editions. Good practice demands that clinical practitioners use *multiple assessment instruments* and *more than one measurement time point* to make firm diagnoses of clinical conditions. Several U.S. laws today protect minority individuals and tested groups from discriminatory and adverse impacts associated with improper diagnostic actions based on assessments (Cohen et al., 2022).

CASE STUDY 3—LEGAL ISSUES AND ADVERSE CONSEQUENCES OF DIAGNOSTIC ASSESSMENTS

A well-known case, dated but still relevant, is that of *Daniel Hoffman v. the Board of Education of the City of New York* (Sattler, 1988, pp. 1–2). Daniel Hoffman was diagnosed as mentally retarded based on intelligence testing performed at a very young age. However, many years later, a retesting showed that the early result had been erroneous due to a confounding of symptoms of a speech impairment with mental retardation. The case illustrated how overreliance on a single testing by the Board of Education, and failure to reevaluate the child within 2 years (as recommended by the psychologist), severely limited future educational and work opportunities for the examinee. Outside the lawsuit, a major validity concern is the misclassification of an early childhood speech impairment as mental retardation. The unnecessary and long-term placement of the misdiagnosed individual in an occupational school for mentally retarded youth led to the lawsuit.

At least three issues concerning the uses of high-stakes clinical assessments in grades K–12 education contexts have similarly engendered heated discussions (Shepard, 1989). First, special needs identification (e.g., a learning disability like dyslexia) has traditionally depended on the use of intelligence tests designed for other purposes—like the Stanford–Binet in the United States. Second, because of the fallibility of commonly used testing procedures, normal children of minorities are often misidentified or overidentified as "handicapped" or learning disabled. Studies have shown that of the students identified as having learning disabilities, as many as half may be wrongly classified because of predictive validity problems of the diagnostic instruments. Many of the tests also show cultural and linguistic biases against minorities as well. A negative consequence is the mislabeling and possible long-term stigmatizing of otherwise normal children as disabled or "deviants" from the mainstream.

2.4.2 Low-Stakes Assessment Uses: Guidance and Counseling Applications

In contrast to the above, relatively low-stakes assessment uses include providing counseling and guidance to individuals based on the results of an array of assessments (Harmon, 1989). Counselors—typically also trained psychologists and social workers—use assessments to help clients explore educational options, develop career and life plans, and support personal development goals. A wide variety of assessment instruments have evolved over time to serve these purposes, ranging from interest and attitude inventories to aptitude and ability tests to personality assessments of individuals. For instance, guidance counselors might employ assessments to determine the intellectual, emotional, and attitudinal profiles of clients to enable decisions on their educational, vocational, and personal goals.

Unlike clinicians, counselors can operate with very few legal constraints in their use of assessments. However, the challenges of inadequately defined constructs, insufficient validity, reliability or utility evidence, and culturally biased assumptions underlying tests and instruments all affect assessment uses for guidance as well. First, the information from any given assessment provides only a small part of the whole picture needed to form conclusions on the best paths for individuals. The counselors' training and knowledge of applied measurement and psychometrics help prevent inappropriate uses of the results of specialized instruments. As always, the tests and assessments should not be used inappropriately. Users should seek adequate documentation of the quality of the measures in the personalized contexts that apply (AERA et al., 2014; see also Harmon, 1989, p. 535).

2.4.3 Assessment Uses in Clinical Training and Program Evaluations

Counselors often work alongside social workers, psychologists, and other clinicians to provide clients with skill-based training programs in behavior change and self-management skills, where assessments may be used to evaluate client-level and programmatic outcomes. Practicing counselors could employ the assessments as classroom instructors would in any skill-based training context. Their curricula would typically focus on personal, social, and emotional areas of development, such as coping with stress, conflict resolution, dealing with personal or family crises, anger management, or managing interpersonal problems at home, work, and school.

Similarly, attitudinal assessments may be employed to evaluate programs, such as by comparing groups of clients on their perceived levels of service quality in a business, hospital, or health care organization. A program's impact evaluation may, likewise, employ pre- and postprogram comparisons of client groups on affective and behavioral construct measures (Rossi et al., 2018).

CASE STUDY 4—ASSESSMENTS AT CROSS PURPOSES?

Consider now Box 2.3 describing corporate uses of the *XQ factor* assessment in a *Time* magazine article. A large number of Fortune 500 companies and business organizations were recently reported to be evaluating entering job applicants with tests of attitudes and personality traits. Depending on the company, the professionals they sought could differ widely. For example, the job openings were varied for management executives, call center employees, Wall Street traders, and a number of other specialized positions. As shown, the companies (or their assessment service provider) adopted a cluster of preexisting personality or attitude survey tools for this purpose, either "as is" or with minor modifications. Three specific traits valued by the organizations, as included in the XQ factor test, are spontaneity, independence, and curiosity.

As described, the overall assessment is an omnibus, multiconstruct measure. What is the *inference* that the companies wish to make from the information generated by the *X-factor* test? According to the news clip

BOX 2.3 High-Stakes Personality Assessments in the Workplace

"How High Is Your XQ Score?"

This question was posed in a 2015 cover story title in the *Time* magazine. A person's XQ factor is a purported measure of "job fit" based on a series of personality and attitudinal measures.

Here is an adapted illustration of an XQ assessment. (For more on XQ items, see *https://time.com/3915807/personality-fits-job.*)

To what extent are the following statements true for you? Use *one* of these response options: (a) Definitely True, (b) True, (c) Not Sure, (d) Untrue, (e) Definitely Untrue.

1. I trust my instincts more than data.
2. I would rather read a book than watch TV.
3. I am a level-headed person at work.

in Box 2.3, the measures purportedly indicate each applicant's "person-to-job fit."

This case raises several alarm bells. Numerous personality and attitudinal assessments are available today. But a vast majority were designed originally for specific uses in clinical, counseling, or mental health contexts, and/or intended for very different populations (Cohen et al., 2022). Individually, the measures may have limited to no validity evidence at all that would allow inferences on a number of different and somewhat specialized "job fit" levels. Collectively, they were certainly not designed for supporting the high-stakes recruitment decisions for markedly different corporate roles. When instruments are multipurposed in this manner, what are the "best practice" recommendations?

Two standards provide specific guidelines for the assessment developers/adopters and the primary users in such scenarios (AERA et al., 2014). For the assessment designers, Standard 1.0 states:

> Clear articulation of each intended test score interpretation for a specified use should be set forth and appropriate validity evidence in support of each intended interpretation should be provided. (p. 23)

Aimed toward assessment users, Standard 1.4 states:

> If a test score has been interpreted for a use in a way that has not been validated, it is incumbent on the user to justify the new interpretation for that use. . . . (p. 24)

In cases like Box 2.3, therefore, the burden falls on the Fortune 500 companies (the instrument adopters) to defend their recruitment actions with the XQ factor tests. Designing entirely new instruments for their own purposes is an option. Alternatively, validating the adopted tools/construct measures *situated* in the new assessment contexts is another.

QUICK RECAP: See Table 2.3. A vast number of the assessment uses in psychology, health, business, and fields outside education tend to focus on *individuals* as the population units for making inferences and decisions. Several of these individual-level decisions carry high stakes and are consequential for those tested. Depending on the case, there may be legal and human rights issues. Elsewhere, program- or organizational-level evaluations could utilize grouped data from assessments, where the inferences would apply to the unit or level of the entity that is evaluated (such as a department with employees). Major threats to validity arise with clinical constructs if there is inadequate scientific knowledge on the diseased condition, disability, or disorder. When existing assessment tools are employed in new contexts, the redesign-validation efforts should be renewed to justify any new score interpretations for different populations and purposes.

Reflection Break 2.3: Objectives 1–4

- List how assessments used for *research or evaluative investigations* differ from assessments used for (1) *clinical diagnosis*, (2) *guidance and counseling*, and (3) *workplace recruitments*. Answer with reference to the inferences, specific uses, units/levels of decision making, and stakes tied to assessment results.
- Why are *clinical diagnosis assessment* uses considered "high stakes" compared to *clinical screening* decisions? Explain.

- Distinguish between *formative* and *summative uses* of assessment results in the following user contexts: (1) mental health or health care, (2) workplace, (3) guidance and counseling, and (4) research and development. Give an example of each.
- See Figure 2.1. Explain the connections between (1) *validity* and *assessment purposes*, and (2) *validity* and the *assessment context.*
- Brainstorm the *positive* and *negative consequences* of using the XQ factor assessments as the Fortune 500 companies did.

2.5 Applying User-Centered Principles to Improve Practices

2.5.1 Consequences of Assessment Uses: Examining the Issues

In modern measurement theory, validating the *consequences of assessment use* refers to formally collected evidence showing that a test or assessment has the intended positive impacts on the examinees or respondents, as well as the concerned stakeholders. The abbreviated label for this class of evidence is **consequential validity**. Consequential validity overlaps closely with the quality criterion of **usefulness** of assessments and construct measures, introduced in Chapter 1 in the utility discussion. Both concepts assume that the developers and primary adopters/users of given assessments aspire to achieve some socially desirable outcomes through uses of the tool. The investigations aim to verify that, when applied as designed, the assessment instrument yields the expected benefits for the persons tested and others in the larger assessment environments. Consequential validity and utility-relevant impact research are essential in all high-stakes testing scenarios, especially to ensure that any undesirable or unintended impacts are absent.

Messick (1989) first proposed that instrument validation include evaluations of the consequences of score uses, recognizing that all assessment applications have some consequences—whether good or bad. The concept, however, was slow in entering the measurement literature. Consequential validity studies are still sparse in practice. The 2014 Standards recommended that large-scale test developers add this specific category of evidence to their validation protocols (AERA et al., 2014).

2.5.2 Primary User Paths

Review Table 2.3 on page 57, alongside Figure 2.1. Based on the literature reviewed in this chapter, the table presents eight main strands depicting the major **user paths** for the assessment uses we find currently across the surveyed fields and sectors. The user paths are (1) science, research and development; (2) professional certification and credentialing; (3) clinical screening, diagnosis, and placement for therapy/treatment; (4) candidate selection in education for admissions, scholarships, or recognitions/awards; (5) personnel evaluations in the workplace for recruitment, coaching and professional development, or promotions; (6) program/policy evaluations, accreditation, and accountability in organizations; (7) classroom teaching and learning; and (8) guidance and counseling.

The user paths summarize the general parameters of the *assessment user contexts* that designers could choose from when beginning the instrument design or selection process (Figure 2.1). In many applied settings, as documented in this chapter, the user paths do not remain discrete. An instrument designed for classroom testing purposes may be also employed for program evaluations (User Paths 6–7). In instances where the primary users desire to multipurpose an assessment tool in more than one path, Table 2.3 may be helpful in alerting designers/users on the potential changes in the population units, measure-based inferences, and the specific uses. This would help set the stage for validation.

2.5.3 *Why Assess?:* Specifying the Assessment Purposes, Primary Users, Measure-Based Inferences, and Uses

User-centered design principles require that we start by specifying the functions and purposes of an assessment instrument before we give it a physical form, shape, and structure (Giacomin, 2014; Lowdermilk, 2013; Norman, 2013; Roozenburg & Eekels, 1995). A first issue to address, therefore, deals with identifying the user paths broadly.

TABLE 2.3. Modern Drivers of Assessment Use: Eight User Paths

User path and assessment purposes	Examples, primary users, and stakeholders	Specific uses and measure-based inferences
User Path 1: **Science, research, and development**	***Example:*** Personality research in Psychology ***Primary users and stakeholders:*** Scientists, researchers, participants, and public users of research	***Specific uses:*** New knowledge production and dissemination ***Measure-based inferences:*** Varies depending on interests of researchers
User Path 2: **Professional certification and credentialing**	***Example:*** National medical board examinations for certifying physician competency ***Primary users and stakeholders:*** Examinees, credentialing organizations, test developers and researchers, organizations that hire professionals	***Specific uses:*** Certification in a profession ***Measure-based inferences:*** Proficiency in specialized skill and knowledge domains
User Path 3: **Clinical screening, diagnosis, and treatment placement**	***Examples:*** Tests used in Psychiatry, listed in the *Diagnostic and Statistical Manual of Mental Disorders* ***Primary users and stakeholders:*** Clinicians, tested individuals and families, test developers and researchers	***Specific uses:*** Diagnosis and treatment of diseases, disorders, and disabilities ***Measure-based inferences:*** Severity of disease or disability
User Path 4: **Admission, selection, scholarships, and awards in education**	***Example:*** College or university entrance examination ***Primary users and stakeholders:*** Examinees and families, decision-makers in organizations, test developers and researchers	***Specific uses:*** Identifying able candidates ***Measure-based inferences:*** Potential to succeed at the next education level
User Path 5: **Personnel evaluations in the workplace—coaching, recruitment, or promotion**	***Examples:*** Cognitive ability tests, personality and attitude surveys ***Primary users and stakeholders:*** Examinees and families, decision-makers in workplaces, assessment developers and researchers	***Specific uses:*** Identifying able candidates ***Measure-based inferences:*** Potential to perform and succeed in the workplace
User Path 6: **Program and policy evaluations, institutional accreditation and accountability**	***Examples:*** Assessments used in evaluating educational programs and institutions ***Primary users and stakeholders:*** Programs/institutions with faculty, staff and leaders, examinees and families, researchers and evaluators	***Specific uses:*** Formative or summative decisions ***Measure-based inferences:*** Quality of programs, institutions, or departments
User Path 7: **Classroom teaching and learning**	***Example:*** Teacher-made tests and assessments ***Primary users and stakeholders:*** Students and families, educators, teachers, leaders, test developers and researchers	***Specific uses (stakes):*** Formative or summative classroom decisions ***Measure-based inferences:*** Quality of teaching, students' learning levels and needs
User Path 8: **Guidance and counseling**	***Example:*** Multiple assessments that yield "profile scores" ***Primary users and stakeholders:*** Individual clients, counselors, psychologists, assessment developers and researchers	***Specific uses:*** Goal setting, counseling and guidance decisions ***Measure-based inferences:*** Best matches of individual profiles to specific educational, career, and/or life paths

A second issue deals with the primary users. To be maximally responsive, the Process Model requires that design–validation processes are integrated with primary users' needs, interests, and capacities, enhancing their overall "user experience" when dealing with the assessments. To conclude, we return to Figure 2.1 and Table 2.3 together, to consider the detailed steps in specifying the *Why assess?* boxes.

2.5.3.1 Specifying the Assessment Purposes

To specify the Assessment Purposes, we ask the following types of guiding questions referring to Table 2.3. Will the assessment's results be used mainly for research purposes, such as to measure the outcomes of an experiment (User Path 1)? Or, for classroom teaching and learning, such as to assign student grades in college courses (User Path 7)? Or, for performing institutional evaluations (User Path 6)? Will there likely be *more than one* user path (and groups of primary users) involved? Should they *all* be taken into account before embarking on the instrument design/adoption process?

2.5.3.2 Specifying the Primary Users

An immediate second question is this: Who are the most likely users of the assessment tool and the information it will provide? What kinds of specific information will they be looking for, given the larger contexts where they operate? The literature on user-centered design distinguishes between primary, secondary, and tertiary users of a product (Giacomin, 2014; Lowdermilk, 2013; Norman, 2013; Roozenburg & Eekels, 1995). For instrument design/adoption purposes, we consider the **primary users** mainly, recognizing that the others are among **stakeholders** in the broader contexts where the instruments are used.

Who are the primary users? Typically, this group includes the direct users of the instruments and the results—that is, the individual test-takers and respondents, the assessment designers, adopters and test administrators, and/or those directly involved in interpreting and using the assessments results for specific decisions. These subgroups are not always mutually exclusive. For instance, teacher-designers are also often the interpreters and action-takers with classroom assessment results; the same holds for researchers or other users.

Appropriate design steps and interpretive guidelines are necessary when the designers and action-takers belong in separate groups or are distanced from the design process, especially when the measures are technically complex or nontransparent. To avert breakdowns in validity afterward, the important question to ask during this step is: Who will likely draw inferences directly from the construct measures and make decisions with the results?

2.5.3.3 Specifying the Measure-Based Inferences

See the box to the right of the Assessment Purposes in Figure 2.1. Exactly how the primary users plan to interpret the results for each separate use must be specified next. Here are some guiding questions for this step: In what formats do the users wish to interpret the construct measures (e.g., individual test scores, aggregated scores for groups, other forms)? What meanings will those measures convey vis-à-vis the construct(s) measured in each application? Will the construct meanings be expected to change for different units of the population or at different levels?

2.5.3.4 Specifying the Assessment Uses, Stakes, and Consequences

The *assessment use* parameter is a loaded one. We would need to clarify three aspects of the uses: the exact decisions that users plan to make with the assessment results, the likely stakes to be tied to those actions, and the consequences anticipated for each use for the test-takers/respondents, users, and other stakeholders.

What the term *high stakes* means specifically could change in different contexts. Furthermore, perceptions of how high the stakes are could vary in the eyes of different actors. A helpful exercise in executing this step is to brainstorm both good and bad scenarios with a selected group of primary users.

Several questions could be asked at this point, such as: At how many levels will the primary users be taking actions with the construct—individuals, groups, organizations, other entities? Will users make formative and/or summative decisions with the measures? At what time points will each type of decision be made?

Are the planned decisions *high-stakes* or *low-stakes*? What benefits do the users expect for the population assessed and other stakeholders, in the short and long term? Could there be any adverse consequences of the proposed assessment uses for any individuals, groups, or society as a whole?

2.5.3.5 Specifying the Assessment Context

The answers to the *Why assess?* questions must be integrated closely with the *What?* and *Who?* questions in Phase I (Figure 2.1). All three aspects complete the specification of the overall *assessment user context*—also called the *assessment context* or the *user context* in this book. The assessment context is a necessary anchor; it is *the* reference point for cycling back to the design, refine, validate, evaluate, and finalize stages of compiling an assessment and its components (Phases II–V). Plus, specifying the organizational or societal ecology where the assessment tool will be used, and the backgrounds of the individuals or groups to be tested, help understandings as to who the stakeholders might be for the assessment tools.

QUICK RECAP: All our intended interpretations and uses of an assessment's results have to be *specified in advance*. The *Why assess?* portal of the Process Model focuses directly on specifying users, uses, and user-desired inferences of assessment results. This final section suggested prompts to guide actions of assessment designers and adopters in Phase I. These actions were linked to Phases II–V in the cyclic process of assessment design, selection, validation, and use. Specified thoroughly and clearly beforehand, the assessment user context serves as an anchoring point for the remaining parts of the process.

Reflection Break 2.4: Objectives 3–6

- Suppose you wish to adopt a previously designed assessment instrument for your own use.
  - Specify the *Why assess?* boxes in Phase I in detail.
  - Specify the overall *assessment user context* in Phase I in detail.
  - Distinguish among the *primary users* and *stakeholders*.
  - Outline the steps you would like to take to maintain *validity* of the interpretations and uses of the assessment results in that context.
- Select a common assessment tool in your profession. How is it typically applied, and what are the expected *benefits* of the specified assessment uses on the populations tested?
- Define the term *consequential validity*. How would you investigate it for a tool that you design.
- List ways in which the *Process Model* can improve practices of (1) assessment designers; (2) assessment adopters; and (3) the primary users and stakeholders of a given tool.

2.6 Summary

Chapter 2 described some of the earliest drivers of assessment use, cutting across research- and practice-based applications in multiple fields. Based on the historical and a more updated literature review, it identified eight broad strands (user paths) where tests and assessments are used today. The chapter emphasized "best practice" guidelines throughout, underscoring the validity, utility, and consequential validity issues that arise when instruments are multipurposed or misused outside the boundaries of the originally intended user contexts.

Several case studies showed the distinctions between formative and summative uses, and high- and low-stakes actions taken with the assessment results. High-stakes assessment uses in health, psychology, and business fields differ substantively from those typical in education.

Upholding validity principles in contexts where tests and assessments are typically used has posed numerous challenges in the past. Threats arise when assessment instruments are applied for more than one purpose, or for a purpose that was originally unspecified for a tool and its measures. Elsewhere, the assessments may be adopted for use in vastly different situations with new populations. Without the requisite evidence, both circumstances could jeopardize construct validity levels of the measures. When adopting and using preexisting assessments, therefore, attention is necessary to the limitations of the tools, and proper interpretation and use of the results situated in context.

Consequences of high-stakes assessment uses require due attention of both assessment designers, adopters, and users. The chapter reviewed several cases of high-stakes assessment misuses, each with different ethical, legal, or societal repercussions. Given a heightened awareness of the negative consequences of some forms of testing on particular social groups or individuals, the 2014 Standards called for formal evaluations of the consequences of test use, fairness, and measurement bias.

The Process Model is a framework that integrates assessment design–validation–use processes. The chapter concluded with guiding questions to help implement the Assessment Purposes box in Phase I.

CHAPTER 3

Whom to Assess? and *How?*

Specifying the Population and the Assessment Operations

3.1 Chapter Overview

3.1.1 Introduction

Building on Chapter 2, this chapter now considers two added foundational questions for assessment design, selection, and use, namely, *Whom to assess?* and *How?* (see Figure 3.1 that follows and Figure 1.4 in Chapter 1). The chapter elaborates on the notion of contextually and culturally responsive assessment design and selection, introduced in Chapter 1, defining and illustrating technical concepts like *measurement bias* in some depth. Operations relevant to four broad assessment modalities are introduced, along with guidelines to inform the choice of operations tied to context specifications. Note that discussions of operations are *brief* in this chapter; Chapters 5–7 will offer more detailed design information.

Figure 3.1 illustrates the segments of the Process Model of concern in Chapter 3, and their connections with the rest of the book. In practice, as Figure 3.1 indicates, the actions we take in the *Whom to assess?* box should be closely interlinked with the *What?* and *Why?* boxes in Phase I. Taken together, these three boxes should influence design-relevant decisions in Phases II–III or the *How?* boxes. As needed, readers may refer back to the complete Process Model in Chapter 1.

3.1.2 Chapter Objectives

After reading this chapter and completing the accompanying exercises, the reader should be able to:

1. Illustrate how key population characteristics and context factors could influence the validity levels of the assessment results in given groups of examinees or respondents.
2. Explain how consideration of the larger *socioecological context* can improve assessment design, selection, and use processes.
3. Identify the relevant sociodemographic, cultural, and contextual factors that could present systematic interferences in given assessment design or selection scenarios.
4. Describe commonly observed forms of *measurement bias* rooted in faulty assumptions about the populations or subpopulations assessed.
5. Specify the boundaries of the intended population, population units, relevant background characteristics, and socioecological context factors prior to initiating assessment design or use processes (Phase I of the Process Model).
6. Compare/evaluate the general features, advantages, and disadvantages of different assessment modalities for measuring a range of constructs in diverse populations (Phases I–II of the Process Model).

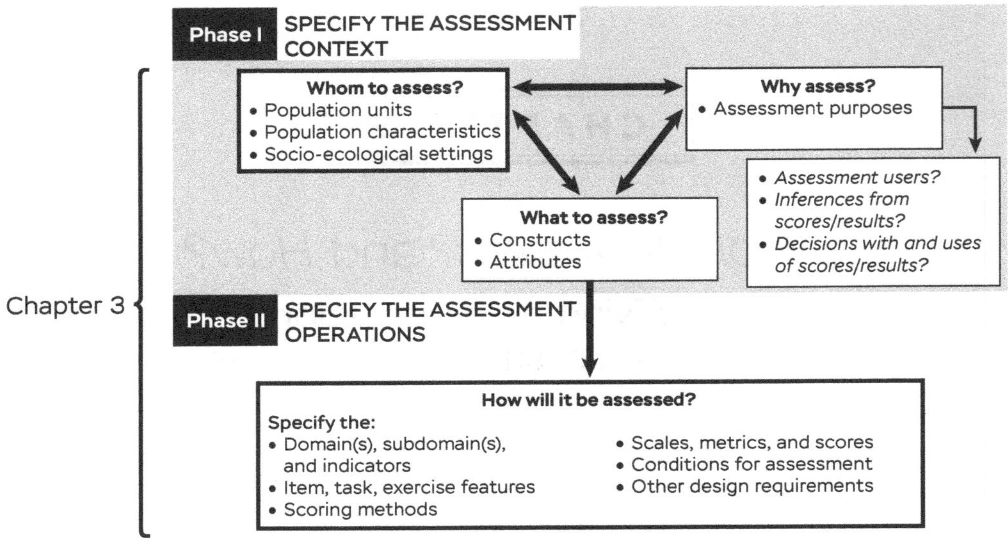

FIGURE 3.1. Connecting Chapter 3 to the Process Model and the rest of the book.

3.2 Why Population Characteristics and the Socioecological Contexts of Assessment Matter

Psychometrists try to make estimates of the "intelligence" of an adult with little or no consideration [of] his race, personality, or economic circumstance. . . . [T]he growing emphasis upon social psychology illustrates the recognition of the influence of many factors upon perceptions [and other construct measures].

—IRVING LORGE (1951)

3.2.1 Population Characteristics, Assessment Contexts, and the Validity of Construct Measures

Let us consider, as we begin Chapter 3, what the term **standardization** means when it comes to assessment design and administration. It refers to the formal practice of applying uniform procedures for *all* potential test-takers or respondents when administering and scoring an assessment instrument, the latter built with exactly the same or highly similar tasks, assessment operations, and scaling methods for everyone. Standardization assumes that everyone in the intended population is essentially similar and will respond in a similar fashion to various aspects of a given assessment exercise. From the test developers' perspective, the standardization procedures help place every test-taker or respondent on an equal plane, making the assessment results more comparable, equitable, and fair (Von Davier, 2013). During standardization, comparability of the measures is typically established with **norm-referenced scores** and scales.

In the quotation from the 1950s, we find Irving Lorge making the observation that the assumptions underlying "standardized" assessments may not be appropriate in all assessment design or selection scenarios. Background characteristics of some members of a population could yield significantly different responses, with differential assessment outcomes for ethnically, socially, or otherwise diverse subgroups and individuals. He was drawing then on new knowledge emerging in the field of social psychology.

While Lorge (1951) was pointing in particular to an observed deficiency in the mindsets of developers of intelligence tests then, he also mentions measuring human perceptions. Researchers and other assessment developers of that period tended to assume that differences in background characteristics of tested individuals, or of specific subgroups within those populations, would not affect the *validity* of the inferences from assessment-based scores in significant ways. The common practice was to overlook variabilities on demographic or intrapersonal characteristics of subgroups within the designated populations for assessment. Such assumptions were especially dominant in the mindsets of "standardized" intelligence test-makers, like those of the Army Alpha and Beta tests (Carson, 1993).

Even today, standardized test developers assume to a great extent that within the boundaries of the intended populations, all individuals are largely comparable and will respond similarly to given assessments with minimal adjustments and accommodations. When such assumptions about "sameness" are not upheld empirically in the response data, we face issues with validity. Recall from Chapter 1 that validity refers to the degree to which the *systematic variability* in the test scores or measures is primarily attributable to the constructs we seek to measure (AERA et al., 2014; Stanley, 1971). When background factors have large or undue influences on the assessment results of specific individuals in systematic ways, the measure-based inferences and uses that follow could become distorted with respect to validity levels.

Recall an educational testing example mentioned in Chapter 2 of an international assessment program involving relatively low stakes for individual examinees, the PISA. Backoff (2013), among many others, reported cultural, linguistic, and curricular background differences that systematically and adversely affected the PISA scores of students from countries like Mexico, complicating interpretations of their performance. Validity issues were observed in these regions despite standardized administration and scoring of the tests, with test items translated into Spanish for non-English speakers. Non-native speakers of English are often found to perform poorly on international educational assessments compared to students of the same age from more industrialized, English-speaking countries. When systematic variabilities due to outside factors interfere with straightforward PISA test score interpretations for regional test-takers, we face difficulties in making valid intercountry comparisons based on the average outcomes—a declared goal of the PISA (Feuer, 2013; Sireci & Faulkner-Bond, 2015).

In 1966, Edmund W. Gordon, an educational psychologist, scholar of human development, and lifelong advocate of equity, made another observation on the inadequacy of "standardized" psychoeducational tests employed to evaluate disabilities in disadvantaged students in schools. Recall from Chapter 2 that disadvantaged groups may be assessed for identifying needs for special education placements or clinical interventions. Professor Gordon (Teachers College, 2021) pointed out that while the existing assessments consistently revealed the mental, physical, or other physiological *deficits* of these children in comparative and numeric terms (usually with norm-referenced measures), most of the instruments failed to shed light on the substantive and qualitative nature of the students' disabilities in a valid manner. His exact words were:

> In order to provide equality of education for disadvantaged children, we must identify the children and *characterize the nature of their disadvantage*. [But] psycho-educational appraisal has more often been directed at establishing the fact and quantity of deficit than at evaluating its quality and nature. (Gordon, quoted in Teachers College, 2021; emphasis added)

Gordon was suggesting that there is an untapped potential in how psychoeducational assessments were being designed and applied at the time for students with special needs. Not only were their needs being missed, the assessment purposes were also not constructive! Inadequate attention was being given to learning about how to help this subpopulation of students develop in an affirmative manner (Gordon & Bridglall, 2007). If instruments were better designed to characterize the disadvantages that the learners faced, he posited, the results could be better used to strategically inform the next steps in the children's development—an entirely different assessment purpose.

In yet another early but influential article in the *American Psychologist*, Robert Ebel articulated in more direct terms as to why the concept of validity in measurement should be viewed as group- and situation-specific. Ebel said, "Validity . . . is specific—specific to a given group of individuals tested, to the treatment given to them, and to a given purpose for testing" (1961, p. 218). From Ebel's perspective, we should expect specific and real variabilities in the response patterns of individuals who are situated in diverse contexts, with different past exposures, treatments, and life experiences. Assuming blindly that every individual is essentially similar, in fact, may thwart the goals of obtaining consistently valid measures for highly diverse persons or groups *within* a population.

In sum, broad or limiting assumptions about background and contextual characteristics of *minorities* within the populations, based on what we observe in the *majority* groups, could diminish validity levels of the eventual assessment results. In groups from racially, socioeconomically, culturally, or otherwise diverse circumstances, actions using the measures could be especially consequential in high-stakes assessment applications. The next section illustrates how general assumptions of "sameness" could lead to issues of **measurement bias** against specific individuals or subgroups.

We will start with the premise that contextual, cultural, and demographic characteristics of individual respondents *do* mediate their responses to given items or tasks on assessments and, therefore, could often alter the assessment outcomes. On any given assessment, individuals with similar background characteristics might respond in one way to particular tasks under the given conditions. Highly dissimilar or diverse individuals from the same designated population who are assessed under the same conditions might respond quite differently. When this occurs, a first challenge for both assessment designers and prospective users of the assessment results is to ensure accurate interpretation of the item response data and overall measures vis-à-vis the underlying constructs. Making appropriate, equitable, and fair uses of the assessment results in action-taking contexts is the second challenge. At the core, both these problems deal with validity (AERA et al., 2014).

3.2.2 Issues in Adopting Preexisting Instruments: Is the Reported Evidence on the Quality of Measures Generalizable?

Suppose we are adopting existing instruments for new applications. Many existing assessment tools are already designed and disseminated, with published evidence available on the **validity**, **reliability**, and sometimes **utility**—along with other technical qualities of the construct measures. Most scientists, practicing professionals, and other assessment users would like to believe that previously "validated" measures and tools are ready for use generally. A common assumption is that of **construct invariance** (also called *measurement invariance*). We want to believe that the construct measures would remain unchanged in terms of meaning regardless of differences in group definitions or variations in the assessment use contexts, where the tools are administered (Gregorich, 2006; Meredith, 1993). The "invariance" assumption basically holds that the construct meanings and demonstrated properties of measures from a given tool, administered in one context, will replicate in another without issues of measurement quality. There is a deceptive logic to this line of thinking that needs to be investigated before we can apply the tools freely.

Recall again the issues with various cases in Chapter 2 with multipurposed assessments in different contexts. There are lessons to be learned from the early-20th-century applications of intelligence tests with new immigrants, African Americans, and other minority populations in the United States. Hence, measurement theorists and psychologists like Ebel (1961) and Lorge (1951) long advanced the conservative position that quantitative estimates of validity and reliability on all construct measures are situation- and group-specific. **Situation specificity** counters the notion of measurement invariance; it means that the empirical evidence on the quality of measures *cannot* be easily generalized from one assessment context or sample of respondents to others without added investigations, especially when groups are very different in composition or assessed under significantly different conditions and altered settings.

The above theoretical stance places a practical burden on future adopters and users of existing instruments. They must now carry out their own validation studies as application contexts change, a position now endorsed in the Standards (AERA et al., 2014).

Two concepts in the measurement literature, **validity generalization** and **reliability generalization**, evolved to ease the problem described above. Validity generalization studies are *evidence synthesis* studies. For any given published or widely used instrument, such studies aim to compile and summarize the available empirical evidence on the validity or reliability of their measures. These "summary" studies are usually performed with specialized statistical techniques like **meta-analysis**. They help determine the extent to which the validity or reliability evidence reported across a set of studies on a given tool, or a set of similar instruments, can be extrapolated and applied in new settings, with new populations (Schmidt & Hunter, 1977).

In an early demonstration, Schmidt and Hunter (1977) performed a meta-analysis for synthesizing "predictive validity" evidence on selected measures from a collection of studies that shared the *same situational characteristics*. The study focused on tools designed for workplace- and employment-related applications. **Predictive validity** evidence, as further elaborated in this chapter, shows the degree to which the measures from given assessment instruments will predict a desired behavioral or performance outcome *in the future* for a defined group of respondents. To obtain better results on generalizability, the researchers kept the situational factors controlled across the studies. Where such generalization was not entirely justifiable, Schmidt and Hunter (1977) stated that the meta-analysis procedure still provided an "average" predictive validity level for the construct measures across many studies, allowing improved data analysis and decision making with the tools. Tammi Vacha-Haase (1998), along similar lines, applied meta-analysis in a reliability generalization study on two widely used psychological scales. A majority of current validity and reliability generalization studies continue to rely on meta-analysis or closely related evidence synthesis methods. Each such synthesis study might have conceptual and technical limitations to which users should carefully attend.

The 2014 Standards (AERA et al., 2014) acknowledge that validity and reliability generalization studies might be useful when the database of existing studies on given instruments is large enough, and the situational facets of the studies on the instruments also overlap sufficiently with what users have in mind. In the studies selected for such evidence syntheses, Chapter 3 recommends that we ensure the groups/subgroups and the overall Assessment Context (see Figure 3.1) are sufficiently alike. Details of these techniques are beyond the scope of this book; hence, interested readers should seek the help of experienced and trained researchers, as necessary.

In the absence of generalizable evidence on validity and reliability, we should attempt to establish reasonable matches of the tool with population profiles and the *socioecological contexts* of the primary assessment users. Guidelines on how to apply the Process Model to improve these procedures before adopting preexisting or published tools follow later in this chapter. As a general rule, we should withhold from applying existing tools in an unfettered manner.

3.2.3 Socioecological Contexts for Assessment Design and Use

The notion of the **socioecological context**, mentioned in the preceding subsection, is borrowed from the literature on designing public health interventions in communitywide settings where one expects high levels of demographic and other forms of diversity (Kok, Gottlieb, Commers, & Smerecnik, 2008; Schölmerich & Kawachi, 2016). Scholars and practitioners in the health fields have long called for health interventions, like the current COVID-19 vaccination education campaigns, to be designed from a socioecological perspective so as to obtain the desired levels of public participation (Kok et al., 2008; Schölmerich & Kawachi, 2016). This perspective holds that individual behaviors in response to given interventions are influenced not just by the persons' demographic backgrounds, but also their *intrapersonal characteristics* and the *ecology* of their larger social environments. Under "intrapersonal" factors, we would include the idea that individuals' prior abilities, cultural values, and attitudes could also influence their responses to an intervention, including assessments.

The above is a useful concept for designing and using culturally and contextually responsive assessments as well. How respondents and examinees engage with assessments is also influenced by outside factors in their larger *socioecological context*. Some influences could stem from the respondent's demographic backgrounds, such as a person's race, sex, age, home language, or culture; other factors could include the values and social norms found within the family, community, or organization where they live, work, or attend school—in other words, their immediate ecological environment. For instance, if within my household's social ecology, family members believe that COVID-19 vaccines are effective, chances are that I will share that belief, too. When interpreting where individuals in a socially diverse or minority community stand on measured beliefs about vaccines, for example, some socioecological context factors may need consideration. Specifically, investigating validity issues would mean that we try to ascertain: (1) how much of the choice of responses, or what individuals say, present, or can produce during an assessment exercise, is systematically determined by the constructs we want to measure and (2) how much is influenced by outside factors tied to their socioecological contexts.

Taking a socioecological approach to assessment design also allows assessment designers and users to view the assessment context as a "system" with different levels (Conley, 1987; Steele, Hamilton, & Stecher, 2010). This helps to identify the appropriate *population units* for inference making with the construct measures and, subsequently, to understand the levels of the system where the assessment results will likely be interpreted and used. For example, to evaluate the effectiveness of a health intervention designed for reducing cigarette smoking levels with a socioecological perspective, the assessment designers may desire to measure changes in adults' attitudes and behaviors at multiple levels of a "community system" after the intervention is delivered. At the individual adult level, they might measure smoking-related behaviors and attitudinal constructs. At the neighborhood level (across all adult residents), they might again measure the same constructs, but now as the average. The average measure of attitudes toward cigarette smoking *in a neighborhood* has a completely different connotation. These are *two metrics*, measured at *two levels* of a socioecological system, for evaluating the public health intervention's outcomes. That is, there are *two units* for making measure-based inferences—individuals and neighborhoods. For each unit and level of the system, there are differences in what the measures would denote. At the individual level, the measures would allow inferences on a person's attitude toward smoking; at the neighborhood level, the average would indicate the effectiveness of the health intervention in curbing smoking. The implications for validity change (other examples appear in Schölmerich & Kawachi, 2016).

For another example, think back on assessments and tests employed for school evaluation and accountability purposes in education (see Chapter 2 case studies in education systems). Here, too, a socioecological perspective is helpful for identifying various levels and units for inference making from the construct measures. At the individual pupil level, the construct measured with curriculum-based tests is usually *achievement*. Users make direct inferences about student achievement levels from the test scores. School-wide performance, using the aggregates of the same test scores, is generally measured at the organizational level. Although the data are from the same instrument, these are two different levels of the system and population units for making measure-based inferences. Each level carries a different construct meaning.

- **Construct I:** Achievement (How much did individual students learn based on their test scores?): *Pupil-level inference*
- **Construct II:** School effectiveness (How effective are the schools, given the average test scores of students in a school?): *Organization-level inference*

In summary, applying a socioecological perspective to assessment design and use can be helpful in two ways: (1) recognizing the sociodemographic and ecological factors that might inadvertently but systematically interfere with responses of particular individuals or subpopulations during the assessment process and (2) identifying the relevant units of the population and levels of the system where measure-based inferences and uses of results will apply. Applying these concepts thoughtfully as we begin the processes of designing or adopting assessment instruments could improve the eventual validity levels of measures and overall quality of the assessment's outcomes.

QUICK RECAP: Given an open, globalized, and interdependent modern world, it is reasonable to expect higher levels of diversity in the populations and subpopulations we assess. The first section provided a theoretical rationale with selected literature sources on why we need to attend proactively to the sociodemographic backgrounds, culture, and ecological contexts of respondent populations for sound assessment design or selection. It pointed to the benefits of recognizing the levels in the larger socioecological systems for identifying the relevant population units to make appropriate inferences and uses of assessment results. Even if we are adopting previously validated or standardized measures, it is helpful to remember that validity and reliability estimates are situation-specific. Assumptions we make about measurement invariance should be investigated.

Reflection Break 3.1: Objectives 1–3

- In your view, is it better to (1) design assessments for specific populations and contexts, and restrict use of the tools to those groups and settings only, or (2) allow assessments, once designed, to be adopted and administered freely to various populations in different contexts, with the onus placed on new assessment users for appropriate application? Evaluate the pros and cons of each approach.
- Given your own experiences with tests and assessments, do you think *validity* is situation-specific? Make an argument for, and against, the notion of *validity generalization.*
- Similarly, given your own experiences with tests and assessments, do you think *reliability* is situation-specific? Make an argument for, and against, the idea of *reliability generalization.*
- What is the *socioecological* perspective as applied to assessment design or selection, and use? Do you agree that it is helpful? Explain.
- What are some assumptions that makers of standardized tests tend to make about the populations tested?
- Give an example of an assessment instrument in your own field where the results are interpreted differently when used at two or more levels of a system.

3.3 What Is Measurement Bias?: Case Studies and Hypothetical Illustrations

Measurement bias is a general term that refers to empirically verified, systematic differences in the responses of two or more subgroups of a desired population to particular items on a test or an assessment as a whole, who are otherwise at the *same level* on the measured construct (AERA et al., 2014). Depending on the assessment purposes and situation, we could encounter a number of specific types of measurement bias. As we will see, most are rooted in inappropriate and unjustified assumptions of designers *or* oversights of users about how specific persons or subgroups will respond during the assessment process, when compared to others in the larger population assessed. This section illustrates four, commonly observed forms of measurement bias with data tables and graphic displays in Figures 3.2–3.4 and Table 3.1. Some new statistical and psychometric concepts are mentioned and described along the way; these will be treated further in Chapters 8–11. The section ends with a summary in Table 3.2 of typical assumptions that may precipitate issues of measurement bias.

3.3.1 Persistent Achievement Gaps or Unknown Sources of Measurement Bias? A Case Study of Student Assessments

Let us examine Figure 3.2 on page 70 first. **Achievement gaps**, initially described in Chapter 2, are not commonly described as instances of "measurement bias" in the educational assessment literature or in technical assessment reports. Rather, mean test score gaps like those displayed in Figure 3.2 are viewed as actual and reliably measured differences between defined student subgroups in a given grade and subject area. This case analysis will question this routinely made conclusion by examining the achievement results for a selected ethnic minority group in the state of Montana more closely. A fairly recent public assessment report from the state provides useful and comprehensive results for this case study (Montana Office of Public Instruction, 2018). The data were gathered in public school settings in both Montana and the nation under the National Assessment of Educational Progress, a federal government testing program (NAEP, 2017).

Indigenous tribes and Native American students (referred to as "American Indian" in the graphs shown, AI hereafter) comprise a significant minority subpopulation in Montana's public schools. Over multiple and successive years, this group has shown persistent achievement gaps as compared to the White majority students on the NAEP tests in grades 4, 8, and 10. A similar pattern of gaps is observed on other standardized educational assessments built with similar procedures and assumptions, including the state-adopted tests of the Smarter Balanced Assessment Consortium (Montana Office of Public Instruction, 2018, pp. 4–5; SBAC, 2018). Over a 12-year period in the two graphs (2005–2017), we see the average scores on the NAEP standardized tests in reading and math for White students at grade 4 in the top two lines (nation above, state of Montana slightly below). Parallel data for AI students are depicted in the two lines at the bottom. We see remarkably similar achievement gaps in the state level and nationwide comparisons. The pattern is replicated, more or less, year after year on both reading and math tests in grade 4 (Montana Office of Public Instruction, 2018).

NAEP tests are expected to be generally aligned with the curriculum goals set nationally in the above two subject areas in given grade levels at schools. The tests are standardized to maximize comparable testing and data-collection procedures. Given that, the common interpretation of the results as presented in the state report is that AI students are well behind their White peers (Montana Office of Public Instruction, 2018). They have not learned enough in school, as measured by the tests. They appear to *not* be learning enough in school consistently, on a yearly basis for over a decade. Although not shown, the pattern is repeated in grades 4, 8, and 10 in both subjects. Seemingly, the schools are also failing to serve the AI students' needs. Why are the gaps replicated on NAEP tests, and other similarly designed and administered tests?

A very different interpretation of the achievement gaps could emerge if the questions are asked differently. We could inquire, for instance: How could AI students be learning *so much less* than their White counterparts as measured by these tests, with such consistent gaps year after year, cohort after cohort, regardless of grade level and subject area? Why is it that their achievement gaps compared to those of their White peers remain the same despite the many reforms, innovations, and resources dedicated specifically to support these minority groups of students at the schools? In the same report, survey and demographic data showed that larger numbers of AI students of Montana who live on Native American reservations or urban areas outside come from economically unstable homes and family environments, as compared to their White peers. More of them report high levels of alcoholism, substance abuse, and mental health issues. Fewer attend school regularly, about 6–15% less depending on how they are grouped. Hence, several socioecological context factors could result in significant differences in the *opportunities to learn* that AI students may receive, as well as their academic and socioemotional readiness to succeed on traditionally designed tests (Montana Office of Public Instruction, 2018).

A possible alternative hypothesis to explain the findings therefore arises (subject to verification locally). Perhaps the assumptions with which the "standardized" assessments are crafted and administered are more closely aligned with the sociodemographic and contextual profiles of White, mostly middle-class students in Montana and the nation? Hence, the tests are inadvertently favoring them over the AI students. Consistently and systematically, in contrast, the assessments may be presenting barriers to AI children and youth *to be able to demonstrate and show* what they have learned. Because what this group of minority students learn at school is not adequately registered on tests of this type, the pattern continues year after year on both the state-adopted and NAEP tests.

In other words, there may be built-in but yet undocumented sources of bias stemming from the larger ecological conditions under which the AI students are attending schools and taking the tests. Here are some background and socioecological interferences that could reasonably and systematically bias the results that should be investigated:

- The topics, content, and skills on the tests are not taught regularly as a part of the coursework and classes that AI students typically take, particularly in middle and high school.
- The topics, content, and skills on the tests are not relevant to the local household and neighborhood contexts where the AI students live and attend schools.
- Use of highly restrictive item-response modalities under strict time limits (with predominantly multiple-choice questions) present barriers for AI students to be able to show what they know and are best able to do.
- AI students at reservations or in urban areas face various barriers in meeting traditional schooling expectations that White students do not; this may be due to stark differences in their home backgrounds, culture, values, norms, home language, and other life circumstances.
- AI students have less involved and educated parents/guardians than their White peers, who are

unable to provide the expected educational supports (e.g., guidance with homework).

- There are fewer accessible supports outside school for AI students to learn and master the material taught in schools in the manner expected, such as libraries, after-school tutoring centers, practice opportunities, and so forth, that lead to poorer performance.

While tests can be standardized to some degree, what cannot be standardized, therefore, are factors in the socioecological contexts of White versus AI examinees/respondents *before* the testing instruments are administered.

To draw firm conclusions on what the observed achievement gaps mean in Figure 3.2, therefore, the suspected sources of "bias" need to be thoroughly investigated and disconfirmed. In theory, formal evidence of measurement bias would be verified when AI students of *similar ability levels* to their White peers are found to perform poorly on a given test. Large-scale, standardized test developers often overlook the investigatory steps on possible measurement biases against AI subgroups because their numbers are too small among test-takers to support the requisite statistical analysis. Nevertheless, suspected issues underlying the observed differential outcomes should be subjected to careful study with *both* qualitative and quantitative methods of research.

The earlier issue raised by Gordon (Teachers College, 2021) on shifting the assessment purposes to support the development of disadvantaged students applies for AI students as well. If the assessments merely show the gaps quantitatively but fail to shed light on what can be done to help the learners, teachers, and primary assessment users in understanding the nature of the AI students' learning disadvantages, how could their needs be met, or the gaps closed? Converging qualitative and quantitative methods to obtain deeper insights on AI students' needs may facilitate greater successes locally (e.g., Creswell & Creswell, 2023).

3.3.2 Investigating Item Bias: Differential Item Functioning

When assessments are designed, we typically assume that *all the items* will behave in a similar fashion with all prospective examinees or respondents in the specified population (the *Whom to assess?* box in Figure 3.1). However, if particular items or tasks function differently for some individuals who otherwise show the *same* measured standing on the construct, we must then address an issue called **differential item functioning (DIF)**. On a scholastic achievement test, for example, DIF occurs when two or more groups of examinees of the same ability in a tested area (say, math in grade 7) are found to show significantly different response distributions to a particular item under similar conditions of assessment.

As a psychometric concept, DIF is easiest to grasp with a **multiple-choice item** as an example. Let us look at the following question from a science test for grade school students, with illustrative data shown in Table 3.1. The data are adapted for illustration purposes from Berk (1982).

Item 1: Which of the following is an example of a *fruit*, based on the definition in your science textbook?

A. Carrot

B. Potato

C. Spinach

D. ***Tomato*** [*Correct answer*]

In Table 3.1, we see response data breakdowns for two hypothetical items: Item 1 (like the one above) and Item 2 (another similar item). In both, the four options A–D at the top are answers that examinees could choose from, with D identified as the correct answer. The cells in the table present counts of examinee responses that fall under each response category. These responses apply to two subgroups: (1) an racial-ethnic "minority" group toward whom the item is suspected to be biased (such as African Americans, Hispanics, or Native Americans in the United States) and (2) the "majority" group for reference, usually the dominant racial-ethnic group to which the minority is compared (such as Caucasian Americans or Whites in the United States). The total number of students in each of the two subgroups is 100, with 200 subjects in all in the DIF analysis.

For identifying DIF, the question to answer is whether the *observed differences* in response counts

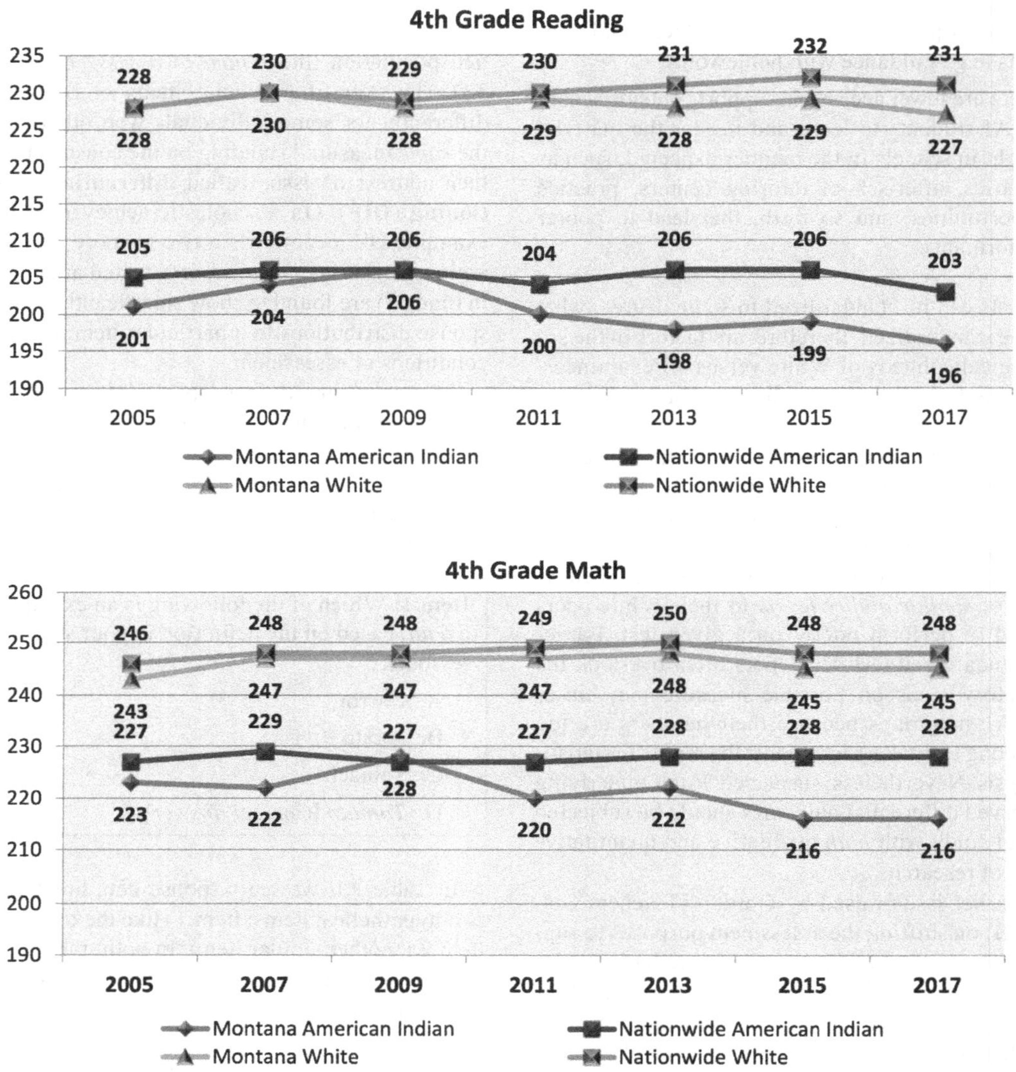

FIGURE 3.2. White versus Native American (here referred to as American Indian) students' achievement gaps on the NAEP reading (top graph) and mathematics (bottom graph) assessments from 2005 to 2017: Comparisons in Montana and the United States. Reprinted with permission from Montana Office of Public Instruction (2018, pp. 4–5).

for the “minority” versus “majority” groups falling under the A–D categories are **statistically significant**, or beyond what we could expect merely by chance. A statistically significant result allows the conclusion that the variability between groups is attributable to systematic outside interferences, within a preestablished tolerable margin of error, usually 1–5% (Best & Kahn, 2016, give a general background on tests of statistical significance). To detect DIF in Item 1, a statistical analysis is performed with an inferential test. An example is a modified chi-squared (χ^2) test with the Mantel–Hansel method, commonly applied in psychometrics. Such tests compare the actual cell counts with the cell counts that would be predicted by chance based on a theoretical probability distribution (Berk, 1982).

In Item 1, we see that 60 in the majority group versus 45 in the minority picked the right answer, D, showing an apparent difference of 15 points between groups. Following the inferential test, the differences in response counts in all the cells were found to be statistically insignificant, or *not* better than what we could expect by chance. The χ^2 estimate is therefore relatively small at 4.92. With no statistical evidence of DIF, we would conclude that Item 1 is *not biased* toward the minority group. The story changes with Item 2, which presents evidence of bias with the same procedure. The between-group difference here is larger for Option D (70 to 33, a difference in counts of 37). The χ^2 estimate stands at 28.73, much higher than 4.92 for Item 1. This, we find, is a statistically significant difference, suggesting that there *is* evidence of DIF.

Note that while DIF evidence serves as the first sign that an item-related measurement bias might exist, one must also ask: What is causing the DIF? Usually, this question is answered with further inquiry into the qualitative causal processes. Depending on what respondents and others close to the assessment procedure have to say, differential outcomes could be caused by multiple and simultaneous factors. Going back to the possible causes for AI achievement gaps, items on tests would show DIF if minority groups find the topics tested to be very obscure as compared to the majority group. Similarly, item presentations using formal, academic English language could pose systematic barriers to a minority group whose dominant language at home is different.

The Item DIF technique in Table 3.1 is just one of many methods for detecting biased items on a test. Commercial and large-scale assessment developers are expected to conduct similar item bias studies as a part of the overall assessment design and validation procedures. Problematic items like Item 2 should ideally be reexamined, removed, or revised before the final assembly of an assessment instrument (AERA et al., 2014; Bandalos, 2018; Crocker & Algina, 2006).

3.3.3 Differential Prediction and Selection Outcomes

A key purpose for many assessment instruments, as Chapter 2 showed, is to yield measures that will enable *prediction* and *selection*. Here, users seek to identify eligible or qualified individuals from a larger group

TABLE 3.1. Differential Item Functioning in Multiple-Choice Test Items: An Illustration

Item no.	Groups	A	B	C	D*	χ^2	Statistical significance	Conclusion
1	Minority	6	8	41	45	4.92	NS**	No DIF (unbiased item)
	Majority	5	3	32	60			
2	Minority	14	41	12	33	28.73	$p < .01$***	DIF (biased item)
	Majority	12	16	2	70			

Note. Cells show counts of examinee responses in each response category, A–D.

*Correct answer.

**NS = not statistically significant.

***$p < .01$ = statistically significant at 1% error level.

for, say, job recruitment, promotions, awards, admission into selective education programs, or placement in specialized treatment and intervention programs. For the individuals assessed in such cases, a given assessment is expected to function as the **predictor** measure, which is then expected to foretell their performance on a **criterion** measure in the future. For the primary assessment users, the criterion is usually a measured outcome they desire to see in the tested individuals at a later point and setting.

In all such applications, a basic requirement is that the predictor instrument's measures have adequate levels of *predictive validity*— essentially, this is correlational evidence showing that the predictor and criterion measures have a sufficiently strong statistical relationship in typical groups assessed. In addition, we would need assurance that the predictive validity levels are similar for all breakdowns in the population. The predictor should be proven to yield *equitable outcomes* in various individuals and subgroups assessed, irrespective of their background differences. Stronger correlations would permit more confident predictive interpretations, justifying the prediction and selection decisions that follow.

The most common example of a "predictor" test is a college entrance examination designed for high school students (Chapter 2). To recap, these test scores are expected to predict students' measured performance in their college coursework—the future "criterion." Similarly, diagnostic assessments used in clinical care settings may serve as predictor measures for identifying individuals with the highest needs for a given treatment. In both cases, we would expect the predictor and criterion measures to both be sufficiently correlated *and* predict the desired outcomes equitably in all individuals, such as males and females, young and old, various racial groups, and so forth.

Now, take a look at Figure 3.3. In prediction and selection scenarios, measurement biases manifest as statistically significant and different levels of predictive validity for different subgroups, as compared with the combined group (Cole, 1981). As shown in Figure 3.3, when the correlations of the predictor and criterion measures are graphed, any differences in the observed relationships are revealed in the slopes and origins of the predictive lines for particular subgroups and the total group. Comparing the slopes and points of origin of the lines visually, and confirming those differences statistically, provide evidence of bias from a psychometric standpoint (AERA et al., 2014; Cole, 1981).

Figure 3.3 illustrates a prediction bias for a hypothetical instrument that favors males over female subgroups. The cutoff score-point for selecting candidates on the criterion measure is set by decision-makers at 500. In the top graph, we that the origins on the vertical axis for all three prediction lines for boys, girls, and total group are the same at 100. But the slopes of the lines vary considerably. On average, girls who get a score of 50 on the predictor would meet the acceptance bar of 500 on the criterion; but for boys, the corresponding average score would have to be much higher at 90. Here, if the predictor score of 70 for the combined group is used by decision-makers instead of the separate prediction lines for girls or boys, fewer girls would be selected who could easily meet the cut point of 500 at a later point. But more boys than may actually be eligible would be selected using the combined group's prediction line.

By contrast, in the bottom graph in Figure 3.3, we see three different points of origin for the prediction lines for girls, boys, and the combined group, at 100, 200, and 300. Regardless, the selection outcomes would be similarly biased against females if users relied on the data from the combined group only. All such possible biases should be investigated so that actions of primary users (the decision-makers and adopters of the assessment) can be corrected in a timely manner.

The results in Figure 3.3 show that the predictor measures tend to underpredict for females, while overpredicting for males. Although this illustration is hypothetical, the issue presented is a controversial and commonly reported one for both the SAT® and general GRE tests—respectively, these two instruments have been applied widely for college and graduate school admissions purposes in American and overseas institutions (see, e.g., Dang et al., 2021). If assessment designers and users choose to dismiss the gender group differences as negligible, thereby relying only on the combined group data, the likelihood of biased actions increases. For instruments intended for prediction and selection purposes, the possibility of differential predictive validity in relevant subgroups should be carefully and thoroughly investigated during validation (AERA et al., 2014).

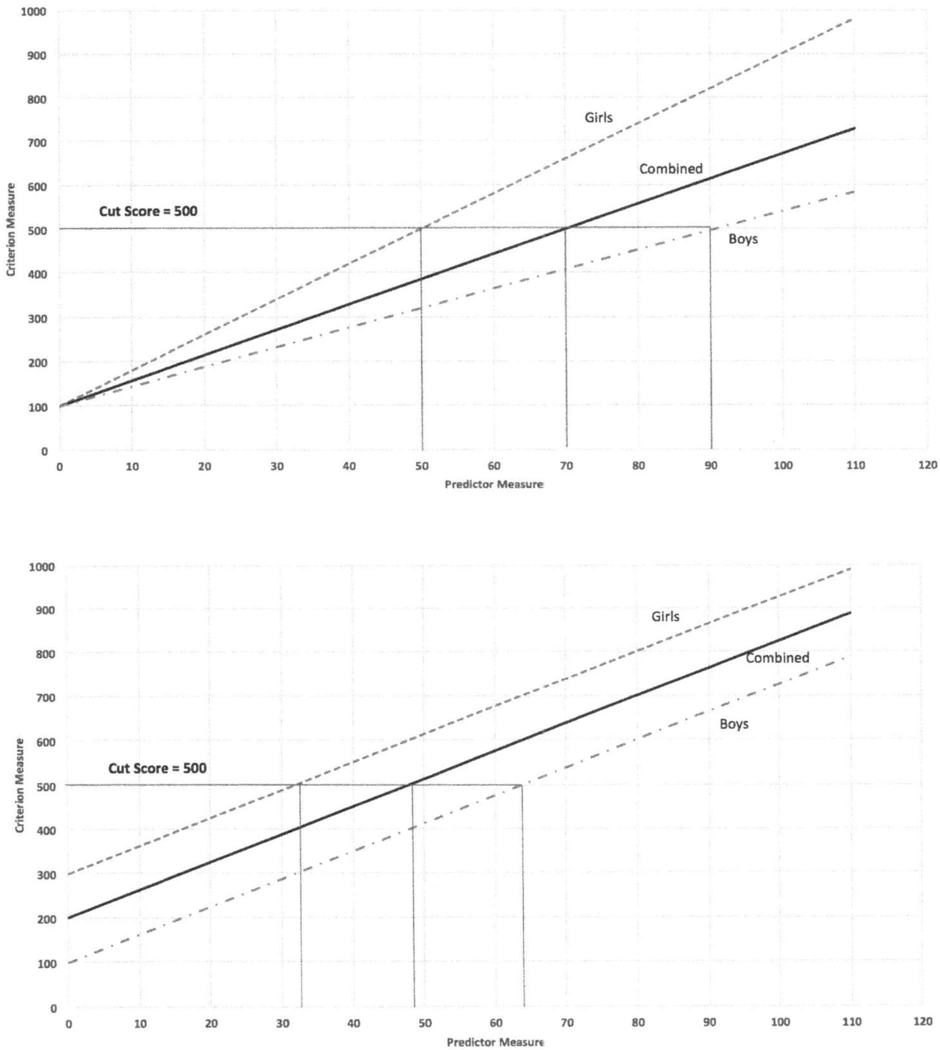

FIGURE 3.3. Differential predictive validity levels: illustrative outcomes in boys, girls, and the combined group.

3.3.4 Biases in Making Norm-Referenced Comparisons

In both research or applied settings, assessment users frequently want to adopt existing *norm-referenced assessments* for selecting individuals for particular programs, treatments, or services using **cut scores** on a scaled construct, similar to the score of 500 we saw in Figure 3.3. Norm-referencing offers a useful comparative perspective; *percentile ranks* are a commonly encountered type of norm-referenced score. However, here, if the norm group used for comparison is not a good match with the populations that interest assessment users, a different kind of measurement bias could result. For an illustration, see Figure 3.4 with the data tables adapted from Wechsler (1989) for illustration purposes.

In Figure 3.4B, we see data on the ethnic composition of a hypothetical norming sample for a standardized, norm-referenced assessment for children in their early childhood years. The demographic breakdowns when the test was developed compare well with that of the U.S. population for the same age group, attesting to the national representativeness of the original sample for comparative interpretation of scores. Now suppose that this same assessment tool is still in use with the same norms (from 1986) and is applied in a re-

	Ethnic Breakdown		
Group	Percent in U.S. population in 1986	Percent in norming sample in 1986	Percent in local sample in 2019
White	70.3	70.1	45
Black	15.1	15.3	20
Hispanic	11	11.2	30
Other	3.5	3.4	5

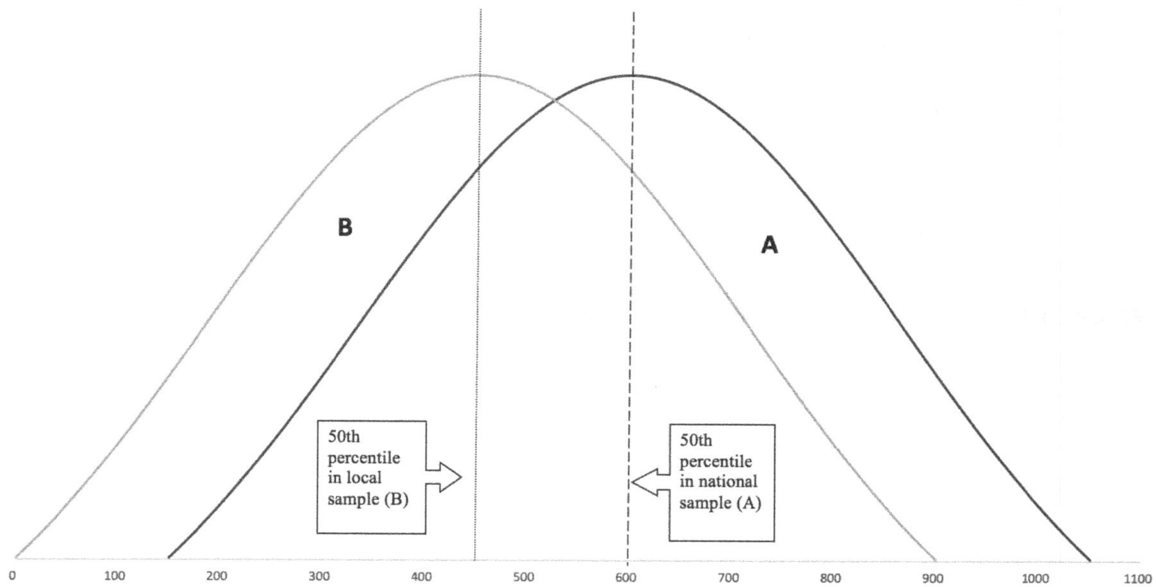

FIGURE 3.4. Mismatches in norms and cut scores with population changes: An illustration.

gion that has seen major demographic shifts, such as a Texas school district. Also suppose that the instrument is currently employed locally for selecting eligible kindergarten children for enrichment programs using a cut score. This hypothetical scenario is not uncommon in real-world applications today.

The tabulated data presented with the graphs show how the demographic differences, if considerable, could distort and bias student selections. Figure 3.4A shows the original norming sample's distribution in graph A contrasted with that of the local distribution in graph B. The average score at the 50th percentile is 600; it serves as the original cut score for student selection. With the local demographic shifts, we find that the score corresponding with the 50th percentile in the local distribution is lower at 450 in 2019 (graph B). Should local decision-makers choose to use the test with the original norms for comparison purposes, biases could result in child selection. As a result of the outdated norms coupled with an assumption that any differences in population changes are irrelevant, fewer demographically diverse local children would meet the old cut score. Fewer would be identified as eligible for the educational opportunities. Essentially, due to oversights of technical properties and limitations of popular instruments in the scenarios, inappropriate assessment *inferences* and *uses* of results could lead to issues of bias.

3.3.5 Anticipating Population-Specific Sources of Systematic Error

The prior examples of systematic biases have assumed we have standardized or semi-standardized instruments. Nevertheless, the issues pointed out could apply to all or most assessment design or selection endeavors, both formal and less formal. Table 3.2 summarizes five common population-specific sources of error tied to flawed assumptions we might make during assessment design or use, leading to systematically biased outcomes. The real-world examples in the table point to possible underlying causes for any observed, differential outcomes in each instance—remember, these causes would remain unknown unless formally investigated. While only a few assessment instruments we design or select will be standardized in a technical sense, it is prudent to anticipate such potential sources of bias beforehand.

3.3.6 "Fairness" versus Measurement Bias in Assessment Contexts

To end this segment, we must consider issues of **fairness** of the assessment results, especially in high-stakes contexts. Unlike measurement biases, fairness is not a statistically determined property of any assessment-generated data. The concept of fairness does not have a technical definition rooted in either empirical or research-based evidence. While public notions of what is "fair" are closely related to the concept of measurement bias, it takes on far broader social meanings due to potential social justice and policy implications. Unsurprisingly, the topic provokes heated social, ethical, and legal debates.

According to the Standards, there are four perspectives on fairness that could apply during assessment design and/or use. These align closely with the topics and examples discussed thus far. They are (1) fairness as equitable treatment of all individuals and groups during the assessment process; (2) fairness as lack of measurement bias, demonstrated with relevant kinds of psychometric or other evidence; (3) fairness as giving all individuals equal access and opportunities to respond to an assessment, regardless of physical or other barriers, so that they are all able to demonstrate their true ability or standing on the construct measured; and (4) fairness as facilitating valid interpretations and uses of assessment results for all individuals assessed, regardless of their demographic backgrounds, disability status, or other characteristics. Numerous standards delineate the responsibilities that should be borne by assessment designers and prospective assessment users, particularly for formal, commercial, or large-scale testing endeavors. Guidelines also speak to making allowances and accommodations during assessment for particular individuals and groups while attending to issues of construct invariance and validity (AERA et al., 2014, pp. 49–61).

QUICK RECAP: While assessment designers and adopters do not seek to intentionally bias the results of an instrument one way or the other, they are responsible for carefully evaluating population-specific factors that could introduce systematic biases in results. We should expect higher levels of diversity in populations today. To design, select, or use culturally and contextually appropriate

TABLE 3.2. Population-Related Assumptions Leading to Differential Assessment Outcomes

Sources of systematic error	Examples of differential outcomes	Flawed assumptions
1. Socioeconomic status (SES)	"Achievement gaps" were found on math assessments in students of similar ability who were from rich and poor neighborhoods. ***Possible cause:*** More of the wealthier students were able to enroll in after-school tutoring programs.	*All members of the population are from similar backgrounds with comparable resources and opportunities to learn in out-of-school settings.*
2. Ethnic, linguistic, and cultural barriers	Treatment disparities were found between Hispanic and non-Hispanic patients at clinics where intake surveys were given in English. ***Possible cause:*** Most Hispanic patients turned in blank surveys. They were then overlooked for follow-ups, diagnostic testing, and placement into care programs.	*All patients will be able to understand and respond similarly to the intake assessments administered in English, the official language of the region.*
3. Developmental or age-related barriers	On a timed, verbal skills assessment for children, the youngest children obtained systematically lower scores despite their fluency levels. ***Possible cause:*** Children ages 3–5 years missed all the fixed-choice items requiring them to answer on a scan sheet by pencil without any help from adults.	*Regardless of age differences, all test-takers will be able to respond independently using pencils and scan forms.*
4. Physical handicap or disability-related barriers	Speech-impaired adults who performed poorly on a cognitive ability interview obtained higher scores on a paper-and-pencil version of the test. ***Possible cause:*** Responses of speech-impaired individuals to interview prompts were slower and more labored and systematically miscoded by examiners as "incorrect."	*All test-takers, regardless of disabling condition, are similar in their capacity to respond to an interview-based assessment.*
5. Sex-/gender-related barriers	On a quantitative skills test used for selecting the most able candidates, girls performed poorly compared to boys on some items. ***Possible cause:*** Females missed questions that included scenarios describing unfamiliar activities in which males typically engage, like playing baseball.	*All members of the population, regardless of sex, will be able to relate to and respond similarly to tasks with comparable outcomes.*

assessments, we should plan to avoid measurement biases and unfairness toward any subgroups or individuals. Most forms of measurement bias are defined in statistical terms. In this section, we reviewed four types, of which Item DIF and prediction/selection biases are those investigated commonly by developers of large-scale assessments. Fairness in assessments is a social construct with more than one definition. Social definitions of fairness matter especially in high-stakes assessment decisions. Responsibilities for assuring fairness and correcting detected measurement biases should be shared by both assessment designers and users.

Reflection Break 3.2: Objectives 1–4

- In what ways are the terms *fairness* and *measurement bias* similar? In what ways are they different?
- *Psychometric definitions of "bias" are specific to assessment situations.* Is this statement true or false? Explain.
- Grade 10 math classes at an inner-city school are required to take an end-of-year assessment. One class of mostly minority students were not taught the geometry portion of the curriculum during the year. Describe a potential source of bias that could yield differential outcomes for the class. How would you verify it? See Table 3.2.
- Explain each term that follows to someone who is not formally trained in measurement: (1) DIF, (2) prediction bias, (3) biased norms, (4) biased cut scores, (5) measurement invariance or construct invariance, (6) achievement gaps.
- In your opinion, would issues of fairness and measurement bias matter more when we use assessment tools for (1) research and scientific studies or for (2) decision making in practice settings? Explain your answer.

3.4 Selecting Assessment Operations for Diverse Populations and Multidisciplinary Constructs

Constructs we choose to measure are specified characteristics of individuals or entities that belong in defined populations. In this section, we shift the focus to Phase II of the Process Model in Figure 3.1 (*How to assess?*) as it relates directly to *What* we want to measure (the specified constructs), and to *Whom* (the specified population). To ensure validity, the operations should be appropriately matched to the constructs we desire to measure. In addition, the ways in which the respondents interact with the tasks in any given assessment exercise must be well matched to their socioecological backgrounds and prior capacities.

The assessment operations, readers will recall from Chapter 1, include all the parts and procedures with which designers build a test, instrument, or assessment system. Decisions on assessment operations could pertain to components like item/task formats, response modalities of subjects, delivery platforms, timing and administration conditions, scoring protocols, and scaling methods (Phases II–III). Information on the distinctive features, advantages, and disadvantages of optional assessment methods is helpful in these decision-making processes. As a preamble to Chapters 5–7, this section offers snapshots of six broad categories of **assessment methods**. While on most occasions, user needs will be well served by one particular assessment method; in others, designers may choose to combine more than one.

Assessment devices can be classified variously based on a number of criteria (Chatterji, 2003). For instance, we find classifications in the measurement literature based on the following aspects of assessment tools:

- Type of construct that is measured (e.g., a cognitive ability test or an attitude scale)
- Item design features (e.g., multiple-choice questions, behavior-based tasks, or self-reported items)
- Scoring method for items (e.g., a binary 0/1 score, or a rating scale, 1-2-3-4-5)
- Procedures for score interpretation (e.g., a norm-referenced test yielding scores like a percentile rank)

- Task and item presentation platforms (e.g., a paper-and-pencil mode or a technology-based interface)
- Participant grouping formats (e.g., large-group, small-group, or individualized assessments)
- Degree of standardization in administering and scoring the tools (e.g., from unstandardized to semi-standardized to highly standardized tools)
- Response modality for subjects (e.g., a written, spoken, or behavioral response mode)

In this section, we use the last bullet or the participant's *response modality* to consider six broad types of assessment methods as optional approaches to measure a range of multidisciplinary constructs: (1) written structured-response assessments, (2) written constructed-response assessments, (3) product- and portfolio-based assessments, (4) behavior-based assessments, (5) survey-based assessments, and (6) interview-based assessments. Each is now described with reference to examples shown in Boxes 3.1–3.4. Table 3.3 provides a brief summary to close the discussion.

3.4.1 Written Structured-Response Assessments:

3.4.1.1 Distinctive Features

See the top two item examples in Box 3.1. Written structured-response assessments include timed tasks in a fixed response or a selected response modality. As evident in these item types, the responses required of examinees and respondents are highly structured. The familiar examples are multiple-choice (Example 1), fill-in-the-blank, true–false, and matching questions/tasks. Individual items in this category typically measure discrete elements of topical knowledge or skill in an area, with only one best or correct answer possible. Partial credit scoring is rare and requires major modifications to the basic structured item design formats. Guessing by respondents could introduce random error in responses to such items.

Modifications of the standard item forms in Table 3.3 are useful on occasion, such as the Cloze passage shown in Box 3.1 (Example 2). The passage shown is intended to measure a reading comprehension skill that requires the use of semantic and context cues to fill in

TABLE 3.3. A Classification of Assessment Methods Based on Response Modalities

Assessment method	Response modality and format features	Example
Structured-response assessments	Highly structured item formats; the correct or best answer is selected by respondents from options provided or filled in with one or a few words	Multiple-choice tests
Constructed-response assessments	Tasks with semistructured or unstructured, open-ended response modalities	Essay examinations
Survey-based assessments	Self-reported items with multipoint rating scales	Attitude surveys and opinion polls
Behavior-based assessments	Behavioral demonstrations that are directly observed and rated as events unfold naturally or in structured formats	Job performance observations
Product- or portfolio-based assessments	Prepared products or portfolios with collections of products, videotaped or audiotaped behaviors, and performances	Art portfolio assessment
Interview-based assessments	Face-to-face interactive interviews of examiner and respondent(s) involving direct verbal communications	Focus-group interviews

BOX 3.1 Written Assessments: Variety in Response Choices and Operations

Example 1. A Multiple-Choice Test Item

Select the best answer from the options given.

Which of the following is NOT an example of a food in the carbohydrate group?

A. Bread

B. Chicken

C. Pasta

D. Rice

Best or correct answer: B

Example 2. A Cloze Exercise

A **Cloze** exercise is a variation of the fill-in-the-blank task format. Here, every fifth word is deleted from running text to test for reading comprehension levels. Examinees use contextual and semantic cues to fill in missing words so as to demonstrate competence.

Complete the following sentences by filling in the missing words using *context and word cues* in the text. Every *fifth* word is deleted.

The Salvador Dali Museum ____________ home to the world's ____________ comprehensive collection of works ____________ the late Spanish surrealist, ____ Dali. This is a place ____________ time flows easily and ____________ are not quite what they ____________.

Best/correct answers (in sequence): *is, most, by, Salvador, where, things, seem*

Example 3. An Essay Task

We have been studying the qualities of strong political leaders during wartime and peacetime. Please select **one** among the following U.S. presidents and make a case for who, in your opinion, was the best peacetime leader. You need to offer at least three (3) arguments for supporting your choice with facts/details to back up your points. Write a two-page typed essay in 12-point font size. Lines must be double-spaced. You will have the full 60-minute class period to complete your essay.

- *Franklin D. Roosevelt*
- *Barack Obama*
- *William J. (Bill) Clinton*

the blanks. Context-dependent structured-response items could also measure higher-order thinking skills tied to a reading passage, a data table, or problem scenarios.

3.4.1.2 Advantages

This assessment method is efficient to administer to large groups. Items can be delivered via a computer interface or in a traditional paper-and-pencil format. Because individual items take very little response time, a large body of content can be assessed in a short testing time. Items can be objectively and efficiently scored with a predetermined answer key or with machine-scoring tools.

3.4.1.3 Best-Measured Constructs

Structured-response items are well suited for measuring a range of *cognitive constructs*, such as knowledge- or skill-based proficiency domains in educational settings, and mental ability constructs in a variety of other contexts. Within limits, items can be designed to measure a range of cognitive levels, ranging from simple recall to higher levels of comprehension, application, analysis, synthesis, and evaluation of the content.

3.4.1.4 Best-Suited Populations

Because of the highly constrained response structures and time limits, assessments that incorporate these item types are better suited for children of at least 8–10 years of age and older individuals. They are unsuitable for very young children, individuals with disabilities, special needs populations, or adults with low levels of literacy in the primary language used for test construction. Errors may result from an examinee's unfamiliarity with the restrictive response formats within allocated time limits—often viewed as a type of "culture bias" toward populations unaccustomed to this test-taking modality.

3.4.2 Written Constructed-Response Assessments

3.4.2.1 Distinctive Features

See Example 3 in Box 3.1. Written constructed-response assessments include tasks where examinees must create a response to an open-ended prompt, either in a semi-structured "short answer" or more open-ended "essay" format. As shown, these are usually timed exercises that could be delivered in a traditional paper-and-pencil medium or via computers. As the example suggests, the better-designed constructed-response tasks provide clear directions with boundaries for acceptable responses.

Because of the time examinees' need to respond to these open-ended exercises, less content can be sampled in a given amount of testing time, as compared to structured-response items. While guessing is not a threat, bluffing by respondents may occur—this is a major source of scoring error for individuals who may use elaborate language and vocabulary to compensate for a lack of content knowledge. Although computer scoring algorithms are now available, most such items are subjectively scored by human raters; hence, the use of structured scoring rubrics and rater training are recommended to avoid rater inconsistencies and biases. Open-ended tasks are lower in utility; multiple tasks, rather than a single task, on given assessments improve the reliability of results but will hamper validity of score-based inferences when examinees cannot complete the test.

3.4.2.2 Advantages

More flexible, partial credit scoring is possible with constructed-response and essay tasks, unlike structured-response items. The items also allow both *analytic scoring* (where the response is assessed in components, each scored separately) and *holistic scoring* (where an overall score is given to the entire response). Each component or the overall response could be scored with rating scales or checklists. These tasks make it possible to accept more than one correct or reasonable answer. In addition, this modality can be efficiently administered to large groups.

3.4.2.3 Best-Measured Constructs

This response modality is highly suited for measuring *complex cognitive constructs* that cannot be captured well with structured-response items or the other assessment methods. For example, we could measure application, organization, problem solving, creative writing, or other higher-order thinking skills involving the making of arguments and persuasive writing (as shown in the example in Box 3.1).

3.4.2.4 Best-Suited Populations

Popular in scholastic and educational settings for older students (age 12+) and adults, this assessment method is unsuitable for nonwriters, young children, individuals with special needs or disabilities, unless suitable accommodations are made.

3.4.3 Product- and Portfolio-Based Assessments

3.4.3.1 Distinctive Features

Box 3.2 provides an example of a portfolio-based assessment for high school students that incorporates a number of creative products in the form of poems of different genres. In this example, each individual poem, produced under a flexible timeframe, could be examined as a *product-based assessment*, with the poetry collection rated together as a *portfolio-based assessment.*

By definition, a product-based assessment is an untimed, open-ended "product" creation exercise. In contrast, portfolio-based assessments are purposeful collections of creative products, recorded performances/behaviors, or work samples prepared by the examinees or respondents with more flexible time limits. Portfolios could be used to either showcase one's talent or proficiency in an area, or to chronicle one's development over time in a given number of areas.

Both product- and portfolio-based assessments are typically untimed, open-ended, and subjectively scored by human raters. Hence, they are lower in utility and vulnerable to the same sources of error as essays and behavior-based assessments. Clear scoring criteria are necessary. Sufficient samples of the behaviors or products are also necessary for higher reliability in

BOX 3.2 A Portfolio-Based Assessment for Students in a High School Creative Writing Class

Directions to students from teacher:

I would like you to include one original poem in each of the following categories in your portfolio:

1. Limerick
2. Haiku
3. Cinquain
4. Diamantes
5. Bio poem

The poems should reflect the use of **one or more** of the following poetic devices: alliteration, personification, onomatopoeia, metaphors, and rhyme.

Show the creative writing process you followed by including your drafts, edits, revised and final versions of poems in publishable form. Include *all* your work in the portfolio.

To complete your portfolio, write a short reflection on your creative process. Your essay should not be more than 1,000 words. In this essay:

a) Identify each poem by type and say why it fits the definition of the type.
b) Identify where you used poetic devices and why.
c) Describe your writing experience and what you learned from this exercise.
d) Describe which parts of the work were the most engaging, difficult, frustrating, or rewarding for you.

Grade: Your final grade will be based on the scoring rubric handed out in class for assessing your poems and your reflective essay as a collection.

the scores. Computerized scoring algorithms enhanced with artificial intelligence technology are now available. These advancements should be carefully evaluated prior to adoption.

3.4.3.2 Advantages

These two assessment methods allow multimedia response modalities from examinees and respondents, including written, audio, video, and live performances. Like the behavior-based performance assessments, vthe methods can be individualized or adapted to small teams/groups. Flexible and partial credit scoring is possible, with weighted and unweighted scores, analytic or holistic scoring, either with rating scales or checklists.

3.4.3.3 Best-Measured Constructs

These assessment modalities are useful in a number of professional fields and subject areas for measuring an array of *cognitive*, *social*, and *behavioral* constructs that lead to specific product development or performance skills, such as producing laboratory reports (in science), writing poetry (in creative writing), playing a musical piece on an instrument (in music), or demonstrating a skill (in any profession or competitive sports). As the example suggests, the methods can be adapted to measure technical skill-based performances and product creation abilities.

3.4.3.4 Best-Suited Populations

While this assessment response modality is often applied in guided projects for young children at school, it is ideal for older students and adults in various professional arenas. The methods are adaptable for various age groups but must be carefully crafted for young children and special populations.

3.4.4 Behavior-Based Assessments

3.4.4.1 Distinctive Features

See Box 3.3 for an example of a behavior-based assessment for anesthesiologists in medical education settings, where respondents are required to demonstrate a medical procedure with obstetric patients in an ex-

BOX 3.3 Behavior-Based Assessment for Anesthesiologists-in-Training

How well can anesthesiologists perform preoperative assessments of their obstetric patients? An excerpt of an observation checklist below shows seven criteria given by Scavone et al. (2010). Each check is awarded 1 point and multiplied by the assigned "importance" weight.

Check if observed.

	Weight
Preoperative assessment	
Introduce self	3
Obtain pertinent obstetric history	4.5
Past medical history	4
Medication history	4
Allergy history	5
Previous anesthetic/family anesthetic history	4
Perform airway exam	5
Preoperative patient care	
Administer sodium citrate	4
Administer 100% O_2 by mask	5
Provide left uterine displacement	5
Ensure working intravenous catheter	5
Apply blood pressure cuff	5
Apply pulse oximeter	5
Apply electrocardiogram	3

Source: Adapted with permission from Scavone et al. (2010).

pected sequence and manner. This assessment method requires respondents to "perform" the behaviors under natural "authentic" settings or more structured task demonstration conditions (as shown). The performance is directly observed by examiners or raters in "real time" as it is occurring. As with constructed-response tasks, we need to sample the behaviors on more than one occasion to obtain higher reliability in the results.

Direct observations demand time for both observing and scoring. Like essays, these tasks are subjectively scored and may be vulnerable to inconsistencies and biases of human observers. This modality is impractical for large-group administration; tasks are usually performed individually in front of observers.

3.4.4.2 Advantages

Like essays, it is possible to accommodate more than one "correct" or acceptable response with flexible analytic or holistic scoring options, using either rating scales or checklists. Similarly, we can allocate partial credit with weighted and unweighted scoring possible. The illustration in Box 3.3 shows a weighted scoring framework in the form of a "checklist."

3.4.4.3 Best-Measured Constructs

Behavior-based assessments are suitable for measuring many *cognitive*, *noncognitive*, and *social-behavioral* constructs, including complex performances and behaviors. The response modality lends itself to measuring the performance of individuals and small groups (e.g., teams at workplaces).

3.4.4.4 Best-Suited Populations

Behavior-based assessments are adaptable for observing planned performances or natural behaviors in various age groups, including very young children and linguistically and sociodemographically diverse or disabled populations.

3.4.5 Survey-Based Assessments

3.4.5.1 Distinctive Features

Survey-based assessments require self-reported responses from participants. These tools include questionnaires with either single-item measures or multi-item "scales" that collectively measure a construct (see Chapter 1 again for the Patient Health Questionnaire). Box 3.4 shows another example, the Rosenberg Self-Esteem Scale. Here, each item has a structured, Likert-type response scale; this is a selected response format but with no correct answer. The items together yield a "self-esteem" score.

The self-report modality is convenient for assessment developers, but vulnerable to various errors from respondents—among them, subjective personal biases,

BOX 3.4 Rosenberg Self-Esteem Scale

Items:

1. I feel that I am a person of worth, at least on an equal plane with others.
2. I feel that I have a number of good qualities.
3. All in all, I am inclined to feel that I am a failure.
4. I am able to do things as well as most other people.
5. I feel I do not have much to be proud of.
6. I take a positive attitude toward myself.
7. On the whole, I am satisfied with myself.
8. I wish I could have more respect for myself.
9. I certainly feel useless at times.
10. At times, I think I am no good at all.

Response scale:

Strongly agree = 3 Agree = 2 Disagree = 1 Strongly disagree = 0.

Scoring instructions:

Responses are scored from 0 to 3 per item, for a total maximum score of 30. Negatively worded items (numbers 3, 5, 8, 9, and 10) are scored in reverse fashion such that a higher total score indicates increased self-esteem

Source: Adapted with permission from Dr. Morris Rosenberg of the Rosenberg family, September 24, 2021.

semantic misinterpretations of questions, providing socially desirable responses, and response faking. The instruments allow a large number of questions to be asked in a short time and yield sufficiently reliable scores with adequate numbers of items included in a scale.

3.4.5.2 Advantages

The self-report modality is quick and convenient, and allows flexible item formats; hence, it is a popular modality in multiple fields of research and practice. Surveys can be administered via a paper-and-pencil format in a large-group setting, or individually by mail, by telephone, or via the internet—the latter is a dominant medium today.

3.4.5.3 Best-Measured Constructs

Survey-based assessments are suitable for measuring a range of *noncognitive*, *attitudinal*, and *social-behavioral* constructs. They are the only method for directly tapping into a person's feelings, opinions/beliefs, values, perceptions, and personal experiences.

3.4.5.4 Best-Suited Populations

Survey-based assessments require respondents to have high levels of verbal literacy in the language in which questions are presented. Respondents are expected to be familiar and comfortable with the self-report modality. The modality is less suited for individuals who may face barriers in responding freely and honestly due to social norms or cultural constraints; other barriers could stem from respondents' first language and literacy levels. Hence, the survey modality is unsuitable for nonreaders, young children, disabled and special populations.

3.4.6 Interview-Based Assessments

3.4.6.1 Distinctive Features

Interview-based assessments also require self-reported responses from participants. But, unlike surveys, these tools require a one-on-one verbal (oral) interaction setting with participants. Interview situations could be flexibly structured to different degrees. Probing questions can be added to improve validity of response recordings. Interviews are time-consuming to administer and score; hence, less content can be assessed in a given timeframe. Expertly trained human interviewers and structured designs can reduce the vulnerability of results to subjective interviewer inconsistencies and biases. Due to their lower utility, applicability of interviews is often limited to constructs revealed best through one-on-one human interactions, such as mental health issues.

3.4.6.2 Advantages

One benefit of interviews over survey-based assessments is the ability of interviews to probe with second-tier questions to improve the validity of self-reported responses. Interviews accommodate more than one answer, with partial credit scoring possible. Similarly, the assessment method allows a great deal of flexibility with weighted and unweighted scoring, and analytical or holistic scoring, and use of rating scales, checklists, or note-taking.

3.4.6.3 Best-Measured Constructs

Interview-based assessments can measure a range of *cognitive*, *noncognitive*, *social*, and *behavioral* constructs. The modality may be ideal when verbal communication is a part of the construct definition (see Table 3.3).

3.4.6.4 Best-Suited Populations

Interviews are the preferred format for very young, elderly, or special needs populations. Often, "surveys" are delivered in interview formats with disabled populations.

3.4.7 Deciding on Optional Operations

A question to ask when making choices about specific assessment operations is: To what degree will the design choices help measure the underlying construct in authentic (real) terms in population members, given their backgrounds, ecology, and sociodemographic characteristics? Particular choices of operations should be guided by considerations of validity, reliability, and utility, keeping the specified constructs and populations at the forefront.

For example, to assess *language skills* (the construct) in *children of 5–6 years* (the population), it would be unreasonable to opt for a 2-hour-long, group testing format with written multiple choice questions. Developmentally, based on the early childhood literature, younger children may not be able to hold their attention for lengthy periods of time, particularly when required to respond independently to highly structured-response tasks in a large-group setting. Given that, a better modality may be an individualized, one-on-one, interactive assessment with a familiar adult examiner like their teacher (Copple, Jerlean, & Tomlinson, 2007).

The choice of an *interview-based assessment* modality would allow 5- to 6-year-old children to demonstrate their spoken and written language skills in a more natural and authentic manner. With a more faithful match of the assessment operations with the specified construct and population parameters, validity levels of assessment outcomes would likely increase. At the same time, we must weigh the pros and cons of this design decision. An interview would increase the burden in terms of utility of the assessment procedure, as it will be more labor-intensive and time-consuming. Furthermore, random rating errors from interviewers could compromise the reliability of the results.

Several of the assessment methods in Table 3.3 allow a more authentic, real-life response modality with minor adjustments to the conditions. For instance, we could assess a person's job performance indirectly through scenario-based structured-response tasks (e.g., simulated, self-report surveys); role-play exercises at work (e.g., semi-simulated, behavior-based assessments); or directly observing on-the-job performance (e.g., a real-life behavior-based assessment).

From a measurement perspective, it is appealing to think of authenticity as equivalent to validity. From this viewpoint, the operational choices in the example in Box 3.3 for assessing anesthesiology skills are authentic. Here, the anesthesiologists-in-training are expected to conduct a preoperative assessment of real patients before the latter undergo surgery. The performance criteria in the checklist and weights assigned to items were determined by consensus among medical educators and subsequently validated by anesthesiology experts (Scavone et al., 2010). The skills tested are valued in medical training curricula; here, therefore, the authenticity of the assessment makes for a more valid assessment.

Elsewhere, the term *authentic* is equated with close-to-realistic assessment criteria but in more contrived settings, such as at school. Wiggins (2011) described tasks or demonstrations in grade school as authentic when they utilize challenging performance criteria similar to real life. By this latter definition, while a test in driving *on the road* would be considered "authentic," a paper-and-pencil test on road rules would be less so. An interesting issue for debate and validation is the following: Can the more "authentic" road test replace a written test of road rules, or are *both* necessary to enable more comprehensive (and valid) measure-based inferences regarding driving proficiency?

QUICK RECAP: No single assessment method is the "best" given the variabilities one typically encounters with respect to populations, constructs, situations, functions, and user needs. The guiding criteria for making selections on assessment operations should be validity, reliability, and utility of the resulting instrument and the measures it yields in given assessment contexts. A careful review of the pros and cons of each of the six assessment methods listed in Table 3.3 will assist in balanced decision making as to the most appropriate method(s) for particular populations, attributes, and assessment purposes.

Reflection Break 3.3: Objectives 1–4 and 6

In a study sponsored by the U.N. High Commission for Refugees, a team of clinical researchers and health care providers were interested in assessing the levels of *psychological functioning* in refugees displaced from Syria, temporarily housed at a refugee camp in Jordan. All or most of the existing screening and diagnostic assessment tools they found had been designed as written surveys for English-speaking individuals and validated with samples of Western patient populations served through hospitals/clinics in the United States and Europe.

- In the above scenario, what *population-specific and socioecological threats to validity* should the team be concerned about when selecting and using the existing assessments?
- Compare and evaluate the *six assessment methods* in Table 3.3, to select the best one(s) for this scenario. You may use more than one.
- A large number of the instruments they found were designed with *paper-and-pencil survey items presented in English.* Given the discussion so far, what should the team do to adapt the assessment operations for the refugees in the new assessment context?

3.5 Steps and Actions: Specifying *Whom to Assess?* and *How?* with the Process Model

In applying the Process Model, review next Table 3.4 and Figure 3.1 together. Let us consider the problem faced by the team from the U.N. High Commission for Refugees to do so. The issue was: *To assess levels of psychological functioning in refugees displaced from Syria and situated at a temporary refugee camp in Jordan, which assessment tools would yield construct measures of the highest quality?* What criteria guided by the theoretical principles for equitable and fair as-

TABLE 3.4. Applying the Process Model to Specify Population Characteristics and User Context Parameters

Timing	What we should do	Process model phase(s)

During assessment design	• Define the targeted population's boundaries
	• Identify relevant demographic and socioecological characteristics of the population and subpopulations
	• Identify the population units for inference-making
	• "Know" population's distributions on key variables
	• Ensure a close match of the assessment operations to:
	  o Population and context parameters
	  o Constructs
	  o Intended inferences and uses of results
		I, II

During assessment selection and/or use	• Identify relevant demographic and socioecological variables of the new population, subpopulations, and user context • Identify the population units for inference-making • Compare the match of the new user setting with the original tool's population and user context • Revise and adapt the assessment operations to match the new user context; be responsive to context and cultural diversities • Make appropriate interpretations and uses of measures in new user context, given validation evidence	**I, II, IV, V**
During validation	• Situate validation studies in "new" assessment user context • Validate revised tasks and assessment, as needed, in new user context • Attend to diversities in population, subpopulations, and user context • Include evidence gathering to rule out possible measurement biases • Keep fairness issues at the forefront • Compare validation results with available evidence on the quality of measures in similar user contexts	**I, IV, V**

Note: Recommendations may change depending on whether the assessments involve informal or more formal, high-stakes applications of assessments.

sessment practices in Chapter 3 could the team have followed?

The team could have approached the problem in three alternate ways:

1. Design new assessments for that specified user context.
2. Select and adapt preexisting assessments, developed for other populations and settings, for use in the new refugee context.
3. Validate the new or existing instruments and construct measures in both scenarios.

Readers should refer back to Figure 1.4 in Chapter 1 with the complete Process Model, as needed, as we examine the options.

3.5.1 Population Parameters When Designing New Assessments

3.5.1.1 Specifying the Population Boundary and Background Characteristics

A first concern in Phase I is to specify the boundaries of the intended population; here, all the Syrian refugees flowing through the camp at Jordan within particular time points. Once a population for assessment is delimited, attention must be diverted to evaluating how individuals in that larger group are distributed on key background variables, identifying any "majority" and "minority" subgroups within. A clear sense of the *most pertinent* population characteristics will assist in selecting the best-fitting assessment operations. The commonly used variables for this purpose are:

- Race/ethnicity
- Gender (self-identified)
- Age
- Primary/native language or first language spoken at home
- Geographic region of origin or nationality
- Socioeconomic status at point of origin
- Disabilities and current health status
- Religion (relevant in some cases)

The list above should not be overly long. The background variables should be realistic with respect to *the observed* or *expected forms of diversity* in the given population and assessment context that might systematically interfere with, or help inform, sound measurement of the targeted construct—psychological functioning.

The *What?*, *Why?*, and *Who?* questions should be answered in an integrated manner in Phase I, as highlighted in Figure 3.1. That is, the constructs and overall assessment purposes should be specified as we prepare the population specifications. For example, to design assessments to *diagnose* (the assessment purpose) levels of *general psychological functioning* (the construct) in *migratory Syrian refugees* at a temporary camp (the population), which background and contextual variables are most relevant? Prior mental health issues and treatment history, alongside diversity with respect to ethnicity, age, gender, and first language, could be deemed as relevant by the researcher and practitioner team in this case.

3.5.1.2 Specifying the Population Units: Individuals, Organizations, or Groups

The second step requires a systems-based lens, or a perspective where we see the potential pool of assessment respondents/examinees situated in a larger socioecological system. For most individuals, the relevant levels of a typical socioecological system during assessment are the following:

- Household/family units where they belong
- Community or neighborhood units where they live
- Institutions or organizational units where they participate, receive services, work, or attend school
- Larger geographic area or regions where they reside
- Other or some variations of the above

When assessment operations are selected in Phase II, awareness of potential socioecological factors will help improve design decisions, averting future issues of bias or mismeasurement. There are questions to answer as we execute this step:

1. Are the *assumptions* about similarities across the families/households, organizations, or larger entities in which the individuals are nested reasonable? Are there any individuals or subgroups in the population where the assumptions will be significantly violated? Will the assessment operations or design specifications be clearly inappropriate for some?
2. At how many different levels, and in which *population units*, of the socioecological system will assessment-based scores or data from members of the population be interpreted and used?

It is critical to recognize the relevant units for making measure-based inferences at these early stages. In a vast number of assessment applications in the social and behavioral sciences, the population unit of greatest interest is the individual. In others, it may also include the household, a community, a team of workers, a classroom of students, a department, or an entire organization. Recall from prior examples, when assessment results are aggregated or averaged at upper levels of a system, that the construct meanings often change. If inferences about the constructs apply to organizational units or groups, similarly, background variables that are relevant could also change.

3.5.2 Addressing Population-Specific Issues When Selecting Operations or Adapting Assessments

Here, review the second panel in Table 3.4 again. Typically, assessment users—researchers and practitioners alike—like to adopt and apply the most easily accessible instruments for groups that are of immediate interest to them, especially if there is some published evidence on validity and reliability. But the population specifications and contexts must be taken into account. Commonsense steps that we could follow are suggested in Table 3.4. These might help address potential contengencies of bias and unfairness *before* we adopt and use existing assessments in a new context.

Essentially, selecting existing instruments for displaced Syrian refugees would require that we evaluate the match of the original population and contextual profiles for an instrument with that of the new one. Moving too far away from the original population specifications increases the risks of systematic errors and biases in the outcomes.

3.5.3 Troubleshooting during Validation for Population-Specific Issues

Numerous methods and techniques are continually evolving to troubleshoot, detect, and mitigate various sources of systematic error that could yield biased assessment outcomes for different persons or subgroups. This section provides selected examples of research and recommendations from the measurement literature that recognize the challenges of diversity, and with a mind toward improving equitable assessment practices. Several ideas could be utilized and built on in local and smaller-scale assessment projects.

In commercial and standardized test development efforts, such work is typically undertaken at two points of the assessment design and validation process: (1) immediately after test construction in completed, whereby expert panelists are invited to conduct "culture bias" or "gender bias" reviews of the items/tasks *before* the assessments are finalized; or (2) *post-hoc* analyses of assessment response data from instruments, similar to DIF and predictive bias studies illustrated earlier (AERA et al., 2014).

In many cases, the population becomes more heterogeneous over time as an assessment tool broadens its reach. How do testing programs address the issues of equity, "fairness," and bias as population parameters shift? Von Davier (2013) highlighted that standardization is one way in which testing organizations assure the quality, comparability, and psychometric equivalence of test scores while allowing test-takers of different backgrounds flexibility in terms of the lengths of tests they take, availability of different test forms, choices for more traditional or computerized modes of testing, and different test-taking times. Regardless, she cautions, test-makers should still remain vigilant and learn continuously about population changes. Specifically speaking to computer adaptive test design, Von Davier recommends that assessment designers keep abreast with the ability distributions of the target population before designing cognitive ability tests. "Learning about the population," in her words, is a key to better test design.

With international testing programs like the PISA, Ercikan and Oliveri (2013) suggest different ways of breaking down groups so as to detect DIF better as the assessment populations reach higher levels of diversity with globalized distribution of tests and testing programs. Consistent with the recommendations in Chapter 3, these authors also recommend that the targeted score-based inferences *and* subpopulations need to be identified explicitly before assessment design begins. This, in their view, would allow examination of DIF issues as a part of validation. It might also prevent misidentification of item bias levels and poor score-based inferences later, when instruments are put to use.

Sireci and Faulkner-Bond (2015) reviewed the literature on how best to validate assessments and construct measures in populations that include a specific minority group—namely, non-native, *English language learners* (ELLs). ELLs comprise a significant-sized minority in American education systems that routinely employ standardized educational tests. The main validity issue for examinees who are ELLs is *construct-relevant variance* in their scores. The primary users of the assessment results should be able to rule out influences of language confidently when making proficiency-related inferences from test scores of ELL students. Endorsing the recommendations of the 2014 Standards on securing five main strands of validity evidence, these authors recommend changing validation requirements to expect higher levels of ELL diversity in school populations (AERA et al., 2014; see also Chapter 1).

Lastly, Montenegro and Jankowski (2017, 2020) speak specifically to designing contextually and culturally responsive assessments for supporting learning in students in the higher education sector, a highly diverse and global enterprise today. They recommend four main strategies: meaningful student involvement in assessments for aiding learning; use of assessment data by faculty, administrators, and students to support pupil growth and development; use of context-specific and sociocultural understandings of learning and cognition in selecting assessment methods and approaches; and embedding transparent assessments throughout the learning process assuming diverse students. Consistent with recommendations in Chapter 3, these authors also emphasize the need for assessments that allow students to demonstrate their learning in various modalities.

3.5.4 Guidance from National Associations

The last two editions of the Standards (AERA et al., 1999, 2014) offer practical guidelines separately for assessment designers—referred to as "test" developers—and assessment users.

An important standard under the section on validity, excerpted below from the 1999 and 2014 editions, asks designers to make population characteristics and boundaries explicit at the start so as to assist prospective users of an instrument in connecting the population parameters with the constructs measured. The correspondences of this particular standard with the *Why?*, *What?*, and *Whom?* portals in Phase I of the Process Model (Figure 3.1) should be obvious to readers. Standard 1.1 (2014) states, "The test developer should set forth clearly how test scores are intended to be interpreted and used. The *population(s)* for which a test is appropriate should be clearly delimited, and the construct(s) that the test is intended to assess, should be clearly described" (p. 17, emphasis added).

Likewise, Standard 1.4 (2014) under validity underscores user responsibilities to justify new uses of existing assessment tools and measures by "collecting new evidence if necessary" (p. 18). Assessment users and stakeholders, as mentioned in the first section of this chapter, are expected to bear the responsibility for assuring validity by applying the tests and assessment instruments they adopt appropriately, with attention to the population specifications (AERA et al., 2014). When an existing instrument is employed in previously untested populations and contexts, the burden falls on assessment users to examine validity issues anew with groups or persons assessed. The assumption is that validation will be followed by mitigation to minimize any potential validity threats in action-taking contexts.

The latest Standards (2014) dedicate an entire chapter to addressing fairness and equity issues in formal testing environments, providing several added methodological and practical recommendations applicable to the design–validation stages, as well as during assessment use. We review a few procedures in Chapters 8–1[illegible].

3.5.4.1 American Evaluation Association's Essential Practices for Cultural Competence

The American Evaluation Association (AEA) is more explicit in recommending culturally competent research and evaluation practice, assuming assessments applications as a part of evaluative inquiry in general. The AEA asks that we (and assessment and evaluation professionals) seek to understand how constructs are defined by different cultures with awareness of the many ways epistemologies and theories can be utilized. We should avoid mindsets or approaches to assessment design or use that may exclude or overlook some members or groups in society; continuous self-monitoring and reflection as we conduct research or evaluation studies might help. Similarly, how assessment data are collected, analyzed, and interpreted, and the diversity of user contexts in which findings can be disseminated and used, could have implications for cultural bias and inequity, of which we should be mindful. Among the AEA guidelines are the following (see www.eval.org/ccstatement):

- Acknowledge the complexity of cultural identity.
- Recognize the dynamics of power of different groups.
- Recognize and eliminate bias in social relations.
- Employ culturally congruent epistemologies, theories, and methods.
- Continue self-assessments and self-monitoring on possible biased perspectives and actions.

QUICK RECAP: Proactive attention to the socio-ecological context, diversity levels, and the relevant inferential units increases the likelihood of valid, equitable, and fair inference making from assessment results, improving uses that follow. Procedural steps for specifying the population and contextual parameters under three scenarios of assessment design—assessment selection, and validation and use—run parallel to one another and align with different phases of the Process Model. The 1999 and 2014 AERA, APA, and NCME Standards and AEA's guidelines for culturally competent assessment and evaluation practices are consistent with recommendations presented in Chapter 3.

Reflection Break 3.4: Objectives 1–6

- Refer back to the assessment problem with Syrian refugees in Reflection Break 3.3. What would be your recommendations on *the criteria* the team should use to compare the profiles and characteristics of the *refugee population* with the *original population* for the previously validated instruments they found?
- Highlight the three most important *guidelines* from AEA and AERA et al. that you would stress they follow. Justify your selections.
- Identify the relevant *levels* and *population units* of the socioecological system of the camp at Jordan at which the team should be measuring and evaluating assessment results. Explain your answer.
- Make three suggestions on steps to adapt the *assessment operations* to best suit the refugee populations.

3.6 Summary

While, traditionally, assessment developers and builders of standardized instruments worked from the assumption that creating "sameness" in terms of the item content, structure, and conditions of assessment across respondents would yield more valid, fair, and comparable results, such design practices must be significantly altered today in light of documentable diversities in a vast number of global populations we assess, and across multiple fields of research and practice. Flawed population-specific and contextual assumptions during assessment design and selection have led to problematic measurement biases and validity issues historically, especially when left unchecked. Instruments so designed have yielded little or no information on the nature of the difficulties that the most disadvantaged or diverse individuals may face, leaving them behind in terms of opportunities in life, work, or education.

Chapter 3 pointed to key validity and quality questions that arise in interpreting accurately the observed differential outcomes in given subgroups we might assess. Once we accept that there could be contextual and cultural influences in the responses of some subgroups and individuals in the populations for assessment, we can proactively design or select the tools and measures to be responsive to these expected diversities. Some systematic interferences stem from the respondent's sociodemographic backgrounds; others derive from cultural and social norms found within the ecology of their immediate environments. The assessment operations we select must be consistent with these population profiles and parameters.

For assessment designers, "knowing" the population's boundaries, contexts, units, and their characteristics is the key to assuring that users make valid measure-based inferences. Issues of invalidity arising from misspecifications of the population units in the early stages of assessment design or selection could avert several validity threats. Biases rooted in gender, culture, language, disabilities, or other conditions could yield differential outcomes in individuals or defined subgroups with serious social and political implications.

Evaluating the advantages and disadvantages of alternate operational choices is a necessary step in the design or selection of assessments for measuring different constructs, populations, and purposes. These choices entail trade-offs with regard to validity, reliability, and utility. As the design and validation process continues, population-specific issues should be detected, mitigated, and minimized to best serve the primary assessment users' information needs.

SECTION II

ASSESSMENT DESIGN

CHAPTER 4

What to Assess?
Specifying the Domains for Constructs

4.1 Chapter Overview

4.1.1 Introduction

Chapter 4 marks the beginning of the methodological sections of the book. It discusses the theoretical foundations and methods for specifying construct domains. Well-specified domains help improve the quality of individual items and assessment instruments that we create, select, or adapt for our own specified assessment purposes, impacting the validity levels and overall quality of the assessment results. This chapter details the major techniques, with applied examples of the procedures from the literature.

Figure 4.1 shows how Chapter 4 connects with the rest of the book and the Process Model, with two boxes. The specific topics deal with the *What to assess?* portal under Phase I, linking directly with the first bullet under the *How to assess?* portal under Phase II: Specify the domain(s), subdomain(s), and indicators. Readers should refer back to Figure 1.4 in Chapter 1 for the complete model, as necessary.

4.1.2 Chapter Objectives

After reading this chapter and completing the accompanying exercises, the reader should be able to:

1. Explain the interrelationships between domain sampling theory, procedures for specifying domains, and the validity of construct measures.
2. Distinguish between instruments conceptualized with simple (nonstratified), stratified, ordered, and/or unordered domain structures.
3. Locate relevant theory, literature, data sources, or knowledge bases to specify domains, subdomains, and indicators for constructs of interest.
4. Write and organize indicator statements when specifying construct domains, using appropriate guidelines and conventions.
5. Apply suitable taxonomies to clarify, categorize, and organize observable indicators of construct domains (e.g., Bloom's taxonomy, the functional taxonomies, or the cognitive-affective-behavior-metacognitive [CAB-M] taxonomy).
6. Validate the construct domains as a step in Phases I–II of the Process Model (using the criteria of content relevance, content representativeness, organization, coherence, and clarity).

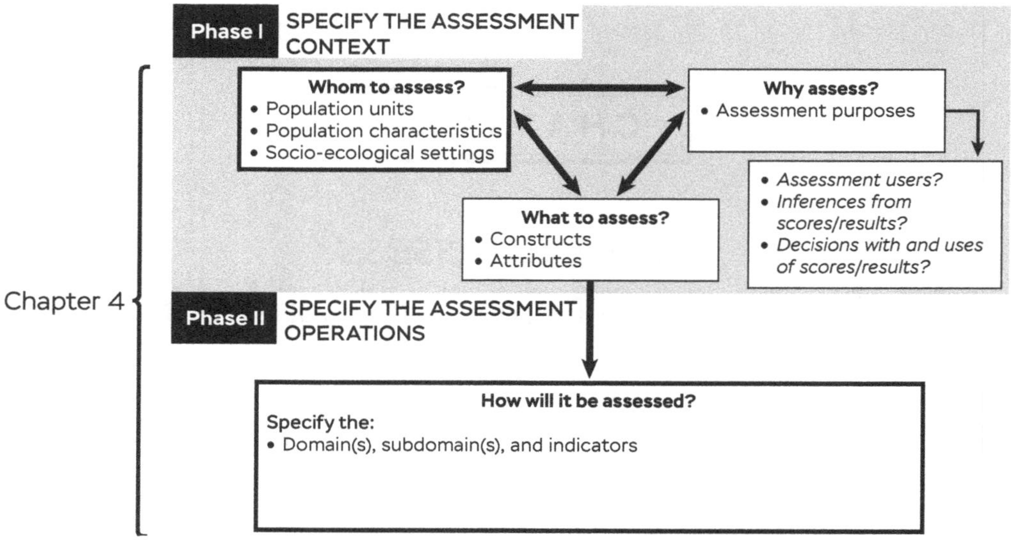

FIGURE 4.1. Connecting Chapter 4 to the Process Model and the rest of the book.

4.2 Domain Sampling and Domain Specification: Foundational Theory and Applied Illustrations

Generosity is ascribed to a person who gives more frequently or regularly than others, or who gives larger amounts or amounts which are larger in relation to his income or other obligations. . . . The actions in each case define the attribute.

—EDWARD E. CURETON (1951, p. 152)

A critical requirement for sound assessment design deals with having clarity about "what" we would like to assess. Chapter 4 focuses on the theoretical foundations and selected techniques for specifying construct domains. Recall that, in the typical case, the constructs we desire to measure are hypothetical and unobservable characteristics of persons, groups, objects, or entities. By measurement convention, we rely on proxy "indicators" that are more directly observable to make inferences about their presence or absence, whether in absolute categories or to different degrees (after Cronbach & Meehl, 1955; see Chapter 1). Specifying construct domains thoroughly and defensibly with observable indicators should be a first concern of all assessment designers seeking to build validity into the instrument design process from the earliest stages. This chapter explains why this procedural step is also informative for adopters and users of preexisting instruments, whether the tools are implemented as is, or excerpted in parts.

4.2.1 Domain Sampling Theory and Beginning Illustrations

Figure 4.2 illustrates an approach for identifying observable descriptors of constructs drawing on a school of thought called **domain sampling theory** (Ghiselli, Campbell, & Zedeck, 1981; Nunnally & Bernstein, 1994; Tryon, 1957). Domain sampling, a recommended approach in this book, could be applied when measuring an array of attributes and constructs in any theoretical or applied field. As forthcoming examples will show, the approach is evident in a vast majority of test development projects in education, both past and present.

Domain sampling theory holds that any given assessment instrument is but a *sample* of all possible items, tasks, or exercises that could be linked theoretically or empirically to the constructs we attempt to measure. It posits that it is possible to operationalize a theoretically proposed construct as a collection of observable responses, behaviors, words, or actions that the respondents would likely display when given the items taken from a larger universe. The "universe" should ideally be grounded in an acceptable body of knowledge with a discernible boundary. It could be drawn from established theories, scientific research, practice-based experiences, or socially accepted norms, but, for the constructs to be measured credibly, it must be relevant, coherent, and defensible (Chapter 1). The observable indicators of a given construct must also share properties in common rooted in that same knowledge base.

For any given construct, this bounded universe of indicators is referred to as the **domain**. Guided by a domain specified with observable indicators, we could then develop or select matching **item samples** to build an assessment instrument.

These theoretical ideas on domain sampling are illustrated with a concrete example in Figure 4.2. We focus on the attitude suggested in the opening quote: *generosity* (a psychological construct) representing an individual's general predisposition and willingness to give to others. Initially, the concept of generosity might appear vague and abstract. There could be various competing theoretical conceptions of it in the literature, with an infinite number of potential indicators. We might question the few indicators offered in the quote (Cureton, 1951), such as "a person who gives more frequently or regularly than others." Importantly, however, we see three observable *actions* indicating what a generous person would likely do, such as the frequency of their giving. These actions serve as a useful starting point to operationalize the otherwise ambiguous construct. To lend credence, however, we must tie these initial indicators to an accepted knowledge base. For any construct, the choice of a knowledge base rests on the judgments of assessment designers or researchers involved. Once identified, we could expand or narrow the depth and breadth of the domain within some clearly set limits, as well as verify its merits with regard to the substance of the indicators. The next steps in defining the construct can then follow reasonably, systematically, and manageably.

The pictorial illustration shows how the domain sampling procedure would proceed for measuring *generosity*. The picture shows different kinds of circles to depict qualitatively different behavioral indicators. Notice the proportionality in the items matched to the distribution pattern of substantively different indicators for the construct domain. We could either create the set of items for inclusion in the assessment tool or select them from elsewhere. As we apply this procedure, it becomes clear why assessments are viewed as "behavioral samples" indicative of the targeted constructs. Because any given test or instrument can include only a limited sample of all possible items, there is always some amount of error in the test scores or construct measures we produce. Errors rooted in item sampling issues are referred to as *domain sampling errors*. During validation, we would evaluate the extent to which these and other sources of error interfere with the quality of the construct measures produced and our intended inferences and uses of the same.

Starting with the domain specification phases in Figure 4.1, how could we ensure we have sufficient levels of **content-based validity** in the measures? Indicators for a targeted construct should specify two components clearly, namely, the *content* and *behavior* dimensions. For example, one observable indicator of a generous person is someone, as Cureton posits, "who gives larger amounts or amounts which are larger in relation to his income or other obligations." Here, the verb "give" suggests an expected action; this is the *behavior* specified for an indicator of *generosity*. The phrase "larger amounts or amounts which are larger in relation to his income or other obligations" is the object of the verb in the sentence; it points to the attitude-specific *content* in that action.

Gives [behavior]	. . . ***in large amounts to others*** in relation to their income and other obligations [content]

Similarly, we could specify the attitudinal content and behaviors in the remaining indicators that Cureton's (1951) quote suggests, as follows:

- Persons who ***give*** [behavior] ***regularly to others*** in relation to their income and other obligations [content].
- Persons who ***give*** [behavior] . . . ***frequently to others*** in relation to their income and other obligations [content].

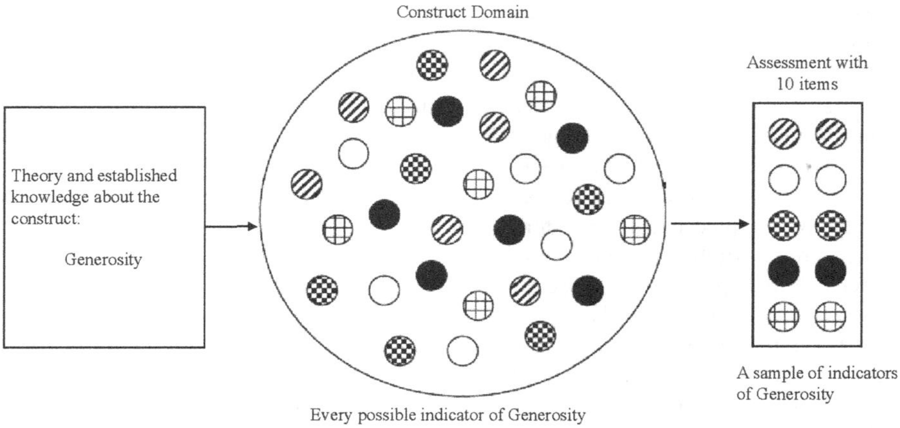

FIGURE 4.2. Domain sampling for content relevance and content representativeness. Adapted with permission from Chatterji (2003). Allyn & Bacon. © Madhabi Chatterji.

The items we design or select must be relevant and representative with regard to the underlying knowledge base for the underlying constructs, from which we would specify the *content* and *behaviors.* Once a domain is adequately specified, it is easier to arrive at a *content-relevant* and *content-representative* sample of items that match the indicators. This is an essential requirement for building content-based validity into the instrument, also referred to as *content-oriented evidence of validity* (AERA et al., 2014). What this brief opening example makes evident is that we often *cannot see* what we are attempting to measure until we have specified the construct domains with action-based indicators that are directly observable.

Adopting a domain sampling approach for instrument design calls for some up-front investments of thinking, time, and labor, but all the assessment operations that follow become easier. Identifying the construct-specific content and behavioral components of indicators, as shown, adds clarity to the indicators. One would typically need multiple indicators—often well more than three—to measure a construct well. The higher the clarity in the content and behaviors of indicators, the better informed the item construction or item selection steps will be during assessment design.

The parallels between the domain sampling theory applied to assessment design and general sampling theory in the social and behavioral sciences may be obvious by now. When applying domain sampling principles, the domain with the specified boundary is analogous to a bounded population of persons or objects, with the indicators replacing the elements within. Unlike probability sampling, however, assessment designers must rely on judgment-based, logical procedures for developing the indicators and then mapping and selecting items to match. In sum, we would apply **purposive sampling** procedures for domain specification and sampling purposes, guided by thoughtful judgments (Creswell & Creswell, 2023; Henry, 1998).

The theoretical ideas on domain sampling are aligned with a good deal of measurement theory on **reliability**. Thinking of the items that are included in an instrument as a random sample of some larger universe allows access to several useful ideas. Mathematical formulations for reliability estimation under classical test theory and generalizability theory draw on domain sampling theory (Crocker & Algina, 2006; Cronbach, Gleser, Nanda, & Rajaratnam, 1972; Shavelson, Webb, & Rowley, 1989). More follows in later chapters.

4.2.2 Applying Domain Sampling Ideas to Build Educational Tests

Table 4.1 illustrates the approach that Ralph Tyler (1949) undertook to map and sample the content and behaviors from a domain of **educational objectives** for a test in a high school course on human biology. As evident, he organized the curricular material in a 2 × 2 table, parsing the instructional objectives into *content* and *behavior* components. The test items were then sampled in a systematic manner from selected cells of the table, marked with an X. Not every cell is marked, suggesting that some parts of the tabulated curriculum were not being tested. These emphases are usually determined by classroom instructors according to their own professional decisions during lesson planning.

Examine the two dimensions of the table in further detail. Like the indicators of generosity, the table specifies (1) a "content" component outlining topics to be taught, learned, and tested in the vertical header (e.g., nutrition, circulation, or respiration) and (2) a "behavioral" component indicating the targeted cognitive behaviors and mental processes in the horizontal header (e.g., show understanding, apply principles, or interpret data). Restated, the objectives from Tyler's (1949) table might look like the following.

Subsequent to instruction, students should be able to:

Apply [behavior] . . .	. . . ***principles in nutrition*** in the unit on foundations of human organization [content]
Interpret [behavior] . . .	. . . ***data on nutrition*** in the unit on foundations of human organization [content]

The parallels in the wording and formatting of indicator statements for the generosity domain and Tyler's achievement domain are not accidental. Formal conventions and widely accepted guidelines now exist for formulating indicator statements along the lines shown. (Readers may also notice the similarities in structure of the Chapter Objectives provided in this book.)

Notice that Tyler formulated educational objectives as the desired ends, or as *outcomes* of the teaching–learning processes, as demonstrable by students at strategic points after instruction. In his view, the objectives defined the curriculum for teachers; hence, they should serve as the common foundation for designing both the instructional plans and classroom assessments (Tyler, 1949, p. 50). His thinking of instructional objectives as **learning outcomes**, or statements that projected the achievement expectations for students, is common practice today, but was an innovation at that early point in the history of American education. An undesirable framing of an educational objective, in Tyler's viewpoint, might specify the activities to be performed by instructors instead. For example, the following would be a poorly framed objective: *Instructors will deliver lessons on nutrition.*

The principle of matching what is tested with what is likely to be taught is the main basis for establishing content-based validity of assessments of educational achievement domains. Tyler's approach set a historical precedence for educational test design efforts (1949,

TABLE 4.1. Domain Sampling with a Table of Specifications

		Behavioral aspects of the objectives						
Content aspect of the objectives	Foundations of human organizations	1. Understanding of important facts and principles	2. Familiarity with dependable sources of information	3. Ability to interpret data	4. Ability to apply principles	5. Ability to study and report results of study	6. Broad and mature interests	7. Social attributes
	1. Nutrition	X	X	X	X	X	X	X
	2. Digestion	X		X	X	X	X	
	3. Circulation	X		X	X	X	X	
	4. Respiration	X		X	X	X	X	
	5. Reproduction	X	X	X	X	X	X	X

Note. Reprinted with permission from Tyler (1949). © University of Chicago Press.

1951; original table in Table 4.1). He illustrated how **domain specifications** laid out in the form of a table could help in the systematic sampling of content and behaviors we desire to measure. That tabulated format is called a **table of specifications** or a *table of test specifications* today. It is an operational standard in all large-scale educational test design projects. For a recent application of similar domain sampling approaches in education guided by the Common Core State Standards reforms, see the mathematics domain with accompanying task and item specifications, released in 2015 by the Smarter Balanced Assessment Consortium (SBAC; see *www.smarterbalanced.org/wp-content/uploads/2015/08/Mathematics-Content-Specifications.pdf*).

4.2.3 Alternatives to Domain Sampling: Empirical Methods of Instrument Design

Another widely used but altogether different approach to instrument development originated in psychology. Referred to as the "empirical method of scale development" (Comrey, 1988, p. 754), the approach departs from domain sampling theory in distinctive ways. It relies on *items gathered from other tools*, and the results of empirical testing and research on those items, for instrument design purposes.

We often see new instruments fashioned with items, tasks, and exercises selected from elsewhere, guided largely by the common sense and interests of the researchers and designers. In the empirical method, the assessment design process starts by assembling or adapting items directly from existing tests and assessment resources based on the judgments of the assessment designers or researchers. Following that, items and instruments are empirically tested with typical examinees or respondents. The statistical properties of the data generated by the newly assembled items and tool inform decisions on which items will be retained or dropped in the final instrument. Many well-known psychological tests and scales were compiled in this manner in personality and social psychology (see studies on the Minnesota Multiphasic Personality Inventory as examples).

A number of statistics and analytic options are available to establish conceptual distinctions among similar and dissimilar sets of items in the empirical approach to instrument design (AERA et al., 2014; see also Briggs & Cheek, 1986; Comrey, 1988). For instance, empirical **correlations** of a newly compiled instrument's scores with external variables could be useful. Here, it is the correlations that designers and users rely on for scale design and evaluation purposes, not any prespecified domain structures. In efforts to identify the latent traits measured by specific groups of items that are compiled, various **factor analysis** techniques are another frequently applied technique.

Although popular, there could be limitations to taking a purely empirical approach to instrument design. A first concern is that designers rely too often on superficial characteristics of items for devising new instruments, such as the wording or language in the original items. Second, when the source instruments are designed for, or previously tested on, very different samples of respondents, the item and score properties often fail to generalize in new contexts. Finally, if we start with originally *untested* items and tools, we could obtain flawed assemblages of items. Other issues with empirical instrument design methods could be:

- Lack of a strong conceptual foundation for the constructs to be measured by items
- Badly designed items to begin with, in the original source instruments
- Improperly balanced item composition in the new instrument
- Inadequate respondent samples or data-collection designs in the original instrument try-outs
- Inherent limitations of the data analytic techniques relied on to assemble items

4.2.4 What Is the Recommended Approach?

This book's approach is to combine the most valuable elements of domain sampling theory with those of empirical instrument development methods. In the absence of a theory-guided domain framework against which empirical results can be referenced or interpreted, errors could enter the instrument design and assembly process—including subjective biases of researchers and assessment designers themselves. The recommended sequence for instrument design is Phases II–III for domain specification and item sampling, and Phase IV for performing the content and empirical validation efforts.

We begin building instruments by specifying the construct domains guided by the principles and procedures of domain sampling theory. The item design, item sampling, and content validation procedures follow accordingly. We continue the iterative design process with appropriate empirical validation studies. Importantly, the design and validation efforts should fit the assessment user contexts. By evaluating the empirical validation results against *a priori* domain frameworks, the aim is to optimize the functioning of instruments and measures in the specified user contexts. For the complete Process Model, see Figure 1.4, Chapter 1.

QUICK RECAP: Domain sampling theory offers useful principles and systematic procedures for specifying domains for hypothetical constructs we might desire to measure. Domain specification should be the first step in operationally defining constructs; it helps create instruments with higher levels of content validity. Regardless of construct type (attitudinal and educational achievement domains were illustrated), we apply similar steps and procedures for specifying the indicators of a domain. Well-specified indicators make the construct "observable" and should be tied to defensible knowledge bases. Empirical methods of instrument design rely on items from preexisting instruments and statistical analyses of item response data for item selection and instrument assembly. Each approach has its merits, utility, and limitations. The Process Model integrates key elements of both, undergirded by the logic of user-centered design.

Reflection Break 4.1: Objective 1

- With an example of an assessment in your area, distinguish between the *theoretical definitions* versus the *operational definitions* of the constructs measured.
- For designing or selecting your own assessment, identify two to three strategies from *domain sampling theory* that you find useful. Justify your answer.
- Compare the *pros* and *cons* of the *domain sampling approach* versus *empirical methods of scale development*, taken individually.
- Outside the two main approaches in Section 4.2, have you seen *other approaches* to assessment design? Describe how the design process was carried out. What are the advantages and disadvantages of that approach?

4.3 Construct Types, Domain Conceptualizations, and Structures

In the social and behavioral sciences, the nature and type of construct often dictate the domain conceptualizations and structures we can reasonably adopt for instrument design purposes. This section provides an overview of the main construct types and domain structures in the literature as a preamble to the sections that follow. See Boxes 4.1–4.3.

4.3.1 Types of Constructs

What are we interested in measuring? Constructs we choose to measure could fall under one or more of the following four categories.

1. **Cognitive constructs:** These constructs were historically classified under the *cognitive domain* by Bloom and colleagues (1956) and deal with one's mental abilities and intellectual capacities in a specified area, both inborn and learned. Indicators in cognitive domains could deal with specific human capacities like concept recall, retrieval and understanding; application of concepts and principles; other types of information processing; problem-solving skills; and proficiency levels in performing mentally demanding procedures. *Examples:* practical intelligence, quantitative skills, decision-making skills, language proficiency, scholastic achievement in science.

2. **Social-behavioral, personality, attitudinal, and affective constructs:** This class of attributes was historically classified under the *affective domain* by Bloom et al. (1956) and are often labeled broadly as "noncognitive" attributes. These are all psychological constructs dealing with one's social-emotional mindsets, proclivities, or dispositions; opinions and values;

personality characteristics; or perceptions, feelings, and social behaviors related to some topic, object, or area. Noncognitive attributes could also be innate or learned tendencies of human beings. *Examples:* attitudes, satisfaction, ethical behaviors, emotional volatility, political beliefs.

3. **Health-related constructs:** Broadly, these constructs deal with various aspects of one's health, well-being, and daily functioning, including one's physical abilities and motor skills; physiological well-being; mental health conditions; or conversely, one's disabilities, diseases, or disorders. Bloom et al. (1956) labeled motor skills learned in school under a *psychomotor domain. Examples:* physical strength, endurance, clinical depression, cerebral palsy, sleep apnea.

4. **Sociodemographic constructs:** These constructs deal with societally defined and agreed-upon background and demographic characteristics of individuals, groups, or entities. *Examples:* nationality, socioeconomic status, religion, race/ethnicity, private versus public sectors.

Sometimes, individual constructs we desire to measure may be determined to belong in more than one category, or a new category that lies outside this taxonomy based on the latest literature or societal perspectives. For example, research in the brain sciences suggests that both cognitive and noncognitive characteristics, as defined above, arise from activities and functions in different regions of the human brain, calling into question the biological basis for the first two category distinctions (see, e g., Naliboff & Mayer, 2006). Readers should treat the four classes of constructs as a practical categorization system useful simply for initiating the instrument design process.

4.3.2 Ordered and Hierarchical Construct Domains

Once we pin down the construct to measure, a first question is: What is the best way to conceptualize and organize the domain's indicators, given the underlying theory? Ordered domains are useful for measuring a person's growth or change on constructs; unordered domains are useful for measuring a person's status on the construct at a given time point.

In one measurement tradition, the construct domains are envisaged as *ordered* and *hierarchical.* Researchers following this tradition have attempted to measure the underlying attributes with unidimensional linear scales similar to a meter rule for measuring the length of objects. In applying this tradition, the domain's indicators and matching items are located in a hierarchy, increasing based on their judged levels of difficulty, value, importance, or intensity on an underlying continuum.

For an example of an ordered domain for a cognitive construct, examine Box 4.1. Here, we see a sample of progressively more difficult indicators in a mathematics learning domain. The construct deals with student abilities in recognizing and reasoning with mathematical patterns. This domain, and others like it, were specified for designing developmental assessments for multi-age groups of students. The students were being schooled in nongraded environments where they were allowed to progress at their own pace through the instructional units in different subject areas. As shown with the examples, the mathematics tasks were developed to match each competency level in that hierarchal arrangement of indicators (the curriculum objectives), clarifying the expectations for both teachers and students in nongraded classrooms (Banerji, 1999; Banerji, Anderson, & Kerstyn, 2000; Banerji & Ferron, 1998; Goodlad & Anderson, 1987).

In music education programs, for another example, we might encounter hierarchical domains underlying assessments to measure levels of competence in playing a musical instrument, like the piano. The expected performances are graduated by difficulty from beginner to intermediate to more advanced levels. For other educational applications, think of hierarchically linked, ordered domain specifications underlying mathematics assessments taken by students at the end of elementary school (grade 4), middle school (grade 8), and high school (grade 10). Ordered cognitive domains are useful in either educational or workplace training contexts to map how individuals develop over time in areas that become progressively more difficult or challenging. Most tests based on hierarchical domains are conceptualized to yield a common multilevel, ordered scale structure that increases in difficulty or intensity level.

Note that sometimes, separately constructed assessments designed for different grade level curricula are "vertically linked" mathematically after the fact (see,

BOX 4.1 Ordered Domain Specifications for a Classroom Assessment: Mathematics Indicators and Items at Three Levels of Difficulty

Assessment Use Context

What to Assess?

Learning progressions in skills and concepts on mathematical patterns

Whom to Assess?

Third- to fourth-grade students in public schools in the United States

Why Assess?

Classroom assessment

- *Measure-based inferences?* Learning gaps and learning progress along the mapped curriculum
- *Specific uses?* Classroom-level formative decisions
- *Primary users?* Teachers, instructional aides, learners, and families

Domain with Indicators and Tasks at Three Levels

General Indicator

- Given problems arranged by difficulty, students will identify and explain mathematical patterns represented by symbols, basic number concepts, and arithmetic operations. (Taxonomic level: *Higher-order thinking*)

Specific Indicators

- **Level 1 Indicator:** *Identify, continue, and explain simple repeating patterns involving shapes, numerals, or letters.*

  Matching-Item Example:

  What is the pattern that you see below? Fill in the last *three* blanks to continue the pattern. Say why your answer is correct.

  ABC, ABC, ABC, ______, ______, ______?

  Explanation:

- **Level 2 Indicator:** *Identify, continue, and explain mathematically increasing patterns using basic number sense and arithmetic concepts.*

  Matching-Item Example:

  What is the pattern in the series of numbers below? Predict the last *three* numbers in the series. Explain the mathematical rule. Show all your work.

  1, 10, 100, 1000, ______, ______, ______?

  Math Rule:

  Explanation:

- **Level 3:** *Identify, continue, and explain mathematically increasing patterns, using intermediate-level arithmetic concepts—for example, multiplication, division, fractions, prime numbers, and squares.*

  Matching-Item Example:

  See the pattern in the series of numbers below. Predict the last *two* numbers in the series. Explain the mathematical rule that helped you find the answers. Show all your work.

  2, 4, 16, ______, ______?

  Math Rule:

  Explanation:

Answers.

1. Rule: repeating series of same letters. ABC; ABC; ABC.
2. Rule = x*10. 10,000; 100,000; 1000,000.
3. Rule = x^2. 256; 65,536.

e.g., Strachan et al., 2020). Typically, these instruments are not based on hierarchically conceptualized domains. Standardized test developers often perform this type of test-linking procedure. But the tests are usually not built from ordered test design specifications, nor administered to large, multigrade samples of test-takers. Hence, the inferences possible from the vertically linked construct measures are limited.

4.3.3 Unordered Domains: Homogeneous and Heterogeneous Structures

In an alternative tradition, the domain is conceptualized as *unordered*, where indicators are not hierarchically arranged, but highly similar and interchangeable with respect to the content and behavior to be measured. Unordered domains often have a **simple (nonstratified) domain structure.** Think of a domain tapping into only addition skills in mathematics with one-digit numbers: 5 + 4 = ____, 3 + 3 = ____, 7 + 8 = ____, and so on. Such a domain would have a simple structure because the items or tasks would focus on one tightly defined indicator, with items linked to that narrowly specified range of content and behavior: *Add* [behavior] *single-digit numbers* [content] *correctly*. Here, we would expect items to be replicable with respect to difficulty level. By design, a simple, unordered construct domain is homogeneous in nature—a property that can be tested empirically with a statistical index, an *item homogeneity index* (more on that in Chapters 10 and 11).

By contrast, think of a construct domain tapping into a wider range of arithmetic skills requiring separate proficiency levels to be measured in addition, subtraction, multiplication, and division. Given the four qualitatively different indicators, this domain would have a **stratified domain structure**. Contrasted to the addition only domain, there would be four heterogeneous strata here. Under a general domain of arithmetic skills, we would have four subdomains corresponding with each stratum. Within each stratum, we could still have unordered **subdomain** structures. Once the indicator-referenced items are compiled, each subdomain could potentially yield a **subscale** or subtest with a separate score. With sufficient overlap in content and behaviors across strata, we could tie together the measures under a common domain framework representing the overall construct.

Graphically, for generosity, Figure 4.2 suggests a similarly stratified, and unordered domain structure. There are five hypothetical strata. The content of indicators is shown graphically (with differently filled-in circles). Implicitly, each subdomain would be defined by observable indicators of generosity that were substantively different. For example, "acts of generosity" as demonstrated in five separate arenas of life could be specified, such as generous acts in the family, the workplace, the neighborhood and community, religious organizations, and political/governmental organizations. As with all unordered domains, the indicators (and items generated) would be treated as equivalent in terms of difficulty, value, or weight, with no implicit hierarchy in the strata.

Take a look at two real-world applications now. Respectively, each served as the foundation for designing cognitive and noncognitive assessments.

The first domain framework is shown in Box 4.2 (Chatterji, Graham, & Wyer, 2009). This domain was specified for designing multiple-choice tests to measure competency levels of resident physicians while they were under training at university hospitals. Similar to Tyler's structure, this domain was also conceived as two-dimensional. Physicians under training were expected to demonstrate their skills in practicing evidence-based medicine (EBM). The four "content" strata are therapy, diagnosis, prognosis, and harm (refers to evaluating harmful side effects of treatments). The content strata are crossed against "behavior" strata corresponding to four EBM skills: ask (asking clinical research questions to gather evidence), acquire (acquiring the evidence), appraise (appraising the evidence), and apply (applying the evidence to patient cases). Items were developed to populate the cells of this table of specifications with weighting assigned to items in the cells, as shown. This is an example of a heterogeneous, stratified domain that is unordered.

In Box 4.3, we see a domain for a noncognitive construct to measure the personality characteristics of effective teachers. This domain is based on a literature review conducted by the authors (Madni, Baker, Chow, Dellacruz, & Griffin, 2015). It is a similarly stratified and heterogeneous domain with four strata: Conscientiousness, Extraversion, Emotional Stability, and Openness to Experience. The developers recognized separate strata that define the overall personality construct, identifying added dimensions to be described

BOX 4.2 Unordered and Stratified Domain Specifications for a Cognitive Competency Assessment

Assessment Use Context

What to Assess?

Competencies in practicing evidence-based medicine

Whom to Assess?

Resident physicians undergoing training at university hospitals

Why Assess?

Program evaluation and accreditation

- *Measure-based inferences?* Competency levels of trainees and overall program performance
- *Specific uses?* Evaluating average trainee competency levels for program accreditation
- *Primary users?* Faculty, program directors, trainees, and mentors

Domain Specifications

General Indicator

Resident physicians will formulate clinical questions to locate, appraise, and apply the best-available research evidence for making clinical decisions relevant to patient needs.

Specific Indicators

- "Ask" skill: Formulate questions to guide information searches on therapies and clinical courses of action for patients.
- "Acquire" skill: Select evidence-based courses of clinical action for patients.
- "Appraise" skill: Critically appraise the quality and applicability of the evidence for individual patient cases.
- "Apply" skill: Integrate the evidence into clinical decisions while taking into account individual patient values and circumstances.

Table of Test Specifications

Behaviors:	*Content:* **THERAPY**	*Content:* **PROGNOSIS**	*Content:* **DIAGNOSIS**	*Content:* **HARM**
"Ask" Skills	10%	5%	5%	5%
"Acquire" Skills	10%	5%	5%	5%
"Appraise" Skills	10%	5%	5%	5%
"Apply" Skills	10%	5%	5%	5%

Note. All items carry equal point weights. Percentages denote item weighting and distribution plan for designing a multiple-choice test matched to the domain.

Source: Adapted with permission from Chatterji, Graham, & Wyer (2009). ©Accreditation Council for Graduate Medical Education.

later. Although not in the original article, each stratum could be represented by a general indicator using the conventions we applied for *generosity*; specific indicators are also added here for illustration purposes. Once specified, all domains should be validated independently to add rigor to the domain specification procedures.

QUICK RECAP: How we conceptualize the domain structure depends on the type of construct, the supporting literature, traditions of measurement that influence the design process, and the assessment purposes. The construct type could be cognitive, noncognitive, health-related, or sociodemographic. Domains could be conceptualized as ordered or unordered. For both, we could opt for either homogeneous or heterogeneous structures. These design decisions should depend on the purposes for assessment, as given by the primary users and assessment designers, and other contextual factors.

Reflection Break 4.2: Objective 2

- Define each broad type of construct introduced in this section: cognitive, noncognitive, health-related, and sociodemographic constructs. Give *new examples* in the four categories.
- How will you deal with any construct ambiguities you find during the instrument design process?
- Distinguish between the following: ordered domains; unordered domains; simple homogeneous

BOX 4.3 Stratified and Unordered Domain Specifications: Assessing Personality Traits of Effective Teachers

Assessment Context

What to Assess?

Personality characteristics of effective teachers

Whom to Assess?

Teachers in public education systems in different localities

Why Assess?

Formative decisions in workplace contexts

- *Measure-based inferences?* Strength of different personality characteristics
- *Specific uses?* Professional development, mentoring, and goal setting
- *Primary users?* Teachers, supervisors, mentors

Domain Specifications

General Indicator. In professional contexts, teachers exhibit the personality characteristics of:

- *Conscientiousness*
  Specific Indicators *(Examples):*
  - Teachers complete all their school-related obligations on time.
  - Teachers prepare lessons carefully to meet diverse students' needs.
- *Extraversion*
  Specific Indicators *(Examples):*
  - Teachers behave in a friendly manner toward colleagues and coworkers at school.
  - Teachers reach out voluntarily to support colleagues and coworkers at school.
- *Emotional stability*
  Specific Indicators *(Examples):*
  - Teachers show calmness in their classroom demeanor.
  - Teachers speak in a well-modulated tone at school.
- *Openness to experience*
  Specific Indicators *(Examples):*
  - Teachers show openness to new methods of teaching.
  - Teachers express open mindsets when teaching diverse students.

domains; stratified, heterogeneous domains. Give examples of each from your experience.

- Describe how you plan to conceptualize the construct domains(s) for your own instrument.

4.4 Domain Specification as a Part of the Process Model: Steps, Techniques, Guidelines, and Conventions

See Table 4.2 next in conjunction with Figure 4.1 presented earlier in this chapter. There are five steps to the domain specification process. This section offers some established guidelines and techniques for specifying construct domains, situated in the Process Model. As we proceed, we refer back to Boxes 4.1–4.3, with added illustrations and discussion.

4.4.1 Five Iterative Steps for Specifying Domains

Specifying Phase I of the Process Model is fundamental to user-centered assessment design. By aligning the indicators with the population characteristics and relevant socioecological factors mindfully, we could specify construct domains in a more contextually and culturally responsive manner. Similarly, keeping the user path, intended inferences, and uses of construct measures in mind alerts designers to the assessment stakes, as well as the interests of the primary users. As a general rule, the higher the stakes tied to assessment-based actions, the more rigorous the design procedures should be—starting with the domain specification and initial content validation processes. Good practice demands that we subject the initially drafted domains to at least one critical review and revision, even for informal assessments. The overall process is iterative rather than sequential. Refer to Tables 4.1 and 4.2 next showing the steps that would follow.

TABLE 4.2. Five Iterative Steps to Specify Construct Domains

Step	Domain specification procedures
Step 1	Identify constructs or attributes to measure with reference to Phase I of the Process Model (*What to assess?*). • Label the construct(s) and set the theoretical limits. • Take into account the population specifications (*Whom to assess?*). • Take into account the assessment purpose specifications (*Why assess?*).
Step 2	Locate appropriate knowledge bases, data sources, or resources for deriving indicators. • Literature reviews, scientific research, curricula, and/or documentary sources. • Expert knowledge and specialist perspectives. • Direct observations, critical incident techniques, or case studies.
Step 3	Write and organize indicators using established guidelines and conventions. • Use standard guidelines to specify observable aspects of indicators. • Organize indicator statements in useful ways.
Step 4	Use appropriate taxonomies for classifying and clarifying the behavioral dimensions of indicators. • Sort and separate indicators in cognitive, noncognitive, health-related, or sociodemographic constructs. • Identify homogeneous clusters of indicators by "behavior" dimensions to be measured. • Develop or select item or task examples to match selected indicators.
Step 5	Validate the specified domains using internal and/or external reviews. Iterate and revise, as needed.

4.4.2 Locating Appropriate Resources for Specifying Domains

Assessment designers should try to locate credible sources from which to derive the construct indicators. For most informal assessment design efforts, a quick Google search might suffice. In more formal applications, added research and alternative data sources will likely be necessary. This section discusses three commonly used data sources and associated research methods for domain specification:

1. **Using existing theory, research, literature reviews, and documentary sources:** Common resources for domain specification are scientific, professional, and academic research articles in relevant fields; documents published by national or international professional associations; mission and policy statements of

organizations, institutions, or programs; and current textbooks or curriculum resources in a given field and education level.

How are indicators extracted? A useful way to identify indicators is by conducting a thematic content analysis of the articles gathered. For example, Madni and colleagues (2015; Box 4.3) desired to measure noncognitive traits of effective teachers. Through a review of the research literature dealing with effective teacher characteristics, they identified four general areas (domains): personality characteristics, motivational attributes, intrapersonal skills, and interpersonal skills. Guided by the five-factor theory of personality (Olver & Moorardian, 2003), they further broke down personality characteristics of teachers into five dimensions: conscientiousness, emotional stability, extraversion, agreeableness, and openness to experience. Box 4.3 is developed from that work, with specific indicator statements added to illustrate how the domain could be specified in further detail.

Similarly, the cognitive competency domain in Box 4.2 was operationalized as shown based on an extensive literature review performed by the authors (Chatterji, Graham, & Wyer, 2009). The research team drew on a variety of documents for the literature review: established standards and guidelines in the medical profession, curriculum goals and criteria set by the accreditation agency for graduate medical programs, and medical research literature and users' guides on EBM (Guyatt, Rennie, Meade, & Cook, 2002). In addition, they sought perspectives of medical and EBM experts to fortify the indicators and subindicators of the construct domain. The table of specifications shown was compiled after the indicators of the domain and subdomains were validated by experts. To build the competency tests, the team designed a large pool of multiple-choice items to match the indicators in the cells. Items were sampled proportionally from each cell based on percentage weights assigned by medical experts on the team.

2. Using expert opinions and perspectives: In situations where the construct to be measured is very new, or the attributes are little known and yet to be formalized in the existing literature, we could utilize the opinions of experts, scientists, or experienced practitioners for specifying the domain's indicators.

How are indicators extracted? There are several qualitative research methods and facilitated group processes for eliciting knowledge from individual experts or expert panels. During the data-collection process, researchers could either take notes or record the chief points conveyed by experts on domain-relevant topics. The data could then be categorized qualitatively by theme and subtheme using content analysis methods. Multivariate statistical methods, like **cluster analysis**, may also be used subsequently to analyze and further interpret the qualitatively coded data we secure. Selection of the "experts" is key for domain specification purposes with these methods; the individuals solicited should be highly knowledgeable and/or experienced professionals, with the necessary insights into the constructs and populations of concern. Widely used in this category are the Delphi method, focus group interviewing, nominal group technique, and concept mapping. Each is described briefly below.

The **Delphi method**, originally developed as a systematic, interactive forecasting method, is based on the principle that consensus-based decisions from a structured group of qualified individuals are more accurate than those obtained separately from each expert (Dalkey & Helmer, 1963). Here, the experts would answer questionnaires in two or more rounds on the hypothetical construct (or topic). After each round, a facilitator would provide an anonymous summary of the experts' ideas along with rationales for those judgments. In the second round, participants would be encouraged to revise their earlier answers in light of the facilitator's feedback on the overall group's perspectives, until the group converges toward consensus.

Focus group interviewing is a form of qualitative research in which a carefully selected group of people is asked for their perceptions, opinions, beliefs, or attitudes about given topics, such as the manifestation of COVID-19 as a disease in different social groups. The interviews are conducted through guided discussions. For market research or political analysis purposes, a focus group is a small but demographically diverse group of people whose reactions are studied to determine their reactions about a new product or policy (Greenbaum, 2000). For domain specification applications, the interviews could attempt to extract opinions and points of view on the indicators of a construct.

The **nominal group technique** is another group

process involving problem identification, solution generation, and decision making in an area. This approach could be similarly useful for arriving at consensus-based indicators of a new construct (Delbecq & Van de Ven, 1971). The method has been used in curriculum design and evaluation contexts, as well as in social policymaking. The expert groups may be of different sizes, but the interest is in making a decision quickly with everyone's opinions taken into account.

Concept mapping is another method that could be useful for grouping ideas on unknown or still undefined constructs with facilitated expert group processes, followed by appropriate qualitative and quantitative analysis of the data (Goldman & Kane, 2014; Rosas & Kane, 2012). Expert participants start by brainstorming a series of descriptive, representative statements on a construct-related question, such as "What are the signs of severe COVID-19 in the elderly?" Next, all statements are clustered, sorted in piles, and quantitatively rated by experts to indicate similarities and dissimilarities. To verify commonalities among indicators based on the ratings, multivariate statistical methods (like cluster analysis) may be employed to identify similar clusters of statements. In a final step, the expert group helps interpret the clusters, thereby creating a domain and subdomain framework for the construct.

An applied example with a combination of the above methods can be found in the work of Graham and colleagues (2009). This research team used a variant of focus group interviews and nominal group techniques to identify the key indicators of a relatively unexplored medical competency area called systems-based practices (SBP), given by the Accreditation Council for Graduate Medical Education. Their goal was to operationally define resident physicians' competence in SBP in terms of observable roles, actions, and behaviors.

The researchers collected data using structured focus group interviews of a total of 88 health care professionals working in various roles in large hospitals and health care systems in New York City—doctors, nurses, technicians, patient care support staff, and administrative staff. Their methodology involved gathering data from group meetings, coding themes obtained from the consensus-seeking procedures, and then conceptually matching and organizing the indicators to define the SBP domain. The domain served as the basis for designing observational assessments to rate physicians' SBP competency levels during their residency training.

3. Direct observations, critical incident techniques, and case study research: Other ways to define domains for constructs that are relatively undocumented or unknown involve observational and case study methods. Three commonly employed practices are discussed next.

How are indicators extracted? The **critical incident technique**, a method based on direct observations and reporting by key informants, is useful for identifying extreme behavioral indicators of a given construct. A key informant is an individual with firsthand knowledge of a topic or situation. An early study by Flanagan (1954, as cited in Crocker & Algina, 2006, p. 68) employed the method by asking job supervisors (the key informants) to define so-called critical behaviors representing outstanding performance on the job in a given workplace setting, contrasted with completely ineffective performance of workers. The identified behaviors served as indicators of the construct.

Case study methods involve detailed reviews and analysis of case records for identifying and cataloging behavioral indicators of constructs. Case study methods are particularly useful in defining health-related constructs for still undocumented diseases or disabilities. Constructs could be defined comprehensively by studying symptoms and behaviors of patient cases via direct observations supplemented with other forms of case data. To enhance credibility, the case data must be collected by appropriately trained professionals and corroborated over multiple cases (Stake, 2015).

See Box 4.4 for an illustration of how case studies could be used to specify domains. The illustration draws on a historical narrative on cures for cancer, describing how early understandings of leukemia evolved from recordings and direct observations of patient cases by committed doctors and cancer researchers (Mukherjee, 2010). Careful observations, documentation, cataloging, and classification of the symptoms from multiple cases led to collective learning about the disease. The most useful observable indicator of the disease was determined to be the count of white blood cells in the patients' blood. This discovery provided the gateway toward developing protocols for measurement and diagnosis of the condition in patients.

BOX 4.4 Using Case Studies to Derive Observable Construct Indicators

Assessment Use Context

What to Assess? "Leukemia," an unknown disease at the time

Whom to Assess? Adult patients

Why Assess? Clinical diagnosis and treatment

- Measure-based inferences? Identification of disease symptoms and characteristics
- Specific uses? Diagnosis
- Primary users? Oncologists, cancer researchers, patients, and families

Patient Case Studies for Indicator and Domain Specification

Case 1: An early case study dated 1845 presented observation records of a 28-year-old slate-layer. The observations were made by John Bennett, as described in Mukherjee (2010, pp. 12–13).

Early stages of disease showed the following external signs in the patient:

- "a mysterious swelling in his spleen . . ."
- "great listlessness on exertion," which continued over a period of 20 months
- "tumor in his abdomen which gradually increased in size," becoming stationary 4 months afterward

In the next few weeks:

- rapid disease progression
- patient had "fevers"
- "flashes of bleeding"
- "sudden fits of abdominal pain, gradual at first, then on a tighter, faster arc . . ."
- then "more swollen tumors sprouting in his armpits, his groin, and his neck . . . ," leading eventually to patient's death

An autopsy revealed:

- patient's "blood was chock full [of] white blood cells . . . [which is] a principal constituent of pus . . ." [but] "Bennett could not find a source for the pus" at that time.

Case 2: Observations of another concurrent case were conducted by Rudolf Virchow. This case concerned a cook in her mid-50s, as presented by Mukherjee (2010, pp. 13–16).

- The patient showed "striking similarities" with the first in that she had a "massively enlarged spleen."
- The patient also presented with "white blood cells . . . explosively overgrown [in] her blood."
- Again, there was a mysterious "absence of any wound" as the source of the excessive white blood cells or "pus."

Inferences

Based on the similarities in indicators in both cases:

- Virchow recognized "the blood itself was abnormal. . . . The blood cells had overgrown in a distorted, uncontrolled fashion with "millions of white blood cells . . . seen under his microscope" after the patient's death.
- Virchow named the disease "leukemia."

Implications for Assessment Design

Based on multiple case records, "leukemia could be counted . . . by drawing a sample of blood or bone marrow and looking at it under a microscope" (Mukherjee, 2010, p. 19). The counts of white blood cells of normal versus diseased individuals became a key diagnostic indicator of the condition. Assessment techniques could be built using this and other indicators derived from added case studies.

QUICK RECAP: Table 4.2 recommended five iterative steps for specifying domains. Once the construct types are identified, specifying indicators immediately follows. Locating the right resources to identify domain-relevant indicators typically requires reviews of existing research or documentary resources. For unknown or novel constructs, researchers could seek expert opinions, or conduct small-scale exploratory studies using key informants, focus group interviews, direct observations, or case study methods to generate construct indicators. These steps fall under Phases I–II of the Process Model, under the *What?* and *How?* portals.

Reflection Break 4.3: Objectives 1–3

- What are the *benefits* of specifying Phase I prior to specifying the domain?
- Compare *three different methods* for locating resources to specify construct domains. List the advantages and disadvantages of each for your own instrument design project.
- Suppose you wanted to measure *teacher attitudes toward technology* (or another construct).
  - Identify the *construct type* based on the four-category taxonomy given.
  - How would you specify the *domain* and *subdomains*? What resources would you use to derive indicators and items? What steps would you take to locate resources? What would be your domain structure?
  - How would you establish the credibility of your domain?

4.4.3 Writing and Organizing Indicator Statements

Because most constructs are big concepts comprising multiple and sometimes layered components, we often start the domain specification process with a collection of brainstormed ideas and broad themes extracted from the data sources we select. Restating the initially brainstormed ideas as formal indicator statements helps bring clarity and preciseness to the themes. Organizing the indicators in coherent clusters adds theoretical integrity and meaningfulness to the assessments we design. Three guidelines now follow building on the earlier indicator illustrations on generosity and human biology.

1. **Use action-oriented verbs to write indicator statements.** Action words convey the directly observable behaviors, acts, or responses that are easily measurable through the tasks or items. As mentioned, by using the verb "give," Cureton (1951) offered action-oriented indicators of generosity. Similarly, for indicators in cognitive domains, we would prefer to use the verbs "write," "state," or "apply" instead of verbs like "know," "understand," or "discuss" that are relatively vague. In the same vein, to measure hand–eye coordination in children with cerebral palsy, a health-related construct, a researcher in biobehavioral studies framed an indicator with the action verb shown below (Sarafian, 2020). Cerebral palsy stems from a neurological condition that begins in the prenatal stages, leading to disabilities in the hand–eye coordination of children.

> *The child picks up* [action-oriented behavior] *objects of different sizes with one hand* [content].

2. **When appropriate, specify the content, behavior, condition, and/or performance criterion in indicators.** Minimally, well-written indicators specify the content and behavior components, as demonstrated earlier. Depending on the assessment purposes and construct type, we might specify *four* distinguishable parts in an indicator: behavior, content, condition, and a criterion performance. The condition in an indicator helps place the behavior in an exact setting where it will be performed, observed, recorded, and measured. The criterion indicates the performance expectation or a mastery level that should be demonstrated by the respondent or examinee.

Continuing with the earlier example, children with cerebral palsy are often placed with occupational therapists who help build their hand–eye coordination skills. To design assessments to measure the progress of children receiving therapy, the domain's indicators might specify the condition and a criterion level of performance, as shown below:

When prompted by the examiner during individual assessments [condition], the *child picks up* [action-oriented behavior] *objects of different sizes with one hand* [content].

When prompted by the examiner [condition], the *child picks up* [action-oriented behavior] *objects of different sizes with one hand* [content] *on three separate occasions* [criterion].

For another example, we could write an indicator in the mathematics patterns proficiency domain with all four parts, as follows:

Students will be able to calculate [behavior] *the sum of a sequence of whole numbers* [content] *without a hand calculator* [condition] *showing 80% accuracy* [criterion performance].

An indicator for measuring the teacher personality attribute of conscientiousness that includes a condition could look like this:

In classroom teaching contexts [condition], *teachers exhibit* [behavior] *conscientious behaviors to ensure student learning* [content].

3. Organize the indicators from general to specific. To bring a domain into sharper focus, indicators are typically organized from general to more and more specific statements, until the domain is as clear as possible for item design or selection purposes. Indicator clustering should be coherent and meaningful, guided by the literature or data sources used. In a domain's schematic representation using tree diagrams, the general indicators are more broadly stated and placed at the upper levels of the domain. Further breakdown of the general indicators to specific indicators that are increasingly more concrete clarifies the definition of the construct. For organizing and presenting indicator statements from the general to more specific levels, Figure 4.3 shows a **tree diagram** arrangement.

Examine the concept of *conscientiousness* with and without the specific indicators provided to see why second- or third-level indicators are often necessary to remove any inherent ambiguities in constructs. Box 4.3 provides only two as illustrations for each general indicator, but the need for more may be obvious. To derive the specific indicators, guiding questions might be helpful, such as "What would a conscientious teacher tend to say or do in professional contexts? How would they act, based on the literature or practitioner reports?" The embedded specific indicators add detail to the content and behaviors to be measured.

The tree diagram in Figure 4.3 depicts a domain that aims to measure historical thinking skills in secondary school students. Graphically, the domain shows one main branch with five subbranches. The general indicators illustrated are rather broad and specify the content dimensions only (not desirable!). But, as each is broken down further with a second-level indicator delineating the behavior (such as "analyze") and the content (such as "multiple causation") of focus, the construct is clarified. Each such indicator could be further broken down by adding branches to the tree, until the operational features of tasks and items are evident for assessment design purposes. The number and levels of branches and subbranches necessary in a tree diagram could vary for different construct domains.

For the mathematics patterns proficiency construct (Box 4.2), a general indicator in the main stem of the tree diagram could be broken down at three levels, with each level further detailing the content and task-specific behavior to be assessed, as follows. Mapping out the domain coherently helps retain the logical, internal consistency of the theoretical foundation on which the assessments and construct measures are built.

General indicator (main branch of a tree diagram):

Solves problems dealing with mathematical patterns and sequences.

Specific indicator (second-level branch):

Selects appropriate arithmetic operations to continue a given mathematical sequence.

Specific indicator (third-level branch):

Calculates the sum of the terms of a given mathematical sequence containing whole numbers, decimals, or fractions.

QUICK RECAP: Domain specification is necessary to operationalize the construct with the requisite levels of clarity, focus, and theoretical coherence

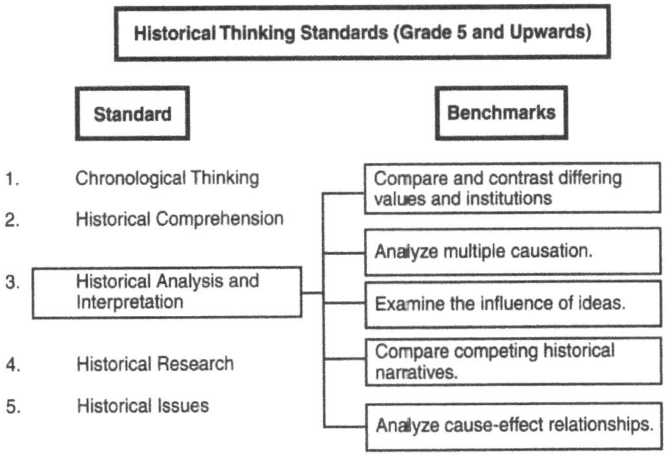

FIGURE 4.3. A two-level tree diagram: A specified achievement domain in history. Adapted for illustration purposes from Chatterji (2003).

to guide item design or selection. By convention, indicators could delineate the content, behavior, condition, and/or the expected criterion performances to be measured. Minimally, indicators should specify the content and behavior dimensions; decisions on the added components should be guided by the larger assessment context, purposes, and construct type. Tree diagrams are useful for organizing indicator statements in a domain from general to more specific levels. Other useful mechanisms for organizing domains are tools like concept-mapping diagrams.

Reflection Break 4.4: Objectives 3 and 4

- For this exercise, think of measuring abilities and attitudes on *driving automobiles* in adult U.S. populations. When specifying the domains, identify the advantages to (1) specifying the construct types, (2) locating appropriate and defensible sources and documents, (3) stating indicators clearly, and (4) organizing indicators from general to specific.
- Write four indicators to assess the construct *automobile driving proficiency*. Specify the content, behavior, conditions, and criterion levels of performance you desire to measure, as applicable.
- Write four indicators to assess the construct *attitude toward driving*. Specify the content, behavior, and conditions in the indicators that you desire to measure, as applicable.

4.4.4 Using Taxonomies to Classify Indicators

Benjamin Bloom and colleagues (1956) began a helpful tradition in assessment design, where the indicators are classified using a selected taxonomy of behaviors that then guides item design or selection. Within the domains and subdomains that define a construct, recall that domain sampling theory assumes that items are similar and homogeneous. A taxonomic categorization of the "behavior" component of indicators enables the production of closely related items tied to the desired indicators, helping achieve homogeneous properties of the items. Classifying indicators using behavioral taxonomies has added benefits in facilitating homogeneous selections of appropriate items, assessment modalities and item formats for differently classified indicators as well. Furthermore, when designing scoring procedures for assessments, the taxonomic level of indicators helps designers with decisions on how much weight (importance in terms of points) to allocate to different groups of items that measure, say, simple recall versus application or higher-order thinking skills.

The literature offers several alternative taxonomies for these purposes, old and new. Each is applicable to a different construct type. This section offers a series of *functional taxonomies* that build on that literature base as optional tools for aiding the assessment design or selection processes for different construct types (Bloom et al., 1956; Chatterji, 2003; Eagly & Chaikin, 1998; Gagné, 1965; Katz, 1960; Krathwohl, Bloom, & Masia, 1964; Marzano, Pickering, & McTighe, 1994; National Research Council [NRC], 2012). Readers are encouraged to review the classic *Taxonomy of Educational Objectives* (Bloom et al., 1956) and more recent taxonomies (NRC, 2012) as a supplement to this section.

4.4.4.1 A Functional Taxonomy for Measuring Cognitive Constructs

The cognitive taxonomy, shown below, recognizes four separate types of cognitive capacities that we could aim to measure (after Bloom et al., 1956; Chatterji, 2003; Krathwohl et al., 1964; NRC, 2012). Each is expected to impose different mental demands on the examinee or respondent. Indicators measuring concept recall and understanding are at the lowest level in terms of expected cognitive demands; application is at the next higher level, with complex procedural skills and higher-order thinking skills at the most demanding levels of cognitive processing. The verbs suggest the cognitive behaviors that the indicators and items would be designed to match. For each level, either structured-response or more open-ended problem-solving tasks could be designed, as appropriate. (See the table at the bottom of this page.)

The categories are cumulative. Application-level tasks will typically also call for concept knowledge and understanding. Likewise, higher-order thinking tasks will typically require both concept recall and understanding, as well as application. A demonstration follows on how to apply the taxonomy for indicators of the mathematical patterns proficiency domain shown earlier dealing with mathematical sequences:

> *Define a "mathematical sequence."* [concept recall and understanding]
>
> *Calculate the sum of the terms of a given mathematical sequence.* [application]
>
> *Solve real-world problems involving mathematical sequences.* [higher-order thinking skills]

Construct type	Levels or types	Definition	Examples of indicator phrases
1.0 Cognitive constructs	1.1 Concept knowledge and understanding	Requires examinee to recall, retrieve, and/or show comprehension of basic concepts, facts, and principles.	State a definition, law, or principle. Describe in your own words. Paraphrase the meaning of. Give examples of. Distinguish between.
	1.2 Application	Requires examinee to apply concepts, rules, principles, tools, or formulas.	Calculate. Solve a problem. Use a tool.
	1.3 Complex procedural skills	Requires the execution of a complex task, involving multistep mental skills and integrative thinking processes, usually following accepted conventions or standards in a field.	Employ a writing process to create a story. Write a laboratory record. Conduct a research study. Develop a blueprint.
	1.4 Higher-order thinking skills	Requires higher intellectual skills involving analysis, synthesis, and/or evaluative judgments.	Analyze, explain, create, compose, compare, contrast, critique, evaluate, defend, or justify.

Apply a multistep procedure to check answers to problems involving mathematical sequences. [complex procedural skills]

4.4.4.2 A Functional Taxonomy for Measuring Noncognitive Constructs

Recall that noncognitive constructs could include attitudinal, personality, and social-behavioral constructs, as well as various interpersonal and intrapersonal domains, including metacognition (NRC, 2012). In the psychological literature, there is a tripartite taxonomy to help organize, classify, and label indicators on attitudes, viewed to have "cognitive," "affective," and "behavioral" (CAB) components (Eagly & Chaiken, 1998; Hovland & Rosenberg, 1960). Note that for noncognitive constructs, the term *cognitive* refers to one's beliefs about something. While this usage is consistent with the literature on attitude measurement (Eagly & Chaikin, 1998), *cognitive* in the context of attitude measurement should not be confused with mental abilities and skills in the cognitive taxonomy given earlier. Rather, it should be interpreted as what a person holds to be true about something. This tripartite taxonomy is broadened below with a metacognitive component with the mnemonic CAB-M. In the demonstrations, the attitude-specific content focus is on childbearing and abortion topics. (See the table at the bottom of this page.)

For more concrete demonstrations, suppose you wish to apply the noncognitive taxonomy above to measure attitude toward childbearing and abortion in adults. The indicators next listed are matched to survey items assuming a Likert response scale: Strongly agree through Strongly disagree. Each item example is designed to measure a different CAB-M dimension.

- **Cognitive (C)** component of attitude toward childbearing and abortion:
  - C-Indicator. *Endorses a woman's right to choose the circumstances for bearing a child.*
  - Item. *A woman should have the right to choose the time when she has a child.*
- **Affective (A)** component of attitude toward childbearing and abortion:
  - A-Indicator. *Indicates feelings about a woman's right to choose on matters of childbearing.*
  - Item. *I am frustrated that my state's laws prevent women from making their own choices on childbearing.*

Construct type	Levels or types	Definition	Indicator or item examples
Noncognitive constructs (affective, attitudinal, personality, or social-behavioral domains)	2.1 **C:** "Cognitive" component of dispositions	What a person *holds to be true* about something; their opinions, beliefs, values, or perceptions about it, including experiences, objects, events, places, or persons	Endorses or communicates beliefs (regarding childbearing). Endorses or communicates perceptions of (childbearing).
	2.2 **A:** "Affective" component of dispositions	What a person *feels emotionally* about social issues, present or past experiences, events, places, persons, or objects	Endorses or communicates emotions or feelings about (childbearing).
	2.3 **B:** "Behavioral" component of dispositions	What a person *would do*, or a person's attitude-governed action and practices would be, in relation to given experiences, events, places, persons, or objects	Communicates doing something or engaging in practices, actions, or behaviors (related to childbearing).
	2.4 **M:** "Metacognitive" component of dispositions	A person's stance on self-reflection and self-evaluation of their own behaviors, actions, mindsets, aimed to self-correct a position.	Communicates self-introspective and self-correcting stances on issues (like abortion or childbearing).

Construct type	Levels or types	Definition	Indicator or item examples
3.0 Health-related constructs	3.1 Physiological indicators of a health condition	Physiological signs or symptoms of a state of well-being or an illness or disorder	Items on heart rate, blood pressure levels, body temperature, etc.
	3.2 Behavioral indicators of a health condition	Behavioral signs or symptoms of a state of well-being vs. an illness or disorder	Items indicating what a person will say or do when well vs. ill (e.g., stutters, forgets details, stumbles, sleeps too much, reports low or high energy levels)
	3.3 Physical appearance indicators of a health condition	Appearance-related indicators of a state of well-being vs. an illness or disorder	What a person looks like when well versus ill (e.g., redness of eyes, paleness of skin, gaunt)

- **Behavioral (B)** component of attitude toward childbearing and abortion:
  - B-Indicator. *Reports practices or acts related to personal stance on childbearing.*
  - Item. *I have participated in anti-abortion protests.*
- **Metacognitive (C)** component of attitude toward childbearing and abortion:
  - M-Indicator. *Indicates engaging in self-evaluations on issues of childbearing.*
  - Item. *I rethink my positions on childbearing based on information I read.*

4.4.4.3 A Functional Taxonomy to Measure Health-Related Constructs

Along similar lines, consider the taxonomy and specific examples next for designing assessments for health-related constructs. (See the table at the top of this page.)

Consider next the health condition of sleep apnea, a sleeping and breathing disorder found in children and adults. The item examples, designed for a caregiver interview for a child, demonstrate application of the behavioral dimension from the above taxonomy.

- Indicator. *Parent or caregiver reports on their child's sleeping habits at night.*
- Item. *How often is your child restless while sleeping at night?*
- Response Options.
  - *Every night of a week—Most nights in a week—Some nights in a week— Rarely—Never*
- Indicator. *Parent or caregiver reports on their child's breathing behavior while sleeping.*
- Item. *How often does your child snore while sleeping at night?*
- Response Options.
  - *Every night of a week—Most nights in a week—Some nights in a week—Rarely—Never*

4.4.4.4 A Functional Taxonomy to Measure Sociodemographic Constructs

Finally, the next taxonomy focuses on attributes and characteristics that are implicitly agreed-upon, societal constructions, typically employed by governments, organizations, and institutions to group individuals broadly. The definitions may vary depending on the cultural, regional, or national context; hence, indicator or item writing should reflect the contextually relevant social norms and construct definitions in given localities where the instrument is applied. Item examples are suggested. (See the table at the bottom of page 117.)

4.5 Content-Validating Specified Domains

Alongside Table 4.2, Box 4.5 provides 10 questions to guide evaluations of initially specified domains for constructs we desire to measure. Content validation is a last step of the domain specification process, accomplished using critical self-reviews, peer reviews, or more formal studies with expert feedback processes. Minimally, the criteria we apply are:

- **Content relevance:** Are indicators well matched and relevant to the construct theory and knowledge bases?
- **Content representativeness:** Do indicators cover all pertinent content strata and levels tied to the construct theory and knowledge bases proportionately?
- **Organization and coherence:** Are indicators organized in a reasonable manner consistent with the construct theory and knowledge base?
- **Clarity:** Are indicators written clearly enough to allow the easy design/selection of items and remaining assessment operations?

Within given domains and subdomains, a *few* items ought to be designed to test the measurability of indicators either taken individually or in coherent clusters. Should assessment designers face barriers with this step, the likelihood is that the domain needs further breakdown or clarification. As provided in Box 4.5, a revision of the indicators and items should follow, using an iterative process, to finalize the domains and continue the design process.

QUICK RECAP: A taxonomic analysis of indicators allows designers to predesignate the exact dimensions to be measured by each indicator or groups of indicators, and as needed, to reorganize the domain accordingly into more homogeneous and logical arrangements. The assessment design literature offers several optional taxonomies for this step. Applications with four *functional taxonomies*, derived from old and new literature sources on the topic, were developed and demonstrated in this section; each taxonomy applies to a given construct type, assuming multidisciplinary assessment design projects.

The final steps in the domain specification process are evaluative, guided by 10 criteria (Box 4.5). The purpose is to correct for persistent ambiguities or major gaps left in the domains (such as oversights in relevant literature or mechanics of indicator specification). Depending on the formality of the endeavor, this step can be more or less extensive.

Reflection Break 4.5: Objectives 4–6

- Classify the construct type for the indicators below. Fill in the blanks with the appropriate functional taxonomy to categorize each type or level of the indicators in italics below. Justify your classification.
  - *Compose a story for children ages 5–7.*
    Construct type: ____________________
    Taxonomic category: __________
  - *Behave ethically in the workplace.*
    Construct type: ____________________
    Taxonomic category: __________
  - *Follow rules while driving cars on main roads and highways.*
    Construct type: ____________________
    Taxonomic category: __________

Construct type	Levels or types	Definition	Indicator or item examples
4.0 Sociodemographic constructs	4.1 Demographic factors	Construct categories based on biological, morphological, or physical characteristics	Sex Race Ethnicity
	4.2 Social class	Construct categories based on one's wealth, income, education, and/or occupations	Education level, socioeconomic status, "white- collar" vs. "blue-collar" workers
	4.3 Geographic, regional, or organizational membership	Construct categories based on membership in a defined country, region, or organized group	Nationality, religion, political party

BOX 4.5 Checklist for Evaluating Construct Domains

Ten Criteria for Domain Specification

1. *What to assess?* Are the different types of constructs identified separately?
   - Cognitive
   - Noncognitive
   - Physical or health-related
   - Sociodemographic
   - Other (clarify)
2. *Phase I specifications?* Are the construct(s) situated in the assessment use and user context?
   - Connected with *Whom to assess*?
   - Connected with *Why assess*?
3. Defensible data sources: Were appropriate data sources used to specify the indicators of the domain?
   - Existing literature and research
   - Curricula
   - Documentary sources, websites, and other knowledge sources
   - Expert viewpoints
   - Case studies, observation records, or other qualitative studies
   - Other (clarify)
4. *Organization:* Were indicators organized from general to more specific statements using a tree diagram format (or another reasonable organization tool)?
5. *Clarity:* Were indicator statements clear? Did they specify the necessary components clearly for each construct: behavior, content, condition, criterion performance?
6. *Coherence and homogeneity:* Was a suitable taxonomy of behaviors (or other appropriate taxonomies) applied to categorize similar types of behaviors to be measured in related groups?
7. *Item design:* Were a *few* examples of items or tasks created or selected to match indicators?
8. *Critical review:* Was the domain validated by the designers themselves, or more formally by peers and external experts?
9. *Revision:* If underspecified or poorly specified initially, was the domain revised using results of reviews?
10. *Quality of domain:* Is the final version of the construct domain defensible, observable, and measurable?

- *Demonstrate 20/20 vision, per optometric criteria, when driving a car at night.*

  Construct type: ____________________

  Taxonomic category: __________

- *Subscribe to the views of a religious sect.*

  Construct type: ____________________

  Taxonomic category: __________

- Which of the above indicators are too vague or broadly stated to allow sound item design or selection? If so, how would you improve it further? Explain.
  - Specify the domain for a construct you wish to measure, using the procedures discussed in Chapter 4.

4.6 Summary

Domain specification is a key step in sound instrument design. Chapter 4 introduced you to domain sampling theory as the main framework for specifying construct domains and subdomains. It presented several guidelines, taxonomies, and conventions to help operationally define unknown, complex, or ambiguous constructs with observable indicators. The chapter demonstrated these methods with examples falling under cognitive, noncognitive, health-related, and sociodemographic construct categories.

Domains could be conceptualized with simple, stratified, ordered, or unordered structures. Five main steps in operationally defining constructs involve locating appropriate construct theories and data sources; writing and organizing indicator statements; applying suitable taxonomies to designate a level or type to indicators and subindicators; creating samples of items to test the quality of indicators; and content-validating and refining the domain prior to item design or selection.

Domain sampling theory espouses the notion that all assessments yield behavioral samples from respondents or examinees, as tied to a theoretically grounded domain. Well-specified domains allow items to be matched to indicators through logical alignment processes. When executed thoroughly, this process builds content-based validity into the items and instrument, maximizing overall validity and reliability of the eventual construct measures. Empirical methods of validation should follow to verify the overall construct validity and quality of the measures.

CHAPTER 5

Designing Assessments with Structured- and Constructed-Response Items

5.1 Chapter Overview

5.1.1 Introduction

Building on Chapter 3, this chapter now focuses on crafting items with highly structured response options or tasks with constructed-response formats that are open-ended to different degrees. Many existing textbooks and reference guides provide as many as 40 guidelines on how to construct these particular item types (see, e.g., Haladyna, 2015; Lane, Raymond, & Haladyna, 2016a). Of these, Chapter 5 selects the most essential guidelines that will permit versatile applications and align with the latest know-how on how humans acquire, develop, and demonstrate intellectual capacities in a variety of cognitive domains. To supplement the information, readers are encouraged to pursue treatments on item-writing topics elsewhere.

Item writing and selection fall under the assessment operations necessary to produce and assemble finished assessment tools under Phases II–III of the Process Model. Figure 5.1 highlights the connections of Chapter 5 with the rest of the book and the overall Process Model.

5.1.2 Chapter Objectives

After reading this chapter and completing the accompanying exercises, the reader should aabe able to:

1. Explain how poor item writing or selection can reduce the overall construct validity levels of an assessment's results.
2. Distinguish among various types of cognitive constructs that are measurable with item formats incorporating highly structured response options or open-ended constructed responses.
3. Apply established guidelines for writing different types of structured-response items with issues of validity, reliability, and utility in mind (i.e., multiple-choice, fill-in-the blank/completion, true–false, matching, and scenario-dependent item sets).
4. Apply established guidelines for writing various types of constructed-response and essay items accompanied with scoring rubrics, with issues of validity, reliability, and utility in mind.
5. Evaluate the implications of advances in the cognitive and learning sciences for effective item and task design.
6. Critically review, revise, and assemble multi-item tests and assessments using an iterative and user-centered process (Phases I–III of the Process Model).

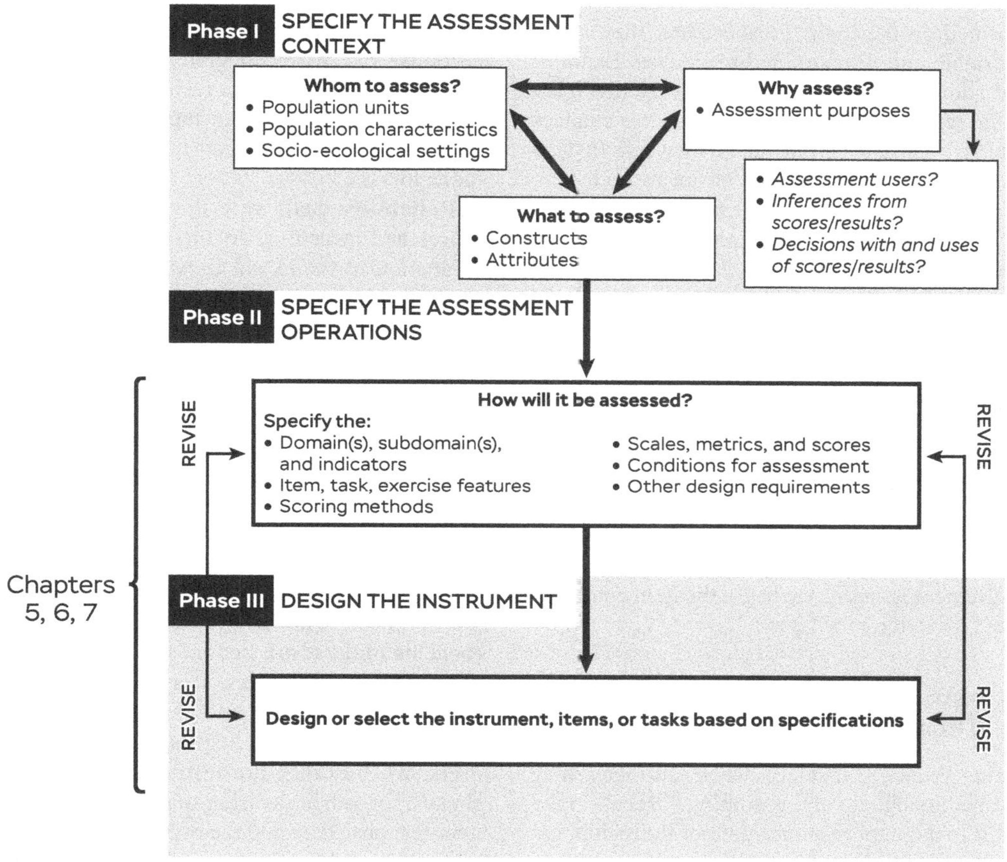

FIGURE 5.1. Connecting Chapter 5 to the Process Model and the rest of the book.

5.2 Why the Mechanics of Item Construction Matter

5.2.1 Item Construction Issues

Good measurement begins with sound item or task designs. A good **true–false (T/F) item** should yield information on what examinees actually know or can do with respect to the content and cognitive processes intentionally targeted by specific items. The wording, the response modality, directions, the item layout, graphics where applicable, and other physical features of the item should not cause respondents to feel a loss of control regarding what they know. Nor should they feel tricked into "falsing"—or giving a response with which they are uncomfortable or feel uncertain. Rather, the question should pose the problem in a clear, direct, and lucid manner. A knowledgeable respondent should be able to select either a "true" or "false" answer confidently, with a deliberate intent to do so. These basic principles apply not only to true–false items, but for all item formats that utilize highly structured response formats.

Similar design principles apply for **constructed-response tasks** as well. Broad, ambiguous, loosely defined essay prompts—such as "Explain World War II"—could perplex examinees who might otherwise be well informed on the topic. Furthermore, they invite highly variable and unrestrained responses. Examinees could address the question from widely divergent angles and reference points, increasing the chances of obtaining "construct-irrelevant" answers. Instead of the domain-specific indicators meant to be tested, examiners or instructors who review such work must now rely on their own personal opinions and subjective judgments when assigning scores. Various biases and sources of error could, therefore, compromise both the validity and reliability levels of the results. By requiring examiners to sort through the irrelevancies in the wide-ranging answers, vague essay items could also slow down the grading process, affecting utility.

Indeed, when items are well constructed, they communicate exactly to examinees what is being tested, allowing self-assessments as to whether or not they are up to the task! Item design guidelines, the primary concern of Chapter 5, are intended to anticipate potential measurement issues as we begin the item construction or item selection processes.

5.2.2 Construct Validity and Item Construction

Item-writing "rules," especially when too many, may appear to be "much ado about nothing." Recall, however, that it is the item response data of individual examinees that eventually yield the test scores and construct measures. Effective item writing increases the likelihood that each item-level response adds to the overall **construct validity** of the assessment's results for individual examinees. Taking a unified view for assuring construct validity means that we attend to issues of validity, reliability, and utility in a holistic and comprehensive manner from the very start of the item or task design processes. Which aspects of construct validity could be impacted during item construction or selection, affecting the ensuing item-level responses? Here are a few to bear in mind (AERA et al., 2014; Bandalos, 2018; Crocker & Algina, 2006; Price, 2018; see also Chapters 1 and 4).

Content-based validity of items and tasks is an essential starting requirement. Building in content-based validity during item design ensures that inferences we draw from the item responses will be meaningful with respect to the specific *content* and *cognitive behaviors* that we desired to measure. A critical corollary to content-based validity is ensuring the **validity of the response processes** by giving attention to the types of mental processing that respondents are expected to utilize during test taking; these should be consistent with the processes implicit in the specified domain's indicators.

Reliability deals with the consistency of the test scores and measures. At the item level, reliability is a function of the extent to which random errors will likely interfere with the responses. As the guidelines that follow will emphasize, random errors are often introduced through poor item wording and task presentation, or sloppy directions. From a domain-sampling standpoint, reliability can also be affected by the total number of items we design or select for measuring a given domain or subdomain. Very short tests or subtests tend to yield less reliable scores; longer tests usually improve the reliability estimates, but up to a point (more on this in Chapters 10 and 11).

Lastly, as elucidated in Chapter 1, utility has to do with both the **usability** (practicality) and **usefulness** (benefits of the test-based information for the primary users) of the assessments. From a user-centered design perspective, we must always prioritize the practical value and feasibility of items and tasks for the primary users, whether they are instructors, students, professionals, or other decision-makers. Furthermore, the item response data and the overall assessment's results must be useful for the specific decision-making needs and priorities set by these groups, which may not necessarily include the assessment designers. Transparency, fairness, and the consequences of using the assessment items and results overall are all important ingredients of the utility aspect of construct validity, especially for high-stakes assessment design endeavors.

QUICK RECAP: Items of high quality are essential to sound assessment design and also improve the quality of the assessment user experience, including test taking. Chapter 5 stresses the key guidelines for writing highly structured response items and constructed-response tasks to help reduce construct-irrelevant variance in test scores. Paying attention to the guidelines during item design or selection improves the likelihood for obtaining high levels of construct validity in the assessment results.

Reflection Break 5.1: Objective 1

- From your own test-taking experiences as a primary user, give examples of poorly conceived or badly presented items. Explain the item problems and how that impacted your test-taking experience.
- Identify three aspects of construct validity that you would prioritize during item design or selection for building a structured-response test for your own uses. Would these priorities be the same for designing an assessment with constructed-response tasks? Explain.
- Is a "tricky" test a good test from a measurement perspective? Explain.
- What does the term *construct-irrelevant variance* in assessment results mean? Explain how the concept is intimately related to the quality of the items we might design or select.

5.3 Cognitive Constructs Measured Best with Structured- or Constructed-Response Items

We turn next to the defining characteristics of typical cognitive constructs measurable with, or best suited for, the highly structured response item structures or constructed-response task formats discussed in Chapter 5. *Cognitive constructs* refer to a broad range of mental ability or skill-based domains, with labels ranging from scholastic "achievement" to workplace "competence" to "intelligence." Each of these is, in fact, a broad construct category in itself where the construct domains are defined in a number of different ways in the theoretical and practice-based literature. There are numerous existing tests and instruments of each that are both standardized and unstandardized, with varied operational definitions.

Regardless, the theoretical basis for each construct conception and the assessment purposes should guide the specific item and task operations we choose. And the goal of the item or task designer is to apprehend and elicit the *maximum* or *best performance* from the respondents to the items of all cognitive assessments. In other words, the items must be written to draw out from examinees what they are maximally capable of performing on the intended indicators, with responses scored based on "correctness."

The traditional medium for item delivery is the **paper-and-pencil format**, but more and more, **technology-mediated assessment** platforms are becoming the standard for item administration for this class of constructs. This latter trend is evident in several illustrative items from the Next Generation Science Assessment Project (*http://nextgenscienceassessment.org*), as well as elsewhere.

5.3.1 Achievement Constructs

Achievement is measurable with the item types presented in Chapter 5. As earlier chapters discussed (Chapters 1, 3, 4), the label *achievement* is ascribed to a defined body of learned knowledge and skills in formal education or training contexts (AERA et al., 2014; Cizek, 1997; Dick, Carey, & Carey, 2022; Good, 1973; Reiser, Reiser, & Dempsey, 2011; see also Tyler, 1949, 1951).

Achievement is measured through curriculum-based tests and assessments, typically administered *after* the delivery of a formal lesson, course, or program of study in K–12 education, higher education, and professional training contexts. In inferential terms, achievement test scores are expected to denote the observed performance level of examinees based on the learning that has *already* occurred following exposure to a curriculum and classroom instruction. For assessment design purposes, achievement domains are typically operationalized with the projected **learning outcomes** serving as observable indicators. In instructional design contexts, this indicator framework reflects the *instructional objectives*, identifying the knowledge and skills that participants are expected to learn through the course of study.

Item design for achievement constructs starts with the assumption that the assessments would be administered toward the end of an educational program, training, or unit of instruction. Collectively, the sample of items should be designed or selected to provide a content-representative and content-relevant snapshot of the domain to be mastered. On occasion, achievement tests are administered *before* instruction—for example, as pretests in classroom practice settings. Regardless, the outcomes focus holds for assessment design and item construction purposes.

From a psychometric standpoint, achievement measures obtained from tests are typically treated as stable indexes at the endpoints of an instructional or educational program. Indeed, the traditional conception of achievement as measured by most standardized tests is that it is a relatively context-free and stable construct, assuming that items are aligned with a curriculum (Crocker & Algina, 2006; Hopkins, 1998). For assessments we produce, these design assumptions have to be verified during validation.

In the typical test and item construction exercise, achievement is also viewed as a "domain-specific" construct. That is, the assessments are built with the belief that achievement in different subject-area domains calls for different types of cognitive processing toward the attainment of domain mastery. This view, called *domain specificity* (or domain modularity), is drawn from a school of thought from the cognitive sciences and developmental psychology (Buehl, Alexander, & Murphy, 2002). It posits that certain regions of the brain and associated neural networks are dedicated purposefully for developing concepts and skills in highly particularized domains that *do not* generalize to other areas. For example, think of the differences in learning specific skills in mathematics versus those in a fine arts curriculum.

There is another school of thought, however, that subscribes to the alternate view of *domain generality*, indicating that human learning and brain development occur cumulatively in broad, generalizable domains. Those general learned capabilities are transferable to learning in other, more specific areas. Despite these two opposing camps, there is an approaching consensus today that both domain-general and domain-specific learning may govern how humans develop, although perhaps in different ways (Buehl et al., 2002; Li, Christ, & Cowan, 2014; Siegler, 2021; Sloutsky, 2010).

For the purposes of achievement test design, subscribing to a domain-specific perspective would influence the *meanings* that the test scores and construct measures will eventually connote. Any interpretations of domain-specific measures would have to link back to the indicators in tested domains and subdomains. By design, the inferences from the assessment results would *not* be generalizable to other domains, subject areas, or professional fields, and not even to subdomains within a given construct domain in some cases. For example, a mathematics achievement test score will not allow direct inferences on, say, a person's achievement in English language arts. For inferential purposes, the item design and response data must be referred back to the particular learning outcome(s) and indicators targeted for measurement, even when the measures are found to correlate statistically later.

5.3.2 Learning and Development Constructs

The above concept of achievement—the more traditional coinage—is differentiated in the literature today from the notion of *learning, learning and development*, and *learning progressions* (NRC, 2012; Pellegrino, 2002; Pellegrino et al., 2001; Pellegrino, Wilson, Koenig, & Beatty, 2014). Like achievement, learning and developmental progressions are typically treated as domain-specific constructs—but beyond this commonality, the concepts diverge with different implications in terms of how we would approach the item design and operational procedures. As Chapter 2 discussed, advances in the cognitive, brain, and learning sciences compel us to rethink and retool traditional item design approaches toward more cognitively informed and often dynamic assessments of human abilities.

In any domain of interest, the literature distinguishes between biological maturation processes and learning in a domain. In other words, learning is not the same as growth in the brain or human body due to natural, biological, or physiological changes. Instead, the concept of learning requires the *active construction of knowledge*, generally conceptualized to occur along a developmental continuum in given domains (NRC, 2012, 2013). Learning is further recognized to be a socially, culturally, and contextually mediated activity (Gauvain, 2005; John-Steiner & Mahn, 1996). We learn continually in a variety of contexts, within the formal environs of classroom settings, as well as informally at home, in the workplace and larger communities in which we live and interact.

To measure learning and development in a domain, therefore, we must envisage the constructs as not only domain-specific, but also as developmental, contextual, and dynamic. Items designed to map learning must follow some developmental paths we expect in learners toward a desired or predesignated goal in a domain. What are the implications for domain specification, and item and task design for a learning and development construct as compared to achievement? A case study follows at the end of the chapter on measuring a learning and development construct in scholastic contexts using the Process Model—the case illustrates several operations concretely.

5.3.3 On-the-Job Competence and Workplace Learning

In workplace contexts, **job competency** domains are measurable with a variety of structured- or constructed-response items treated in this chapter. Job competency constructs are tied to valued aspects of performance on the job in given occupational or professional settings, sometimes (albeit not necessarily) also linked to formal educational or professional training curricula. Typically, the indicators reflect demonstrable knowledge and skills pertinent to job-related functions and roles of different categories of employees in specific organizations or job sectors.

Assessments of job competency domains, similar to achievement constructs, can be designed as outcomes-focused, point-in-time measures. For example, competency tests for employee promotions or periodic performance evaluation purposes often employ this model. Alternatively, we could also think of assessing domains of **workplace learning** in organizational learning and evaluation contexts along some dynamic and developmental continua (Russ-Eft & Preskill, 2009). For the latter, cognitively informed developmental assessments could be useful. Workplace learning assessments, for instance, could identify training needs and professional development trajectories of employees toward desirable performance goals and proficiency levels in job-specific domains. Results may be used for formative feedback and coaching purposes. As with learning and development constructs in education, the item design operations must shift to learning processes, learning progress maps, and short- and long-term outcomes toward reaching designated performance goals in the workplace.

5.3.4 Aptitude

Aptitude is another cognitive construct measurable with the item types discussed in Chapter 5. This concept is traditionally defined as a person's *future potential* to succeed in specific domains relevant to a proposed future career or educational path. Aptitude is predicted based on current assessments of an individual's knowledge and/or skills in given areas. As such, the results of **aptitude** assessments must allow for prognostic inferences about the examinees' expected successes at a future point on suitable criterion domains (AERA et al., 2014; Cohen et al., 2022; VandenBos, 2007).

In theory, aptitude constructs are not connected to the specific competency foci of formal educational curricula. Rather, item design focuses instead on indicators reflecting general intellectual capacities relevant to being successful in *future* tasks in the criterion domains. Aptitude can be measured as a domain-specific or domain-general construct. Most domain-general aptitude tests rest on the psychometric assumption that the construct will remain stable over time.

A familiar example of a standardized, domain-general aptitude test used for entrance into graduate degree programs in higher education is the general Graduate Record Examination (GRE). We consider this example, noting that many colleges and universities are currently rethinking their entrance testing and admissions policies. The most recent version of the general GRE, a computer adaptive assessment administered online, aims to measure the verbal, quantitative, analytic reasoning and writing abilities of examinees at the end of their undergraduate degree programs. The goal of the GRE test is to predict their later performance in graduate school, regardless of degree programs they enter and majors they choose. Items on the GRE verbal reasoning test, for instance, are intended to measure passage-dependent information processing and analysis skills that are expected to be broadly relevant to a wide range of graduate degree programs of interest to members in the examinee pool (see *www.ets.org/gre/test-takers/general-test/about.html*).

5.3.5 Intelligence

Finally, human intelligence is another construct measurable with item types highlighted in this chapter. The definitions of, and theories on, the concept of **human intelligence** are continually evolving. In concert, how we specify the domains and select item/task features must be reconsidered. Emerging conceptions today force us to lean toward defining it as a multidimensional construct that could develop and change over an individual's lifetime.

Intelligence has been measured as both a developmental and fixed construct in the past. Historically, as Chapter 2 discussed, Binet viewed intelligence as a developmental construct, while Goddard saw it as a genetically inherited and fixed concept. The old conclusion that human intelligence was governed by a fixed, inherited, and domain-general capacity—the Spearman *g*-factor—is being replaced by several alternate modern conceptions.

For instance, Davis, Christodoulou, Seider, and Gardner (2011) have proposed a theory of multiple intelligences with eight distinct types of human intelligence, with a possible ninth dimension. Gardner's theory enjoys a following among both psychologists and educators but is sometimes questioned due to inadequate empirical validation. Yet another multidimensional conception of intelligence is that of a triangulate theory of successful intelligent thought (Sternberg, 2018). According to Sternberg's triarchic theory, humans seek to understand, adapt to, and master the world with three basic kinds of information processing: the meta-components, performance components, and knowledge acquisition components. Most intelligent thought, in this latter view, is directed toward one's attempts to adapt to the environment, shape the environment, or select environments that provide optimal survival conditions (Sternberg, 2018).

A more widely accepted "omnibus" definition holds that intelligence is a multifaceted set of mental capacities that changes and manifests itself in different ways across the life spans of individuals. In a general sense, this conception refers to the capacity of individuals to gain and apply knowledge, to reason effectively, to think logically, to have sound judgment, to have a facility with words, and to be a mentally alert, perceptive problem-solver who can adapt to new situations in life (Cohen et al., 2022).

QUICK RECAP: All cognitive constructs call for eliciting the maximum performance of examinees or respondents with item formats we choose and could be conceptualized either as domain-specific or domain-general constructs. This chapter differentiated among the constructs of achievement, learning and development in education, professional competence, workplace learning, aptitude, and intelligence. Differences in the theoretical definitions of these cognitive constructs should dictate the particular properties of items we design or select. Specific item types could utilize a variety of media or delivery platforms. Before starting the item design or selection procedures, a key question to resolve is whether the construct is best represented as changing and developmental, or as a stable and static domain.

Reflection Break 5.2: Objectives 1 and 2

- Based on this chapter and related readings, distinguish between each of the following pairs of terms with an example of an instrument or test measuring each.
  - Achievement versus learning and development constructs
  - Job competence versus workplace learning constructs
  - Intelligence versus aptitude
  - Any other cognitive construct of your choice, for example, COVID literacy or Spanish language proficiency
- What is a *domain-specific* versus a *domain-general* conception of a construct? Give an example of a test or instrument reflecting each approach.
- Do you agree with this statement below? Explain. *Construct definitions should guide the choice of item and task features.*

5.4 Writing Structured-Response Items: Principles, Guidelines, and Applied Examples

A highly structured response item could take the form of a multiple-choice item; true–false item; completion or fill-in-the-blank item; a matching-item set; or a complex, multi-item exercise tied to a scenario. For creating any of these, we should begin by attending to six general principles. Refer to Items A–M shown as illustrations in Boxes 5.1–5.7 and Tables 5.1 and 5.2 as we proceed.

Specific guidelines for writing each subtype of item follow the general guidelines, with added item examples embedded in the text. To make the item examples relatable, the focus is on basic subject matter typically taught at the primary or secondary school levels. The functional taxonomy for cognitive constructs detailed in Chapter 4 is applied in all the item illustrations, building on Bloom et al.'s (1956) taxonomy and the NRC (2012) report.

5.4.1 General Guidelines for Structured-Response Items

When constructing any highly structured response item, we should follow six general principles. Each item should:

1. Match the specified aspects of the indicator(s) to be tested, namely, the content, behavior, conditions, and/or criterion performance level.
2. Be presented in a direct and clear manner, at the appropriate reading level for the intended examinees/respondents.
3. Focus on a single, well-defined concept, principle, or topic (i.e., measure one indicator at a time, or when necessary, a coherent and connected set of indicators).
4. Have *one* correct or single best answer.
5. *Not* provide any clues to the correct answer.
6. *Not* be biased, nor have the *appearance of bias* toward any potential test-taker or subgroup, considering the full range of background characteristics and diversity in the population.

Principle 1: Match the item with key specifications of the indicator.

Good item writing begins by specifying clearly what is to be measured in the targeted indicator and constructing items to match each relevant component. The indicator, whether very narrowly or more generally stated, must be measurable with a single structured-response item. Broken down, three components specified in the indicator in Box 5.1 are relevant: the content focus (mathematical patterns using basic arithmetic operations); a taxonomically categorized level of the cognitive behavior to be tested (here, application); and the condition under which the examinee would respond (here, without a calculator). The performance criterion specified for the indicator is "with 70% accuracy," meaning that 70% of items written or selected to match the indicator shown must be answered correctly for making determinations of competency. This criterion is not relevant for the item-writing processes per se, but it is necessary when users desire to make **criterion-referenced interpretations** of the assessment's results.

Box 5.1 shows three illustrative items of varying quality designed to measure the indicator. Three different item formats are illustrated: completion/fill-in-the-blanks (Item A), true–false (Item B), and multiple-choice (Item C). To identify and revise any areas of mismatch during item writing and selection, the item, item-level instructions, any graphics, or other material linked to the item must be reviewed as a whole.

The item evaluations suggest that Item A aligns with the key aspects of the indicator best. Item B falls short with respect to the cognitive behavior tested; it is measuring concept recall and understanding (defining a number pattern), placing a lower cognitive demand on examinees. While Item C is written to test application, the question does not fit the primary content focus of the indicator (number patterns); it is testing application of arithmetic operations instead, specifically, multiplication. Item directions show that both Items A and C match the conditions specified. Matching the item with each key aspect of the indicator, content, taxonomic level, and conditions helps assure content-based validity during the item-writing process.

Principle 2: Ensure that the language in the item and item instructions is direct, clear, and at the appropriate reading level.

The importance of Principle 2 is illustrated in Item D in Box 5.2, which violates this rule. Here, the true–false item seemingly matches the content and cognitive level of the indicator, but it is presented in a somewhat convoluted manner, elevating the chances of respondent errors. In comparison, Item B in Box 5.1 is a better true–false item matching the same indicator.

There are several ways by which we could improve the clarity of items with a tighter presentation, and more lucid, succinct, and on-point instructions. For instance, with Item D:

BOX 5.1 Items That Match Indicators to Different Degrees: Examples

Indicator

Without the help of a calculator [**condition**], the student will identify the mathematical rule in a given series of numbers [**cognitive behavior**] and continue the pattern correctly [**content**] with a 70% accuracy rate [**performance criterion**].

Taxonomic Level

Application

Item A

See the number pattern below. Continue the series by filling in the next <u>*two*</u> blanks. You may <u>*not*</u> use a calculator to find the answer.

15, 20, 25, 30. ____. ____. [Answer: 35, 40. Rule: Add 5 to last number to find the next.]

Explain how you got the answers [Space provided].

Item Evaluation

Acceptable item! Item matches all three requirements in indicator: content focus (number patterns with basic arithmetic operations); cognitive behavior; and taxonomic level (application). Instructions comply with the condition (no use of calculator).

Item B

Circle whether true or false.

A <u>*number pattern*</u> is a group of numbers in a sequence that are related to each other by a specific math rule.

a. True [Correct answer]
b. False

Item Evaluation

Poor. Although the content focus of the item matches the indicator (math patterns), the item measures concept recall (state the definition of a math pattern). It does not match the cognitive behavior and taxonomic level specified in the indicator. Conditions are irrelevant to the cognitive level tested. Revise or drop item!

Item C

Solve the problem given next, <u>*without*</u> using a calculator:

$175 \times 8 =$ ____?

Choose <u>*one*</u> correct answer from the answers given below. Show your work on the scratch sheet.

a. 1,000
b. 1,200
c. 1,400 [Correct answer]
d. 1,600
e. None of the above

Item Evaluation

Poor. Revise or drop item! Item does not match the content focus on number patterns. While it requires application and matches the condition (without a calculator), its focus is computation skills in multiplication.

- Removing the first sentence containing extraneous or superfluous information would allow examinees to focus immediately on the question asked (definition of patterns).
- Removing the sentence on calculator use would remove an irrelevant instruction when testing concept knowledge. It is a distraction and could mislead examinees into doubting their answers, even when they have full knowledge of the concept.
- Rewriting the item as a direct proposition will improve clarity of communication. See Item B, Box 5.1, as an example: "Circle whether this statement is true or false. A number pattern is. . . ."
- Removing use of language that is too complex will ensure that a math item is not testing reading vocabulary or comprehension skills instead! Reader-friendly language, accessible to examinees at *all* reading levels in the targeted population, will remove any systematic, language-related interferences during assessment.
- Asking, "Is this statement correct or incorrect?" when the only answer options are true–false is a verbal distraction—examinees who know the material may doubt their responses. A better item framing here would simply be "Is the statement true or false?" Aligning question framing with the response options improves the clarity of item presentation.

In sum, items should attempt to elicit the desired performance in as direct a manner as possible, without "tricky" language or off-topic information that could add error variance to the results. Item instructions should be kept short and pertinent to the question. Highlighting, capitalizing, italicizing, or bolding keywords or instructions is helpful for this purpose (e.g., "Choose only <u>one</u> response" in Box 5.1).

Principle 3: Focus on a single concept, principle, skill, or topic per item.

The highly structured response format does not lend itself to testing multiple concepts, topics, or ideas at once with individual items. Doing so with "double-barreled" or "triple-barreled" items could make the item presentation complex and confusing for respondents. Multibarreled items also make it difficult to infer from the response the precise status of the examinee's knowledge or skill on the topic tested. An exception to Principle 3 applies only when we want to intentionally design a single structured-response item to measure a *closely connected set of indicators*. For an example of the latter, see Item G in Box 5.4.

BOX 5.2 Items with Different Degrees of Clarity and Succinctness

Indicator

The student recognizes the correct definition [**cognitive behavior**] of a "number pattern" [**content focus**].

Taxonomic Level

Concept recall and understanding

Item D

Last week, we learned about mathematical reasoning with number patterns. In this sentence, "patterns" refers to a sequence of increasing or decreasing numbers that have a mathematical relationship to one another bound by an underlying mathematical rule. Is this statement correct or incorrect? You may <u>not</u> use a calculator to find your answer.

a. True

b. False

Correct answer: a

Item Evaluation

Poor item. Too wordy; uses confusing and redundant language in instructions making it an unclear item. Stem should be revised to be consistent with true–false choice given. Revise!

To appreciate this guideline, see Box 5.3 with two multiple-choice items, E–F, measuring student recognition skills of different parts of speech used in sentences. Both items match key aspects of the indicator, focusing on recognizing parts of speech in sentences; however, Item E attempts to test students' knowledge of verbs and adverbs together, confounding the measurement of each separately. Furthermore, the item is problematic because the answer options, as presented, include a completely correct answer (a, verb and adverb); an incorrect answer (d, only noun); and two partially correct answers (b, with verb and noun, and c, with noun and adverb). With only one correct answer possible, this design prevents the separation of students with full knowledge of the tested concepts from those with partial knowledge or no knowledge at all.

Item E is also weak on Principle 2—item clarity. Directions and layout, as given, could mislead younger respondents. For example, the reference to the "next sentence . . ." does not point directly to the intended sentence for examinees to consider, given in italics. In contrast, Item F is an improvement on Item E, as it tests students' knowledge of *verbs* only, with a cleaner presentation. Instructions and layout are also improved.

Now, consider applying Principle 3 with regard to Item G in Box 5.4. This is a scenario-based "story"

BOX 5.3 Items Focusing on Single versus Multiple Concepts

Indicator

The student is able to identify **[Cognitive Behavior]** the different parts of speech **[Content Focus]** in given sentences **[Condition]**.

Taxonomic level:

Concept Recall and Understanding

Item E

Read the next sentence. Which answer shows the **verb** *and* the **adverb** in the sentence? Choose only **ONE**.

She arrived at the bus station slowly.

(a) arrived, slowly

(b) arrived, bus station

(c) everyone, slowly

(d) by, the, she

Correct answer: a

Item evaluation:

Problematic item. Item is confounded; it will not yield separate information on respondents' ability to distinguish between verbs and adverbs. Response options include two partly correct answers. The bold font and underling help, but instructions could be improved.

Revise or drop item!

Item F

Instructions: Read the next sentence shown in *italics*.

She arrived at the bus station slowly.

Which of these answers, (a)–(d), shows the **verb** in the sentence? Choose only **ONE** answer.

(a) arrived

(b) bus

(c) slowly

(d) station

Correct answer: a

Item evaluation:

Acceptable. Better-written item than E!

BOX 5.4 Measuring Connected Indicators with One Item

General Indicator

Given real-world "story" problems in math appropriate for the grade, **[Condition]** students are able to solve each problem **[Cognitive Behavior]** by using the appropriate arithmetic operations (addition, subtraction, multiplication, and division). **[Content Focus]**

Subindicators

- Reads the scenario (story) with understanding.
- Identifies relevant information.
- Selects the correct arithmetic operation(s).
- Executes computational steps completely and correctly (applies long-division steps, applies multiplication facts, applies place value concepts, shows work, and evaluates the answer).

Taxonomic Level

Higher-Order Thinking and Problem Solving

Item G

<u>**Directions:**</u> Read carefully the story problem *in italics* below. Then solve the problem. Show all your work on the scratch sheet.

There are 252 students altogether in the grade 4 classes at my school. I would like to give <u>one</u> (1) chocolate chip cookie to each fourth grader on the last day of the school term. Chocolate chip cookies are sold in packets, with 12 cookies in each packet. How many packets should I buy so that every fourth grader gets 1 cookie, with none left over?

Choose only <u>*one*</u> answer from a to e.

a. 12
b. 21
c. 24
d. 252
e. None of the above

Correct answer: b

Item Evaluation

Acceptable item! Measures a coherent set of indicators with only one correct answer.

problem requiring young students to execute a simple long-division procedure by applying several skills in unison. However, as these are closely connected, the general indicator is measurable with a single multiple-choice item. The embedded concepts and skills falling under the broader, more complex indicator are also typically taught and practiced as an integrated set in scholastic settings. The item design aims to test a higher cognitive level of the taxonomy, as specified in the indicator. There is only one correct answer possible. Hence, Item G (or another like it) is acceptable here. It is reasonable to employ a single structured-response item for assessing similar, coherent groups of indicators.

Principle 4: Ensure that each item has only *one* correct or *single* best answer.

This principle follows directly from Principle 3. Items A, F, and G demonstrate this principle best. A major advantage of structured-response item formats is afforded by the property of one correct or best answer. Users can specify the correct item response beforehand, making it time-efficient to score items either by hand or computer with an answer key. To avail of this benefit, there has to be *only* one correct or best answer possible to each question. Importantly, therefore, the "correct" answer must be verifiable, corroborated against authoritative sources such as textbooks, the professional or scientific literature, or by peer-review and expert consensus.

Principle 5: Ensure that there are no clues to the correct answer.

Clues can be introduced into structured-response items in several ways without the designer's intent. We should screen items for clues before finalizing the assessment. **Test-wise** examinees are those who may not have sufficient domain-specific knowledge or skills but are skillful at detecting clues or built-in writing signals that suggest what the correct answer is likely to be for the items. Indeed, this source of error is common enough for some high-stakes test-coaching programs to emphasize clue-detection strategies for participants.

Common clues fall into four categories. Item issues with each type of clue will follow in Section 5.4.2.

- *Grammatical clues linking question stems with correct options.* An example of this occurs when a multiple-choice question might use an article like "an" in the stem with the one correct answer among the options starting with a vowel (e.g., "orange"). Such problems are easily corrected with careful edits or using "a/an" in the question stem.
- *Predictable location of the correct response in an item series.* This could occur, for example, when the same correct option tends to occur in a repeated pattern on the items of a test, such as the "true" answers are mostly the "a" option on a true–false test.
- *Wording-related, pictorial, or context clues as so-called clang associations.* Clang associations are clues that appear via the use of exactly the same words, expressions, terms, or graphics in the question stem and the only correct answer of the options given. These clues lead examinees to select the correct response option simply by association, rather than knowledge of what is being tested.
- *Response choices to prior questions or the item instructions providing clues to the correct answer for items.* In multi-item tests, item-writers may overlook that answers become obvious in questions based on related content tested elsewhere on the same examination or in the item instructions provided.

Principle 6: Avoid inherent item biases, or the appearance of bias, toward any subgroup or members of the intended population.

Biases toward any individuals or minority subgroups can be introduced unknowingly through the content, language, pictorials, or supporting materials of an item or assessment exercise. The "appearance of bias" in items could occur toward individuals or groups based on issues of gender, race, culture, religion, disability, sexual orientation, affluence/poverty, or other diversity characteristic.

For example, items could appear to be biased, or actually be biased, when they reflect:

- Activities relatable only to the dominant group of examinees from a single region in the test-taking population, disadvantaging others (e.g., affluent suburban households).
- Media or technologies accessible to only some but not all potential examinees or groups.
- Language or role portrayals that could undermine or offend a given gender, religious, or another minority group, affecting their performance—referred to as an **inflammatory bias**.

TABLE 5.1. Checklist for Critiquing Structured-Response Items

Six General Criteria

- *Match:* Does the item match the specified content focus, taxonomic level, conditions, and/or performance criterion, as given in the indicator(s) to be measured?
- *Clarity:* Is the item presented in a clear, succinct, and direct (not confusing) manner?
- *Single-concept testing:* Is there only *one* concept, skill, or idea tested in each question, or a tightly linked set of concepts and skills, as aligned with indicator(s)? Are items with double-, triple-, or multi-barreled content revised or removed?
- *Single best answer:* Does the item have only *one* best or correct answer?
- *Lack of clues:* Is the item free of any clues, such as grammatical clues, clang associations, predictable response patterns?
- *Lack of apparent biases:* Is the item free of any apparent biases in the language, content, pictorials, or other material that could inflame or place subgroups or individuals at a disadvantage?

- A content focus in an assessment that is entirely new or largely unfamiliar to significant subpopulations as compared to the majority groups, called an **opportunity-to-learn bias** in educational assessments.

To detect and remove biases at the item level, designers could invite critical reviews by diverse peers or external experts before an assessment is finalized. Field-testing early drafts of items with appropriately diverse respondents from the intended population, followed by appropriate item revisions, may preempt some of the issues listed (see Chapters 10–11).

5.4.2 Guidelines for Specific Types of Structured-Response Items

For this section, refer to Table 5.2 as we consider different item formats with specific guidelines for each. New item examples are embedded in this section's narrative or illustrated in Boxes 5.5 to 5.7, as applicable to each item type. As before, we will review poorly designed and improved items of each type to appreciate the point of the guideline.

5.4.2.1 Writing Good Multiple-Choice Items

The **multiple-choice (MC) item** format is the most widely used, selected response item type. The popular perception, one well supported by common practice, is that structured-response items are useful for measuring the lowest cognitive levels, such as the recall of facts. This myth can be effectively dispelled with skilled and creative use of the MC item format.

The basic MC format uses an incomplete statement or a question as the *stem*, followed by a fixed number of response choices. As indicated earlier, only one option should be the best or correct answer. This basic format can be enhanced with several modifications as Box 5.5 shows in item examples H–K with a content focus on basic high school–level statistics. As we proceed, we will again consider Items C, F, and G in Boxes 5.1–5.4 that also use the MC format.

Item H demonstrates the standard MC format; Item I uses an analogy form; Items J–K is a context-dependent item set, to which several more items could easily be added, varying the cognitive complexity of the exercise. Depending on domain-specific indicators, the items could be written at various cognitive levels, ranging from concept recall and understanding, to application, to higher-order thinking, and complex procedural skills under the functional taxonomy. If accompanied with short-answer questions requiring explanations or justification of answers, MC items could tap into reasoning, making generalizations, as well as analysis, synthesis, or evaluation levels in Bloom et al.'s taxonomy (Chapter 4). Scenario-dependent MC items like Items G and J–K can be varied by using a reading passage, a data table, information box, pictorials, or graphs to which a series of MC questions can be tied. To be effective, scenario- or context-dependent items should *require* examinees to use the information given in the scenario to arrive at the correct responses, rather than rely on automatized recall or prior knowledge.

The number of answer options in MC items usually varies from three to five, with the probability of simply guessing the answer by chance decreasing as the number of alternative answers increases. For example, the chance of a guessed correct answer drops from 33% in a three-option MC item (one correct out of three choices) to 20% in a five-option MC item (one correct out of five choices). When thoughtfully constructed, the incorrect response options—called *distracters* or *foils*—could increase item difficulty levels. Studies have shown that with effective distracters, five choices provide optimal measurement outcomes. In a compiled set of MC items, the correct answer position should be varied in some random order that is not predictable.

Performing item evaluations concurrently while designing the items is a useful practice. Table 5.2 offers criteria to distinguish between poor and better-composed MC items. To claim content-based validity, we must first begin with a match of the item with the specified content, the taxonomically categorized cognitive level, conditions, and performance criterion, as applicable. On this guideline, Items G and H–K are all acceptable, but Item C could be improved, as suggested earlier. Second, the verbal load of MC items should be in the *stem*. This desirable characteristic is demonstrated in all the item illustrations and helps the designer frame the problem in complete terms for examinees.

As we review the specific guidelines in Table 5.1, consider two added MC items on mathematical patterns below, adapted from Item A written for elementary school children.

TABLE 5.2. Critiquing Different Types of Structured-Response Items

Criteria for different item types

A. Multiple-choice items

- Is the verbal load in the item stem?
- Are the distracters plausible?
- Are response options to an item of about equal difficulty?
- Are the responses similar in length, format, language structure, and content?
- Are "All of the above" or "None of the above" used sparingly and with judgment?
- Are responses to items listed in some logical order? Does the correct answer position vary in a list of items?
- Are response options listed vertically?

B. True–false items

- Does the propositional statement focus on *one* important idea, principle, or concept?
- Is the proposition indisputably true or false? If knowledge of an opinion is tested, is the source identified?
- Does the item avoid trivia testing or testing of "commonsense" material?
- Are verbatim excerpts from textbooks or common subject matter resources avoided?
- Are T/F items listed in some logical order, without predictable patterns of correct responses (e.g., TFTFTF)?
- Are true and false statements of approximately equal length?
- Are there approximately equal numbers of true or false answers on the test or T/F assessment exercise?
- Is the item free of "specific determiners" or language-related suggestions, such as use of "always," "generally," or "never"?
- Is the length of the T/F exercise suitable for the intended population?

C. Matching exercises

- Is the set of items homogeneous in terms of content?
- Are the premises (in Column A) longer than the response options (in Column B)?
- Are there more response options than premises? Are the distracters plausible?
- Are responses listed in some logical order, such as alphabetically?
- Does the list of items in the exercise fall within the ideal range of 5–15?
- Does the complete exercise fit on one page or one screen of a computer?
- Do the directions indicate whether the answer options can be used only once or more than once?

D. Completion items

- Are blanks used to test *key* concepts or *main* ideas?
- Are verbatim excerpts of language or text from readings avoided in items?
- Do individual items have *one* blank? If there are multiple blanks in an item, are they appropriate and used with judgment?
- Is the blank placed toward the end? If the indicator requires an earlier placement of the blank, is it located appropriately?
- Are the blanks for words or phrases of approximately equal length?

E. Context-dependent exercises

- Is the contextual material likely to be new to examinees and suitable for the socioecological contexts and age range?
- Is the material clear (uncluttered and easy to read)?
- Do individual items or item sets measure higher levels of thinking?
- Are all items tied to the contextual material?
- Are the items balanced in terms of space usage?

Item with correct answer and instructions
Look at the <u>*increasing series*</u> of numbers below. What are the next three numbers in the series? Choose only **one** answer from the options A–E.
12, 60, 300, ________, ________, ________. A. 12, 60, 300 B. 348, 396, 444 C. 1500, 7500, 35500 **D.** 1500, 7500, 37500 [Correct answer: 12 × 5 = 60, 60 × 5 = 300, 300 × 5 = 1500, etc.] E. None of the above

There are several desirable properties in the above MC item. The item stem ends with a clearly framed question and is just long enough to pose the problem fully. Generally, the use of the question format adds clarity to the communication compared to an incomplete statement, although both formats are acceptable. Item instructions are adequate, with boldface, underscoring, or capitalization used to highlight requirements. To avoid giving inadvertent clues that might help examinees rule out the wrong answers easily, the distracters are similar in difficulty, with parallel form, length, and construction parameters—a common issue found in MC items is that the correct answer is often the longest! Also, answer options are presented in a sensible order—an ascending numeric order in this case, with the numbers getting larger in options A–D. So as to not provide clues, a consistent ordering of answer options for all selected response items on a test is another desirable property. The answer choices of an MC item could be arranged either in ascending, descending, alphabetical, or other logical order.

Additionally, of the five choices, the correct response (option D) is balanced against three *plausible distracters* that reflect common errors made by elementary grade students on the topic. Ensuring that the foils are plausible is a major characteristic of an effective MC item. Test-wise examinees are usually able to identify implausible options without much knowledge of the topic; this lowers the difficulty and validity levels of MC items. In contrast, plausible foils look like the right answer to examinees with partial understandings or limited knowledge of the content, or those with deeper conceptual misunderstandings or no knowledge at all. For example, typical math mistakes at the elementary level include not being able to distinguish between a "repeating number pattern" and an "increasing number pattern" (option A in the example above), or choosing arithmetic operations incorrectly but being unable to continue the pattern (option B, subtracting 12 from 60 to get 48 and adding it to 300 in trying to solve the problem), or making other computation errors (option C). "None of the above" is also a plausible answer option here, as it may capture unanticipated student errors or confusions on the topic.

In contrast, an entirely *implausible* response option in E would have been "All of the above." Given that the answer requires only three blanks to be filled in, all five options cannot be logically correct or reasonable. "All of the above" and "None of the above" should appear as choices with thoughtful judgment. The goal should be to improve measurement by separating respondents with different degrees of knowledge. Tapping into their typical mistakes is good practice, rather than simply adding a superfluous distracter. A weak set of distracters for the same item may look as follows:

A problematic MC item
Look at the <u>*increasing series*</u> of numbers below. The next **three** numbers in the series are:
12, 60, 300, ________, ________, ________. A. 7500 B. 5 C. 348 **D.** 1500, 7500, 37,500 [Correct answer] E. All of the above

The distracters A–C above could give away the answer because they are logically inconsistent with the stem, which asks for *three* numbers in the series. Plus, the answer options are of mixed digit lengths (5, 348, 37,500), or unreasonable in other ways. Lastly, the longest option is the only one with three numbers and happens to be the correct answer. All of these features make the item a poorly constructed one. Items C, F, and G referenced earlier are better examples.

BOX 5.5 Multiple-Choice Item Formats: Standard-, Analogy-, and Scenario-Dependent Exercises

Indicators

The student/examinee will:

Define [**cognitive behavior**] key concepts in descriptive statistics [**content focus**]. *Taxonomic Level: Concept recall and understanding*

Calculate [**cognitive behavior**] selected descriptive statistics correctly [**content focus**] in given datasets [**condition**]. *Taxonomic Level: Application*

Interpret [**cognitive behavior**] descriptive statistics correctly [**content focus**] in given datasets [**condition**]. *Taxonomic Level: Application*

Item H: Standard Format

Directions: Complete the statement in *italics* by selecting the **best answer** from the choices given.

The difference between the highest and lowest score in a data distribution is called the:

a. *frequency.*

b. *mean.*

c. *range.*

d. *standard deviation.*

Correct answer: c

Item I: Analogy Format

Directions: The next question asks you to complete an analogy. Select the **best answer** from the choices given.

Mean is to central tendency as standard deviation is to:

a. *frequency.*

b. *median.*

c. *normality.*

d. *skewness.*

e. *variability.*

Correct answer: e

Items J–K: Scenario-Dependent Item Set

Directions: Read the scenario described in *italics* to answer Items J–K.

A math teacher obtained the following distribution of test scores from her class on the final exam:

10, 12, 12, 17, 18, 19, 19, 19, 20, 21, 22, 23, 24, 24, 25

J. *What is the calculated* **mean** *of the distribution, rounded to the nearest hundredths? Choose only* ***one*** *response from the following:*

a. *15*

b. *19*

c. *20*

d. *285*

e. *None of the above*

How did the student with a score of 17 perform compared to the rest of the class?

a. *Below average*

b. *Average*

c. *Above average*

d. *Cannot be determined*

Correct answers: b, a

Negative wording and language, shown in the MC item embedded below, should be underscored or highlighted when used. Use of *double negatives* should be avoided, as these items often create ambiguity (e.g., "Nobody doesn't like Sara Lee" in the popular old commercial is unacceptable in item-writing practice!). See the modified MC item example that follows, where the negative term is underlined:

Which of the following series is **not** a number pattern? Choose only **one** answer from the options A–D.
A. 1, 2, 3; 1, 2, 3; 1, 2, 3 B. 5; 20; 80; 320 **C.** 20; 150; 767; 959 [Correct answer] D. All of the above are number patterns. Explain your answer.

In the above example, we see *three* desirable characteristics of MC items. This item draws attention to "not" or negative language; a short-answer justification component is included, raising the item's cognitive demand while eliminating possible errors due to guessing; and the explanation segment also allows a mathematically reasonable, alternative answer to be accepted outside the keyed response, C. Again, options A and B above are effective distracters that show either a repeating number pattern or one increasing by a factor of 4, appropriate to the indicator being tested and level of the examinees. Note that "All of the above" is actually a plausible response here—it may help differentiate among respondents with varying levels of concept understanding. C is the only correct answer; it is not a demonstrable number pattern.

Finally, a vertical presentation of answer options will typically improve an MC item's readability. It may also avoid clutter. Options presented *horizontally* can be confusing for young examinees or those with special needs or disabilities. Items J–K and G–I show desirable presentation formats, where answer options are presented *vertically*.

DISADVANTAGES OF MC ITEM FORMATS

Even when the subject matter aligns well with the format, high-quality MC questions are difficult to design with a single indisputably correct or best answer. The format is unsuitable for examinee populations who tend to think more deeply or are able to find reasonable solutions that lie outside the answer choices provided, such as exceptionally gifted respondents or adult learners in graduate-level or professional education settings. Without significant accommodations, MC items (and most other structured-response formats) accompanied with scan sheets for "bubbling" in answers with pencils are not ideal for respondents with special needs, disabilities, the very young, or developmentally challenged respondents.

5.4.2.2 Writing Good True–False Items

Examine the criteria for writing high-quality **true–false (T/F) items** given in Table 5.2, alongside the general principles in Table 5.1. A typical T/F item consists of a propositional statement that the examinee must affirm or negate with a "Yes" or "No," a "True" or "False," or a "Right" or "Wrong" response. The statement can be posed in question form or as a direct statement. For item examples, see Item B again in Box 5.1 and a new item set shown in Box 5.6. For an efficient design strategy, T/F item sets should consist of 5 to 15 propositions with common directions. The T/F format can be used in original form or slightly adapted form. Skilled item-writers can use the T/F format to test a range of performances beyond concept knowledge, including computational skills, making generalizations, identifying causal relationships, or making comparisons and evaluations (application and higher-order thinking levels in the functional taxonomy).

As with all items, a first rule for a sound T/F item requires verifying a match of the item with the selected domain-relevant indicators. We find that although Item B violates this first principle, it complies with most other guidelines for good T/F item writing. In comparison, the T/F item set in Box 5.6 aligns better with the problem-solving and reasoning skills it is intended to measure in elementary school students. As shown, T/F items can be easily modified to include "Yes" or "No" options tied to a problem-solving scenario, with an explanation component added, whereby the examinees must defend the responses they choose. With T/F items, the chances of getting a correct answer due to random factors are elevated to 50%. As a rule, requiring explanations can help contain guessing and also raise the difficulty level of the item or an item set.

It is important for a T/F proposition to be indisputably true *or* false. Double- or triple-barreled propositional material makes for weak T/F items, especially if an item is partially true (and hence partially false). Consider the two-part T/F item below:

> *Indicate whether the following is true or false:*
>
> Albany is the capital city of the state of New York with the largest population.

The first half of the item above is true, but the latter half is false, confounding the measurement of the intended concept knowledge. Here, two separate items should be constructed for each proposition.

When the intention is to test knowledge drawn from different publications, points of view, or opinion-based issues where positions can vary, the source should be clearly identified. See the following examples of fact-based propositional statements testing recall:

> *Indicate in the blank whether each statement is true or false.*
>
> 1. According to state data reports of 2016–2017, the population of Albany, New York, was about 97,000. ____________
> 2. The city of Albany, New York, has a population of 80,000. ____________

Population counts depend on the census year and dated data records. Without a year and source, it is impos-

BOX 5.6 Context-Dependent Exercise with a Variation of a True–False Item Format

Indicators

Given a novel scenario [**condition**], the student will demonstrate problem-solving skills [**cognitive behavior**] by:

- sorting relevant from irrelevant information [**cognitive behavior**].
- justifying choices in writing with reasonable explanations [**cognitive behavior**].

Taxonomic Level

Higher-order thinking and problem solving

Item L

Directions: Read this story given next to answer Questions 1–8.

*Karen lost her library book on her way to school. She asked the other students in class to help her find it. She put a notice up on the bulletin board to help them, with **8 (eight)** things listed about the book. Which of Karen's sentences say something that could help locate the book?*

Circle YES if the sentence has useful information, or NO if it does not.		
1. The book has a hard cover.	YES	NO
2. It was a very warm day.	YES	NO
3. The English teacher had asked the students to read the book before class that day.	YES	NO
4. The book's title is *A Christmas Carol.*	YES	NO
5. The English teacher is very kind.	YES	NO
6. The book is interesting.	YES	NO
7. The book's cover is red.	YES	NO
8. Karen stopped by at Maria's home before school that day.	YES	NO

Explain why you chose your YES or NO answers in a few sentences.

Explanation: [Space provided]

sible to categorize the second statement as either true or false. As the population was reported to be ~97,000 by the state in public reports dated 2016–2017 on the website, the first item is an acceptable T/F item.

As with all structured-response items, negatively oriented words should be used sparingly or highlighted when used, to avoid ambiguous communications. Double negative wording should always be avoided, as shown next, as it creates interpretive barriers unrelated to the indicators.

Indicate whether the following are true or false:

1. According to the 2016–2017 state database, Albany, New York, did **not** have a population of 80,000. [*Acceptable item*]
2. There are **no** records on whether Albany, New York, **does not** have a population of 80,000. [*Confusing item with double negatives and two propositions. Item is undated.*]

Clues can be avoided by keeping both true and false statements of approximately equal length in terms of number of words, distributing T/F answers randomly in a list of items, using approximately equal numbers of T/F answers on the assessment, and avoiding language with embedded *clang* associations. See the two item examples next, where the clang is shown in bold font. The topic focuses on testing and measurement concepts for educator training, a focus of this book.

Indicate whether the following are true or false:

1. **Content-based validity** in classroom assessments deals with the degree of match of the **content** of a curriculum with the **content** of the test items. [*Correct answer = True. Unacceptable item providing clues via clang associations of the term "content."*]
2. **Content-based validity** in classroom assessments deals with the statistical correlation between the test scores and future criterion behaviors of examinees. [*Correct answer = False. Better item!*]

Other T/F clues are called *specific determiners* and include catchall words such as "usually" or "generally," or absolute words such as "always" or "never." Item-writers tend to use specific determiners in T/F items to ensure a statement is completely true or completely false. However, such language could serve as semantic clues to the correct answer for verbally adept examinees.

Statements should also not be lifted verbatim from textbooks or material sources that emphasize rote memory. Similarly, measuring trivia or common knowledge with T/F items makes the assessment process inefficient. For example:

Indicate whether the following are true or false:

1. Teachers employ classroom tests to measure what students have learned.

[*Poor! This T/F statement is obvious, trivial, and redundant for testing purposes.*]

2. According to the 2014 National Research Council report (Insert title), new assessments in science should measure students' learning progressions toward meeting curriculum goals.

[*Better, as this statement presents a substantive opinion with a specific documentary source.*]

DISADVANTAGES OF T/F ITEM FORMATS

As evident, competence in writing effective T/F items is contingent on locating suitable propositional material in the domains for assessment. This might be viewed as a drawback. Too often, T/F items test the lowest levels of the cognitive taxonomy (namely, concept recall). To counter this tendency, we should remember that it is possible to design creative variations of T/F items to assess more complex cognitive capacities, especially with scenario-dependent item sets (see Box 5.6).

5.4.2.3 Writing Good Matching Exercises

In its typical form, a **matching exercise** is made up of two adjacent columns of information that must be matched by the examinee through association. Column A presents the item prompts or *premises*, while Column B lists the *response* options. Although traditionally verbal exercises, words, numbers, pictures, tables, and graphs could also be used effectively.

Review the example in Box 5.7, dealing with matching statistical terms and definitions for a high school course. The items are numbered, and answer options identified with letters.

Common applications of matching-item exercises utilize the following types of lists for Columns A and B.

A	B
Inventors	Inventions
Authors	Quotations
Problems	Solutions
Scientific theories	Applications
Principles	Applications
Parts	Functions
Rules	Examples
Terms	Definitions

The following matching exercise is meant to measure concept recall and understanding in elementary-level science, focused on the functions and parts of green plants, as an illustration.

BOX 5.7 Matching-Item Set from a High School Statistics Test: Standard Format

Indicator

The student/examinee will identify correct definitions [**cognitive behavior**] of statistics concepts and terms [**content focus**].

Taxonomic Level

Concept recall and understanding

Item M

Directions: Column A provides **definitions** of statistical terms. Column B provides a list of **statistical terms.**

Match each term with the correct definition by filling in the blank next to the item in Column A. Each letter response (a–i) can be used ***only once or not at all.***

Column A: Definitions

____ 1. The difference between the highest and lowest score in a distribution.

____ 2. The most frequent score in a distribution.

____ 3. The sum of the scores divided by the number of units in the sample or group.

____ 4. The positive square root of the variance.

____ 5. The score in a distribution that is the 50th percentile.

____ 6. The point in a score distribution below which 25% of the scores fall.

Column B: Statistical Terms

a. Frequency
b. Mean
c. Median
d. Mode
e. Normal distribution
f. Percentile
g. Quartile
h. Range
i. Standard deviation

Directions: Column A shows the **functions** of the main parts of a green, seed-bearing plant. Column B shows the **parts**. Match each function (1–6) with the correct part (a–g) by filling in the blank next to the item in Column A. **Each part can be used <u>only</u> once or not at all.**

Column A: Functions	Column B: Parts
____ 1. Carries water and food to other.	a. Flower
____ 2. Anchors the plant to the ground.	b. Fruit
____ 3. Grows into an adult plant.	c. Leaf
____ 4. Manufactures food using sunlight.	d. Seed
____ 5. Protects the seed.	e. Stamen
____ 6. Attracts insects to help pollination.	f. Stem
	g. Root
	h. Pollen

Although the taxonomic level measured most typically is concept recall and understanding, not all matching exercises need be at rote learning levels. For example, a matching exercise on problems versus solutions in mathematics could be devised to assess application or even complex procedural skills. Similarly, coupled with an elaboration or a justification component, scientific theories versus applications could be used to test higher-order thinking. As with other structured-item formats, open-ended explanations increase cognitive demands of the task.

Table 5.2 presents format-specific guidelines for this item type. First, as with multiple-choice items, the reading load should be in the premises. This guideline helps item-writers pose the question clearly and completely to examinees. The premises *are* the items of a matching exercise and should be presented in Column A. Longer premises should be balanced against short or shorter response options in Column B. Ideally, the exercise should fit on one page, or one screen on a computer interface, to prevent interrupting the flow of thinking for the exercise as a whole.

Second, heterogeneous item sets or response options make a matching exercise too obvious or easy. Consider the following as an alternate list of heterogeneous answer options (Column B) for the exercise shown in Box 5.7:

Column B:

a. Mean
b. Hypotenuse
c. Median
d. Standard deviation
e. Equilateral triangle
f. Range
g. Quartile

Here, "Hypotenuse" and "Equilateral triangle" (terms from geometry) are nonhomogeneous distracters that may be easy for examinees to strike with little or no knowledge of statistics. Instead, distracters such as frequency and percentile (shown in Box 5.7) belong within the content specifications in the indicator; hence, they are more plausible for the indicator being tested.

Next, giving more response options than prompts increases the item difficulty levels by adding distracters. To evaluate the merits of this guideline, compare the six-item exercise in Box 5.7 with only the following six answer options:

Column B:

a. Mean
b. Median
c. Mode
d. Standard deviation
e. Range
f. Quartile

As with multiple-choice items, the responses should ideally be listed in some logical order that is consistent for all items or item sets on a test to prevent giving inadvertent clues to any answers. In Box 5.7, the verbal items are organized alphabetically per this recommendation.

As with the rest, we should always begin by evaluating matching exercises vis-à-vis the general criteria in Table 5.1, including alignment of the items with the targeted indicators and screening the exercise for any potential biases and clues. Other standard guidelines pertain to the clarity of a matching exercise with a clear presentation of items and directions, with key terms highlighted to draw examinees' attention to relevant information.

DISADVANTAGES OF MATCHING-ITEM SETS

The common criticism is that the matching format is mostly suited for testing recall of concept knowledge by association. This format may be adaptable for some subject areas and cognitive domains, for example, when testing basic concept knowledge and application in younger populations. But, as noted, varying the premises could help in assessing concept sorting, computing, interpretation, application, or higher taxonomic levels.

5.4.2.4 Writing Good Completion Items

Refer back to Tables 5.1 and 5.2. The **completion-item** format, also called **fill-in-the-blank items**, is another structured form of item that is relatively easy to build and could be quite versatile. It is different from the selected response variety in that examinees must supply an answer on their own. The response is usually required in a single word, short phrase, a number, symbol, or formula. The common presentation formats are (1) the incomplete sentence; (2) a direct question; or (3) a statement of the problem in a complete sentence, each followed by the blank(s). See Item A in Box 5.1.

The supply format opens up the possibility of examinees coming up with a range of answers that might be partially correct or nearly correct, but not a perfect match with the response in the answer key. This introduces potential ambiguity and possible subjective errors when scoring completion items. It is therefore important that item-writers specify the *exact range of answers that they consider to be fully correct*, as opposed to partially so or incorrect altogether. The overall assessment design specifications should delineate these boundaries. If scoring rubrics are used (discussed later), relevant parts of a task response with the allocated point values for each should be specified in advance.

To begin, the general principles in Table 5.1 should first be addressed with a mind toward revising items, as necessary. Well-constructed completion item formats could be useful for tapping concept recall and understanding, as well as application and higher-order thinking levels. To measure the different indicators shown previously in Box 5.5 on the statistics topics, for instance, we could write completion items with different demands, as follows:

1. Given the above test score distribution (data supplied), the range is ____________ [Answer can vary based on data. *Cognitive level: Application*]
2. What is the score in a distribution with the highest frequency called? ____________ [Answer: *Mode. Cognitive level: Concept recall and understanding*]
3. Compute the **mean** in the score distribution given (data supplied). Write down your answer and the formula you used.

   Mean: ______ Formula used: ____________
   [Answers can vary. *Cognitive levels: Application, concept recall*]
4. Compute the **standard deviation** in the score distribution given (data supplied). Write down your answer and the formula you used.

   Standard deviation: ______
   Formula used: ____________ [Answers can vary. *Cognitive levels: Application, concept recall*]
5. Interpret the calculated mean and the standard deviation in the dataset. Why do we need both statistics to understand the data distribution better? Explain in one to three sentences. [Space provided. *Cognitive level: Application*]

Table 5.2 underscores that well-written completion items could present a problem either in question form or as incomplete statements. However, the blank should test *important* concepts, keywords, or principles that are directly relevant to the content or skill specifications in the indicators. Verbatim lifting of text from books or required readings leads to testing of rote learning and memorization, rather than deeper understandings—therefore, we should avoid doing so. Multiple blanks in a completion item add to ambiguities in the question being asked and could lead to an array of responses that are difficult to score. Consider the four versions of the item next illustrating common issues with poorly constructed completion items. The indicators measured are again from Box 5.5.

1. In a data distribution, the score ____________ the highest frequency is called the mode.

   [Answer: with. *Poor item! The missing preposition "with" is trivial, not a key concept tied to the indicator, or worth testing.*]
2. In a ______ distribution, the _________________ the ______ frequency is ______ the ______.

   [Answers: data, score, with, highest, called, mode. *Poor item! Multiple blanks make the question very unclear. The mix of trivial words, contextual details, and key concepts that are missing obstructs measurement of what is being tested.*]
3. In a data ____________, the score with the highest frequency is called the mode.

   [Answer: distribution. *Still a weak completion item. Although "distribution" is a related concept, the blank is situated in the beginning of a sentence, preventing clear question framing. Multiple reasonable and correct answers are possible, such as table, graph, or chart.*]
4. In a data distribution, the score with the highest frequency is called the ____________.

   [Answer: mode. *Much better completion item! Key concept is tied to the indicator, question is framed clearly with verbal load in front, and with a single blank placed at the end.*]

In sum, the better-designed completion item in traditional form has one blank placed at the end. Directions are also important. For instance, here are directions appropriate for a completion exercise to measure the statistics indicators in Box 5.5:

> *Directions for Items 1–6 below:* Complete each of the following statements by filling in the missing blank(s). Some items will require calculations using the data supplied; others will not. For all calculations, show your computational steps clearly on the attached sheet. Do **not** use a hand calculator or the computer to find answers.

Finally, a **Cloze exercise** is a variant of the completion-item format, where multiple blanks in a passage are acceptable (Taylor, 1953). These passages incorporate deliberately situated blanks are employed to test reading comprehension levels; Chapter 3 provided an example. When first invented, words from a body of running text were deleted at fixed intervals, for instance, every fifth word in a passage. Respondents were expected to fill in the blanks by using context cues in the passage they read, thereby demonstrating reading comprehension skills. When testing comprehension of concepts in other domains, Cloze exercises can be adapted by deleting *key terms*, rather than random words at particular intervals.

DISADVANTAGES OF COMPLETION ITEMS

The recognized limitations of all structured-response items apply to completion items as well. But, as the illustrative items suggest, completion exercises could be designed productively to measure multiple levels of the cognitive taxonomy. Situating the items in contextual material, such as a passage, dataset, or scenario, could assist in increasing the cognitive level of the task.

5.4.2.5 Writing Good Context-Dependent Item Sets

As pointed out throughout, structured-response items organized in a coherent item series tied to a common passage, graphic, data table, or scenario are more useful for tapping into multiple levels of the cognitive taxonomy than stand-alone items. Their utility was illustrated in Items G, H–K, and L. But, to do so well, it is important that the items are truly *dependent on* the contextual material. Scenario-dependent items, like all other item formats, should be an appropriate fit for measuring the domain or subdomain indicators we intend to measure, as well as the level and socioecological backgrounds of expected examinees. For challenging examinees while reducing task construction errors, the contextual material should be:

- Novel and unfamiliar to examinees
- Clearly presented, visually uncluttered, and easy to read
- Not too long—should ideally fit on one-half page in print or on a computer screen

The use of audio presentations for older seniors, the disabled, or very young children may be appropriate. Printed material should be short enough for readability. Adaptations should fit the needs of anticipated examinees.

A question to settle beforehand is whether context-dependent items should be designed as *content-free*, meaning there are no expectations about examinees having any particular subject matter knowledge or expertise, such as knowledge of American history, general science, or algebra. A *content-dependent item set* is one where examinees are expected to draw on prior knowledge of specific subject matter when responding. When employed effectively, complex interpretive exercises may be designed to assess the following types of higher-level indicators from a variety of domains (Miller, Linn, & Gronlund, 2013):

- Discerning the relevance of information for a purpose
- Evaluating arguments presented in contextual material
- Recognizing, or distinguishing between, valid and invalid conclusions from contextual material provided in tables, graphs, pictures, or text passages
- Interpreting patterns or relationships in data tables or informational text passages.

QUICK RECAP: Good item writing requires strong writing abilities and practice. There could be many creative variations to the basic item formats described. With some thought, items could be designed to measure the full range of the cognitive taxonomy. Problematic items of any format should be improved iteratively through critical review and revisions, guided by the general principles and specific item-writing guidelines (Tables 5.1 and 5.2). The coded correct answers should also be verified during the review process or through pilot testing of the drafted items with typical examinee groups.

Reflection Break 5.3: Objectives 3–4 and 6

- There is no such thing as a perfect item! Review the illustrative items in Boxes 5.1–5.7 again. Identify any item *flaws* you see based on the guidelines provided. Describe specific actions you'd take to improve the item issues. See Tables 5.1 and 5.2 for reference.
- Specify indicators in *any* cognitive or proficiency-based domain of your choice that are measurable with one or more structured-response item formats in Chapter 5. Justify your answer.
- Create *two* items or item sets in each of the following formats: multiple-choice, true–false, completion, matching, and context-dependent items.
    - Evaluate the quality of your items using the criteria in Tables 5.1 and 5.2.
    - Which issues did you identify? How would you revise the items?
- Identify preexisting structured-response tests in common usage in your profession or field of study.
    - Critique the items using item-writing guidelines in Tables 5.1 and 5.2.
    - Identify any clues in the items reviewed.
    - Suggest specific ways to correct the flawed items.

5.5 Guidelines for Designing Constructed-Response Tasks and Essays

The constructed-response item format includes **short-response tasks** or **essay questions**. These formats assume that respondents are capable of focused, written communication. Most constructed-response tasks are timed exercises. Their design requires a written prompt, with examinees *supplying* a response in writing either on an answer booklet or via a word-processing program on a computer interface. Most such tasks are better suited for older students or adults, rather than very young children, the very elderly, disabled, or special needs populations comprising non-writers. An open-ended item structure that calls for very lengthy responses or independent writing over long time periods may pose barriers to some respondent groups, especially non-native speakers of the primary language of the assessment.

Table 5.3 provides the essential design guidelines for this class of items. Task construction is improved considerably by following three general criteria in Table 5.3, namely: task-to-indicator match; task clarity; and ensuring that items are free from apparent biases.

5.5.1 Criteria for Constructed-Response Tasks

Now, see Box 5.8 and Tables 5.4 and 5.5 in tandem with Table 5.3. The box illustrates a multicomponent short-response task series; examples of essay tasks follow in the narrative. Both short-answer and essay formats are particularly well suited for measuring higher-order thinking and problem solving, but the entire range of the cognitive taxonomy could be assessed. Short-answer items are usually accompanied with a quarter- to half-page writing space; essays may incorporate response spaces with one, two, or multiple pages. In Box 5.8, we see an example delimiting the content and length of the expected responses with mathematical patterns tasks and directions appropriate for younger, elementary school students.

Essay items should be thought-provoking, measuring indicators not well measured with other item formats. Some of these could be:

- Integrated sets of indicators (such as skill sets in writing a letter for a purpose and audience; constructing and interpreting a data table or graph for a purpose; interpreting artwork; critiquing a poem or literary passages/excerpts; or solving multistep problems in given subject areas)
- Indicators that involve skills in reasoning, argumentation, defending, justifying, or explaining an issue (such as skills in writing a persuasive communication)
- Use of complex cognitive processes and *process indicators* falling under complex procedural skills of the functional taxonomy (such as applying a *writing process* to prepare a polished communication, involving the steps in outlining, drafting, editing, and revising of the work)

Because open-ended tasks are costly in terms of time and effort needed for scoring, we should reserve the format for only those indicators that cannot be measured otherwise.

TABLE 5.3. A Checklist for Evaluating Constructed-Response Items and Essay Tasks

A. General criteria

Match

Does the item match the specified content focus, taxonomic level, conditions, and/or performance criterion, as given in the indicator(s) to be measured?

Clarity

Is the item presented in a clear, succinct, and direct (not confusing) manner?

Lack of apparent biases

Is the item free of any apparent biases in the language, content, pictorials, or other material used that could inflame or place some subgroups or individual members at a disadvantage?

B. Specific criteria for constructed-response tasks or essay items

- Does the task measure indicators that *cannot* be measured by other assessment modalities and structured item formats?
- Is the task thought provoking? Does it foster deeper thinking?
- Are instructions and tasks presented in a manner that matches the socioecological contexts of typical examinees?
- Is the task written at a readability level suited to typical examinees?
- Does the prompt clearly delimit the task? Are there clear parameters for responses expected, such as length, scope, and criteria for acceptability?
- Will the task parameters help prevent bluffing or off-topic answers?
- For short-answer tasks, is the number of tasks adequate for yielding a reliable sampling of the domain?
- Are there scoring rubrics to accompany the tasks?
- Are the scoring rubrics of high quality?
    a. *Validity:* Do rubrics match the specified domain's indicators in a meaningful way?
    b. *Validity:* Are rubrics aligned to the users' inferential needs and assessment purposes (e.g., formative vs. summative)?
    c. *Reliability:* Are there anchor papers and sample responses for the expected performance levels of examinees?
    d. *Utility:* Are the tasks and rubrics easy to use by examiners and other users, including learners? Will they yield information that benefits *all* users?
- Are the assessment conditions adequately defined (e.g., time limits, space limits, provisions for special needs, supporting materials)?
- Is the task designed to allow examinees at all levels to produce their best work?

Table 5.3, section B, provides specific criteria for evaluating and refining this class of items. Delimiting open-ended tasks with clear parameters is key to assuring measurement quality. Vague task prompts, associated with ambiguous and open-ended directions, are ineffectual in focusing respondents on the expected performances. As indicated in the opening section, without parameters, such tasks could generate a wide array of responses that are difficult to score with the requisite meaningfulness, accuracy, or consistency.

For another real-world example for secondary school students, see the next essay prompt. This initially crafted prompt led students to provide the following range of responses:

BOX 5.8 A Multistep Constructed-Response Task on Number Concepts and Patterns

Indicator

The examinee will identify, continue, and explain [**cognitive behaviors**] increasing number patterns involving basic number concepts and arithmetic operations [**content focus**].

Item N

Directions: Read each part (A–D) of the next question carefully and enter your answers in the spaces provided. The four parts will be scored together using the rubric attached.

A. See this number pattern below. Continue it by filling in the last two blanks.

15, 30, 60, ______, ______.

B. What math rule did you use to get the answer? Show your work clearly below [*Space provided*]

C. Suppose the same pattern was continued by someone up to 1920. What two numbers would come next?

1920, ______, ______.

D. Explain in no more than five (5) sentences why your answers are correct. Use math words when it makes sense to do so.

[*Space provided*]

Scoring Rubric: See Tables 5.4 and 5.5.

TABLE 5.4. Holistic Rubric for Rating Elementary School Student Performances on Mathematics Tasks

Score	Description of expected performance
3 (highest level)	*All* parts of answer show *full* understanding of the mathematical series or patterns • Continues the pattern by applying a correct or reasonable math rule, number concepts, and arithmetic operations • Shows all necessary computations • Gives clear and complete explanations • Answer shows *no* mathematical errors or gaps with only minor issues unrelated to the mathematical content tested.
2	Fills in *all* or most blanks and parts of problem showing *satisfactory* understanding of number patterns, number concepts, and/or operations • Continues the pattern with mostly accurate computations and/or identification of math rule • Gives acceptable explanations • Uses some math vocabulary • Answer shows some issues, omissions, and errors (1–5)
1	Shows *limited* understanding of number patterns, number concepts, and/or operations • Attempts to answer *most parts* using some number concepts, math patterns, and/or arithmetic knowledge and/or explanations • Makes several or repeated errors pertinent to the content tested (6–8) • Leaves few to several blanks
0 (lowest level)	Shows *very little or no* understanding of number patterns, number concepts, and/or operations • No responses; too many gaps in answers or incomprehensible and unreasonable responses • Answer shows many and repeated issues, omissions, and errors pertinent to the math content tested (>8)

TABLE 5.5. An Analytic Scoring Rubric: Rating Elementary School Student Performances on Mathematics Tasks

	Rating scale			
Performance indicators	**0 Unsatisfactory** (No response or incomprehensible inaccurate answers with multiple omissions, errors, or issues)	**1 Satisfactory** (Acceptable response but with multiple omissions, errors, or issues)	**2 Good** (Mostly reasonable answers, some errors or issues)	**3 Excellent** (Complete and reasonable answers, no errors)
1. Identified and continued the number pattern.		X		
2. Used an effective strategy to solve the problem (e.g., trial and error).		X		
3. Selected appropriate arithmetic operations (addition, subtraction, multiplication, and/or division).		X		
4. Performed computations correctly, also showing mastery of prerequisite skills (e.g., place value, multiplication facts).	X			
5. Followed all item instructions.		X		
6. Showed a sense of math patterns, as applicable to the task.		X		
7. Explained answers reasonably, using mathematical language appropriately (e.g., increasing series, decreasing series).	X			
Total score for student = 5				
Maximum possible score = 21				

Note. Ratings are for an imaginary student.

Initial essay prompt

Based on your readings, explain the problems of climate change and global warming.

Answers obtained

- A list of major facts on climate change (one page)
- A description of a recent major climate event (less than a page)
- A very lengthy, five-page historical review of global warming and climate change, with definitions of relevant terms
- A two-page opinion statement on possible causes and effects of climate change
- A three-page call for environmental policy changes on climate change
- A combination of the above, with different factual errors and unsupported claims

To correct the measurement issues posed by the above, item designers would first need to rewrite the task prompt, referring back to desired domain-specific indicators to be tested. Next, adequate directions would be necessary to set clear boundaries for response expectations, as suggested below:

Revised essay prompt

Directions: This is a closed-book essay exam. Respond to this four-part essay question on *global warming* and *climate change*, based on scientific facts and readings we reviewed in class.

- Define each of the two terms *global warming* and *climate change*.
- Describe a recent event that is being attributed to global warming and climate change. Respond in no more than two paragraphs.
- Explain three steps that the scientific community is recommending to slow down the above processes. Cite your sources accurately and respond in no more than three paragraphs.
- State how you would persuade leaders in your neighborhood or locality to support policies to control global warming and climate change. Justify your answer. This segment should be three to five paragraphs long.

Note. Locate your designated computer station. Your essay should be typed on the computer using MS Word. It should be between 1,000 and 1,200 words long and organized in the paragraphs suggested above. You will have 120 minutes of class time to complete the essay. Your work will be scored using the attached rubric [Attachment]. No points will be deducted for English-language or spelling mistakes, but please try your best to follow formal writing conventions and spell words correctly.

To design effectual essay tasks, we should ask: "What would high performance look like on this exercise? How could we control for redundant, extraneous, or irrelevant responses?" The prompt(s) and directions should be crafted accordingly. Notice that the length of the expected answer, the scoring criteria, the expected contents of the essay, and conditions under which the student must respond (e.g., time limits, closed book, on a computer) will together set the parameters for the response. Inclusion of scoring rubrics further communicates the performance expectations explicitly and clearly to respondents.

Poorly conceived essay or short-answer prompts encourage bluffing. Bluffing, or the practice of "faking" a response in a clever manner to camouflage what examinees *do not know* or *cannot do*, could be a major source of systematic error in essays. Test-wise examinees who bluff like to use sophisticated writing skills or other distracting information to impress examiners or readers. Tightly designed rubrics could curtail or even eliminate the influences of bluffing.

5.5.2 Types of Scoring Rubrics for Constructed-Response Tasks

The topic of scoring rubrics is introduced here, with added discussions in Chapter 6 in connection with rater errors found in performance assessments. Review again, closely, the two rubrics in Tables 5.4 and 5.5.

Well-designed scoring rubrics are a critical component of both essay and constructed-response tasks. Giving examinees and examiners access to rubrics prior to assessment improves communication of performance expectations and could change the overall assessment outcomes in educational and training contexts.

Holistic scoring rubrics for given tasks allow a review of each response *as a whole*, with the assignment of a single overall score (Table 5.4). **Analytic scoring rubrics** allow a *task breakdown with a series of separate scores* assignable for each relevant part (Table 5.5). Both types could employ a multilevel rating scale or a binary checklist to denote levels of quality. Regardless of type, content-valid rubrics are tied to the key components in the domains specified for assessment.

As evident, holistic rubrics like that in Table 5.4 help rank-order performances by their overall quality. These protocols are suitable for making summative decisions in educational settings. The multistep task in Box 5.8 calls for examinees to identify, continue, and explain patterns with a specific mathematical content focus. Each constructed response to the task is rated as a whole with a scoring rubric to match. This rubric incorporates a four-level rating scale, ranging from lowest (0) to highest (3). Each performance level is defined by descriptions of the response expected. As illustrated, this particular rubric would allow faster grading and yield a summary score denoting the overall proficiency level of each respondent on the skills that the task demands.

Contrast the above to the analytic rubric presented in Table 5.5 for the same domain and type of task. Analytic rubrics offer intraindividual diagnostic profiles useful for formative decision making in educational, training, clinical intervention, or coaching contexts. Often, as shown, a student or examinee might show a stronger performance on some indicators than others. In designing an analytic scoring system, the specified domain dictates what aspects are to be scored and how the scores will be weighted. The unnamed candidate in the table receives an overall low score of 5, with a diagnostic profile denoting mostly 0's and 1's. Such information could be useful in shaping the next actions of the primary assessment users. Well-designed analytic rubrics also reveal interindividual competency differences on the selected criteria. While it is always possible to sum the ratings across all the indicators to obtain a total score, it is the property of describing differential performances within and across individuals that gives the rubric its analytic character and diagnostic utility. The score of 5 for the illustrative student is based on unweighted ratings on seven indicators.

Although not shown here, designers could specify how each indicator-based score will be weighted. Different indicators might be weighted differently depending on their relative importance to users or instructors. For example, the indicator on following instructions in Table 5.5 might have the lowest weight of 1, with the indicator on showing a sense of math patterns weighted at 2, and the indicator on explaining the answer weighted the highest at 3. If these weights are accounted for in the illustration, the imaginary student would receive 2 weighted points for Indicator 6, instead of 1 (*Rating of 1* × Weight of 2).

5.5.3 Designing Scoring Rubrics

What is an acceptable answer to a given open-ended task, especially when one is confronted with ambiguous responses? Expertise with both the population and the domain helps in the rubric design process. For tasks that share common design features and properties, the goal is to devise a standardized procedure for scoring the full range of responses possible. Loosely defined or vague scoring criteria are often easier to compile. On the other hand, very extensive but cumbersome scoring procedures could be equally problematic, lowering utility levels.

One starts the rubric design procedure by selecting the valued indicators in the construct domain aligned with specified expectations for the tasks, keeping in mind the assessment purposes. Clearly written domain and indicator specifications are imperative for supporting the rubric design process (Chapter 4). The rubrics are initially drafted aligned with the task-based indicators.

Once the tasks or items are designed, the choice of a holistic versus an analytic rubric is dependent on whether the assessment purpose is summative or formative, or a combination of the two. As already suggested, holistic rubrics enable quicker assessments for summative purposes; analytic rubrics enable better diagnosis of needs.

The most appropriate rating scale or checklist for point allocation must be decided on by the designers based on the expected variability in the examinee responses. Binary checklists are often used with analytic rubrics when the expected responses are likely to vary at two levels for each indicator. When degrees of quality need to be differentiated, rating scales are more useful.

Conducting a small-scale pilot test or try-out of the tasks with typical examinees is often a useful exercise for finalizing the rubric and the point allocation method. A review of sample answers helps in formulating the descriptive statements that represent different levels of quality in task performances. A detailed cataloguing of common errors is also often the best means for refining the rating scales, checklists, or a combination of point allocation schemes that may be used for different parts of a response. Reviews of actual responses also help in fine-tuning the task prompts, instructions, and sometimes, the indicators in domains. To differentiate among responses of differing degrees of quality—that is, those that qualify for a score of 1 versus a 2 or 3, the assessment designers, instructors, or domain experts may all need a collective review to arrive at a consensus.

Selecting actual answers as "anchor" papers could also help in containing errors during the scoring process when the rubrics are applied. Serving as a reference point for raters, anchor papers help establish the range of possible performances to expect at each score point or rating level. When applied effectively, anchors can significantly reduce both systematic and random rater variabilities.

5.6 Instrument Assembly

Item and instrument assembly is an important step of assessment design. Test compilation should be user-oriented and guided by the assessment purposes. This phase is best completed after validation is completed. What is minimally necessary?

- **Title of the test:** Assessments should have a succinct title that clarifies the assessment's purpose and main topic. This is useful for priming examinees and other stakeholders on the purposes of the assessment tool.
- **Item layout:** A reasonable plan for item layout and organization is necessary. Items may be organized randomly, alphabetically, by subdomain, or otherwise. This plan should be a part of the assessment design specifications in Phases I and II of the Process Model and, preferably, specified in advance.
- **Presentation platform or medium:** The platform or medium for item presentation and delivery should be carefully selected so that it is well suited to the domains, respondent population, primary users, and assessment purposes (Phases I and II of the Process Model).
- **Item-level instructions:** There should be clearly written item-level instructions, as well as directions for the overall test or test segments, as needed. The instructions should help curb respondent confusions and user errors during test taking and administration.
- **Scoring procedures:** Scoring keys or scoring rubrics must be appropriately designed, tested, and verified to have optimal levels of functionality with users.
- **Supporting materials:** All supporting materials for an assessment should be prepared according to the design specifications. The materials should be pilot-tested for usability and found to be accessible for examinees, as well as the scorers, proctors, and other assessment users and administrators.

QUICK RECAP: Constructed-response tasks and essay items are appropriate for measuring higher-order indicators in cognitive domains that cannot be assessed in other ways. These task formats should be deployed judiciously, as they can challenge reliability and utility levels of assessments. Well-prepared items define the task expectations clearly for examinees. Each should be accompanied with an appropriate scoring rubric, as suited to the specified domains and assessment purpose. To facilitate consistent scoring, rubrics should be clear, unambiguous, and supported with samples of answers showing typical errors and ranges of performance. For all assessments, the final test assembly procedures should be consistent with the overall design specifications.

Reflection Break 5.4: Objective 4

- In a construct domain of your choice, formulate indicators best suited for measurement with essays or constructed-response tasks.
- Design *five* constructed-response tasks with a rubric of your choice to measure your chosen indicators. Self-critique and improve your assessment tasks and rubrics using Table 5.3.
- Review the item illustrations in this chapter requiring examinees to *supply* answers or explanations. Would those components be better measured with a rubric instead of a fixed answer key? Justify your answer.
- Evaluate the quality of essay items from an existing assessment using the criteria in Table 5.3. What issues or omissions did you identify? How would you revise the items? Be specific. Defend your revisions.
- Identify five criteria you would prioritize for assembling a test in finished form? How would these criteria differ for structured-response versus constructed-response tests? Explain.

5.7 Applying the Process Model: Cognitively Based Item Design to Measure Learning Progressions

"Cognitively informed item design" could be approached in more than one way. The chapter presents a case application of the Process Model for designing cognitively based *diagnostic assessments* for supporting students' *learning and development* in a specific math skills domain (long division) in elementary school classrooms. This particular effort utilized several of the item types discussed in Chapter 5 and draws on six theoretical principles derived from the combined literatures in the cognitive sciences, educational assessment, instructional design, and human learning. The domains were operationalized along the lines discussed in Section 5.3.2 and earlier in Chapter 4 for specifying hierarchical domains to map growth and change in an area.

To supplement this section, which builds on the historically evolving literature on test development from a cognitive science perspective first referenced in Chapter 2, interested readers should also consult added articles on newer theoretical and mathematical approaches (see, e.g., Barret, 2017; Bennett, 2010; Lane et al., 2016a; Mislevy, 2006, 2019; Pellegrino et al., 2001, 2014). Each foundational idea utilized in the project is presented next, followed by the corresponding implications for assessment design (after Chatterji, 2012; Chatterji, Koh, Choi, & Iyengar, 2009b; Chatterji & Lin, 2018; Gordon et al., 2014).

5.7.1 Cognitively Based Assessment Design: What It Means in Theory and Practice

5.7.1.1 Changing Knowledge Structures in the Human Brain

To begin, the literature suggests that the human brain's architecture is made up of both the short-term working memory and the long-term memory. The organized knowledge of the world is stored for the most part in the long-term memory. These knowledge structures are basically the neural networks in the brain that govern an individual's **cognitions** (what we know about different aspects of the world) and **emotions** (how we feel about those aspects). As human brains are not static, individuals are continually building and rebuilding these "knowledge structures." For different people, the brain's knowledge structures may develop through different pathways and at different times (Lane et al., 2016a; Pellegrino et al., 2001).

When faced with a new problem or task to be learned, an individual's level of success depends on how well that person can *retrieve* and *use* appropriate information from the long-term memory and bring it to bear in the responses and attempts at learning the new tasks. To help explore and reveal existing knowledge structures in relation to new task learning, the literature recommends the use of strategies like *probing questions*. Probes help delve into a person's prior knowledge levels, learning gaps, misconceptions, and readiness to learn something new or find solutions to novel problems.

IMPLICATIONS FOR ASSESSMENT DESIGN

When attempting to measure learning in new areas, the knowledge structures of learners should be a main focus of item construction efforts. To reveal what the domain-specific learning gaps and learning progression needs may be, **probing question** designs should seek to map the underlying knowledge structures along some developmental continua. Given that the structures may vary in different individuals, effective assessment items and tasks would anticipate and accommodate that human variability, helping in making visible the differences in prior knowledge levels, gaps in cognition, and readiness levels to advance along the domain continuum.

5.7.1.2 Metacognition

Second, humans possess and can continually develop the abilities to reflect on and monitor their own learning in different areas. This capacity is called **metacognition**. When pursuing a desired goal, thinking about one's specific successes, challenges, missteps. and failures is useful information for self-regulating and correcting course. Experts in a domain tend to engage in greater levels of metacognition and self-regulation than do novices.

IMPLICATIONS FOR ASSESSMENT DESIGN

Item designs should include self-assessments to guide the development of metacognitive skills, alongside assessments of the knowledge and skills in given domains. As learning progresses in the domain, differences in metacognitive capacities will enable differentiations of varying levels of developed expertise in individuals.

5.7.1.3 Contextually Situated Cognition and Learning

Third, much of what humans know, learn, and can do is gained through interactions with others in particular social and cultural contexts, including the classroom, family, organizations, and the community. Deeper understandings of the world develop in context, and the meanings particular objects carry could vary for diverse individuals operating in different social and cultural contexts.

IMPLICATIONS FOR ASSESSMENT DESIGN

Knowledge-acquisition and knowledge-testing experiences must be made contextually relevant for the learners. Tasks should be situated in relatable contexts applicable to given domains. In addition, the items and tasks should be relevant for a diversity of contexts suited to learners who might belong in dissimilar social and cultural groups.

5.7.1.4 Transfer of Learning

Fourth, knowledge transfer is not automatic, and individual capacities to transfer knowledge and skills from situation to situation can vary. However, the use of *scaffolding* techniques, such as providing explicit suggestions, guidance, or support, facilitates the transfer of knowledge from one setting to new situations and to different types of problems.

IMPLICATIONS FOR ASSESSMENT DESIGN

Transfer of knowledge can be facilitated through item designs that embed scaffolding techniques with tasks that suggest, guide, or teach as they test. Items or tasks that serve as "scaffolds" could deliberately connect prior knowledge with new information in a problem situation, or guide respondents toward success by suggesting or demonstrating the connections. Item scaffolds could enable the transfer of basic skills to more complex, problem-solving skills.

5.7.1.5 Need for Error Detection, Mediation, Feedback, and Practice during Learning

Fifth, the research shows that to learn and grow, all individuals need to make mistakes and need chances to learn from their mistakes. In this process, goal-directed coaching, feedback, and practice play important and helpful roles. In educational or training contexts, learning is facilitated with cycles of feedback and coaching to correct any errors identified while teaching and learning are ongoing. To consolidate new neural networks and cognitive bonds, timely mediation and practice opportunities are essential. Skills that individuals practice more often become more automatic and efficient over time. Such efforts could be initiated and reinforced in formal school settings, as well as at home or in other community contexts (Chatterji, 2012; Chatterji & Lin, 2018).

IMPLICATIONS FOR ASSESSMENT DESIGN

To measure learning and development constructs, assessment and item designs should facilitate error detection and diagnosis, opening up possibilities for corrective coaching and feedback to be provided by teachers, parents, or coaches. Tasks that motivate learners to engage in goal-directed practice can be similarly helpful for promoting learning and improvement. Diagnostic and formatively oriented assessment designs will likely lead to greater levels of expertise building in any given domain.

5.7.1.6 Interdependence of Human Cognitions and Emotions

Finally, positive affect is associated with learning and mastering any domain. Cognitions and emotions are all interconnected and learned reciprocally through human experience in given areas. When attitudes and self-beliefs are positive in learning something new, individuals tend to undertake more difficult tasks; furthermore, they tend to take risks in persisting at the tasks, even if they fail initially (Barret, 2017; Chatterji, 2012; Chatterji & Lin, 2018).

IMPLICATIONS FOR ASSESSMENT DESIGN

Assessment designs must acknowledge the reciprocity of cognitions and emotions during the learning process. Creating an affirming culture is a necessary part of designing the overall assessment environment with "learning and development" constructs. Learners should feel encouraged and comfortable as they engage, take risks, make mistakes, improve and gain mastery in given domains. In contrast, assessment conditions that engender negative forms of competition, fears, or anxieties (e.g., of being embarrassed or punished for failure) are not conducive to fostering growth and development in a domain.

5.7.2 Designing Diagnostic Learning Assessments for Classroom Use with the Process Model—A Case Study

A description of the project incorporating the theoretical ideas above now follows. To set the stage, let us first consider the project's rationale and larger context.

PROJECT RATIONALE

Why a focus on long division? In U.S. public education settings, elementary school students in grades 3–5 are expected to become proficient in multiplication and division skills before they start middle school. Yet, many struggle, with learning gaps exacerbating as the demands for using advanced mathematics skills increase in higher grades. In middle school (grades 6–8), students are required to apply long division with automaticity, especially when performing "real-world" problems, or relating division to fractions and decimals, taking a square root by hand (the long-division method is the standard procedure), or manipulating basic algebraic equations. As the gaps accumulate, students face more difficulties in learning mathematics generally.

PROJECT CONTEXT

An informal "needs assessment" at the project's district site had shown that large numbers of children in grades 4–6 were falling behind their math preparation levels in three specific units, including long division. To address the needs, the project's team set a goal to reduce the students' learning gaps in long division by implementing a specific model of diagnostic and formative classroom assessment practice with teachers and schools. The participating teachers on the team received training in a research-based approach that built on the six principles just discussed. This model involved the ongoing use of diagnostic assessment tasks and short learning assessments, coupled with timely mediation, feedback, practice, and coaching activities with students. To support the practices, the project's team and participating teachers designed an *item bank* of cognitively based diagnostic items and short learning assessments that were made accessible to all.

The project itself was a relatively low-stakes research and development effort intended to pilot-test and fine-tune the new cognitively based approach to diagnostic classroom teaching and assessment. Simultaneously, there was a larger districtwide, high-stakes testing program in operation, with standardized tests administered annually by the state for accountability purposes. Given the latter, there was some pressure on the project's participants to show student gains on the external tests at the end of each school year. Each phase of the Process Model, as implemented in designing the item bank and short assessments for the long-division unit, is described next.

PHASE I OF THE PROCESS MODEL: SPECIFYING THE ASSESSMENT USE AND USER CONTEXT

- *What?* **Construct:** Learning and development in a long-division skills domain.
- *Who?* **Population:** For assessment design purposes, the population included the students enrolled in grades 4 and 5 in four elementary schools at the school district. The families of these children were primarily African American (over 80%), with most enrolled in the free or reduced-cost lunch program, indicative of the high levels of poverty in the district. When the project began, these learners were at widely different places with respect to their proficiency in long division.
- *Why?* **Assessment Purposes:** (1) Teaching and learning and (2) research and development.

There were two user paths relevant to the project's purposes that were closely overlapping (see Chapter 2 for definitions). The first dealt with *teaching and learning in classrooms*—the teachers and students were expected to use the diagnostic items, assessments, and the results on a day-to-day basis to inform teaching and learning activities according to the specific model of formative assessment practice that was being pilot-tested. The second dealt with *research and development*—the project's researchers and district's leaders were interested in using the assessment results (and added data) for evaluating the viability, utility, and early effectiveness of the approach for detecting and closing the documented learning gaps in students.

Measure-Based Inferences. The main inferences from the assessment results dealt with detecting students' cognitive gaps, learning barriers, learning progressions, and proficiency levels in the long-division skills domain along a developmental continuum.

Specific Uses of Assessment Results. The learning assessment results were used by teachers to make domain-specific diagnoses of students' needs during ongoing classroom activities. At the end of each project year, the assessment results were collected and reviewed for improving aspects of the model of classroom practice.

Primary Users. The primary users of the assessment results were the participating teachers, students, and the university-based research team that initiated the project. Among the secondary assessment users and stakeholders were the school district's leaders and district constituents, including the children's families.

PHASE II: SPECIFYING THE ASSESSMENT OPERATIONS

The design process was guided by the six undergirding principles of cognitively based assessment design (Section 5.7.1). See Box 5.9 for an example of a diagnostic learning assessment from the project.

Specifying the Domain. The initial domain was ordered with indicators at progressively higher taxonomic levels ranging from very basic to more complex skills, as follows. The expected learning progressions were mapped along a projected developmental path, leading up to mastery of culminating tasks similar to those of Item G (Box 5.4).

Culminating Learning Outcome

- The student will be able to solve real-world "story" problems using long division and supporting arithmetic operations, show all work, and explain all the parts of the solution. [higher-order thinking, high-level difficulty]

Selected Developmentally Ordered Indicators

- Recall multiplication facts. [prerequisite skill, concept recall and understanding, lowest difficulty level]
- Paraphrase the long-division problem in the story, using own words. [concept recall and understanding, lowest difficulty level]
- Set up the long-division problem in the story, with the dividend and divisor identified correctly. [application, midlevel difficulty]
- Perform all the steps of the long-division computation correctly, showing all work:
    - Compute with one- or two-digit dividends and single-digit divisor (e.g., 25 ÷ 6 = ____). [application, midlevel difficulty]
    - Compute with three- and four-digit dividends and single- or double-digit divisors (e.g., 125 ÷ 11 = ____). [application, high-level difficulty]
    - Recognize remainders correctly. [application, high-level difficulty]
- Check all computation steps by using reverse operations. [complex procedural skills, high-level difficulty]
    - Identify mistakes along the way.
    - Correct errors along the way.
- Explain parts of the computation procedure and answers, situated in the scenario. [higher-order thinking, high-level difficulty]

The culminating outcome and short-term expectations were specified as *product indicators*, denoting the desired endpoints of the learning process. Others were specified as *process indicators*, such as checking and correcting the computational steps on the way to arriving at answers. Classroom teaching and assessment processes were closely aligned with and guided by this ordered domain.

Item and Task Design Specifications. The item design specifications are evident in the item series for the learning assessment in Box 5.9. For example:

- Items are arranged developmentally on the short assessment exercise.
- For enabling deeper and more fine-grained diagnoses, the assessments include several probing items.
- Items incorporate typical errors and error reviews.
- Items guide students in metacognitive activities.
- Items scaffold the steps in the learning progres-

BOX 5.9 A Diagnostic Assessment: Probing Knowledge Structures

Long-Division Learning Assessment-1

Grades 4 and 5

Directions: This test is to help you learn and improve your long-division skills. Try every problem, even if you are not sure of the answers. You will not be given a grade on this test. Your answers will help your teacher guide you further. Read the instructions for each question set carefully. When asked, show all your work or write your answer in your own words in the spaces provided on the test booklet. Be neat. Take your time, relax, and enjoy the exercise!

Start here ↓

See the problem below to answer Questions 1–4.

$$5\overline{)175}$$

1. Choose **<u>one</u>** answer from *a–e* to answer Question 1.

   The problem is asking me to ____________

   a. Multiply 5 and 175.

   b. Divide 175 into 5 equal parts.

   c. Subtract 5 from 175.

   d. Add 5 and 175 to find the sum.

   e. Do something else (explain). [*Space provided*]

2. Circle if true <u>or</u> false.

   Another way to say what the problem is asking is: Find out how many groups of 5 there are in 175.

   a. True

   b. False

   Explain. [*Space provided*]

3. Now, solve the problem. Show all your work. Write the answer clearly. Show the remainder, if there is one. [*Space provided*]

4. If you did not find a remainder, say why. Write your answer here. [*Space provided*]

5. Now, see the **<u>next</u>** problem that I completed. Check all my work carefully. Then, answer Questions 6–12.

$$\begin{array}{r} 610 \\ 5\overline{)552} \\ \underline{-54} \\ 12 \\ \underline{-9} \\ 3 \\ \underline{-0} \\ 3 \end{array} \text{ (Remainder)}$$

6. I know I made mistakes. Are my errors with the multiplication facts?

   Say "Yes" or "No." ______

7. Are my errors with place value?

   Say "Yes" or "No." ______.

8. Are my errors with the "bring down" steps?

   Say "Yes" or "No." ______.

9. Is my error with the remainder?

   Say "Yes" or "No." ______.

10. Please use **backward operations** to find and circle **<u>all</u>** my mistakes. Say in your own words where my answer is wrong. [*Space provided*]

11. Please **<u>redo</u>** the problem correctly. Show **<u>all</u>** your work here. [*Space provided*]

12. Say what you did to make sure your answer was correct. [*Space provided*]

Your Feedback

Did you enjoy doing this math exercise? [*Space provided*]

Did you find the math problems easy? [*Space provided*]

Did you want to stop, get tired, or give up before you finished all the problems? [*Space provided*]

Which parts or questions would you like more help with? [*Space provided*]

What would you like to learn next? Anything else you want us to know? [*Space provided*]

Source: Adapted from Chatterji (2012).

sions to help guide student thinking toward mastery and transfer of knowledge.

- Items and assessments acknowledge the affective and cognitive aspects of learning.
- Items use mixed-item response formats to obtain richer data on students' cognitive processes and status.
- Items measure both learning process and product indicators.
- Items are situated in meaningful and age-appropriate scenarios.

For practicality, each diagnostic learning assessment was specified to be short in length, no more than 10–20 items long. The tests could be compiled by teachers as desired from the item bank produced by the project teams, and used for classwork, homework, mid-unit practice, or end-of-unit exercises. Along the way, teachers were trained to add new and validated tasks to the item banks. As a part of the practice model, teachers were requested to summarize, share, and discuss the results in a timely fashion, with corrective feedback communicated to students in meaningful ways. Easy-to-use analytic checklists linked to the initial domain of indicators accompanied the long-division tasks (shown next).

PHASE III: DESIGNING DIAGNOSTIC ITEMS ON LEARNING ASSESSMENTS

Compare the items in Box 5.9 with the item in Box 5.4. Instead of stand-alone and unrelated items on a test, the diagnostic learning assessment incorporated a connected item series. This series was designed to match progressively ordered indicators in the intended domain that led to a proximal outcome (long-division computation), suggesting a developmental path that teachers and the project teams arrived at by consensus. By design, Items 1–5 were easier than Items 6–12 in Box 5.9. Although not reaching the culminating outcome yet (Item G), a logical learning progression toward similar tasks is mapped in the item series.

To differentiate among very specific or different learning needs, probing items were frequently embedded in the test. For instance, Items 1 and 2 probe students' skill levels in paraphrasing what a problem is asking and include an explanation component intended to reveal added information on their thinking processes.

The items encouraged metacognitive skill building by directing students to monitor and think more deeply about each step. See, for example, Items 6–12 for evaluating each possible oversight or error during the computation process. To help learners become more proficient at the next step, the same items served as scaffolds, priming and suggesting to students how they should be thinking to arrive at the correct solution.

To reveal children's thinking processes more comprehensively, the assessment incorporated both structured-response and constructed-response items. Finally, the "story" in the culminating item reflected a realistic problem context for the typical learners, indicative of common student experiences at schools (Item G).

Several design strategies were intended to encourage students to engage in the learning process without fear, avoidance, or anxiety. In an attempt to create a positive assessment environment, the assessment instructions clarified the assessment's formative purposes at the start to students, who were recognized to belong among the primary users of the assessment's results. The assessment instructions and open-ended items at the very end gathered data on students' feelings and affect pertinent to their learning experiences, as well as gaining mastery of long division.

Designing a Scoring Rubric. To facilitate metacognition during learning, the project teams designed a student- and teacher-friendly analytic rubric with "Yes/No" scoring, mimicking the typical steps and agreed-upon processes that teachers were expected to reinforce during teaching, as follows:

I can:

read a story problem and say in my own words what the problem is asking me to do.

plan the math operations I need to solve the problem.

find the dividend and divisor in the story for the long-division problem.

set up the long-division problem correctly.

use multiplication facts correctly when doing long division.

use place value correctly when doing long division.

finish all the steps of the long-division computation.

say what the answer and remainder mean in the story.

PHASE IV: VALIDATION AND ITERATIONS

All the tasks and assessments were generated in teacher workshops; the items were critically reviewed internally and *content-validated* by members of the research team and teachers not involved in the design using standard criteria and the literature (Tables 5.1–5.3). As instruction began, the initial collection of items, practice tasks, and long-division domain's indicators were also pilot-tested with students and teachers in participating classrooms, shedding light on their *usability* and *usefulness* (see Chapters 1 and 4).

A vast number were revised, adapted, and refined by the teachers and the research team based on the information collected. Detailed task analysis and error cataloguing during instruction, along with student interviews, informed many of the revisions necessary to arrive at final versions. Based on common errors, for example, the following two *process indicators* were added to the domain and analytic rubric:

- Locate the digit in the dividend with the highest place value to start the long-division computation.
- Think aloud each computational step and predict the next step.

Teacher experiences and feedback also showed that several student blocks dealt with poor work habits, beliefs, and attitudes. Changes to the rubric were made accordingly, with new *affective process indicators* added. See the following:

I can:

keep my scratch work neat so that I do not get lost when doing a math problem.

look at my mistakes without feeling sad.

look at my mistakes to help me grow.

not give up before I finish the problem fully.

PHASE V: USING THE DIAGNOSTIC CLASSROOM ASSESSMENTS FOR FORMATIVE PURPOSES

Once the design and validation processes were completed, the participating teachers and students were given access to all the assessment materials and rubrics. Most of the local stakeholders were positive about continuing the efforts on their own beyond the funded project's timeline. Early research on the cognitively based formative assessment approach yielded several positive outcomes with students and teachers. Further research and development on the classroom model for designing learning assessments are continuing, informed by the project's findings.

For example, the teams learned that the observable indicators of any learning domain must be developmentally organized with a justifiable defense of the same. Some of this justification was derivable from existing math curricula, literature, and theory; the rest must be obtained through empirical evidence collected directly from classrooms with the participating teachers and students in action.

Second and importantly, items that yielded both qualitative and quantitative types of data were more useful in shedding light on the classroom-level learning dynamics. Useful items were those that were designed along a developmental path and targeted several aspects of learning long division, as follows:

- **Learning process indicators:** We could measure, as desired, the fine-grained cognitive processes employed by learners during task learning, by operationally defining these as "process indicators" of the domain.
- **Learning progressions:** With documentation of learner responses to developmentally ordered tasks in a domain, such as their successes, typical errors, and number and nature of tries with tasks at different levels of difficulty, we could track and map the pathways that different learners may take toward acquiring mastery.
- **Short-term learning outcomes:** We could also measure, if desired, any short-term learning outcomes, or the *proximal milestones* attained by learners along the way, leading up to a longer-term learning outcome.
- **Culminating learning outcome(s):** As with achievement measures, we could also measure the

culminating learning outcome as the main end-product of the learning and development process as a "product indicator."

In sum, with learning and development constructs (like the long-division skills domain), item construction must allow for the progress paths to be mapped for different individuals, describing any dissimilar learning trajectories. From the domain specification procedures to the item design and selection approaches, several of the assessment operations need to be different from those we would typically employ for measuring achievement.

The case showed that the timing and uses made of the item response data and overall construct measures for learning and development constructs must also change in applied settings. To shape learning formatively in the desired directions in educational contexts, the primary users (here, both the teachers and learners) would need to collect and jointly review such assessment data at frequent intervals and dedicate the information purposefully to supporting learner growth in the desired directions. These complex processes are by no means automatic. For the primary data users, it calls for systematic training, practice, coaching, and changing of classroom habits (see Chatterji, 2012; Chatterji et al., 2009; Chatterji & Lin, 2018).

5.7.3 Dynamic Assessments

Historically, a method of *dynamic testing* accompanied with affirming and immediate examiner mediation was also shown to be effective in improving capacities of institutionalized, mentally retarded adolescents (Feuerstein, Rand, & Hoffman, 1979). These early dynamic assessment studies relied on traditionally designed items and existing intelligence tests of that period; however, the supportive, guided feedback altered the measured outcomes of examinees. Developmental and cognitively based assessments coupled with appropriate feedback could be similarly helpful for individuals requiring rehabilitation, for example, those with brain injuries or other compromised mental or motor functioning levels.

QUICK RECAP: The literature to date on cognitively based assessment design provides insights and innovative ways to map the complexities of "learning and development" constructs more effectively, suggesting strategies for adapting or revamping the standard item formats discussed in Chapter 5. The case study on applying the Process Model demonstrated the design of domain-specific, learning assessments with mixed-item formats for classroom and school-based applications. Added ways to design effective cognitively based items and tasks are suggested in the literature sources cited.

Reflection Break 5.5: Objectives 3–6

- Summarize three (3) ideas from the latest research from the cognitive sciences that you find most useful for assessment design purposes? Explain your position.
- Which item design approach, cognitively informed or traditional, would be better for an instrument you want to design or use? Explain.
- Distinguish between *product indicators* and *process indicators*. In a cognitive domain of your choice, identify examples of each type of indicator. Create separate items to measure product indicators and process indicators in the domain.
- When measuring a learning and development construct, what is a *learning progression*? What is a *learning pathway*? Explain these terms with examples.
- The Process Model stresses *user-centered assessment design*. Who were among the *primary users* in the case study reported here? How well were their specific information needs addressed as a part of the assessment design process in the case? Refer to both User Paths to explain.

5.8 Summary

Chapter 5 dealt with designing structured- and constructed-response items for a range of cognitive constructs. While most mental abilities and proficiency-based constructs are measurable with the item formats discussed, we should be mindful of the theoretical underpinnings for each construct type and choose the most apposite item modality and measurement approach.

Alongside the domain's properties, user needs, the intended functions of the assessment's results, and the population's characteristics, should all guide the choice of item response formats. Validation of assessments and items with user involvement is a necessary part of a user-centered design process. The case study with the Process Model attempted to highlight these points.

The chapter provided the major guidelines for writing, selecting, and critically reviewing items of different types. The most commonly observed pitfalls during item construction can be minimized by attending to the guidelines during item writing, selection, and assembly of the tests in final form.

Traditional versus cognitively based item design approaches are grounded in different assumptions and research foundations. Both can be useful for measuring cognitive constructs, but one or the other might be better suited for different assessment purposes. The chapter reviewed cognitively based item design approaches in some depth, showing the usefulness of these techniques for measuring "learning and development" constructs in school settings.

CHAPTER 6

Designing Behavior-Based, Product-Based, and Portfolio-Based Assessments

6.1 Chapter Overview

6.1.1 Introduction

Historically, the term *performance assessment* refers to an array of different assessment techniques (Berk, 1986). Of these, Chapter 6 provides background theory and guidelines for designing *three* types of performance assessments, namely, behavior-, product-, and portfolio-based assessments. Broadly defined, interview-based assessments may be viewed as another type of performance assessment; these devices are discussed alongside other self-report instruments in Chapter 7.

Looking back, Chapter 3 introduced readers to the general characteristics, advantages, and limitations of performance assessments generally. Chapter 6 builds on that information, elaborating now on their history, added properties, and implications of the "performance" modality on design-related decisions that could impact the properties of measures. Readers are encouraged to pursue relevant readings elsewhere to bolster the information in the chapter. To connect this chapter with the rest of the book and the Process Model, see Figure 6.1.

6.1.2 Chapter Objectives

After reading this chapter and completing the accompanying exercises, the reader should be able to:

1. Identify the distinctive features, advantages, and typical applications of three performance assessment modalities—namely, behavior-, product-, and portfolio-based assessments.
2. Select appropriate performance or response modalities and task operations for measuring a range of cognitive, noncognitive, health-related, and other constructs.
3. Identify relevant facets of a performance assessment for supporting the planned inferences and uses of scores desired by primary users.
4. Identify potential errors from various sources when designing observation protocols and scoring rubrics for performance assessments.
5. Apply established guidelines/criteria to design behavior-, product-, and portfolio-based assessments.
6. Critically evaluate the quality of performance assessments for meeting the specified information needs of assessment users in given contexts (guided by the *What?*, *Why?*, and *Whom?* portals of the Process Model).

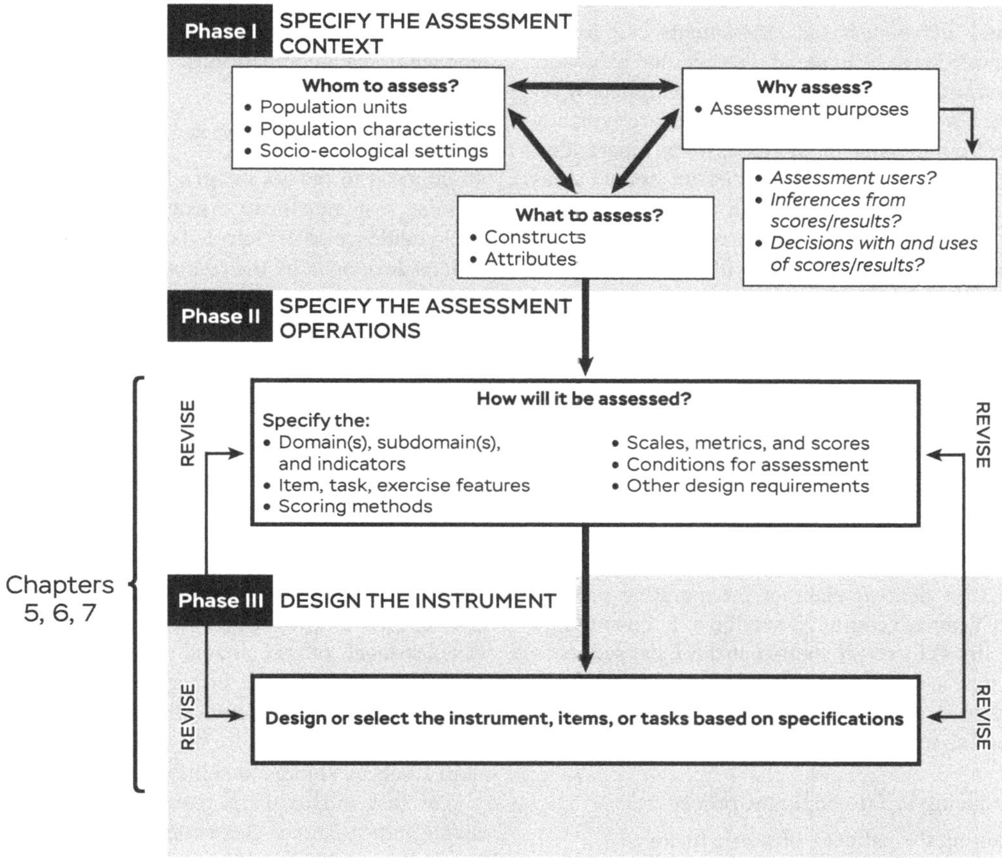

FIGURE 6.1. Connecting Chapter 6 to the Process Model and the rest of the book.

6.2 Behavior-, Product-, and Portfolio-Based Assessments: Definitions, Examples, and Origins

Performance assessments . . . require [human respondents] to generate rather than choose a response. . . . Exhibitions, investigations, demonstrations, written or oral responses, journals, and portfolios are examples. . . .

—JOAN L. HERMAN, PAMELA R. ASCHBACHER, and LYNN WINTERS (1992, p. 2)

6.2.1 Performance Assessments: A General Overview

Let us begin with definitions, descriptions, and examples, some old and some new. The three assessment types of concern in Chapter 6 are clearly distinguished from each other based on the specific response modalities each requires of human respondents. In high-stakes educational assessments, these respondents are none other than the examinees themselves; elsewhere, they could be students, patients, workers, candidates for competitive awards or recognitions, or service clients. In experimental and research settings, the respondents are typically the subjects of the investigations.

6.2.1.1 Behavior-Based Assessments

Known also as **observational assessments**, this type of performance assessment requires individuals to exhibit the targeted behaviors under natural or "live" conditions. For obtaining evidence of the underlying construct(s), behavior-based assessments call for direct observations to be made of the specified behaviors while these are being demonstrated or exhibited by respondents. External observers, therefore, are typically an integral component of the assessment operations. Individual instruments could focus on spontaneous behaviors that are recorded in an informal manner, or more formally enacted performances that are observed, recorded, and/or scored with tightly designed protocols. Construct-relevant indicators could deal with valued cognitive skill or ability domains, noncognitive or attitudinal areas, health-related conditions, or physical abilities and motor attributes. Occasionally, a combination of constructs may be measured, as desired by the primary users.

Refer back to Box 3.3 in Chapter 3 for an example of a **behavior-based assessment** in medical education. This instrument is intended for examining the readiness of anaesthesiologists in administering anaesthesia to a defined class of preoperative patients (pregnant women needing C-sections). Focusing on a very specific skill set, it spells out the ideal sequence of steps that a competent and trained medical practitioner should display while serving individual patients. For example:

- Introducing self (to begin the procedure)
- Obtaining the patient's obstetric history
- Obtaining the patient's medical history
- Gathering data on allergies
- Performing an airway examination, and so forth

Each step in the expected sequence would be checked off as observed during the performance examination. Observers in this case would be the medical examiners (usually, the supervising doctors at university hospitals). Examinees would be assigned scores according to a weighted point-allocation system while they performed the procedures (Scavone et al., 2010). Other examples of behavior-based assessments could include assessing the technical and artistic quality of ballet dancers' stage performances; examining the effectiveness of a manager's negotiation skills while in action with clients; observing everyday behaviors of elderly patients to identify early signs of dementia; assessing the professionalism levels of workers in action; or rating high school students' debating skills as they engage in team competitions.

6.2.1.2 Product-Based Assessments

In contrast to the above, **product-based assessments** require respondents to create tangible products that yield evidence of the selected constructs. It is the product, as developed by the respondents, that is scored for measurement purposes. Unlike the usually timed and more structured essay testing formats, product-based assessments may incorporate less constraints, typically allowing generous time limits. We should remember that even when the domains involve process-based indicators, it is the *product* generated eventually that is the focus of the assessment exercise. (Refer to Chapters 4 and 5 for definitions of process and product indicators in cognitive ability domains.)

See Boxes 6.1 and 6.2 next for an example of a product-based assessment accompanied with a holistic scoring rubric. This tool was developed for assessing the competency levels of specialized trainers in the health care industry who would be providing training to medical staff located at various clinics/hospital systems. The assessment aims to measure the trainers' knowledge and skill levels in a biomedical informatics domain.

The task in Box 6.1 is intended to be administered as an end-of-course classroom assessment where the "trainers under training" are expected to have received relevant coursework beforehand at community colleges. The product that trainers are asked to prepare is an instructive handout or document that could be usefully incorporated within a typical training session.

The specific content tested focuses on standards applicable to the electronic health records (EHRs) of patients. This is a highly specialized biomedical informatics domain that deals with maintaining and giving health care providers access to patient data electronically, in compliance with laws and data standards relevant to protecting information security and patients' privacy rights. The larger project, described in further detail later in this chapter and Chapter 12, is one where the design teams applied the Process Model to design a tri-partite training curriculum for community college instructors, including (1) domains of expected learning outcomes, (2) matching instructional materials, and (3) domain-referenced classroom assessments. One

BOX 6.1 A Product-Based Assessment Task

Task Description

Directions to examinees.

In this scenario, imagine you are training a group of medical professionals to meet public health information standards when using a new electronic health record system at your hospital or clinic.

With specific examples, prepare a document that explains in a convincing manner why each of the following **six** aspects of public health information standards will reduce errors and improve patient care. Point out the consequences of noncompliance or oversight.

Prepare a finished document (not a draft) for distribution to trainees during a training session. The statement must be one to three typed, double-spaced pages in length. List three to five key literature sources. You may take 24 hours to complete this task. Submit your finished document via the online portal.

Public Health Information Standards

- Clinical data representation
- Medication terminology
- Organizational context
- Grammar data standards
- Notice of privacy practices
- Health Insurance Portability and Accountability Act security requirements

Note. See Boxes 6.2 and 6.4 for two different scoring rubrics to accompany this task.

of the assessments is displayed in Boxes 6.1 and 6.2 (Chatterji et al., 2017).

Other examples of product-based assessments could variously include items such as laboratory reports (the product) for assessing *science proficiency* levels of students on particular topics (the construct); assessing published works of writers/scholars in given academic disciplines for measuring their *merit or impact levels*; assessing the annual financial reports prepared by company managers to determine their *productivity levels*; or examining the quality of lesson plans prepared by classroom instructors to ascertain their *teaching competence*.

6.2.1.3 Portfolio-Based Assessments

Portfolio-based assessments are distinct from the preceding two types in that they draw on *collections* of work samples, creative products, behavioral observation records, or some combinations of such items for evidence on the constructs and characteristics we elect to measure. The items are compiled intentionally in the portfolio, and by design, the portfolios may contain domain-relevant personal reflections from the respondents themselves, as well as of examiners and other participants (such as parents of school-goers). Similarly, depending on the assessment purposes and design specifications, the items could be collected at one or a number of time points. In portfolios for measuring growth—for instance, see Table 6.1—items may be gathered at multiple but designated time points within a given time period. In other applications, an end-of-grade portfolio could "showcase" an individual student's best works in a curricular domain at a single time point only. To enable construct-relevant inferences, portfolio-based assessments typically require users to integrate information collected via more than one data source or assessment method, setting, or observation time point (Butler, 1997; Klenowski, Askew, & Carnell, 2006; Santos, 1997).

Although useful at all education levels, portfolios are often a preferred assessment method in professional and higher education systems that prefer to move away from traditional marking systems and grade point averages (GPA). One or more of the following reasons could guide that choice (Herman et al., 1992; Klenowski et al., 2006; McMullan et al., 2003).

1. Appropriately designed portfolios could serve several different assessment purposes in education systems—instruction, assessment, program evaluation, or other forms of administrative decision making.
2. Work samples in a portfolio could provide measures of cognitive process indicators (e.g., *using scientific reasoning when preparing a laboratory record*), as well as product- and outcome-based indicators (e.g., *reporting results of an experiment in a laboratory record*).
3. Portfolio-based assessments may easily be integrated with daily classroom instruction so that testing is not a one-time procedure, but an ongoing process.
4. Portfolios can be designed collaboratively with the involvement of various participants outside the instructors, such as the students, educational professionals, or parents.
5. Finally, portfolio-based assessments could facilitate ongoing **metacognition** by participants via embedded self-reflection and self-evaluative exercises.

BOX 6.2 Holistic Scoring Rubric for a Product-Based Assessment Task

Product: A training document to promote compliance with selected public health information standards

Product quality score	Description of performance
4	A. The training document and list of references show that trainer is well informed of the selected *six areas* of public health information standards. Reasonably argues for all six aspects of standards and highlights the importance of each. Examples of noncompliance or violation are realistic and meaningful. Concepts, definitions, and terms are accurately presented in a coherent, compelling, and well-written statement useful for training purposes and audience.
3	B. Argues reasonably for *most* aspects and the document meets task instructions and criteria. Accurately describes and highlights the importance of standards when implementing electronic health records, but there are *minor errors or omissions*. Specific examples are appropriate. Statement is well written overall and useful for training purposes and audience.
2	C. Argues for *at least three* aspects of standards. Meets *some* task instructions and highlights the importance of standards. Some examples are specific and applicable, but there are *several errors or omissions* that make the statement less compelling or incomplete for training purposes. Statement may be descriptive rather than persuasive even when well written.
1	D. Fails to address standards completely or overlooks *more than three aspects*. Fails to explain or argue for the importance of standards. Examples are missing or limited and/or there are *major inaccuracies, errors, or omissions* that make the statement unacceptable or inadequate for training purposes.

Source: Adapted from Chatterji et al. (2017).

Table 6.1 shows a portfolio designed to map the growth of young children ages 4–8 years in selected handwriting and English-language skills at the elementary school level (adapted from Chatterji, 2003). In the example, teachers collected a fixed number of writing samples at three time points during the academic year. At each time point, a child's performance is rated using a set of developmentally ordered indicators. As evident, some are behavioral process indicators, calling for direct observations of children as they work (e.g., demonstrating directionality while writing). Others are outcome-based indicators, reflecting the expected end-products of learning (e.g., knowledge of upper and lowercase letters in print). The observed evidence from the writing samples collected is rated with a multipoint scale. The rating method is a choice made by the designers; as children develop, each individual's rated profile is expected to shift rightward with greater evidence on the more advanced indicators (e.g., writing in cursive).

Other examples of portfolio-based assessments could also include assessing a professional photographer's portfolio of selected works to mark a career milestone; examining a student's portfolio of original written compositions to evaluate end-of-term performance in a creative writing course; or measuring worker development in professional areas valued at the workplace.

6.2.2 Historical Examples of Performance Assessments

Looking back at Chapter 2, we learned that uses of performance assessments in China date as far back as 1000–2000 B.C.E. The Chinese conducted very high-stakes civil service examinations to select promising officials to the highest ministerial positions. Their tests included subject areas like arithmetic, music, horsemanship, geography, the practice of civil law, writing, applying Confucian principles, and demonstrating knowledge of public and private ceremonial practices; however, not much documentation exists on *how* these examinations were constructed (Allen & Yen, 2002; Cohen et al., 2022).

Similarly, there is evidence that performance assessments were prevalent among early **progressive education** enthusiasts in the United States (Cremin, 1961; see Chapter 2). While little consensus existed on the exact definition of progressive education when the concept originated, recall that the movement emphasized the principles of *learning by doing*. These teaching and learning ideals emphasized students' problem-solving, creative, and critical-thinking skills. Progressives, therefore, leaned toward student-developed projects and products for evidence of student learning and achievement (Aikin, 1942; Dewey, 1897, 1902; Smith & Tyler, 1942; see also *http://education.stateuniversity.com/pages/1947/Eight-Year-Study.html*).

Education reforms in the 1990s revived **alternative assessments** in American public education as a protest against the overuse of multiple-choice tests to measure basic skills (Jaeger & Tittle, 1980; see Chapter 2). In contrast to the **behaviorist view** that had dominated earlier testing approaches, American educational reformers shifted toward **constructivist views** of teaching, learning, and assessment, with many emphasizing the usefulness of performance assessment modes (Herman et al., 1992). Modern standardized testing programs continue to include constructed response tasks in grade K–12 assessments (see item examples at *www.smarterbalanced.org/assessments/sample-questions* and PARRC at *https://parcc.pearson.com/practice-tests/*).

Finally, recall that Binet (1909) created one of the earliest performance tests of human intelligence, incorporating a combination of verbal and nonverbal tasks for multiage children. Three historically recorded tasks on the original test were (Crocker & Algina, 2006, pp. 9–10): *Point to eyes, ears and nose* (age 3); *Indicate omissions in this drawing and repeat with five different figures* (age 7); and *Criticize sentences containing absurdities* (age 11). The tasks were individually administered to each child. The original Binet test was intended to measure the so-called educability levels of children for placement in appropriate educational settings. Binet's age-referenced **norms tables** for interpreting their responses to tasks were something of a breakthrough then in the measurement of children's intelligence (Du Bois, 1970; R. M. Thorndike, 1990; Ward et al., 1996; see Chapter 2).

QUICK RECAP: Performance assessments are a broad category of instruments that utilize a variety of optional response modalities and techniques,

TABLE 6.1. Portfolio-Based Assessment for Mapping Longitudinal Progress

Writing Development Summary Form

Child's Name: ______________________ Grade: __________

Note to the Teacher: *This checklist must be completed by the teacher based on observations made of the child in class, as well as reviews of informal or formal writing samples in the child's portfolio. Please share with the student, parents, or guardians at appropriate times.*

Checklist codes: Y = Observed N = Not observed U = Unable to determine or not applicable

	Work sample description (alphabet writing, creative writing, informal notes, journal writing, etc.)	Date reviewed	Teacher comments
1.			
2.			
3.			
4.			
5.			

Items:	Semester 1	Semester 2	Year-end
1. Holds pencil properly when writing.			
2. Shows left to right directionality when writing.			
3. Shows correct posture when writing.			
4. Has correct paper position when writing.			
5. Prints uppercase letters correctly (How many?).			
6. Prints lowercase letters correctly in print (How many?).			
7. Writes uppercase letters correctly in cursive (How many?).			
8. Writes lowercase letter correctly in cursive (How many?).			
9. Spaces correctly between words in sentences.			
10. Demonstrates mastery of the complete alphabet in writing samples.			
11. Uses basic punctuation marks when writing (period, comma, question mark).			
12. Uses capital letters correctly.			
13 Prints words and short sentences legibly.			
14. Writes words and short sentences legibly in cursive.			

Please fill in this section based on discussions with the student and parents/guardian.

Other indicators (teacher comments):

What can we work on next?

deployable under a wide range of conditions. Depending on user needs, the assessments may be designed with different degrees of structure. A vast majority of these procedures incorporate subjective judgments of external observers and/or judges and, hence, are vulnerable to human errors. The tools are useful for measuring a range of constructs, including those relevant to educational, workplace, social, or clinical contexts. Centuries-old examples of these assessment methods exist to this day.

Reflection Break 6.1: Objectives 1 and 2

- A. Review the measurement scenarios in *italics* (Items 1–6) next. For each, identify the specific performance assessment modality and the targeted construct(s). Choose from the options (a–e) given.
  - a. Behavior-based?
  - b. Product-based?
  - c. Portfolio-based?
  - d. A combination?
  - e. Other? (Explain.)
    1. *Measuring a health professional's history-taking abilities with adult clients and patients, before they prepare their treatment and service plans*
    2. *Measuring the comprehensiveness and accuracy of a psychologist's formal written report after diagnostic testing of a client*
    3. *Measuring a teacher's pedagogical abilities based on a prepared syllabus*
    4. *Measuring a worker's ability to lead culturally diverse teams based on personal journal records and observations made by supervisors*
    5. *Assessing a doctoral student's depth of knowledge of a topic based on their oral presentation and defense of the dissertation*
    6. *Your own assessment scenario (describe the assessment type(s) and identify the constructs being measured, as may apply)*
- B. For each scenario, is the specific performance modality (or modalities) well matched to the suggested construct(s)? If not, how would you improve the assessment operations to better measure the same? Explain your answers.

6.3 Advantages of the Performance Assessment Format

In comparison with structured-response tests explored in Chapter 5, performance assessments could add several design-related complications and burdens. Yet, the performance format is necessary in some circumstances. When the fit is close with the specified indicators of the construct domains, a performance response affords several advantages from an overall construct validity standpoint. Importantly, the format allows us to:

- See the construct differently and sometimes more comprehensively than may otherwise be possible.
- Gain insights into situation-specific aspects of a construct that may otherwise be elusive or overlooked during measurement.
- Incorporate key facets of a complex construct into the design and scoring procedures, allowing improvements to the intended inferences and uses of measures.

6.3.1 Seeing Construct Complexity

To maximize validity of measures, we must be able to "see" the intended construct as fully as possible. Performance assessments of different types afford new and more comprehensive ways of seeing, or being able to see, aspects of constructs that we might otherwise not be able to reach and, therefore, measure. Selecting the best-fitting response or performance modality for different parts of a complex construct domain is central to good assessment design. For illustration purposes, we look at competency domains in selected professional fields that encompass indicators from multiple constructs or dimensions, most of which are deemed important by their respective assessment users.

Consider the measurement of classroom teaching abilities as operationalized in the Performance Based Teacher Education (PBTE) program of the

1990s (Mayher, 1990). The PBTE assessment designers viewed teaching ability as "a mental state which underlies and is enacted in performance. . . ." Their procedures therefore required direct observations of live teaching events, targeting a complex set of indicators that could only be marginally addressed with traditional structured-response tests. Simultaneously, the designers recognized that "the structure of [teaching] competence is so complex, as are the contexts which influence and affect how it is employed, . . . [that one] cannot determine the competence by only observing performance" (Mayher, 1990, pp. 278–279).

Similarly, for assessing the demonstrable aspects of medical expertise of physicians on a developmental continuum, George Miller (1990) delineated a general, hierarchical framework that expert physicians would display on-the-job once they progressed from being novices under training to practising experts in clinical settings. Shown in Figure 6.2, Miller's now famous pyramid has easy-to-remember labels at each level of expertise without specifying the exact content knowledge and skills that physicians would display (i.e., the domain-specific indicators would change for doctors in various medical specialty areas, like internal medicine, paediatrics, orthopedics, etc.).

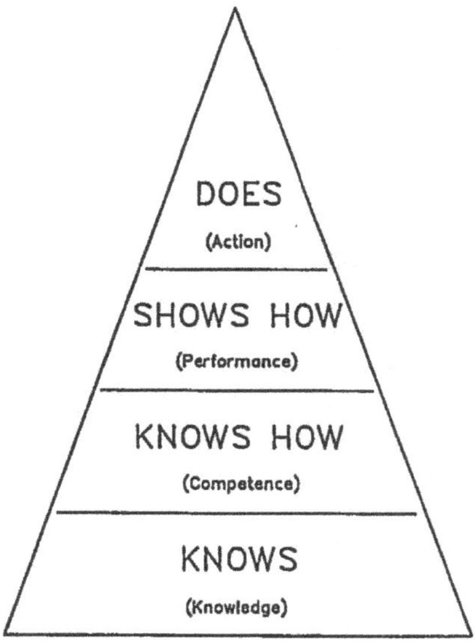

FIGURE 6.2. A hierarchical taxonomy: Four levels of expertise for designing competency-based performance assessments. Reprinted with permission from Miller (1990). © Wolters Kluwer Health, Inc.

As we see, the levels progress from a beginner-level performance ("knows," a level expected minimally of junior medical students), on to the intermediate level ("knows how"), leading to the next higher level ("shows how," expected typically in resident physicians undergoing graduate-level training), and peaking at the highest expertise level ("does," expected in fully trained doctors). Miller concluded that "no single assessment method could provide all the data required for judgment of anything so complex as the delivery of professional services by a physician" (Miller, 1990, p. 563).[1] He also observed that medical assessments often fall short in sampling the three highest levels of his pyramid adequately, and in practice settings, the total number of observational assessments of medical students and resident physicians is too few (Miller, 1990, pp. 563–565).

Each level of Miller's pyramid might require designers to select a different assessment modality that is best matched to it. While "knows" and "knows how" levels could be measured satisfactorily and efficiently with structured-response or constructed-response testing formats (Chapter 5), one or more of the performance formats in Chapter 6 might be desirable for measuring the "shows how" and "does" levels demanding complex cognitive processes and hands-on skills. Note that Miller's pyramid is general enough to be applicable for the measurement of teaching competence, as well as competency domains in other applied professions.

For a final example, consider another multilayered domain, *management competency*, as theorized and operationalized in workplace contexts. According to the vast literature on this topic, able leaders of organizations should embody and display a complex and diverse array of abilities, skills, and traits (see, e.g., Freeman, 2010; Northouse, 2018; Sedera & Gable, 2010; Thornton & Byham, 1982). Of these, *communication skills* is a subcompetency area, common to

[1]Chapter 4 presented several taxonomies akin to Figure 6.2 to classify indicators in various domains, such as Bloom's taxonomy and its derivative, the functional taxonomy, as offered in this book. Miller's pyramid may be viewed as a similarly useful taxonomy for domain specification purposes; applications will follow in the design sections of this chapter.

most theoretical formulations of management competence.[2]

Minimally, according to this literature, communication skills involve the subskills of listening, reading, writing, speaking, and responding (Jackson, 2014; Palmer, 2014; Smith, 2005). Written communication skills could also be assessed directly through essay-types of exercises, or indirectly in this instance, via opinion surveys of an organization's employees. But performance assessment formats afford a different and more authentic lens for "seeing" the construct couched in the actual conditions of a workplace. For example, two competency indicators that would make performance assessments a better match than any other alternative, would be the following:

- Competent leaders frame a vision in writing for the company through easy-to-access, meaningful, and inspirational publications. [*product-based assessment*]
- Effective leaders articulate the company's vision to employees via stimulating speeches and formal presentations, as well as informal conversations held at the workplace. [*behavior-based assessment*]

6.3.2 Situation-Specific Performances

Another advantage of the performance format is that it affords the measurement of **situation-specific performances**. Situation specificity means that some parts of the targeted domains must be exhibited in a particularized setting, often authentic or "real-world" contexts. To maximize validity, we must see the performance *in context*, such as in actual schools, work organizations, homes, or communities. Situation-specific performances raise the demands and difficulty levels of tasks, as compared to assessments couched in artificially structured or simulated settings. On the other hand, they are less controllable exercises, exposing the measurements to various external sources of error—a topic we will review in the next section. Consider next examples of *authentically situated* versus *simulated* performance tests falling under situation-specific performance assessments.

6.3.2.1 Performances in Authentic Contexts

When the construct domain is defined by conditional action-taking skills, a situation-specific performance mode in a real context is preferred for optimizing validity. Say, in an application of Miller's pyramid, doctors-in-training are required to "show how" to perform physical examinations of patients in hospitals and communicate those findings to real patients in lay terms. Here, an authentically situated assessment may be the best match. In a situation-specific performance test, the doctors would have to demonstrate the requisite skills competently amidst the dynamic, unpredictable day-to-day conditions of a hospital or clinic—a more difficult task that closely matches the real conditions of a medical practice setting.

Similarly, given the complex construct in the PBTE program (Mayher, 1990), the observation measures were taken while the teachers taught real classes of students. The unscripted and natural school environments added context-specific challenges, increasing difficulty levels of teaching tasks and altering the construct definition. The designers deliberately selected a situation-specific, performance assessment method as the most apt technique in this case.

Consider another, more recent assessment design case that focuses on measurement of subject matter competence of teachers. Here, Gitomer, Phelps, and colleagues (2014) and Gitomer and Zisk (2015) decided on situation-specific performance assessments instead of an alternative testing mode. These authors started by specifying what teachers with greater mastery of subject matter would be *able to do while teaching* their classes in mathematics and English language arts. Adopting this conception of teaching competence would mean that we have to observe teachers in action in classroom situations to infer their levels of subject matter mastery.

Table 6.2 shows an excerpt of their situation-specific domain with a sampling of indicators. In this operational definition, teachers with greater subject matter knowledge are expected to:

[2]Up-to-date job analyses in different industries may reveal sector-specific variations in definitions, but some other domains, according to the management literature, are initiative, leadership, stakeholder and customer orientation, motivation and energy levels, budgeting and planning, organization, delegation, negotiation, nimbleness and learning agility, knowledge and information management, recruitment and hiring, resource management, and judgment and decision making.

- Anticipate student misconceptions.
- Tackle student challenges and questions ably.
- Explain concepts in multiple ways to improve student understandings of a topic.
- Perform the academic tasks they expect of their students in a competent way themselves, and so on.

The authors defined subject matter competence with the similar sets of situation-specific indicators in both subjects, as shown (Gitomer & Zisk, 2015, pp. 22–23).

6.3.2.2 Simulated Performance Assessments

Not all performance assessments can be realistically situated in actual or natural settings. Here, designers could craft "simulated" performance assessments by creating artificial environments where the conditions mimic actual events and conditions, but with controls instituted deliberately. Two examples follow.

The business management literature introduced the notion of **situational testing** at so-called assessment centers, where workers took performance tasks in simulated organizational situations (Bass, Burger, Doktor, & Barrett, 1979). The skills assessed, such as negotiation skills, were demonstrated under conditions carefully orchestrated at the centers while allowing direct observations to be made—either through glass partitions for one-way viewing by external observers or the presence of human observers at the assessment centers.

In modern examples of simulated but situated performance testing, we find designers capitalizing on video and Web technologies. One example, emerging in the medical education literature, is called a *serious game* or *serious video game*. The technique involves interactive online exercises that test a doctor or trainee's responses to a simulated medical scenario, usually a patient-in-crisis case. Typically, serious games are accompanied with built-in behavioral checklists or rating systems that track responses entered by trainees as they engage in the game, bypassing the need for external observers. The resulting assessment data can then be used formatively for feedback and debriefing purposes, or in a summative manner for end-of-program certification, research, or evaluation purposes (see, e.g., Blum, Muret-Wagstaff, Boulet, Cooper, & Petrusa, 2018; Lee, Chen, Landau, & Chatterji, 2019a; Lee et al., 2019b, 2023).

6.3.3 Measuring Key Facets of Performance

Lastly, performance formats afford the design of **many-faceted assessment systems**—this may be viewed as an advantage for both assessment designers and users. The logic of a many-faceted assessment system has been applied traditionally in psychometric analysis related to **generalizability theory** and **many-faceted Rasch measurement** methods (see Brennan, 1984; Linacre, 2006; Linacre & Wright, 2002; Shavelson et al., 1989; see Chapters 10 and 11 for further discussion). While many-faceted data analyses techniques are usually applied *post hoc* (or after the assessment data are collected), it is useful for designers to think about the important "facets" of a performance proactively during the assessment design phases.

The term **facet** in an assessment design context refers to the identifiable parts of an assessment that are systematically intended to interact and influence the variance of numeric measures of respondents. Conceptualizing a performance assessment as a many-faceted assessment system in a deliberate manner helps give structure to the ensuing operations and scoring procedures. It also alerts us to the controls that we would need to build into the instrument to manage anticipated sources of error.

To elaborate, let's start with an illustration of a two-faceted knowledge test made up of multiple-choice items. Implicitly, most assessment designers conceptualize such a test with two systematically interacting facets: the *items* on the test and the *examinees*. When taking the test, each examinee (Facet 1) is logically expected to interact with each item (Facet 2) and respond based on their ability level in the domain. Barring any outside interferences, the two-faceted *Examinee* × *Item* system is expected to produce item-level responses for each test-taker, which then yield the scaled construct measures thereafter.

Two-faceted system of a multiple-choice test

Examinees × Items = Score (all else held constant, controlled, or managed)

TABLE 6.2. Measuring Content Knowledge of Teachers with Behavior-Based Assessments: Classroom Actions and Indicators

Indicators	What teachers of mathematics would do	What teachers of English language arts would do
1. Anticipates student challenges, misconceptions, partial misconceptions, alternate conceptions, strengths, interests, capabilities, and background knowledge.	• Anticipate student challenges in reasoning about and doing mathematics due to the interplay of content demands and students' understanding. • Anticipate likely misconceptions, partial conceptions, and alternate conceptions about particular mathematics content and practices.	• Anticipate the impact of limited English-language proficiency on students' comprehension of text and speech and on their written and spoken expressions. • Anticipate how students' background knowledge, life experiences, and cultural background can interact with new ELA concepts, texts, resources, and processes.
2. Evaluates student ideas evident in work, talk, actions, and interactions.	• Evaluate student work, talk, and actions in order to identify conceptions in mathematics, including incorrect of partial conceptions. • Evaluate nonstandard responses for evidence of mathematical understanding and in terms of efficiency, validity, and generalizability.	• Evaluate student work, talk, and actions for evidence of strengths and weaknesses in reading, writing, speaking, and listening. • Evaluate discussion among groups of students for evidence of understanding ELA concepts, texts, and processes.
3. Explains concepts, procedures, representations, models, examples, definitions, and hypotheses.	• Explain mathematical concepts or why a mathematical idea is "true." • Interpret a particular representation in multiple ways to further understanding.	• Explain literary or language concepts, using definitions, concepts, and analogies when appropriate. • Explain processes of reading, including why certain processes are appropriate for particular texts and/or tasks.
4. Creates and adapts resources for instruction (examples, models, representations, explanations, definitions, hypotheses, procedures)	• Create and adapt examples that support particular mathematical strategies or to address particular student questions, misconceptions, or challenges with content. • Adapt student-generated conjectures to support instructional purposes.	• Create and adapt examples or model texts to introduce a concept or to demonstrate a literary technique or a reading, writing, or speaking strategy. • Create and adapt analogies to support student understanding of ELA concepts, texts, and processes.

Note. Adapted with permission from Gitomer and Zisk (2015). © Sage Publications.

Note that if the test is designed well (i.e., with well-written items, directions, etc.), other external errors and interferences are expected to be minimal, thus yielding scores that reflect the true ability levels of the examinees as closely as possible on the tested domains. Typically, the test scores will present as a **variable** (Chapter 1). That is, the scores will vary from person to person as their individual ability levels also vary.

If we turn now to designing a performance assessment, minimally, we would require the involvement of observers or judges as a part of the assessment operations. The typical performance assessment, therefore, would yield scores that are governed by *at least* three facets instead of two: (1) items in the domain or the *performance tasks*, (2) the human respondents, and (3) the human judges/observers. Most performance assessments are conceptualized as three-faceted assessment systems, as follows:

Three-faceted system of a performance assessment

Examinees × Tasks × Observers/Judges = Score (all else held constant, controlled, or managed)

Here, by the intention of the designers, a well-designed assessment would yield scores moderated systematically by the above three facets. For this to occur with minimal errors entering the assessment process from elsewhere, we need to take a number of design-related actions—such as prepare clear and user-friendly task instructions, institute controls in the environmental conditions, create well-written observation and scoring guidelines, and orient judges so that they comply with the guidelines during assessment, and so on.

How might specific design-related actions on **key facets** of a performance tool affect validity, reliability, and utility of measured constructs? See Table 6.3 for an illustrative four-faceted assessment in science education, where students are asked to show what they know in two settings: the classroom (simulated) or laboratory (authentic). Table 6.4 reviews how each design action we take—not an exhaustive list—may be tied to the concepts of validity, reliability, and utility. By building in effective controls during design, we could equip an assessment to yield scores that vary as closely as possible as the true levels of respondents in a domain, with minimal errors or issues.

TABLE 6.3. Four-Faceted Performance Assessment in Science Education: Evaluating the Design Implications

Key facet	How many? (number of elements in the facet)	Will the facet directly impact the measures?	Assessment design implications? (examples of actions to improve validity, reliability, and/or utility)
1. Students/ respondents	20 students	Yes	• Provide clear instructions and rubrics to students on task requirements. • Ensure students had prior opportunities to learn and practice with similar tasks.
2. Tasks	5 problems	Yes	• Align tasks and scoring rubrics with construct domains. • Match the conditions and materials to curricular requirements and student needs. • Adapt task conditions and instructions to meet diverse or disabled student needs.
3. Settings	2 classroom (simulated) versus laboratory (authentic) task demonstration sites	No	• Set common task demonstration parameters at both sites. • Standardize observation conditions and protocols at both sites.
4. Observers/ examiners	10 instructors	Yes	• Provide clear guidelines and rubrics for observers. • Provide observers with illustrative models, training, or practice in assessing.

TABLE 6.4. A Checklist for Improving Validity, Reliability, and Utility of Performance Assessments

Quality criteria	Steps to take	How it helps
1. *Validity* *Meaningfulness of the measures with respect to the constructs in the specified population units and for the specified inferences and uses*	• Match performance tasks with indicators in the construct domains • Match scoring rubrics with indicators in the construct domains • Match situation-specific task conditions with construct definitions • Ensure respondents have prior exposure and/or practice with similar tasks (with rubrics), including diverse or disabled individuals • Consider diverse or disabled respondent needs when writing instructions and setting up task conditions	Ensures that systematic interferences are kept to a minimum
2. *Reliability* *The extent to which the measures remain consistent and free from random disturbances*	• Provide clear task instructions to respondents, assessment users, and judges • Include a sufficient number of tasks or task demonstration opportunities for respondents (up to a point) • Provide clearly written scoring rubrics, observation guidelines, and/or training for judges, examinees, and assessment administrators • Standardize assessment conditions at different sites (time, equipment, materials, quiet environment)	Ensures that random measurement errors are kept to a minimum
3. *Utility* *Usefulness—The extent to which the instrument and measures benefit the primary users, as intended* *Usability—The extent to which the instrument and measures are practical and easy to implement*	• Pilot-test the tool to evaluate user access levels, transparency, and barriers to implementation • Ensure that assessment is not too lengthy, time-consuming, or costly for primary users • Evaluate the consequences of assessment use on primary users • Revise the assessment based on feedback from respondents and primary users	Ensures transparency, practicality, and benefits for primary users

In many scenarios, there could be *more* than three or four facets to a performance, or nuances to the facets of performance, that we must consider. Using the previous medical example again, suppose we wanted to develop a situation-specific performance assessment of medical school students on their skill levels in diagnosing the health needs of patients, as before. Suppose also that the trainees are examined in *two* settings on this task: independently in unsupervised settings of hospitals, and in supervised settings at university clinics. Here, assessment users (say, the academic instructors and program directors) might desire a separate score from each setting, leading to *four* relevant facets, as follows:

Four-faceted system of a medical performance assessment in two settings

Examinees × Tasks × Observers/Judges × Settings (Hospitals vs. Clinics) =

Score 1 (Setting 1: supervised performances in clinics)

Score 2 (Setting 2: unsupervised performances in hospitals)

(all else controlled, managed, or held constant)

In another scenario, there could be two or more independent groups of judges, such as senior trainees (peers) and supervising physicians (instructors), each awarding a different score type under each setting. The data from peer assessments might be used for formatively oriented feedback and teaching, and results from the instructor assessments for summative performance decisions. Depending on user priorities, each situation would alter facets of the assessment system that are key to consider during design.

Note that the key facets we *do* identify will impact the construct conceptualization; and the corresponding operations and controls we implement must follow accordingly. For example, more rigorous design procedures would be necessary if summative decisions with the assessment results are a user priority, rather than formative.

> **Four-faceted performance assessment with two groups of observers**
>
> *Examinees* × Tasks × Settings × Observers/Judges (Peers, Instructors) =
>
> *Score 1* (peers: formative assessment, all else controlled or held constant)
>
> *Score 2* (instructors: summative assessment, all else controlled or held constant)

Bear in mind that in different assessment scenarios, the number of relevant facets could vary widely by type and number. Facets could include demographic variables, for instance. Building on Facet 1 (examinees) in the medical example, we could add gender of trainees or year of training as additional facets. Inclusion of a higher number of facets adds greater complexity to the design; but too many facets may also pose implementation burdens, cost barriers, adding other sources of error later. Hence, we should strive for a practical balance between validity, reliability, and utility guided by user interests when selecting facets (Tables 6.3 and 6.4).

Once the key facets are identified, a many-faceted grid like that shown in Table 6.3 is useful step in setting up the **assessment design specifications** for performance assessments. To arrive at Table 6.3, an important question for designers is: "Which facets should count in producing the score, keeping in mind the user-desired inferences and uses of the assessment results?" In the medical assessment scenario from before, we might have several facets to begin with that we would wish to narrow down:

- **Facet 1:** Respondents/examinees (the trainees)
- **Facet 2:** Tasks (patient problems, comprising the range of health issues presented)
- **Facet 3:** Settings (clinics, hospitals)
- **Facet 4:** Judges/examiners (peers, supervisors)

A score could be produced based only on examinees and tasks (Facets 1 and 2), as suggested in Table 6.3, assuming potential errors stemming from the remaining two facets will be adequately controlled as a part of the design process. Suggested actions to shape the assessment design procedures would be similar to the "Implications for design" column.

Reducing a potentially many-faceted system into a simpler two-faceted one (as shown in Table 6.3) is a common approach to designing a performance assessment system. If we take this approach, only one score is produced from the assessment per examinee. The main question for users opting for a two-faceted performance assessment, with conditions in the two settings (clinics vs. hospitals) managed to remain consistent, would be:

> *How did the respondents (trainees in medical scenario) perform across the range of tasks (patient problems), assuming that the judges applied the observation and scoring guidelines as designed, behaving in a consistent and interchangeable manner while observing?*

In an alternate scenario, users may desire separate scores from each setting (Facet 3)—a score under hospital settings and another score in clinics, assuming observers (Facet 4) will not add error variance. Here, the user question would change to:

> *How did the examinees perform across the full range of patient problems in the domain, sorted by type of setting, assuming any error variability on the remaining facets is controlled or negligible?*

In either case, designers would need to take deliberate actions to address potential issues. The **validation** burden for both assessment designers and users, of course, will be to show empirically that the levels of error from various sources *outside* the key facets are tolerable for the assessment purposes. (Later in the chapter, Case Study 3 illustrates how the validation phases might be implemented with the Process Model.)

Finally, multifacted grids like the one illustrated in Table 6.3 could help prevent an assessment from becoming too unwieldy, resource-dependent, or impractical. Because they are time-consuming and resource-dependent, utility is an important consideration with all performance assessments. For example, to optimize reliability of scores—which depends on the number of performance opportunities a respondent is given—designers would need to specify a minimum number necessary. Three task demonstration opportunities for each candidate are more practical than, say, 5 or 10; it is also likely to yield higher reliability estimates than just one or two. Once the instrument is designed, these issues could be investigated during validation.

QUICK RECAP: Performance modalities afford the advantages of revealing aspects of constructs that are typically not obvious and could be overlooked. More than one performance mode may be necessary to measure complex domains. As needed, we could design situation-specific performance assessments in actual, simulated, or structured environments. Recognizing in advance which performance facets will intentionally influence the assessment's scores/results assists in crafting the design specifications, selecting the operations, and building necessary controls within the assessment tool. The key facets we select should be guided by user needs. In choosing a performance modality, one should balance validity, reliability, and utility issues purposefully and judiciously.

Reflection Break 6.2: Objectives 1, 2, and 4

- Identify constructs or complex domains that are better "seen" with one or more of the performance assessment methods in Chapter 6.
- Identify your own examples of a situation-specific *authentic* or *simulated* performance assessment found in (1) workplaces, (2) health care systems (3) education systems, or (4) other settings. Which *context factors* are critical to defining the construct(s) in each example?
- Identify the facets you would value in a performance assessment you might design. Explain why those facets would be "key" in systematically causing the scores to vary.
- Select the best-matched performance assessment mode(s) to measure some of the indicators shown in Table 6.2. Justify your selection using validity, reliability, and utility reasons (see Tables 6.3 and 6.4 for reference).
- Suppose teachers in a music department are designing a performance assessment to test how well students can read and play written music on a piano. They would like to compile three separate measures in a portfolio on each student from (1) informal classroom assessments, (2) an end-of-year examination, and (3) a concert performance. Name each facet that you consider as "key" in this assessment design scenario and explain why. Create a many-faceted grid that could serve as part of the assessment design specifications.

6.4 Disadvantages of Performance Assessments: Human Vulnerabilities, Errors, and Biases

6.4.1 Issues with Task Instructions, Observation Guidelines, and Scoring Rubrics

Recall from Chapter 5 the discussions on *scoring rubrics* for constructed-response tasks, distinguishing between **analytic scoring rubrics** versus **holistic scoring rubrics**. Critical structural components of a performance assessment are the task instructions, observation guidelines, and scoring protocols, the latter typically also called "rubrics." Without guidelines and rubrics for judges and other assessment participants, a performance assessment is incomplete and will be exposed to a number of sources of error. This section describes some of these issues and common solution strategies. We refer again to Boxes 6.1 and 6.2 and Table 6.1 with an added example for illustration purposes.

1. **Rubrics and guidelines tethered clearly to specified construct indicators help contain levels of subjectivity and human error.** No matter their levels of expertise, judges tend to fill the gaps in assessment guidelines and rubrics with their own personal opinions and criteria, leading to invalid, inconsistent, and sometimes unfair scores. To assist judges in remaining faithful to the substantive nature of the constructs, a well-designed task and rubric must be **domain-**

referenced. Tighter alignment with domain specifications raises the **content-based validity** levels of the assessment's results. This design practice is evident in Boxes 6.1 and 6.2. Here, the task, instructions, and rubric were intentionally tied to the user-valued indicators of the domain (e.g., see the bulleted points in the rubric). Similarly, we see the key developmental components from the domain listed in Table 6.1 to draw the teacher's focus to relevant aspects of children's work.

The educational assessment literature recommends that instructors share scoring rubrics with students in advance as a part of their instructional routines. Such practices have been shown to improve student learning, motivation, and self-regulation levels. Rubrics are useful tools in communicating educational expectations clearly and transparently to learners (Brookhart & Chen, 2014).

2. **Observation and scoring guidelines aligned with the desired assessment purposes lower levels of subjectivity and human error.** Inconsistencies arise with observer judgments if there is ambiguity of purpose in designing the observation guidelines or scoring rubrics. For example, when the purpose is to diagnose fine-grained needs of respondents, but the rubric is too general, vague, and holistic in orientation, we are likely to encounter higher levels of subjectivity interfering with the judgments. The opposite could also be true, although analytic rubrics tend to have more flexible properties.

Generally, the holistic approach is useful when summative decision making and efficiency are a user priority. In Boxes 6.1 and 6.2, the tool was designed for end-of-course summative assessment purposes. Holistic scoring, called **global scoring** because of its focus on the whole performance rather than its parts, yields rank-ordered, overall judgments of performance quality. Guided by the rubric in Box 6.2, instructors could assign either a 1, 2, 3, or 4 in the ranking system to the left. A single global rating is generated for summative evaluations of each product's quality.

In contrast, view again the analytic scoring profile in Table 6.1. Although meant for measuring children's growth over time, its purpose is to diagnose strengths or weaknesses along the way on each indicator, facilitating more granular types of formative decision making by teachers. At a given time point, a child could show stronger performance on some, but not other indicators. Well-designed analytic rubrics reveal such differences, carrying diagnostic and formative utility for users to take the next steps. The number of ratings/scores the analytic rubric yields should link directly back to the valued parts of the work sample, performance, or product that users wish to separately assess. Depending on the purposes, it is also possible for an assessment exercise to be scored in part analytically and in part holistically. That is, the item-level ratings/checks may be totalled to obtain an overall score by domain or subdomain. In sum, an advantage of analytic rubrics is that they could be designed to serve both formative and summative purposes. The assessment uses that the primary users prioritize should guide these design decisions.

3. **Well-conceived point allocation schemes lead to less subjectivity and human errors.** In developing scoring guidelines, a major design decision deals with the point allocation schemes that judges will apply for each item or part of a performance. The point allocation choice is usually either in the form of a **checklist** or **rating scale**, with combinations of these also possible for different sets of items on an instrument. Ideally, the scheme should map the expected levels of variability in the quality of products, task performances, or behaviors to be observed as closely as possible. Cataloguing the types of observed misconceptions, omissions, and errors that respondents at different levels typically make is a useful method to calibrate the scales. Subjective variations in judgments arise when the scheme we design or choose overlooks the possibility of unusual but correct responses, or judges encounter unexpected errors or response patterns, such as omissions of specific behaviors or added elements in performances that they deem notable.

As we know, commonly used checklists have two levels, such as

Yes = 1, No = 0

Present = 1, Absent = 0

Observed = 1, Not observed = 0

For a relatively poor checklist allowing subjective variations of judges, descriptors might be

Consistent = 1
Inconsistent = 0

Although widely employed, notice that the more generic descriptors often carry different meanings for different judges. Unless they are defined with explicit and observable descriptors, the use of broad terms like "good," "average," or "consistent," therefore, are ill-advised from a measurement standpoint. We also need to ask the following: "What does each scale point above represent vis-à-vis the domain being measured?"

Rating scales allow for 3-, 4-, 5-, 7-, 10-point, or an even wider range of quality differentiations. Here are two popular, but relatively weak, rating scales:

Poor	Fair	Good	Excellent
1	2	3	4

Below Average	Average	Above Average
1	2	3

Point values on checklists or rating scales function better when anchored with *unambiguous descriptors* that are tied to domain-referenced indicators *and* closely reflect the possible ranges and types of responses we might actually see, thereby promoting more consistent interpretations of performance by judges. An improvement to the 4-point *Poor to Excellent* rating scale shown above could look like this:

Poor: Score 0
Did not attempt to perform the task or omitted significant parts of task, **failing to meet all or most** minimally required professional standards for acceptability.

Fair: Score 1
Performed task in **partial compliance** with several criteria but failed to meet some key professional standards for acceptability.

Good: Score 2
Performed task in **full compliance** with a majority of professional standards and met expectations for acceptability on key indicators.

Excellent: Score 3
Performed task thoroughly in **full compliance** with all professional standards and **exceeded expectations** of acceptable task performance on several indicators.

The standardization of observable error ranges in numeric terms (e.g., "*Examinee demonstrated at least 60% of indicators*") could remove any added ambiguities by defining each performance level with greater clarity. Finally, anchor papers or products tied to each level of a rating scale can further help judges control their subjective variability. With performance assessments, anchors are simply samples of videotaped behaviors, products, or work samples from respondents that vary in terms of quality.

4. Subjectivity from judges is reduced when protocols and guidelines match the observable elements of a performance or product. When there is an ideal order for carrying out a complex task or procedure, or if respondents must engage with specific objects, equipment, or materials to generate products under particular conditions, the guidelines should reflect every observable element and contingency, as these are expected to occur, during the assessment. Consider an assessment illustration next on this point. This assessment was designed to measure how quickly physicians are able to tackle changing conditions in the workplace when dealing with simulated patient crises (excerpted again from Blum et al., 2018, p. 11, Appendix 2, with minor adaptations). The developers offer descriptors of actions that observers should see, with an expected flow of physician activities that would be checked off, such as

- Shows situational awareness.
- Performs rapid and frequent reassessments.
- Prioritizes among multiple tasks.
- Is decisive.
- Is adaptable.
- Manages time, personnel, resources, and so on.

The more closely the instructions and items in rubrics like this match typical respondent behaviors, the expected activity flow, task conditions, and the like, the less room there will be for subjective variability in the recorded observations of judges.

In sum, in the performance assessment environment that designers create, the tasks, instructions for judges and task administrators, as well as scoring rubrics, must all cohere and fit together as one piece. In areas where these alignments are weak, or there are too many oversights, greater levels of subjectivity will tend to occur from judges.

6.4.2 Added Sources of Human Error

Despite our attention to crafting the exercises and scoring rubric well, we must remember that judges may still succumb to other subjective biases and random disturbances. The research literature on issues with judge behaviors, drawing mainly on essays, isolates at least five added threats to which performance assessments are also vulnerable. These are discussed next with counterstrategies to employ (after, e.g., Chatterji, 2003; Hopkins, 1998). Performance assessment results may be compromised due to the following:

1. Halo effect
2. Item or task carryover effect
3. Test or performance carryover effect
4. Order effect
5. Writing/language mechanics/presentation effect

6.4.2.1 Halo Effect

The *halo effect*, a kind of subjective bias, is evident in circumstances where the judge's impression of the respondent on characteristics unrelated to the construct affects the score or rating. This influence usually occurs in a positive direction, although the reverse could also be true. In an Olympic figure skating championship, we would conclude that the halo effect is operating if we found that the U.S. judge tended to award higher ratings to the U.S. skaters, irrespective of their performances. Similarly, teachers are vulnerable to the halo effect whenever they award higher ratings on work produced by their favorite students, regardless of its quality. Conversely, a poor general impression of some students, say, in behavioral areas, might lead teachers to give them unnecessarily harsh ratings on their academic work.

It is possible to control for halo effects by using qualified, external judges who are unknown to the respondents or who have no vested interests in the assessment outcomes for individuals. Blinding names of candidates, or keeping the work anonymous in product-based assessments and essay tasks, also helps reduce this source of error.

6.4.2.2 Item or Task Carryover Effects

This error occurs when the judgment on the first task or performance of a given examinee or respondent carries over to the next task by the same person, influencing the overall score. In the Olympics figure skating championship, if a judge's score of an ice skater's performance on the "short program" influences their judgment on the same person's "long program," we would have an *item* or *task carryover effect*. We encounter the same issue in classroom assessments, when the teacher's rating on the first problem influences the scores on problems that follow on a given student's paper.

To counter task-to-task carryover effects, a useful strategy is to provide guidance to judges to observe/rate a given task for *all* respondents/examinees before beginning on the next task. For example: "Complete the observations on Task 1 for each candidate and, as you proceed from one to the next, assign the score. Next, continue on Task 2 in the same manner. Continue until all tasks are reviewed and scored one at a time, for all the candidates."

6.4.2.3 Performance Carryover Effect

Educational researchers have found that essays of average quality tend to be rated much higher when they are rated after two very poorly written essays, rather than well-written papers. This type of contamination, where the judged performance level of one examinee carries over and influences the scores on the next examinees' papers, is called a *performance* [quality] *carryover effect*. With behavior-based assessments, a performance carryover effect would occur if judgments of the first person's performance colored the judgments of the performers who immediately followed them.

To combat the impacts of the performance carryover effect, examiners are advised to take breaks between observation and scoring sessions, and periodically shuffle products or papers in a random order to alter their mindsets. Similarly, observation sessions should be randomly distributed for individuals observed and reshuffled periodically.

6.4.2.4 Order Effects

The order in which performances, papers, or products are reviewed or individuals observed has also been found to result in inconsistent or poor rating patterns. For instance, prolonged judging sessions and repetitive work can lead to a gradual decline in the quality of ratings on papers at the bottom of a pile, or for a set or observations scheduled at the end of a long day. Typically, this downward slide occurs because of observer or examiner fatigue.

To reverse order effects, judges should take breaks to rejuvenate themselves during long scoring or observation sessions. Again, periodic and random reshuffling of the distributions of observations or papers can similarly counterbalance the order effect.

6.4.2.5 Writing, Speaking, Language, and Presentation Effects

In performance assessments, more polished speaking, crafty visual presentations, or clever language usage and writing skills may interfere with the construct domains being measured. Research shows that judges tend to be influenced by spelling, vocabulary, punctuation, grammar, length of the answer, neatness, or effective presentation skills of respondents. Say, in a world history course examination, test-wise students with little knowledge of the topics bluff their way into earning higher-than-warranted scores by writing very long and creative essays. Here, they are capitalizing on this known vulnerability in human judges who stray away from domain-referenced criteria even when supplied with rubrics.

To address the issue at the source, task instructions should direct examinees to specific content-related expectations and limits of expected responses for a task. In the same vein, rubrics and accompanying instructions for judges should be designed to maximize validity during observation and scoring. Again, the use of "anchors"—samples of videotaped behaviors or products of different quality—are a useful way to keep judges focused on domain-referenced expectations of performance. Providing judges with ample practice and training with the assessment guidelines and rubrics are other ways to limit random issues that may contribute to unreliability.

6.4.3 Diversity Issues and Sources of Systematic Bias

As with all assessments, designers must try to avoid problems of giving unequal levels of access, opportunity, or accommodations to some respondents but not others, resulting in a *conditions bias* or *materials bias*. Typically, vulnerable groups of a population are those belonging to diverse religious, ethnic, or linguistic minorities; developmentally younger children; the aged; or individuals with particular disabilities. To start, the demographic profiles, developmental levels, ages, or special needs of individuals and subgroups in the population to be tested must therefore be explicit in the population specifications (*Who?* in the Process Model, Chapters 1 and 3).

In addition, three potential issues to which we should be alert are **readability bias**, where the verbal barriers—such as very high reading or vocabulary levels in the assessment materials—may exclude some respondents from being able to understand and participate fully in an assessment exercise; **inflammatory bias**, where particular words, graphics, or examples used by designers may inflame or disturb respondents of an identity or demographic group, adversely affecting their performance; and **opportunity-to-learn bias** in educational or training contexts, where a systematic lack of curricular exposure to some groups may lead to their poor performance on assessments. Differential opportunities to perform could arise if technologies or equipment assumed to be available to everyone are actually not. These are labeled as *systematic* sources of error as the interfering factors tend to lower measures predictably in the affected persons or subgroups, undermining validity.

On occasion, designers must allow specific accommodations for disabled individuals, such as use of large print for the visually impaired. Field testing of the assessments with all minority subgroups in advance, and validating and carefully improving the assessment materials, equipment, and so forth, are helpful strategies to avoid such issues and better meet differential needs of diverse respondents.

QUICK RECAP: Performance assessments typically incorporate human judges, increasing the chances for subjectivity and human errors. Disadvantages stemming from the human factor can be addressed with specific design-related actions, such as domain-referencing assessment materials; standardization of the task observation parameters, examiner guidelines, and scoring rubrics; use of specific strategies to counter issues of judge fatigue, personal biases, or erratic behavior patterns. With diverse subpopulations and individuals, designers should strive to avoid systematic biases and issues of differential access or opportunities to perform. These issues usually stem from oversight of a subgroup's profile.

Reflection Break 6.3: Objectives 1–4

- Identify *three* distinguishing features of an *analytic* versus a *holistic* scoring rubric. Which would you prefer for a performance assessment you design? Justify your answer.
- Distinguish between the following for a performance assessment: *task instructions*, *observation guidelines*, and a *scoring rubric*. Why should designers attend to all three areas? Explain.
- *Point allocation schemes should map the expected variability in the types and quality of responses.* Give an illustration to show what this statement means. What design-related actions would you take to apply this principle with a performance assessment? Explain.
- Define each source of error: *halo effect*, *task carryover effect*, *language or presentation effect*, *readability bias*, *inflammatory bias*. Provide an example of each.
- Describe scenarios in which one or more *diversity-related biases* could lead to unfair performance assessment outcomes. Be specific in your answers.
- Human judges who are "experts" in the domains frequently have strong opinions that vary. Do you believe their expertise poses a major threat to generating valid and fair results on performance assessments? Explain what you would do to address this issue.
- List the main *disadvantages* of performance assessments of which designers should be mindful.

6.5 Three Case Studies: Applying the Process Model to Design or Validate Performance Assessments

The chapter now presents three cases in designing and validating performance assessments. It begins with a case study of a behavior-based assessment, followed by one of a product-based assessment, the latter already described partially in Boxes 6.1 and 6.2 in Section 6.2. It concludes by presenting a validation study of a performance assessment for measuring movement disorders in young patients with cerebral palsy. The design of portfolio-based assessments is not treated separately in this section, but the five phases and procedures demonstrated in the other cases would be replicated, as illustrated.

6.5.1 Case Study 1: Designing a Behavior-Based Assessment

Review Boxes 6.3–6.5 and Table 6.5 together. The original instrument in this case, presented with minor adaptations here, was developed by a faculty member affiliated with a hospital-based, educational program in physical therapy (PT) located at the Mount Sinai Medical Center in New York City (P. Belarmino, Jr., personal communication, 2002–2003; Chatterji & Freda, 2003). The *construct* deals with a PT competency domain. The trainees in the case received their training in cardiac care units where the hospital's patients are also housed.

BOX 6.3 Case Study 1: Specifying the Assessment User Context for a Behavior-Based Assessment

Process Model: Phase I. Specifying the Construct, Assessment Purposes, and Population

What? **Construct:** Physical therapy competencies in hospital-based cardiac care units

Why? **Assessment Purposes:** To evaluate (1) individual trainees' proficiency levels in the specified competency domain and (2) program effectiveness.

- *Primary Users:* Faculty, student-trainees, program administrators, leaders, and support personnel of programs

  Specific Uses of Assessment Results:
  - To make summative decisions on trainees' merit levels
  - To make ongoing formative coaching decisions on trainees
  - To evaluate program performance

  Score-Based Inferences:
  - To infer trainees' learning needs and proficiency levels
  - To infer program effectiveness levels

  Trainees' Learning Needs and Proficiency Levels
  - Formative coaching decisions on individual trainees based on the first three (3) of six observations
  - To evaluate program effectiveness based on the average score gains made by the trainees, as compared to previous cohorts

  Program Effectiveness

Who? **Population**

- Enrollees in physical therapy training programs of cardiac care units of university-affiliated hospitals.

  Socioecological Profile:

  Urban setting; includes diverse adult trainees in terms of nationality, race/ethnicity, age, sex, socioeconomic status, first language, disabilities, prior education, and work experience.

Source: Adapted from P. Belarmino, Jr. (personal communication, 2002–2003); Chatterji and Freda (2003).

6.5.1.1 Phase I: Specifying the Assessment Use Context and Primary Users

To begin, the *Why?*, *Who?*, and *What?* questions of the Process Model were answered as shown in Box 6.3. Phase I specifies the *context of assessment use*, identifying the *primary users* of the tool. The primary users belonged to two main groups, with some overlap: the PT program's students, faculty, and leaders; and the institutional administrators responsible for program quality reviews, both internal and external. The faculty planned on making proficiency-based inferences with the assessment results with two decision-making needs at the individual trainee level. They hoped to use scores formatively for teaching purposes or for improving their own instructional methods; and they desired to assign midterm and end-of-program summative grades to each participant. Administrators, in contrast, were interested only in the program-level average performance for each cohort, to be collected at the end of each academic term. Their main interest was in performing internal program evaluations or supplying the assessment data to external auditors for program reviews. The User Paths were 6 and 7, respectively (Chapter 2).

6.5.1.2 Phase II: Specifying the Assessment Operations

Phase II began with specifying the PT domain, subdomains, and a many-facet grid as a part of the assess-

BOX 6.4 Case Study 1: Specifying the Assessment Operations for a Behavior-Based Assessment

Process Model: Phase II

Domain Specifications: See Section 6.5.1.

Assessment Method(s) and Performance Modality: Behavior-based assessment

Task Administration Conditions: This is an individual demonstration exercise for physical therapy trainees. It is accompanied with an analytic rubric that yields total domain scores, subdomain scores, and item-level ratings. Each item is rated on a 3-point scale (0–2) to denote competency levels. The assessment should be conducted after a trainee completes induction at a hospital or clinic. Each observation session should be 30 minutes long.

Situation-Specific Requirements: Skills must be demonstrated while students are serving cardiac patients in hospital-based care and rehabilitation programs. Tasks should be performed with at least six different patient cases that meet parameters in the manual.

Key Facets:
Domain (Subdomains × Items) × Examinees × Instructors

Score Types:
Score 1: For summative decisions, a *domain score* will be produced based on all 25 items.
Score 2: For formative decisions, *subdomain scores* and *item-level rating profiles* will be produced.

Weights: Table shows number of items by indicator. Subdomains 1.1 and 1.2 will carry 10/25 points (40%) weight, while Subdomain 1.3 will carry 5/25 (20%) of the domain score.

Table of Design Specifications Showing Number of Items by Indicator

Subdomain	Taxonomic levels				Points
Indicators	Complex procedural skills	Application	Higher-order thinking—evaluation	Higher-order thinking—analysis synthesis	(Weighted by number of items)
Indicator 1.1	2	4	4	0	***10***
Indicator 1.2	2	4	1	3	***10***
Indicator 1.3	0	3	0	2	***5***
Total points	***4***	***11***	***5***	***5***	***25***

Who Assesses? Clinical instructors
Instructors will be provided with observation manuals and two (2) practice sessions in observing trainees.

Source: See Box 6.3.

ment design operations (Boxes 6.4 and 6.5). To compile a complete set of assessment design specifications, the designer consulted with a number of PT faculty and domain experts in the program. Several clarifications were necessary in the following areas:

- Who will participate in the assessment design procedures?
- Which work or behavior samples are to be included?
- What is the number of times that behaviors will be observed and when?
- How many rubrics should accompany the assessment?
- Who will participate in the selection of work or behavior samples to be rated—only PT instructors, program leaders, students, student peers?
- Who will rate the work or behavior samples, and when will the scoring occur to meet the assessment needs of primary users?
- Under what situation-specific conditions should the student behaviors be demonstrated?
- How can we assure that the assessment is not a burdensome process for instructors, administrators, or others?
- What kinds of training or orientation are necessary for instructors, assessment administrators, or other users to ensure observations are of high quality?

SPECIFYING THE DOMAIN

The domain (an excerpt is shown below) included three subdomains and assumed that trainees had prior mastery of the requisite content knowledge; hence, recall or understanding of concept knowledge level indicators were not represented.

Subdomain 1.0

Culminating training outcome: Physical therapists will present a therapeutic plan after taking the medical history of cardiac patients and conducting a thorough evaluation of each patient's present medical condition.

Embedded Indicators

1.1 Investigate the medical status and past medical history of each patient prior to a physical evaluation. [complex procedural skills]

1.2 Perform the tasks of a PT evaluation safely and systematically following established guidelines. [complex procedural skills]

1.3 Create a comprehensive plan of care for each patient based on evaluated medical condition, PT evaluations, and needs/life circumstances of individual patients. [higher-order thinking]

In each subdomain, the culminating outcomes were classified at the complex procedural skills level using the functional taxonomy and broken down further into embedded indicators to allow the design of sufficiently detailed observation protocols. Several documentary sources provided the current, best practice guidelines relevant to PT and rehabilitation techniques that would apply (e.g., American College of Sports Medicine's exercise prescription guidelines; American Heart Association's exercise guidelines; American Physical Therapy Association's Standards of Practice Act and Code of Ethics; *Guide to Physical Therapy Practice of American Physical Therapy Association* [2nd edition, 2001; see the "Cardio-pulmonary" section]; New York State's Physical Therapy Practice Act). Each subdomain was further broken down to enable detailed observations, as illustrated below for Indicator 1.1:

1.1.1 Compile information on individual patient histories and findings from physical exams. [application]

1.1.2 Evaluate the pathophysiology of the disease process using relevant information from patient files—such as preadmission notes, medical history, consultation notes with doctors and medical staff. [higher-order thinking skills]

1.1.3 Make specific PT service decisions with information gathered on each patient. [higher-order thinking skills]

The designers and users placed an almost exclusive emphasis on more advanced levels of mental processing and skill demonstration, deemed to be a greater priority in the curriculum. Applying Miller's taxonomy (Figure 6.2), trainees were expected to perform at the "shows how" level in each subdomain. Once trained, they would be unsupervised when working with actual patients—an outcome expected of each trainee nearing the end of the training program.

SELECTING THE MOST APPROPRIATE PERFORMANCE MODALITY

An in-depth review of the domain by faculty experts suggested that a behavior-based modality afforded better coverage of a greater number of locally valued indicators of the domain. Four logical steps were necessary in making the selection:

1. Clarifying indicators that defined the construct domain(s) in terms of the embedded content, taxonomic levels, and situation-specific conditions
2. Separating the cognitive process versus product indicators
3. Matching individual indicators or *sets of indicators* with best-fitting performance modalities
4. Evaluating the chosen performance and response modalities by weighing validity, reliability, and utility considerations

OUTLINING THE DESIGN SPECIFICATIONS AND A MANY-FACETED GRID

The design specifications included details on user-desired *facets*, *score types*, *rating scales*, and *weights* to be allocated for different scores generated by subdomain and overall domain. Users prioritized competent demonstration of PT skills by domain and subdomain the most, with an equal emphasis on diagnostic rating profiles and overall scores of trainees. Situation-specific parameters were set for clinical situations under which participants would be observed when in action. A minimum of six observation points were set, with observations beginning after each trainee was inducted. Faculty observers were required to receive some prior training and orientation in the assessment protocols and materials.

Four facets were identified, of which three were prioritized, as shown. Two scores would be generated for formative versus summative decisions, respectively. As there would be multiple program faculty involved in carrying out instruction and assessment duties, the design allowed for some flexibility on the instructor facet.

6.5.1.3 Phase III: Designing the Assessment Instrument

Box 6.5 and Table 6.5 together show an excerpted portion of the final instrument. The assembly and compilation of behavior-based assessment exercises and an accompanying instructor manual required attention to several details:

1. Describing in writing (or selecting) *task scenarios* tied to the competency domain
2. Identifying any *situation-specific conditions*, *materials*, or *equipment* necessary for performance of PT tasks
3. Developing guidelines to establish a standardized system for faculty, students, and assessment users to follow
4. Developing rubrics to generate the item-level diagnostic ratings, subdomain scores, and overall domain scores for user-desired decisions

Table 6.5 presents an excerpt of the tool. The initially drafted instrument had 25 items in all, with a maximum rating of 2 for each item. The analytic rubric generated item-level data, a separate summed score for each subdomain, and the overall domain score. The maximum "total score" on the domain would be 50 (or 2 × 25). The scores would be reported as a percentage of the maximum score possible. A score of 40/50 (80%) is interpreted as the competency level in the overall domain.

INFORMAL REVIEWS, TESTING, AND REVISIONS

The PT faculty-designer reviewed the early drafts of instrument protocols himself and field-tested the rubric informally with a few of his own students; these steps, followed by revisions, were essential to the iterative design process. The initial rating scale had required each trainee to be rated on both *competency* and *consistency* on each indicator. This caused confounding and inconsistencies. The final version retained the

BOX 6.5 Case Study 1: Designing a Behavior-Based Assessment for a Physical Therapy Training Program

Process Model: Phase III

Instructions for Assessment Administrators and Observers

Name of trainee: ______________________________

Name of the hospital/school/program: ______________________________

Name of the clinical instructor (observer): ______________________________

Date of assessment and observation no.: ______________________________

1. Please complete all parts of this form. Rate individual trainee performance based on your judgment of their competence, as observed, with the rating scale provided.
2. See the instructor training manual for definitions of terms and added guidelines.
3. Individual observation sessions should be 30 minutes long.
4. Skills must be demonstrated while students are examining cardiac patients in hospital-based care and rehabilitation programs, using appropriate equipment and materials as needed. Items should be checked separately at each session.
5. To interpret level of competence, please sum the ratings across items by subdomain and domain to compute a total score and percentage score out of the maximum possible score.
6. For the first three (3) formative assessments, trainees may be observed directly or videotaped during the task demonstration and rated afterward. Coaching should be provided soon after using results.
7. Please use only the <u>last three</u> (3) observations of a total of six on each trainee for making summative decisions. Communicate the summative purposes to trainees in advance.

Source: See Box 6.3.

competence dimension only and elaborated the descriptors. The revised observer instructions, shown for a rating of 2 only, read as follows:

> *Performs competently (Rating =2) means that during observation . . .*
>
> - A behavioral task, when performed, complies with standards and guidelines of the American Heart Association, American Physical Therapy Association's Standard of Practice Act and Code of Ethics, and the *Guide to Physical Therapy Practice of American Physical Therapy Association* (2nd edition, 2001; see the "Cardio-pulmonary" section).
> - A behavior is observed that is appropriate for the patient case.
> - A clear pattern of the learned behavior is developing.

6.5.1.4 Phase IV: Validating the Items, Instrument, and Construct Measures

On a more formal level, the designer conducted an internal **content validation** by clinical PT faculty and administrators at the Mount Sinai Medical Center next, whereby the domain specifications and revised instrument guidelines, and the scoring rubrics and situation-specific items, were all reviewed again. The validation inquiry was guided by five criteria:

1. *Content representativeness and coverage.* Does the instrument adequately sample all the important indicators and subdomains in the PT curricular domain?
2. *Content relevance.* Do the instrument's items and subdomains/domain reflect the most up-to-

TABLE 6.5. Case Study 1: Behavior-Based Assessment Showing Ratings for a Hypothetical Trainee

Link to domain Indicators 1.1	Behaviors observed.	Rating categories Very competent (points = 2)	Competent (points = 1)	Not observed or incompetent (points = 0)
1.1.1	Reads medical chart of cardiac patient before performing the PT evaluation.	X		
1.1.1	Discusses with medical staff any medical issues concerning the patient.	X		
1.1.1	Reads the preadmission notes of each patient during the review process.	X		
1.1.1	Takes a medical history of patient and records past and current medical status.		X	
1.1.2	Reads available laboratory reports of the patient, such as blood tests or routine tests. during the review of medical history.			X
1.1.2	Reads current progress notes written in the medical chart of patients while reviewing the medical history.		X	
1.1.2	Consults the medical literature for the specific signs and symptoms of the disease before performing the patient evaluation procedure.			X
1.1.2	Correlates current medical problem(s) against the past medical history of patient.			X
1.1.3	Confirms with the medical staff the etiology of the disease process and rules out possible alternate causes for observed medical conditions.		X	
1.1.3	*Reports (to the clinical instructor) the medical disease process of the patient concisely and correctly based on the steps taken, before a PT evaluation.*		X	
Maximum score (10 items × 2 points) = 20	**Subdomain 1.1 score =** **Percentage score =**	**10** **10:20 (50%)**		
Decision: Formative	**Observer feedback:**			

Note. Adapted with permission from Chatterji and Freda (2003). © Madhabi Chatterji.

date know-how and research in PT techniques for cardiac care patients?

3. *Clarity.* Is the language used in instructions and assessment materials clear?
4. *Usability.* Are task instructions, rubrics. and protocols easy to use? Are the items instructor- and student-friendly? Will the specified number of observations be burdensome for program faculty?
5. *Reliability.* Are there sufficient observation opportunities required to produce reliable measures of PT competence of each trainee at the end of the program?

An external content validation was performed by measurement faculty experts and graduate students at a North American university with which the PT faculty-designer was affiliated. Several added improvements to the instrument followed. For example, additions and revisions made to the faculty guidelines for rating scale interpretation are illustrated next.

Performs competently (Rating =2) means that during observation . . .

- **No change:** A behavioral task listed on the rubric, when performed, complies with standards and guidelines of the American Heart Association, American Physical Therapy Association's Standard of Practice Act and Code of Ethics, and the *Guide to Physical Therapy Practice of American Physical Therapy Association* (2nd edition, 2001, see the "Cardio-pulmonary" section).
- **Added:** Each behavioral task was performed in the recommended order for the specific type of patient case (*Guide to Physical Therapy Practice of American Physical Therapy Association*, 2nd edition, 2001; see the "Cardio-pulmonary" section).
- **Added:** Each behavioral task was done *independently*. Only a few reminders (<3) or leading cues were necessary during task execution.
- **Added:** The candidate did not omit any steps in the sequence of tasks.

As there was some urgency in beginning classroom implementation locally, no **empirical validation** studies were undertaken. However, a second try-out of the tool with two added trainees helped further revise and standardize the item breakdown, patient scenarios, faculty instructions, and scoring rubrics, removing ambiguous areas.

6.5.1.5 Phase V: Evaluating Readiness of the Tool for Use

Although conducted on a small scale, the content validation and local try-outs of the instrument pointed to several issues that were deemed to be satisfactorily resolved by the designers and primary users. The revised tool was therefore disseminated to the clinical instructors for incorporation in their training courses.

6.5.2 Case Study 2: Designing a Product-Based Assessment

6.5.2.1 Public Health Policy Context for the Project

Let us revisit Boxes 6.1 and 6.2 and the accompanying description again as we proceed, alongside Boxes 6.6 and 6.7 and Table 6.6 that follow. Case Study 2 also involves the design of workplace competency assessments, but in the health information technology field.

In 2009, the U.S federal government implemented an initiative called the Health Information Technology for Economic and Clinical Health under the American Recovery and Reinvestment Act. This national initiative called on hospitals and health care systems to maintain electronic health records (EHRs) of patients, and for health care professionals to begin using EHRs meaningfully for improving patient care. To prepare doctors and health care staff in EHR use, the Office of the National Coordinator for Heath Information Technology funded five curriculum development centers at major universities, charging each with designing instructor-friendly curricular materials for delivering in-service training courses to health care professionals. The courses, with instructional modules and classroom assessments, were to be delivered by community college instructors affiliated with the centers. Once finalized, the materials were uploaded onto an online system for national dissemination.

The center established at Columbia University in New York applied the Process Model to guide the overall design processes for 10 curricular modules.

The effort was led by a team of biomedical informatics specialists, measurement-evaluation faculty experts, and public health faculty. We now review the design processes for a product-based assessment from a selected instructional module to prepare student trainers (Chatterji et al., 2017).

6.5.2.2 Phase I: Specifying the Context of Assessment Use and Primary Users

See Box 6.6. This particular assessment focused on measuring trainer proficiency levels in content knowledge and skills relevant to health data standards—the *construct*. The targeted *population* comprised student-trainers who were to be assessed prior to their placement in various health care systems and hospitals. The end-of-course assessment results would be used for certifying trainers as ready for placement, a high-stakes summative purpose. The domain and task specifications were intended for supporting the everyday classroom needs of instructors-at-large.

The *primary users* of the assessments and results were hence prospective course instructors and student participants affiliated with the five university centers. As with the first case, there was also interest here in using the course participant data for conducting national project evaluations. These *secondary users* were the decision-makers/leaders located at the national curriculum centers and federal government sponsors.

6.5.2.3 Phase II: Specifying the Assessment Operations

Again, this product-based exercise was *one* of several tasks and assessments that could have been designed to match the domain excerpted next and design specifications displayed in Boxes 6.6 and 6.7. For this module, the culminating learning outcome required student-trainees to be able to demonstrate their knowledge of data standards and guidelines, as well as develop training materials that could alter practices of health care professionals in accordance with guidelines.

SPECIFYING THE DOMAIN

The domain was specified using a broad literature base in health information technology, and patient privacy

BOX 6.6 Case Study 2: Design Specifications for a Product-Based Assessment in Health Information Technology

Specifying the Assessment User Context

What? **Construct:** Trainer competence

Why? **Assessment Purposes:** To evaluate (1) individual trainer proficiency levels in the competency domain and (2) national project quality

- *Primary Users:* Instructors, student-trainers, national project leaders at university-affiliated curriculum centers

  Specific Uses of Assessment Results:

  - Summative certification decisions on each student-trainer at the end of the course
  - Formative decisions on student-trainers during course delivery
  - National project evaluation at the end of the project

  Score-Based Inferences:

  a. Proficiency levels: To what extent did individual trainers demonstrate competence in the domain?
  b. Knowledge and skill gaps: What are the observed areas of weakness in trainers that could be addressed with feedback, mediation, or revised instruction?
  c. Project quality: To what extent did the project achieve its goals based on the performance of the entire group of trainers on the assessment?

Who? **Population:** Trainers-in-training for the health information technology workforce.

Source: Adapted from Chatterji et al. (2017).

and information security laws. The taxonomic levels of the exiting outcome and three indicators, labeled as course objectives for the module, are shown next.

Exiting Outcome

1.0 Trainers will be able to convince health care professionals to comply with, and apply, health data definitions and standards while upholding patient privacy and confidentiality rights. [higher-order thinking]

Embedded Indicators

6.4 Describe all aspects of EHRs, data definitions, and standards in accurate terms, delineating the role and importance of each. [concept recall and understanding]

6.5 Demonstrate applications of health data definitions, data standards, and patient privacy and confidentiality laws during training sessions in health care systems. [application]

6.6 Prepare compelling communications and training documents to convince professionals to comply with health data definitions and standards. [higher-order thinking]

SELECTING THE APPROPRIATE PERFORMANCE MODALITY

The functional taxonomy was again applied in this case. Two optional assessment formats were selected for the domain tied to this instructional module; online multiple-choice tests were deemed a better match for measuring the concept knowledge indicator. For the culminating outcome demanding a situation-specific performance, the project team selected a student-developed product. This format was viewed as more utilitarian and instructor-friendly than a behavior-based mode.

DESIGN SPECIFICATIONS AND A MANY-FACETED GRID

See the design specifications in Box 6.7. Three facets were identified as key to tighten the design: *Examinee × Tasks × Score Type*. Although instructors could serve as the fourth "judge" facet, as with the first case, the design allowed for adaptability and flexibility on it so

BOX 6.7 Case Study 2: Assessment Operations for a Product-Based Assessment in Health Information Technology

Phase II

Domain Specifications: See excerpts in Section 6.5.2 in Chapter 6.

Assessment Method(s) and Performance Modality Selected: Product-based assessment

Task Administration Conditions: Multiple product-development tasks can be designed to match different content and skills in the domain.

Each task is a take-home product development exercise. It an individual assessment, allowing 24 hours for completion. Each task is accompanied with two domain-referenced rubrics for rating product quality. The holistic rubric is for summative decisions; it should be applied at the end of the course. The analytic rubric is for supporting ongoing formative use by instructors and students.

Situation-Specific Requirements: The products should be suited for training needs and typical conditions found in hospitals and clinics.

Key Facets:
Domain (Subdomains × Items) × Examinees × Instructors/Observers

Score Types:
Score 1: A single product quality score will be produced using the holistic rubric.
Score 2: Item-level quality rating profiles will be produced using the analytic rubric.

Weights: All items will be equally weighted in the total score.

Who Assesses? Health information technology course instructors at community colleges

Source: Adapted from Chatterji et al. (2017).

as to maximize access and usability of the tool in the field.

6.5.2.4 Phase III: Design the Tasks, Assessment Materials, and Rubrics

Now, see Boxes 6.1, 6.2, and 6.7 and Table 6.6 together. Classroom assessments, if designed externally, should be adaptable to local instructor needs (Shepard, 2006). However, some degree of standardization was necessary in the assessment administration and use areas. Parameters were set for the domain indicators, time limits, and "take-home" exercise conditions. Tasks were required to be accompanied with dual rubrics for supporting both formative and summative decision making by classroom instructors. For the particular task shown focusing on six selected data standard topics, summative scoring was supported with a holistic rubric (Box 6.2), while an analytic version was designed for formative scoring (Table 6.6).

6.5.2.5 Phase IV: Validating the Assessment and Construct Measures

Empirical validation efforts lay beyond the scope of the project. However, for meeting the project's national dissemination goals, an external content validation of all curricular materials was considered essential by the design teams. These studies began by carefully selecting teams of qualified *internal* and *external validators* and designing a content validation survey. The validators consisted of subject-area experts, classroom instructors, and public health stakeholders who were already working in health care training or education settings. Validators conducted two rounds of validation, and revisions followed to arrive at the final version of the assessment iteratively.

TABLE 6.6. Case Study 2: Analytic Rubric for a Product-Based Assessment Task

Examining competence of trainers-in-training in health care systems
Product: A training document to promote compliance with selected public health information standards

	Rating scale		
The training document	Points = 3 "Yes," fully or to a great extent	Points = 2 "Yes," to some extent, with minor errors or omissions	Point = 1 "Yes," slightly or not at all, and with several errors or major omissions
1. Discusses *all* required aspects of public health information standards.	X		
2. Highlights the importance of each aspect of standards when using EHRs of patients.			X
3. Provides realistic examples of noncompliance or oversight of standards.			X
4. Provides compelling examples (e.g., consequences to hospital, staff, or patents are clear).	X		
5. Presents concepts, definitions, and terms accurately.		X	
6. Presents information in a coherent manner.			X
7. Is clearly written.			X
8. Is appropriate for the purpose.	X		
9. Is appropriate for the audience.		X	
10. Is compelling (lists authoritative references and is likely to change habits and practices of health care professionals).		X	

Case Study 2 applied similar validation criteria to those in Case Study 1, but with definitions of terms adapted to the project. Namely, these were *content representativeness*, *content relevance*, *usability*, *clarity*, and *reliability*. To evaluate *content relevance*, project teams prioritized the relevance of the assessments to specific workforce roles in addition to verifying the alignment of course objectives, instructional materials and assessments. Pilot testing of the assessment followed at a local community college.

6.5.2.6 Phase V: Evaluating Readiness of Tools for Use

The external validator surveys yielded numeric ratings suggesting largely positive perceptions of the product-based assessment and the curricular products overall. The qualitative comments identified new issues where further enhancements were necessary. One area, for example, was to ensure a tighter connectivity of theory to practice and workforce roles in the assessment. The pilot tests of the assessment with student-trainers in community college classes revealed issues with the holistic rubric as well, showing that scores were restricted to the upper levels (with mostly ratings of 4)! This limitation was attributable to low cognitive demands of the earlier version of the task and better-than-expected prior preparation levels of student-trainees. The domain's indicators were revised thereafter to add application and higher-order thinking levels, as shown, and the difficulty level of the rubric was raised to be more consistent with typical course participants. Following a third round of revisions, the assessment and design specifications were released for classroom use.

6.5.3 Case Study 3: Validation of a Clinical Performance Assessment

For a final case study, we turn to the design of a clinical performance assessment, the Hypertonia Assessment Tool (HAT). The original study presented here did not use the five-phase Process Model as given in this book, but the authors followed several of the recommended steps. This section discusses their reported empirical validation results on the HAT situated within the framework of the Process Model. See Box 6.8 (based on Jethwa et al., 2010).

BOX 6.8 Case Study 3: Validating Item-Level Measures of a Behavior-Based Assessment

The Hypertonia Assessment Tool (HAT)

Results of test–retest reliability, interrater reliability, and validity studies on HAT items and subscales

Subscale	Kappa coefficient
1. *Spasticity*	
Test–retest reliability	1.00
Interrater reliability	0.65
Validity (Physician 1)	0.74
Validity (Physician 2)	0.57
2. *Dystonia*	
Test–retest reliability	**0.43**
Interrater reliability	**0.30**
Validity (Physician 1)	**0.30**
Validity (Physician 2)	0.65
3. *Rigidity*	
Test–retest reliability	1.00
Interrater reliability	0.91
Validity (Physician 1)	1.00
Validity (Physician 2)	0.91

Next steps when applying the Process Model?

Review kappa estimates against criteria for acceptability. Continue improvements until validation results support the intended uses of all subscale measures in clinical contexts.

Source: Adapted with permission from Jetthwa et al. (2010). © John Wiley & Sons.

6.5.3.1 Context for the Study

The HAT is a behavior-based assessment intended to measure *hypertonia* in young children—a syndrome of observable posture and movement disorders that are thought to be rooted in paediatric neurological disturbances. Most common among these is cerebral palsy (CP). Children with CP develop movement and posture difficulties of different types, causing activity limitations that are attributed to damages that may have occurred in the brain during their infancy or fetal development in the womb.

6.5.3.2 Phase I: Specifying the Context of Assessment Use and the Primary Users

Applying the Process Model to the third case, we see that the *construct* measured is hypertonia (*What?*), defined as a preexisting neurological condition in children with CP. In designing the HAT, the researchers specified a broad *population* of North American children aged 2 months to 3 years (*Who?*). In the sample selected for the validation studies, children with both "positive" and "negative" symptoms of CP were included so that the tool's performance could be gauged with a range of normal and non-normal manifestations of the condition.

The instrument was designed for clinical assessments and intervention purposes, as well as for conducting research on children with movement disorders; these were the main *assessment purposes* suggested in the report (*Why?*). The specific clinical inferences to be made from the measures dealt with the severity levels of hypertonia in children with CP and diagnosed three subtypes of movement disorders called dystonia, spasticity, and rigidity. Given the above, the *primary users* of the HAT measures were doctors, researchers, and other clinical professionals involved in studying and caring for children with hypertonia.

6.5.3.3 Phase II: Specifying the Assessment Operations

The report presents a range of observable symptoms of hypertonia, with specific behavioral indicators organized under the three subdomains of dystonia, spasticity, and rigidity, presumably derived from the clinical literature and based on expert knowledge. Given that children's movement and posture issues are observable, a behavior-based response modality seems the most apt. Although the facets are not indicated by the authors, we can infer that there were four (Box 6.8).

- **Facet 1:** Subjects [children in the specified age groups regions]
- **Facet 2:** Items [observable behavioral symptoms] and
- **Facet 3:** Clinical examiners [clinicians]
- **Facet 4:** Score types [item and subscale scores for dystonia, spasticity, and rigidity]

6.5.3.4 Phase III: Designing the HAT

The authors conducted systematic item design work to construct the multi-item observational checklist. To begin with, they developed 14 items grouped under the three **subscales** of spasticity, dystonia, and rigidity. During assessment, individual children were observed in hospital-based care settings, and items were checked by clinically trained professionals (physicians). Each check led to a point. The summed score from all items could generate a total hypertonia score, but this score was not investigated. The focus of the study appeared to be item-level data organized by subscale. A few illustrative items were:

Dystonia (two of nine items)

a. Involuntary twisting movements
b. Variable abnormal postures

Spasticity (two of three items)

a. Presence of spastic catch
b. Hyperreflexia

Rigidity (two of two items)

a. Equal resistance to passive stretch in a bidirectional passive movement of a joint
b. Maintenance of limb position after passive movement

6.5.3.5 Phase IV: Validating the Assessment and Construct Measures

To evaluate whether individual items and subscales could correctly classify CP children as symptomatic versus not, the researchers employed percentage agreement levels between the designers and expert observers. The statistic reported is called the **kappa coefficient**. For interpretation, a kappa value of 0.60 denotes a 60% agreement between pairs of observers on a given child, statistically adjusted for chance factors (including the low prevalence rates of the disease and random bias). The authors used several samples of children to conduct validation studies on the HAT, shown in Box 6.8.

Once designed, the 14 items were first content-validated by two expert physicians (Physician 1 and Physician 2 in Box 6.8). Seven items of the initial set were eliminated through this process as being problematic. On the investigations of validity, agreements ranged from low (0.30 or 30%) to the maximum possible (1.0 or 100%). The problematic subscale appeared to be dystonia, with the remaining two subscales yielding high to very high agreement levels.

The researchers examined reliability levels as well to answer the questions listed below. Again, they employed kappa agreement estimates to yield three separate agreement indices.

1. *Internal consistency reliability index*. Did the item-level checks agree for individual children on all items on a given subscale, indicating *within-person consistency* of the item data by subscale?
2. *Test–retest reliability index*. Did the item-level checks agree for individual children on before and after assessments with a 2-week time gap, indicating stability over time?
3. *Interrater reliability index*. Did the item-level checks agree for individual children across different pairs of observers, suggesting raters were interchangeable?

Results on reliability, as seen, were robust on all items but those on the dystonia subscale.

6.5.3.6 Phase V: Evaluating the Readiness of the HAT for Use

Because the authors conducted validity reviews combined with reliability evaluations, these **empirical validation** results were useful in pinpointing areas in which the tool could be further developed and improved. The overall results (at the time of the study) suggested that the issues identified with the dystonia subscale needed attention. Using a minimal cut point of 50% agreement for acceptability, we see that items were problematic on the dystonia subscale. Added concerns may be raised about the few remaining items (only seven!) on the overall hypertonia scale and subscales, which may be significantly compromised on content relevance and content representativeness. A more comprehensive validation on the HAT might, therefore, be a logical next step to further the instrument's development.

QUICK RECAP: Applying the Process Model to develop performance assessments requires the execution of five iterative phases, Phases I–V, that are replicable regardless of the response modality we choose. Section 6.5 discussed two case studies in designing competency-based performance assessments intended for use in the health care sector. The third case study focused on behavior-based measures of movement disorders in children; the latter illustrated selected steps of the model with results of an empirical validation. Each case study showed different types of evidence useful for content validation or empirical validation purposes.

Reflection Break 6.4: Objectives 4–6

- Based on this chapter, create a checklist to evaluate the quality of a performance assessment that you might adopt from elsewhere.
- Ask a peer to content-validate a performance assessment of your choice. Prepare the steps and guidelines for the content review.
- Teach someone to design a scoring rubric for an open-ended performance assessment task. Which principles did you consider as most essential? Explain.
- Critically evaluate an existing scoring rubric for a performance assessment.
- For a performance assessment you would like to design:
  - Specify the primary users and the context of assessment use.
  - Specify the domain for the construct(s).

- Apply a suitable taxonomy to classify indicators.
- Briefly describe the assessment operations and facets you selected.
- Justify your selection of performance modality using validity, reliability, and/or utility reasons.

6.6 Summary

This chapter focused on behavior-, product-, and portfolio-based assessments. Illustrations with several examples showed the applicability of each modality in measuring a wide range of constructs, from relatively simple to more complex and situation-specific domains. The case studies demonstrated how to apply Phases I–V of the Process Model for behavior- and product-based assessments. The approach emphasizes designing, validating, and improving the usefulness of measures iteratively to optimize their functionality for the specified users in given contexts. The chapter introduced a new taxonomy to specify indicators in competency-based domains that require demonstrations, adding the "shows how" and "does" levels (after Miller, 1990).

The chapter discussed the literature on known vulnerabilities and typical sources of error encountered with performance assessments and the accompanying scoring criteria. Because human judges serve as a major facet of most performance assessments, conceptualizing the instrument as a multifacted assessment system can be advantageous during the design process. Ideally, the facets should be specified in advance to help designers incorporate the necessary controls into the assessment tasks, conditions, materials, and scoring procedures.

CHAPTER 7

Designing Survey-Based and Interview-Based Assessments

7.1 Chapter Overview

7.1.1 Introduction

Chapter 7 is devoted to creating high-quality self-report measures. It focuses on background theory and guidelines for designing various types of survey-based scales, opinion polls, questionnaires, and interview-based instruments. The chapter builds on the introductory information in Chapter 3, treating in greater depth the distinctive features, advantages/disadvantages, and item construction and instrument assembly techniques.

Figure 7.1 connects this chapter with the rest of the book and the overall Process Model. Throughout, readers will encounter examples of a number of construct types measured with self-report instruments; the case study focuses on a noncognitive construct, detailing Phases I–IV for designing a survey-based and an interview-based instrument, respectively.

7.1.2 Chapter Objectives

After reading this chapter and completing the accompanying exercises, the reader should be able to:

1. Identify the distinctive properties, historical applications, and scale development traditions of various types of self-report assessments.
2. Identify constructs best measured with the self-report modality, identifying the specific inferences and uses prioritized in different user contexts.
3. Apply established guidelines for constructing or selecting different types of *survey items* and assembling a finished instrument for given user contexts.
4. Apply established guidelines for constructing or selecting different types of *interview items* and assembling a finished instrument for given user contexts.
5. Classify the major vulnerabilities of self-report tools, and methods for ameliorating biases and errors during the instrument design process.
6. Critically evaluate the quality of a self-report assessment tool in specified contexts of use, guided by the *What?*, *Who?*, and *Why?* portals of the Process Model.

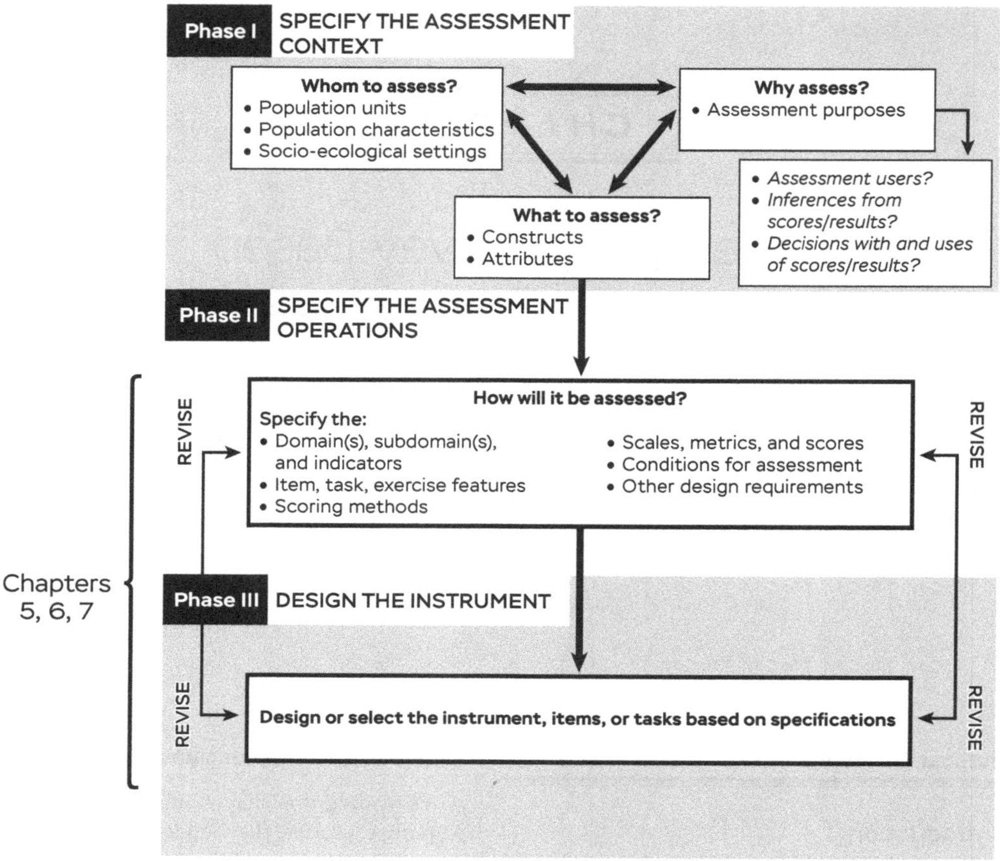

FIGURE 7.1. Connecting Chapter 7 to the Process Model and the rest of the book.

7.2 Self-Report Instruments: Their Defining Properties and Common Applications

> Everyone in the United States [has] been affected by surveys. Politicians launch or scuttle campaigns and dreams based on voter surveys. Manufacturers discontinue or mass produce products. . . . Federal aid programs hinge on the results of population surveys. . . .
>
> —EARL R. BABBIE (1998, p. xvi)

7.2.1 What's in a Question?: In Search of Eden

Often, the easiest and most practical way to learn more about a place, person, phenomenon, condition, or a novel construct that we might hypothesize about is to put the question directly to people who might know about or have some experience with it. According to Babbie (writing in 1998), survey-based research—relying entirely on the self-report methodology—was the most widely used research method in the social sciences at the time. Not much has changed today. For those interested, a quick online search would yield numerous online "survey builder" templates, signaling their utility across academic fields and professions, as well as with the general public (see, e.g., *https://zapier.com/learn/forms-surveys/best-survey-apps*). Although interview-based instruments are also employed widely in research and professional practice, of the two, surveys remain the more favored instrument type.

Yet, a good self-report question is more difficult to create than one would expect. Furthermore, a vast number of survey tools presently in use are known to yield data with major limitations (see Becker & Gözütok, 2022). Consider the brief telephone survey exchange that follows in a place called "Eden" to appreciate some of the challenges an assessment designer might face:

INTERVIEWER: Would you say that Eden is a good, average, or poor place in which to live?

INTERVIEWEE: Oh, I'd say it is a good–average place.

To start, think about how you might have responded to this same question. The keyword in the question, "Eden," could carry multiple meanings for different respondents. If one interpreted it with reference to the first chapter in the Bible, *Genesis*, it would prompt one kind of answer. The Garden of Eden in a biblical sense lies outside the realm of direct experience of human beings in the modern world. This fact in itself might cause confusion in some minds; those individuals could respond with an ambiguous "I don't know" or "What do you mean?" or "This doesn't apply to me." Alternatively, they could provide no response at all. Others who view religion as a private and personal matter may be offended by the query and also avoid giving a response. Note that already the blank responses pose an interpretive dilemma for prospective assessment users and analysts—and furthermore, we find a range of responses that fall outside the three options suggested in the original question.

The item's structure seems to require respondents to pick just one of three possible choices the interviewer presented: (1) good, (2) average, or (3) poor. Yet, all the hypothetical responses we have considered thus far—all plausible— fall outside those parameters. Response-based inferences lie at the heart of the **construct validity** of self-report measures; hence, this pattern in the data should immediately raise the concerns of any serious assessment designer. At the same time, we still need to deal with the meaning of the initial response, "good–average." How should that response be coded, summarized, and interpreted?

A number of reasons could lead to outside-the-box responses like "good–average," some of which are overlapping:

- **Semantic and linguistic barriers:** The respondent may have issues with word meanings or language used in parts of or the entire question. Semantic barriers usually stem from the designer's choices in item wording, grammatical or sentence construction, wording of the directions, language used in the response options, or the overall item or instrument presentation format. Vague words in self-report items of the kind illustrated with the word "Eden" often pose interpretive issues.
- **Limited response options:** Other issues could come into play with the number of response choices given to the respondents in a structured item (like the one in the example). If individuals find the question offers *too few* response options in light of their personal position on the topic, or their answer cannot be accommodated within the available choices, the obtained response will fall outside the expected range.
- **Unclear or otherwise problematic item construction:** Related to semantic ambiguities, some respondents may find that an item is unclear, or otherwise confusing and problematic. For instance, an overly analytic respondent might wonder: Does "good" stand for "above average," "well above average," or something else? Why are the answer options not in a logical progression, as from "below average"? "average"? "above average"? Is there some hidden meaning in the answer choices that I'm missing? Self-report items that instigate too many speculations are a warning signal from a measurement standpoint.
- **Nonserious respondent:** Other respondents may simply not take the telephone survey exercise seriously. They could provide a clever in-between answer to unsettle the interviewer or the interview process.
- **Random errors:** Alternatively, the response could simply be a random event, highly unlikely to be repeated even if the same person were to be interviewed again.

While this is not an exhaustive list of potential issues, the inherent validity problems with self-report methods are already evident.

For those survey-takers who initially interpreted the word "Eden" with reference to a *real place*, namely, a specific town in the state of Arizona that currently bears that name, the same question is more directly answerable. Furthermore, given a few language edits to the item, and by allowing the interviewer to make clarifications and elaborations during the interview exchange within set parameters, the same item might now generate more meaningful and useful information. For example, adding a "Not applicable" response option for individuals who had never lived in Eden would rule out potential nonresponses on that account. These were all probably the original item writer's intentions, but without very deliberate and concrete design changes, the original item remains issue-ridden.

Self-report tools are popular because of their perceived **utility**—they *seem* deceptively easy to put together and administer. But, while anyone could ask a question or count the answers to a series of questions, there is a formal logic as well as skill to designing high-quality self-report items and instruments. The problem for designers is to determine the potential sources and seriousness of errors and preempt such issues through careful design work.

Two vulnerabilities of self-report items should be immediately clear from the opening example. First, when different individuals interpret given words or language in items with their own individualistic frames of reference (e.g., Eden), person-to-person results will vary due to factors lying outside the targeted construct. Second, when structured-response items fail to anticipate the answers that a typical member of the target population is likely to provide, we will find unexpected responses like "good–average" or high nonresponse rates. Both issues lead to undesired levels of variability in the assessment results, or more *error variance* than *construct-relevant variance* in the item responses.

Regardless of who might take a survey or interview-based assessment, then, the designer's goal should be to craft questions that engender more or less *consistent interpretations* by every respondent. As with all instruments, we should aim to design self-report tools that yield the highest quality of information on the construct(s) that interest the primary users, given their prioritized populations and assessment purposes (Figure 7.1).

7.2.2 Item Types, Best-Measured Constructs, and Definitions

Let us now explore some illustrative self-report items. See Box 7.1 and Figures 7.2 and 7.3 next.

Box 7.1 displays two structured-response items (Questions 1–2) adapted from a census questionnaire. In this type of item construction, each individual item stands alone; each is designed to elicit a specific "fact," or a piece of descriptive information on the background of each respondent. The term is given in quotes here because the *implicit intent* of the assessment designer is to extract facts. With self-report items aiming for "fact-based" information, there is always a risk of faking, exaggeration, avoidance, or underreporting by respondents (Curran, 2016; Rees & Metcalfe, 2003). Nevertheless, background items like the ones shown are necessary on a vast majority of self-report instruments used in research, policy, or practice environments; hence, they demand the attention of assessment designers.

Going deeper, the first item in Box 7.1 deals with the *size of households*. To control for possible ambiguities in the terms "home" or "people," notice that the item prompt incorporates detailed directions to respondents on the time period to consider, and procedures for counting other residents like foster children. These details are essential to ensure that the item elicits the most accurate information possible on the fact sought, with every survey-taker reading the item in the same way. The second item is similarly "fact-based," focusing on *education level*. To enhance clarity of the communication in this case, we find parenthetic elaborations to each response choice. Most fact-based items yield categorical data, usually on a **nominal scale** (see Chapter 1 or 8 for more on scales).

Question 3 in Box 7.1 differs in that it is *opinion-based* by design. This last item example would yield **ordinal** data.

In contrast, see Figure 7.2 showing an excerpt of a **multi-item scale** embedded in a survey instrument; readers have seen several like it in previous chapters (e.g., in Chapters 1 and 3). The items are all theoretically or logically related and cohere to measure a sin-

BOX 7.1 "Fact-Based" versus "Opinion-Based" Items

Question 1

How many people were living in your home during the previous calendar year? Select the best response. Include any foster children, newborn children, roommates, or temporary guests in your count. If you/your family resided elsewhere (such as overseas), select 0.

a. 0
b. 1–3
c. 4–6
d. 7–10
e. 11 or more

Question 2

What is your current level of education? Choose **one** response that applies best to you.

a. primary school level or less (up to grade 3)
b. middle school level (up to grade 8)
c. high school level (up to grade 12)
d. 2 years of college or vocational/technical training
e. 4-year college, master's, professional, or advanced degree

Question 3

The United States should allocate a portion of its national budget toward addressing climate change and global warming issues. Indicate if you agree with this statement by choosing **one** response that best reflects your opinion.

a. Strongly agree
b. Agree
c. Uncertain
d. Disagree
e. Strongly disagree

gle **latent construct**. Designed to be administered in service provider settings by counselors, this particular scale aims to measure clients' "satisfaction" levels, a psychological construct.

In a similar vein, we might encounter a multi-item **social index** on a questionnaire for summarizing information on a single construct, usually related to a respondent's background. For example, socioeconomic status (SES) is frequently measured with a logically connected cluster of self-report items dealing with one's education level, job type, and income level (Babbie, 1998, 2021). For another example, the Home Educational Resources index on the student background questionnaire is a commonly derived index by Trends in International Mathematics and Science Study (TIMSS) researchers (see, e.g., Lin, 2018). It is constructed using self-reported data from a number of interconnected items, such as:

1. Number of books the student has at home
2. Whether the student has a study desk for their own use
3. Whether the student has a computer for their own use
4. Whether the student has a dictionary
5. Father's education level
6. Mother's education level

(See the TIMSS student and teacher questionnaires at the International Association for the Evaluation of Educational Achievement website, *https://timssandpirls.bc.edu*, not shown in Figure 7.2.) In applications with social indices and latent construct measures, the designer's intent is typically to create continuous variables on **interval scales** (see Chapter 1 or 8).

Finally, in comparison to the preceding examples, examine Figure 7.3. Here, we see an excerpt of an interview-based assessment instrument intended to assess the competency levels (the construct) of health care professionals in a technique called *motivational interviewing* (MI). MI is an approach applied in many health care settings today to motivate patients to care for themselves (Alrqiq, 2020; Rollnick, Miller, & Butler, 2008). Interview-based tools are unique in that they permit the use of **item probes**. This tool uses a combi-

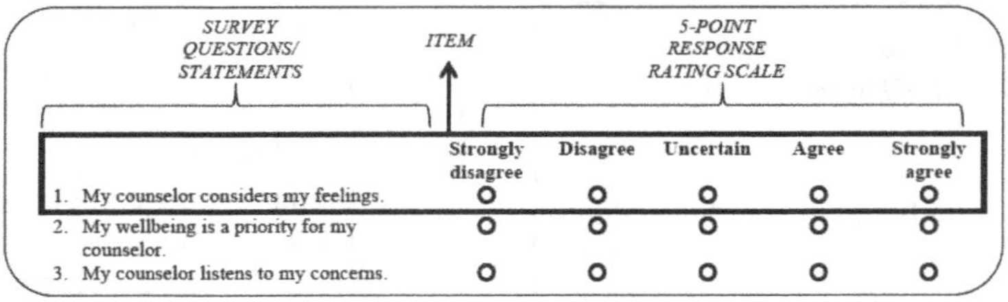

FIGURE 7.2. Closed-ended survey Items with a Likert response scale: Measuring client satisfaction with counselors.

nation of item formats. As shown, probes appear in the form of questions that help interviewers clarify or confirm the responses that interviewees provide to other items. In Figure 7.3, the item probes are employed for deeper assessment of competency levels on specific MI performance indicators.

Taken together, we see that **self-report assessments** are measuring tools whereby individuals respond directly to a set of questions presented to them in either oral or written form. The term *self-report* applies to any method that involves asking a participant directly about their own background, perceptions, recollections of experiences, feelings, attitudes/beliefs/values, or skill-specific behaviors about something with which they are expected to be familiar or knowledgeable.

7.2.2.1 Typical Constructs

Most self-report instruments are designed to measure cognitive, noncognitive, health-related, or personal-social constructs, often more than one. We should remember that the construct measures apply to the **population units** of focus, be it individuals or groups (Figure 7.1), as desired by the primary users. Although surveys predominate, many personality, attitudinal, and psychological constructs have been measured with interview methods. With constructs like *suicidal tendencies* measured in psychiatry and mental health fields, interview-based assessments have been successfully implemented for both clinical screening and diagnosis purposes (Shea, 2017; see *https://suicideassessment.com*). Broadly speaking, readers

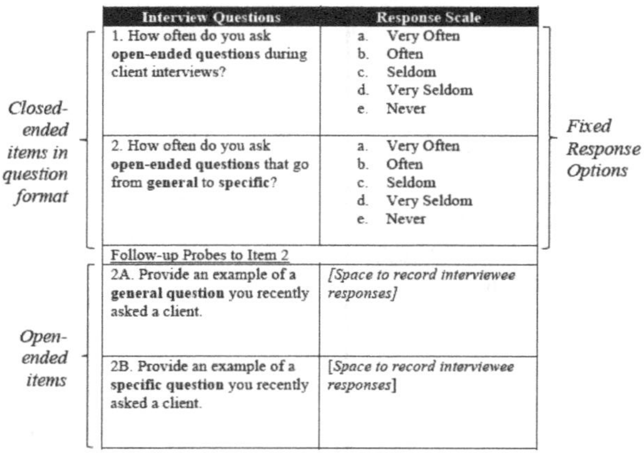

FIGURE 7.3. A combination of open- and closed-ended items on an interview-based assessment: Measuring counselor competence in motivational interviewing.

will recall, **noncognitive constructs** include interests, social-emotional attributes, attitudes and dispositions, and personality characteristics.

Interview-based assessments measuring knowledge and skill-focused domains or various cognitive abilities, such as the MI competency domain shown, could also include *viva voce* examinations administered to students in various scientific disciplines; tests of speaking skills, such as the TOEFL iBT Speaking Test developed by Educational Testing Service (see www.ets.org); or tests of cognitive abilities for early childhood, disabled, geriatric, and populations with special needs.

7.2.2.2 Administration Formats

Traditionally, survey-based instruments are presented in a written paper-and-pencil or online mode; they could be administered in individualized, small-group, or large-group settings. Elsewhere, self-report tools may be presented verbally in one-on-one settings, either via in-person or telephone interviews, or interviews that are computer-mediated or presented through internet-based platforms (e.g., Zoom or Webex). In typical assessment settings, respondents answer on their own, without guidance, interference, or involvement of the assessment administrators, researchers, practitioners, or the media through which the questions are presented.

7.2.2.3 Item Structures

In terms of structural format, self-report tools could utilize **closed-ended items**, as illustrated in the structured-response items in Figures 7.2 and 7.3 and Box 7.1. Here, each question or statement offers a *fixed set of answer options*, out of which respondents must select only one. Similar to that in the opening example, these highly structured self-report items are analogous to a multiple-choice or true–false question one might find on a cognitive test (Chapter 5).

We see the key components of closed-ended survey and interview items marked in Figures 7.2 and 7.3. These include (1) the item, presented either as a statement or direct question; (2) a fixed number of response options or a multipoint rating scale tied to each item, of which respondents are directed to select only one; and ideally, (3) verbal descriptors (sometimes called *anchors*) clarifying what each response category or point on the response scale denotes, such as "Very often" or "Strongly agree."

Alternatively, self-report instruments could allow free responses within the given limits by using **open-ended survey item** formats. An advantage of open-ended items is that they could yield deeper insights into issues investigated, such as the reasons for responses that particular persons or groups provide to closed-ended items. As in the interview-based assessment in Figure 7.3, designers could purposefully combine open- and closed-ended items. To rate or score the quality of open-ended answers when assessing proficiency-based domains, **scoring rubrics** are required. The guidelines for rubric design were discussed at length in Chapters 5–6 and will not be repeated in this chapter.

In noncognitive or other domains, narrative text data gathered through interviews must be coded and analyzed systematically using appropriate qualitative research methods, such as discourse analysis. Generally, the goal is to extract the keywords in context, or the predominant themes and subthemes in such data, with reference to the underlying construct theory and instrument application context (Creswell & Creswell, 2023).

Because of their dependence on data gathered from live exchanges, the interview-based assessment format is less utilitarian than the survey. Often incorporating a training component for interviewers, this assessment method can be costly to deploy in terms of time demands and standardization requirements. For designing a high-stakes diagnostic interview to identify a serious health condition, for example, the standardization levels could parallel those for similar performance- or constructed-response assessments discussed in Chapters 5 and 6. A benefit, however, is the probing component of interview-based tools, affording a means for clarification, verification, or contextualization of a recorded response.

QUICK RECAP: Survey- and interview-based instruments utilize the self-report response modality. Writing or selecting well-performing self-report items is a challenging task unless designers are aware of potential threats and sources of error. Individual instruments could focus on multiple constructs, yielding several measures. While attitude measurement applications are the most common, these tools could be designed to measure a range of cognitive, noncognitive, or health-related constructs and personal-social (background) characteristics, using a number of different question formats.

Reflection Break 7.1: Objectives 1 and 2

- Identify a widely used or published *self-report tool* from any of the following fields: education, psychology, health professions, or another field. Analyze/discuss the items and instrument with your class or colleagues.
- Explain why the instrument interested you. Given the items on the instrument, what are the main constructs or variables that the authors are attempting to measure?
- How many different self-report modalities and question formats are evident? Are the item formats appropriate, given the implicit intentions of authors?
- Identify an item or two aiming to measure a "fact-based" construct. Name it. What, if any, potential issues do you see with the items?
- Identify a set of items that try to tap into a "latent construct" and/or a "social index." Name these. What, if any, potential issues do you see with the items?

7.3 Historical Origins of Questionnaires and Attitude Surveys

7.3.1 Questionnaire Use in Public Policy Surveys and Censuses

Some of the earliest uses of the questionnaire format are documented in public censuses and government surveys (Babbie, 1998; 2021; Dillman, 2011; Dillman, Smyth, & Christian, 2014; Rossi et al., 2018). Reportedly, the first questionnaires for censuses were invented by the Statistical Society of London (Hilts, 1978; Willcox, 1934). Today, the U.S. government's Census Bureau administers similar questionnaires every decade or so (see *www.census.gov/history/.html*; also Box 7.1). The concept of a public policy survey originated within a broader context of questionnaire-based research conducted on a large scale to inform governmental actions and policies.

In technical terms, the typical census is a counting exercise focusing on variables like age, occupation, income, taxpayer status, education, or housing status of individuals. By definition, a **census** is intended to gather descriptive data on *every individual* of a defined region on variables that interest government-level decision-makers. In contrast, **survey research,** also called **sample survey research**, is designed to gather descriptive or opinion-based data more efficiently from a smaller group of persons taken from a defined population, with the intent of extrapolating the results to the larger population within a tolerable margin of error. In common usage, the term *survey* simply refers to the data-gathering instrument employed in such studies (for more, see *www.census.gov* and *https://news.gallup.com*).

Census and survey data may be compiled simply to display descriptively how different variables are distributed. For example, with data from items like those in Box 7.1, decision-makers could simply wish to know the following: "What is the percent of three-person households in the United States?" Elsewhere, the interest may lie in investigating relationships among different variables—for example, "Is the household income of families in the United States related to the number of minor children living in the household?"

7.3.2 Traditions in Measuring Human Perceptions and Attitudes

The early seeds in applying self-report techniques to measure psychological constructs were planted in 19th-century Germany, where the study of psychology first began as an experimental science (Wundt, 1873/1948). The psychoacoustics work of scientists like S. S. Stevens, discussed in Chapter 1, was influenced by this early research on **psychological scale development** (Stevens, 1946, 1968).

Historically, as Chapters 1 and 2 discussed, we find two distinct psychological scaling traditions that influenced modern measurement practice. The goal in a vast majority of these studies was to create continuous scales with equal or equal-appearing units. One tradition involved scale construction methods where the *items are deliberately ordered* by their intensity on a number line representing the scale; this technique builds on scale development traditions begun by L. L. Thurstone and his colleagues. In the second approach developed by Rensis Likert and others, the emphasis is instead on *placing individuals on a scale continuum* based on each person's measured overall strength on an underlying construct. Likert's method, referenced a number of times in earlier chapters, is one with which readers will most likely be familiar. While there are other traditions in attitude scale building, this section will narrow the discussion to these two historical models that dominate present-day applications, alongside another that might interest readers, called the **semantic differential scale** (Osgood, 1964).

To consider the design implications of each tradition, review Boxes 7.2 and 7.3 alongside the three graphic illustrations A–C given in Figure 7.4. The six attitudinal items shown are borrowed from Thurstone's (1930) scale on *attitude toward the movies*.

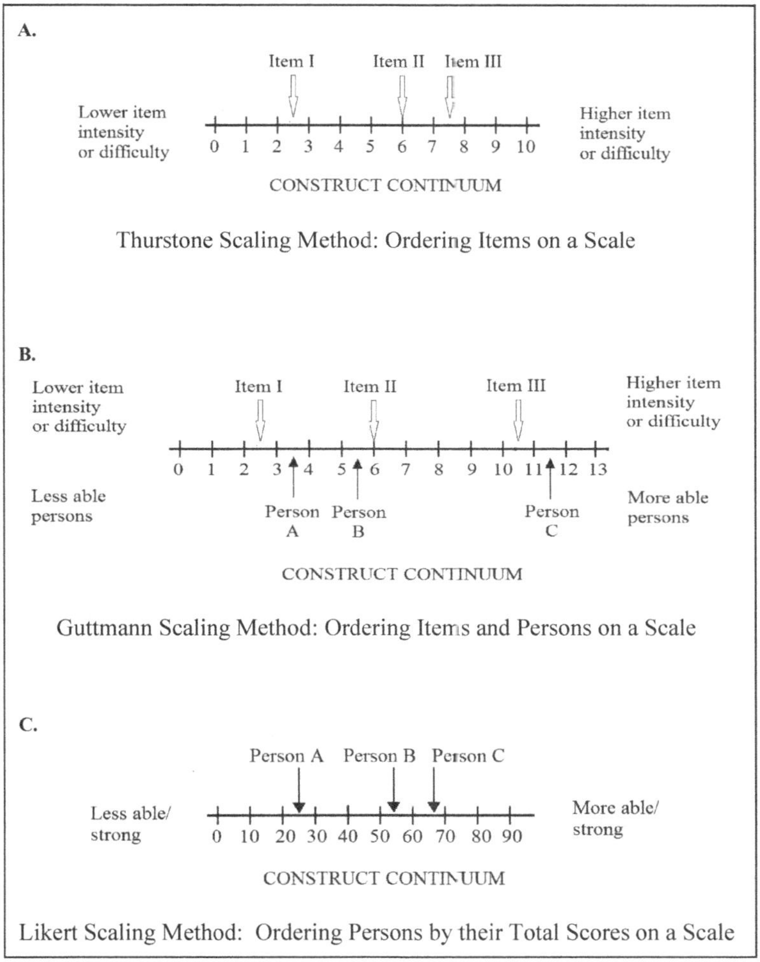

FIGURE 7.4. Graphic illustrations of three scaling techniques.

7.3.2.1 Thurstone Scales

Thurstone's attitude scaling studies relied on human discrimination processes to place items at specific points along a construct continuum (Thurstone & Chave, 1929). Each scale was developed with the help of human judges who applied principled procedures, integrated later by the authors into the *law of comparative judgments*. In one study, Thurstone and Chave (1929) created a scale on the human-perceived *seriousness of crimes* using this method. Different crimes were first presented to the judges, such as assault, theft, or homicide (the items). The judges were then guided to implement a paired comparison method, whereby they rank-ordered and placed the items on a numbered line by comparing the content of each item against that of the others. To identify intensity levels, the judges might be asked: "How *serious* is this crime (item) in your judgment as compared to the others?" To measure the difficulty of an item in an ability domain, they might have asked: "In your judgment, how *difficult* is it to execute this task as compared to the others?" As illustrated in Figure 7.4A, the items thus ordered by their relative "intensity" or "difficulty" levels were then placed on the scale continuum. From the judges' assigned score values on that scale, a numeric "weight" was then derived mathematically for each item.

For another example, examine a portion of Thurstone's (1930) scale on attitude toward the movies shown in Box 7.2, as developed with the same procedure. Notice the differences in the relative numeric "weights" against each item denoting the strength of the targeted attitude along a positive-to-negative continuum. As in the last study, each item's assigned intensity level was determined by the judges. Demonstrated for a hypothetical respondent (Person X) in Box 7.2, the item weights could be applied for obtaining a "weighted score" from the completed questionnaire, as shown.

Figure 7.4B shows graphically another conceptually similar scaling method (Guttman, 1941). This method attempted to order both items and persons jointly on a single scale continuum based on the strength of each. Details of Thurstone's and Guttman's complex theories and mathematical procedures lie outside the scope of this discussion. Modern developments in item response theory (IRT), for example, Rasch scaling models, subsequently offered useful computer-based psychometric tools for designing scales along these lines. These and other scaling methods continue to evolve today (see Yen & Fitzpatrick, 2006; see also Andrich, 1978; Wright & Masters, 1982; Wright & Stone, 1979).

From a construct validity perspective, the scaling choices we make should be consistent with the way in which we conceptualize individual constructs and specify their domains. For hierarchically organized or developmentally arranged domains, ordered scale structures like Thurstone's would be an appropriate conceptual match. Refer back to Chapter 4 for examples of ordered domains.

7.3.2.2 Likert Scales

Also a psychologist, Rensis Likert (1932) was a contemporary of Thurstone and Chave (1929). To illustrate the contrasts in Likert's method of attitude scale development, the same six items from the Thurstone (1930) scale are presented again in Box 7.3. The last graphic, C, in Figure 7.4 shows how individuals would be placed on a scale using Likert's procedure. While Likert also relied on the self-report technique for attitude measurement at the item level, he approached the scale construction problem quite differently.

Likert started the design process by collecting a series of attitudinal statements toward a given object, topic, or issue. All the items were accompanied with the same **bipolar rating scale** comprising the now familiar five response options: Strongly disagree, Disagree, Uncertain, Agree, Strongly agree. Abbreviated to SD-D-U-A-SA in Box 7.3, the Likert responses range from the most negative to the most positive stance on a given subject or issue. Each response option carried a preset numeric value on an increasing gradient, generally ranging from 1 (SD) to 5 (SA), as shown. Once items are written or selected to operationally define a multi-item scale, a *total score* is generated by simply summing an individual's rated responses to the items. For items worded to depict a negative attitude toward the object or topic, the numeric weights for SA-A-U-D-SD responses are reversed to compute the score, as shown in Box 7.3 for a hypothetical Person X. The total score thus obtained represents each respondent's location on the scale continuum, denoting the overall strength of the attitude at that point. Examine again the Likert-scaled item examples in Figure 7.2 and Box 7.1.

BOX 7.2 Thurstone Scale: Measuring Attitude toward the Movies

Directions to Survey Respondents

Below you will find six statements (Items 1–6) expressing different attitudes toward the movies. Enter your response in the space in the column to the extreme right next to the statement:

Mark an A if you *agree*.
Mark a D if you *disagree*.
If you *cannot decide*, place a question mark (?).

There are no right or wrong answers.

Item No.	*Intensity weight*	Item	*Person X's responses*
1	*0.0*	It is a sin to go to the movies.	*D*
2	*1.3*	Going to the movies is a foolish way to spend your money.	*D*
3	*2.0*	I don't find much that is educational in current films.	*D*
4	*3.4*	A movie once in a while is a good thing for everybody.	*A*
5	*4.3*	The movies are the most vital form of art today.	*A*
6	*4.7*	The movies are the most powerful influence for good in American life.	*A*

How to Score

1. To score, each response entered by a person is first assigned a point value, as follows:
   - An item with an Agree (A) response receives 1 point.
   - An item with Disagree (D) receives 0 points.
   - Items with Undecided responses are dropped from scoring.
2. For each item answered with an Agree or Disagree, the point value is multiplied by the corresponding item weight.
3. The total score is calculated by summing the weighted scores for items. To obtain a mean score, divide the total score by the number of items.

Person X's score calculation

Score on Item 1 to Item 3 (D marks entered) = [0 (0) + 0 (1.3) + 0 (2.0)] = 0
Score on Item 4 to Item 6 (A marks entered) = [1 (3.4) + 1(4.3) + 1 (4.7) = 15.7
Total score on attitude toward the movies scale (6 items) = 0 + 15.7 = 15.7
Mean score on attitude toward the movies scale (6 items) = 15.7/6 = 2.61

BOX 7.3 Scoring Likert-Scaled Items: Measuring Attitude toward the Movies

Item Examples (statements excerpted from Thurstone, 1959)

1. I find much that is educational in current films. [positive orientation]
2. Going to the movies is a foolish way to spend your money. [negative orientation]

Item response options	Abbreviation	Numeric weights for Items 3–6	Reversed numeric weights for Items 1–2
a. Strongly disagree	SD	1	5
b. Disagree	D	2	4
c. Uncertain (neither agree nor disagree)	U	3	3
d. Agree	A	4	2
e. Strongly agree	SA	5	1

Calculating a Total Score

Person X's total score is based on a sum of the responses recorded below. Items 1 and 2 are reverse-coded.

Item no.	Item	Person X's selected responses and item scores
1.	It is a sin to go to the movies.	c. 3
2.	Going to the movies is a foolish way to spend your money.	b. 2
3.	I find much that is educational in current films.	e. 5
4.	A movie once in a while is a good thing for everybody.	e. 5
5.	The movies are the most vital form of art today.	d. 4
6.	The movies are the most powerful influence for good in American life.	c. 3
	Total Score for Person X	**22**
	Maximum possible score on a six-item scale	*30*

Likert posited that all items tapping a construct are essentially replications of each other and, therefore, interchangeable in terms of their intensity. The simple sum of an individual's responses to a random group of items could therefore yield the total "scale score" for a construct, adjusted for positively and negatively worded items, as shown. These scores would allow the individuals to be scaled, or placed in order, from high to low on the underlying attitude (Figure 7.4C). Likert's scaling approach lends itself acceptably to all nonhierarchically conceptualized domains and is equally applicable to both stratified and nonstratified domain structures. See the examples and discussion of domain sampling theory in Chapter 4 again, as necessary.

7.3.2.3 Semantic Differential Scale

Finally, another useful historic technique when measuring noncognitive, health-related, or social constructs is Osgood's approach to designing a **semantic differential scale** (Osgood, 1964). Osgood developed the approach to answer the question: "What kinds of *meaning* do people attribute to different societal concepts, such as government, schools, corporations, and so forth?" To address this question, his technique employed a series of bipolar items tied to a socially relevant concept, each anchored with adjectives carrying opposite meanings at each end. Each item series is accompanied with a common 7-point rating scale, as shown next in two illustrative items on the theme of government:

Government

Weak 1 2 3 4 5 6 7 Strong

Bad 1 2 3 4 5 6 7 Good

Through **factor analysis** of large semantic differential datasets (a relatively novel psychometric procedure in his time), Osgood's research identified three recurring dimensions in individuals' perceptions of words tied to given social concepts: an *evaluation dimension*, which suggested the value judgments that respondents assigned to a concept; a *potency dimension*, indicating the respondents' perceptions of a concept's influential power; and an *activity dimension*, pointing to perceptions of dynamism/movement inherent in the concept. Osgood's approach (like Likert's and unlike Thurstone's) did not specify any underlying order to the items based on the strength of a construct. Nor did he attempt to ascertain item-level intensities in numeric terms. However, Osgood (1964) recognized that self-report data were inherently subjective and mediated by culture and language. His method for scaling individual perceptions and attitudes has been widely applied since in psychology, linguistics, anthropology, sociology, and market research.

The challenge during item construction is locating a sufficient number of paired, bipolar adjectives that operationally define each dimension effectively. For this purpose, online thesauri or dictionaries might serve as useful resources. Here is a possible application.

Dubious attitudes of the public toward vaccinations under the COVID-19 pandemic has been described as the problem of *vaccine hesitancy* in the public health and medical literature (Horowitz, 2022; Larson, Gakidou, & Murray, 2022). To learn more about perceived barriers to vaccination, we might study the subjective attributions of individuals toward the concept of "vaccines" with a semantic differential scale. Drawing on Osgood's theory and factor analytic research, we could design, sort, or organize a group of semantic differential items by the three dimensions, as follows:

Vaccines			
1. Bad	1 2 3 4 5 6 7	Good	(Evaluation)
2. Slow	1 2 3 4 5 6 7	Fast	(Activity)
3. Static	1 2 3 4 5 6 7	Dynamic	(Activity)
4. Weak	1 2 3 4 5 6 7	Strong	(Potency)
5. Effective	1 2 3 4 5 6 7	Ineffective	Reversed Item (Evaluation)
6. Uncertain	1 2 3 4 5 6 7	Certain	(Evaluation)
7. Powerless	1 2 3 4 5 6 7	Powerful	(Potency)

To avoid thoughtless or arbitrary responses, occasional items may be oriented in a reverse direction, as with Item 5. The purported item links to each dimension must be verified through **empirical validation** studies. Once validated, each dimension would yield a **subscale** score lending insights into public perceptions of a concept on each dimension. Modern developments in factor analytic techniques offer several optional analytic tools to carry out such investigations (see, e.g., Isitan, 2021).

QUICK RECAP: The self-report modality has been utilized variously for measurement purposes historically, and the past applications offer ideas for developing new items, scales, and instruments. Different scaling traditions differ conceptually and operationally, using both ordered or unordered item and person arrangements. During the instrument design process, the scale structure we choose should be consistent with the way in which we specify the construct domains. How meaningfully the scale performs for different constructs is an empirical question; this should be checked with appropriate qualitative, statistical, and psychometric methods during validation.

Reflection Break 7.2: Objectives 1 and 2

- List the *similarities* and *differences* you see among different historical approaches to designing self-report items, tools, and measures: (1) early census questionnaires, (2) Thurstone's scales, (3) Likert's scales, (4) Osgood's scales, or (5) another method you may find.
- Which method(s) would you lean toward for designing a self-report tool of your own? Why? Name the constructs you'll measure and your assessment purposes.
- Why should an assessment designer ensure that the scaling choices are appropriate for the construct domains of interest? Explain with examples.
- *Likert assumed that all items tapping a construct were essentially replications of each other.* Would you adopt this assumption? Explain.
- Review a few interview-based items on the latest version of the Stanford–Binet Intelligence Scale for young children. Are the scaling operations more like Thurstone's, Likert's, or Osgood's? Explain your answer.

7.4 Measurement Issues with the Self-Report Modality

Despite their popularity, self-report instruments are treated dubiously by many users and researchers. At question is often the trustworthiness of the data at the item-level and from measures overall. This section reviews the most common measurement problems we could encounter and some established methods to address these.

7.4.1 Item Construction Issues, Semantic Ambiguities, and Built-In Biases

Poor item construction is the first barrier to sound measurement with the self-report modality. A lack of attention to subjective frames of reference, idiosyncratic responses, semantic ambiguities, poor question-to-responses matches, weakly articulated instructions, and other problems *within* the items or the instrument often cloud the quality of self-reported data.

7.4.1.1 Response Rates and Missing Data

Survey-based instruments are known to produce very low return rates (30–40%), especially mailed and online questionnaires (Dillman, 2011; Dillman et al., 2014). When users intend to examine group differences, large numbers of missing responses from one group or another introduce **selection biases**; this problem can result in misleading inferences about the inadequately represented persons (see, e.g., Greenacre, 2016). Assuming that the self-reporting gaps are simply random could be incorrect; such assumptions need to be verified before software-based statistical algorithms are employed to fill in missing data after a self-report tool is used.

Often, individuals who *do* return the complete surveys are those who desire to have their opinion heard, have the time and resources to do so, or have extreme views on the issue or topic. Other systematic factors built into an instrument that could yield missing data include:

- A lack of Don't know, Not applicable, or Unable to respond options on closed-ended items when these legitimately apply to some participants
- Respondents running out of time due to an overly lengthy instrument
- Reading, interpretive, or other difficulties of respondents during the assessment
- Respondent fatigue, either due to an overly lengthy or overly taxing self-reporting exercise
- Item avoidance due to religious, cultural, or personal background factors
- Respondents not having (or being excluded from) the expected experiences to which the questions pertain

7.4.1.2 Biases within Items or Instruments

Built-in biases of self-report assessments, applicable to all forms of instrumentation, could explain some of the response gaps and missing data as well (AERA et al., 2014):

- *Readability bias.* A bias caused when the reading or vocabulary level is too high for some or most of the participants
- *Inflammatory bias.* A bias in the use of words, examples, or graphics that is belittling or inflammatory to certain groups or sects
- *Stereotypical bias.* A similar bias that makes false assumptions about certain persons or groups, perpetuating social stereotypes, such as females being the "weaker sex"
- *Materials or conditions bias.* A bias introduced through the assessment conditions, format, materials, technology, or platforms used that systematically favor some or prevent others from participating fully in the assessment

Many of these issues arise inadvertently; however, pilot testing, screening, revising, and, as needed, deleting items when biases are detected represent good design practice.

7.4.2 Respondent-Specific Issues in Self-Report Data

7.4.2.1 Faking, Exaggeration, and Underreporting

As discussed in the opening section, self-report measures can be falsified in either the positive or negative direction by respondents, especially on private or sensitive topics. For example, one person might choose to present their home environment as supportive even when a family member is abusive toward them; another might choose to make their home environment look more abusive than it actually is. Faking also occurs when respondents wish to present themselves in the best possible light to the external world (see the next section, "Social Desirability Bias"). Whether motivated by privacy or personal reasons, faked responses in self-reported data reduce validity levels.

7.4.2.2 Social Desirability Bias

A primary type of respondent-specific bias in self-reported results is when participants say socially desirable things. The **social desirability bias (SD)** reflects the tendency of people to say things that will meet with social approval. It is "the tendency to give answers that make the respondent look good" (Paulhus, 1991, p. 17). Usually influenced by the prevalent social norms and standards, social desirability tends to affect the measurement of certain psychological or personality constructs more, especially on topics such as racism, sexual activities, and illegal behavior (Krumpal, 2013). For example, if asked whether we like working in places with people of diverse racial backgrounds, we might be tempted to say, *Strongly agree*, when we know that promoting diversity is a declared policy of the organization conducting the survey. In theory, we could address the issue statistically by correcting the results obtained from a self-report tool for measured levels of SD bias. To do so, there are tools like the Marlowe–Crowne Social Desirability Scale, available now in both short or long form (Fischer & Fick, 1993). Purported to measure the levels of SD bias present in self-reported data, the Marlowe–Crowne scale must be administered to individuals alongside the self-report tool being investigated. However, as the Marlowe–Crowne scale is itself a self-report tool, its results must be found to demonstrate acceptable levels of validity and reliability first before the next analytic steps are taken.

7.4.2.3 Acquiescence and Response Sets

The **acquiescence bias** is a human tendency to readily agree, rather than disagree, with statements. **Response sets** are similar and refer to the tendency, conscious or unconscious, to mark a particular response choice repeatedly without giving due consideration to the content in the items (Dodou & de Winter, 2014). For example, a person might demonstrate an Agree or Uncertain response bias when asked to fill out a Likert-scaled questionnaire. Both biases mask the true standing of a person on the constructs, compromising validity.

7.4.2.4 Biases due to Forgetfulness of Respondents

Self-report assessments are inherently biased by the person's mental status *at the time they fill out* a questionnaire or participate in an interview. When participants feel poorly for reasons other than the issue of focus, they could select or provide more negative responses; the reverse pattern emerges when the same individuals feel better generally. Subjects may also forget pertinent details of the topics on which they are questioned. Unconscious mental blocking of details of unhappy experiences, or symptoms of pain or trauma following a crisis, are similarly common.

7.4.3 Tackling Measurement Errors with Self-Report Tools

The answer to the various measurement errors lies first in giving due attention to the instrument design process, followed by field testing, validating, and making improvements to aspects of the self-report tool that show limitations—whether they be the items, scales, assessment conditions, or directions. These efforts should be undertaken before a tool is applied.

Assurance of anonymity, confidentiality, and open communication about the exact purposes of the instrument with participants is a strategy for combating many of the other problems discussed. Ethics review boards for sensitive research studies often require that respondents feel no external coercion to participate (and could drop out at any time they choose). Participants should also know how to access their own and other results of a data-collection effort with self-report tools (see also AEA, 2018; AERA et al., 2014).

Lastly, specific psychometric and statistical methods are available for checking and estimating the quality of items and scales from different types of self-report tools. Outside expert reviews and cognitive interviews (see the case study in this chapter), we could use a variety of analytic tools to detect issues of validity, reliability, respondent-related, or built-in biases, as well as utility issues. Focusing on survey item and instrument evaluation, Maitland and Presser (2016) recommended that assessment designers and researchers take a *multimethod approach* to evaluating and improving self-report assessments.

The instrument application contexts should guide our selection of appropriate validation approaches and analytic techniques. For example, the Survey Quality Predictor software was built specifically for evaluating surveys and survey items in cross-country sociological studies. This program defines the quality of a survey question as the "strength of the relationship between the latent variable of interest and the response to the survey question, the observed variable" for those assessment contexts. The software employs an updated *multitrait–multimethod* approach, examining validity levels through correlation matrices of self-reported item data linked to multiple latent constructs (see SQP at *https://sqp.upf.edu*; after Campbell & Fiske, 1959). Definitions of different validity and reliability indices, methods of evaluating the same, and assumptions/limitations of different methods will follow in Chapters 10 and 11.

QUICK RECAP: Measurement issues with the self-report modality could be due to problems with item construction and assessment design (e.g., nonresponse rates); built-in biases within the instrument (e.g., stereotypical bias); or biases of respondents themselves (e.g., social desirability bias, acquiescence bias). Many of these issues can be investigated and addressed with specific actions taken during the instrument design and validation process. For sensitive and high-stakes uses of self-report tools, attending to established standards of ethical practice, including the assurance of confidentiality and anonymity of results, can help avert some of these issues.

Reflection Break 7.3: Objectives 1–3

- Explain how each of these problems could arise with self-report items and tools. Define each concept.
  - High nonresponse rates
  - Built-in stereotypical biases
  - Socially desirable responses
  - Acquiescence biases
  - Forgetfulness in responses
  - Other kinds of issues
- For the issues above, explain how you would address the problem.
- Identify ethical practice guidelines that are most important to remember during the design of self-report tools? Why?

7.5 General Design Guidelines for Self-Report Instruments

We turn now to the major principles for designing self-report tools, building on existing background theory and research. What are some general guidelines to follow? And how could we attend to validity, reliability, or utility issues when implementing these? Recall that *systematic errors* affecting the **validity** levels of measures are typically introduced from identifiable and predictable sources. When *random errors* arise from unpredictable or unknown sources, **reliability** levels of measures are compromised. Issues of **utility** arise when the tools or measures are overly lengthy, complex, or difficult to implement.

7.5.1 Nuances to Applying Domain-Sampling Methods with Self-Report Measures

Domain sampling techniques apply to self-report tools in the same way as they do with other assessment modalities, situated within the framework of the overall design process shown in Figure 7.1. Recall that the method involves two main steps: (1) specifying the domains and subdomains for the key constructs with well-supported *observable indicators* and (2) designing or selecting a *sample of items* that closely matches the content and taxonomic levels specified in the indicators. The methodological literature stresses the need for homogeneity of the items organized by domain or subdomain, as it is these item groups that eventually define the scales and subscales of an instrument operationally (see Chapter 4; Ghiselli et al., 1981; Nunnally & Bernstien, 1994).

Sampling self-report items in a content-relevant and content-representative manner assures **content-based validity** of the construct measures we plan to interpret and use. In practice, this validity principle basically means that we develop, select, and distribute the self-report items in a balanced manner to match all the relevant indicators of each domain or subdomain. In the same vein, we could build **internal consistency reliability** into self-report measures by including a *sufficient number* of items from the construct domain and subdomains. This logically executed step ensures that the behavioral samples we obtain are large enough to reduce domain-sampling errors (Chapter 4, Figure 4.2). Importantly, we need adequate numbers of *homogeneously clustered items* by domain or subdomain. A general rule of thumb is to include three to seven well-designed items per subdomain. A useful practice is to create a few more items per indicator than we need. This will enable deletion of poorly functioning or redundant items after item evaluations are completed. In the end, the self-report tool cannot be too long or cumbersome to reduce utility levels desired by users (more on validation in Chapters 10 and 11).

7.5.2 Nature of the Construct(s): Typical Response or Maximum Performance Response?

Prior to beginning item writing or selection for a self-report instrument, we must have clarity on the fundamental nature of the constructs and variables to measure. This step helps determinations as to whether we seek a *typical response* or *maximum performance response* from respondents with different item types. To do so, it is first necessary to identify each construct and construct type to be measured separately with individual items or item sets as part of specifying *What* to measure (see Figure 7.1).

For illustrations, take a look at Box 7.1 again. Most background characteristics of individuals tapped by self-report items are preexisting, such as their education levels. Others may be demographic characteristics that are naturally occurring variables, such as a person's biologically determined sex. In both these instances, the item responses cannot be reasonably categorized as correct or incorrect. Rather, the goal with such items is to obtain the *actual status* of individuals on the background variable and depict the most typical response distributions on the people measured.

Similarly, see the satisfaction scale in Figure 7.2 again. When measuring noncognitive or opinion-based constructs with self-report items, likewise, there are no right or wrong answers. The intent is to depict the individuals' actual positions on a subject, issue, or topic at that given point in time, and obtain the typical distributions for those persons on the measures. To test this premise, consider again the opinion-based Question 3 in Box 7.1. Here, there are no correct answers; hence, we would attempt to elicit typical responses to such items, whether they stand alone or are a component of a scale.

Item instructions on attitude surveys, therefore, often request respondents to be truthful. Or, as we saw on the Thurstone scale presented in Box 7.2, the directions underscore that there are no correct or incorrect answers. Such steps are taken to free respondents from feeling any undue pressures of responding "correctly" as they would with items on a knowledge test, where their answers would be judged. The aim, rather, is to obtain the most honest and *typical response distributions* on the item, or as the case might be, on a group of items defining a scale.

In contrast, review again the last two open-ended questions on the interview-based assessment with the probes (Figure 7.3). A group of these items are designed for measuring a candidate's skills in employing proper MI questioning techniques situated in clinical practice settings. For each of these, there *is* a correct or acceptable response based on widely held standards in the profession or academic field. In this instance, by design, the self-report items must be structured to elicit a person's *maximum performance response*.

For self-report items aimed to gauge knowledge, skill, or ability levels in a tested domain, it is thus necessary to set up appropriate instructions and environmental conditions during the assessment process to control for possible random or systematic interferences. In an ideal application, individual respondents would be alerted beforehand that their responses will be interpreted as their best possible performance. These priming steps maximize the chances for valid inference-making afterward.

7.5.3 Matching the Specific Response Modality to Diverse Population Profiles and Needs

Depending on the diversity of persons to be assessed, the choice between a survey- or interview-based modality could either enhance or impede construct measurement (Chapter 3). Assessment designers often make assumptions about the verbal literacy levels, cultural backgrounds, and basic capacities of respondents to engage effectively with self-report items and assessment delivery platforms. To optimize validity levels, it is necessary to choose a self-report modality that is most appropriate for the specified populations. Systematic interfering factors could include a person's racial-ethnic, cultural, and/or religious background, age, primary or native language, prior education, special needs such as physical or mental disabilities, or degree of access to technology, resources, or equipment required for the assessment (Chapter 3).

Questionnaires and survey-based instruments generally expect respondents to be literate, independently functioning adults, with at least an eighth-grade level of education (see, e.g., *www.pewresearch.org/topic/methodological-research*). Many tools are therefore designed to be relatively rigid, assuming that all respondents know how to speak, read, and write fluently in the language in which questions are presented. For this reason, the *survey modality*—whether in written, telephone, computer, or Web-based form—should ideally be selected after population and subpopulation profiles are carefully considered. Pilot-testing the items and instruments with a smaller but representative group beforehand could help verify how closely the assessment method fits typical respondents. Adjustments can follow to accommodate any observed issues.

In contrast, the *interview-based mode* can accommodate greater variability with respect to individual needs. For example, interviews are adaptable for very young children, individuals with low literacy levels and/or cultural differences, the disabled, the ill, and the elderly. Regardless, added interpretive or translational support may still be necessary with subpopulations with highly specialized needs.

Fitting the best self-report modality to the population profile should logically flow from the early phases of the assessment design process (Figure 7.1). Specifying the population boundaries carefully helps in identifying the major subgroups and groups for whom the instrument is intended. A study of relevant background characteristics, keeping in mind the population units on whom measure-based inferences and uses would apply, will further assist in assuring validity of the measures (Chapter 3).

7.5.4 Selecting the Best Item Response Formats

Thoughtful indicator specification facilitates the selection of the best-aligned assessment methods, in this case, the most appropriate self-report question formats and item response modes to match. The nuances of these design steps differ with cognitive and noncognitive constructs. Each is elaborated separately next, using the item examples shown previously in Figures 7.2 and 7.3. As necessary, readers should refer back to relevant sections of Chapters 4–6 for more on domain specification and task design guidelines.

7.5.4.1 Best Self-Reported Item and Response Formats for Cognitive Constructs

When measuring cognitive domains, we are seeking maximum performance responses (Section 7.4.2). Interview-based item formats, as indicated, could be varied in several ways for this purpose:

- Open-ended interview items, with or without item probes
- Closed-ended interview items, with or without probes
- Mixed interview item formats

The interview items could stand alone or be grouped in connected sets tied to the specified domain. Each must also be accompanied with a domain-referenced **scoring key**, or an **analytic** or **holistic scoring rubric**, for scoring purposes. Again, guidelines on rubric design will not be repeated in Chapter 7; readers are referred back to Chapters 5 and 6 for this purpose.

Note that Likert-type survey items on an agreement scale or modifications thereof (Question 4 in Box 7.1) are entirely inappropriate for measuring maximum performance responses that will be scored as right versus wrong; however, these may be applicable for measuring perceptions or degrees of *perceived knowledge* on a topic. In educational or professional training contexts, such deliberations must be left to the primary users, usually the course instructors and education program directors.

To illustrate the procedure for selecting the best-matched item and response formats, consider the mixed-item set in Figure 7.3 again on the MI competency domain. Let us say that this item series was designed to match the following *MI competency indicator* that health professionals must demonstrate for certification purposes:

- *Indicator.* With real patient cases (competent professionals) can elaborate how the major steps of the MI technique would be executed to yield the desired patient outcomes.
- *Taxonomic level.* Higher-order thinking.

Analyzing the indicator with the guidelines given in Chapter 4, we would have the following breakdown:

- With real patient cases
[*conditions under which knowledge/skill would be demonstrated*]
- The major steps of the MI technique
[*content knowledge to be demonstrated*]
- Elaborate how MI would be executed to yield desired patient outcomes
[*cognitive processing behaviors to be demonstrated*]

Given that designers assigned a higher-order thinking level to this indicator, what are the best item and response formats that could optimize validity of competency-based inferences from the assessment results? And how could we justify that selection? Note that for item design purposes, the functional taxonomy for cognitive domains is applied above (Chapter 4, Table 4.2). Although not shown above, Box 7.4 illustrates how other indicators of the MI domain could be specified similarly to measure four progressive mental processing levels using that taxonomy.

In Figure 7.3, the designers selected an interview-based assessment method with items that cascade and build on one another. To begin the interview, they used two closed-ended items (Items 1–2). These helped gauge the frequency with which examinees actually applied MI questioning techniques. The follow-up question probes were open-ended, allowing deeper examinations of patient-specific applications. This design choice allowed flexibility for different candidates to answer based on their own patient experiences. To continue probing, more open-ended items could be added to delve deeper into the thinking processes of candidates (not shown in Figure 7.3). For example:

Item 2: How often do you ask **open-ended questions** that go from general to specific?

[fixed-response options in Figure 7.3]

[open-ended item probes 2A–2B in Figure 7.3]

Added item probes:

2C. Please provide more details of the patient case you are remembering.

2D. Was the patient motivated to change their health habits and behaviors after the MI session with you?

2E. What helped you confirm that this patient's behavior was moving in a healthy direction? What did they say they were doing? What steps did you take to follow up with the patient?

Together, the progressively built, mixed-item set enables a more complete and comprehensive measurement of the competency indicator. Consistent with the higher-order level specified, the difficulty of the exercise is above the two lower taxonomic levels in Box 7.4.

Of the assessment methods and item response formats, then, the mixed-item interview appears well suited for measuring the general indicator. Although lower in utility than a multiple-choice test, the layered probing enhances content-based validity levels. Effectively deployed interview probes can also detect falsified or exaggerated answers. By requiring examinees to contextualize explanations with specific patients, and elaborate exactly how the MI procedure was executed, the cognitive demands increase.

BOX 7.4 Measuring Motivational Interviewing Skills

Four Levels of Cognitive Processing: A Functional Taxonomy*

1. *Concept Recall and Understanding.*

   Indicator:

   Recall and/or show basic comprehension of motivational interviewing (MI) concepts and principles.
2. *Application*

   Indicator:

   Apply MI concepts in simulated problem scenarios.
3. *Higher-Order Thinking*

   Indicator:

   Justify answers to problem scenarios dealing with MI, showing deeper thinking processes.
4. *Complex Procedural Skills*

   Indicator:

   Demonstrate multistep MI procedures that meet professional standards in clinical contexts.

*See Chapter 4, Table 4.2, for details.

In comparison to other assessment options, a short interview is less time-consuming and hence more utilitarian as well. Had the indicator been specified at one of the lower cognitive levels, it could have been more efficiently measured with a paper-and-pencil test, either with multiple-choice or short-answer items. Complex procedural skills are better measured with a behavior-based assessment, as the latter permits direct observations of examinees as they demonstrate a learned procedure.

7.5.4.2 Best Self-Reported Item and Response Formats for Noncognitive, Health, and Other Constructs

To apply the same procedures with noncognitive domains, examine again the excerpt of a client satisfaction scale in Figure 7.2. Given that it deals broadly with attitudes toward counselors, the tripartite "CAB" theory of attitude measurement is applied here for illustration purposes (CAB-M taxonomy, Chapter 4). This theory holds that attitudes toward any given object or persons are manifested either through one's beliefs (cognitions), feelings (affect), or behavior (Hovland & Rosenberg, 1960). An indicator to measure the *belief dimension* pertinent to counselors or the counseling experience follows, to which the items in Figure 7.2 are aligned. As before, to select the best-aligned item and response formats, it is helpful to first specify the taxonomic levels appropriate for each of the noncognitive indicators, along with the conditions and attitudinal content to be measured. For example:

> *Indicator:* Clients endorse/rate their experiences with counselor(s) from positive-to-negative, given their best recollections of a recent counseling session.
>
> *Taxonomic category:* Belief-specific and value-expressive component of dispositions.
>
> *Analyzed indicator:*
>
> - Given their best recollections of a recent counseling session . . . .
>   [*conditions in which the attitude is situated*]
> - Clients endorse/rate from positive to negative.
>   [*belief dimension of attitude to be measured*]
> - . . . experiences with their counselor(s).
>   [*content—the person, object, or event to which the attitude applies*]
>
> *Matching items:* See Figure 7.2 (e.g., *My counselor considers my feelings*).

Here, assuming that the item instructions call for respondents to think back to their most recent counseling experience, we find a close match of all three items with the major components of the indicator, as specified. By definition, a belief-based attitudinal category indicates what individuals hold to be true in their minds about a past experience, using what they remember. Each item in Figure 7.2 is constructed to present a belief pertinent to the counselor, as follows: [I believe that] *My counselor considers my feelings.* The items share a common five-option, ordered agreement scale allowing a person to endorse the strength of that belief.

In theory, we could design or select self-report items matched to any dimension of the tripartite taxonomy. Or, alternatively, the four categories of noncognitive processing in the functional taxonomy building on the tripartite model could be useful for measuring various noncognitive, personal-social, or health-related constructs. To illustrate, see Box 7.5; in it, each category is applied to indicators from a hypothetical client satisfaction domain with items to match. Items tied to given indicators could be positively or negatively worded, as shown. To remove ambiguities in communication, it is good practice to highlight or underscore the negative wording in items, as Box 7.5 demonstrates.

Returning to Figure 7.2, we see that using common response options for an item set is more efficient, but all the items must be homogeneous. Homogeneity in an item set is achieved by focusing on the same taxonomic category and/or content to be measured (Section 7.4.1). By design, related items should generate responses that "hang together," showing within-person consistency levels when the response data are analyzed statistically. The items shown could be further improved by applying more specific writing guidelines for closed-ended items, which are presented in the next section.

7.5.5 Response Scale Options, Number of Scale Points, and Scale Descriptors for Closed-Ended Items

A number of modifications to the standard Likert response scale with variable numbers of scale points offer design possibilities for closed-ended self-report items. Fink (1995) offered four general classes of response options, shown next in Box 7.6, with suggested applications for each. Poorly matched responses to item statements or questions can reduce the quality of the item-level data and overall measures. Outside logical and linguistic considerations, item try-outs with the respondent groups permit further evaluations of the best-suited response scales.

Compare the following six optional choices to arrive at an appropriate response scale for the next item stimulus (item stem) to measure the behavior dimension of *Attitude toward counselors*. Deliberative criteria in brackets are suggested for performing item evaluations.

> **Closed-ended item stem:** *I attend the scheduled therapy sessions with my counselor.*

BOX 7.5 Four Types of Attitudinal Processing: Measuring Client Satisfaction

Functional Taxonomy of Attitudinal Behaviors

- *Belief-specific and value-expressive component of dispositions:*

  What a person holds to be true about something, reflecting beliefs, opinions, values, and/or perceptions about some present or past experience, event, place, person, or object.

  A "belief" indicator: Clients endorse/rate the quality of their experiences with counselor(s), based on their recollections.

  Items to match:
  My counselor is helpful.
  *My counselor is **judgmental**.*

- *Emotional component of dispositions:*

  What a person feels about some present or past experience, event, place, person, or object.

  A "feeling" indicator: Clients express positive or negative personal feelings about their counseling sessions.

  Items to match:
  I am satisfied with my counseling sessions.
  *I **dislike** participating in my counseling sessions.*

- *Behavioral component of dispositions:*

  What a person does or tends to do, in terms of social behaviors, responses, actions, or practices in relation to some experience, event, place, person, or object.

  A "behavioral" indicator: Clients indicate specific actions they take in relation to the counseling experience.

  Items to match:
  I attend the scheduled weekly sessions with my counselor.
  *I **avoid** the scheduled weekly sessions with my counselor.*

- *Metacognitive component of dispositions:*

  The tendency to self-evaluate one's own mindset, feelings, and behaviors and self-correct course or make adjustments to alter attitudes.

  A metacognitive indicator: Clients indicate self-evaluating their behaviors after sessions with the counselor.

  Items to match:
  I think about how to change my behaviors after counseling.
  *I **do not** think about improving myself after counseling.*

Note. Classified using the Functional Taxonomy.

Response scale 1:

a) *Every week,* b) *Most weeks,* c) *Some weeks,* d) *Only when I can,* e) *Never*

[**Item Evaluation:** Good item. It focuses on a respondent behavior ("attend"). The response choices are frequency-based and an appropriate match with a possible "schedule." The use of a time-based unit, "week" adds greater specificity.]

Response scale 2:

a) *Always,* b) *Almost always,* c) *Sometimes,* d) *Rarely,* e) *Never*

[**Item Evaluation:** This is also a good item, but the response choices are more general. The item would improve if the wording is specifically linked to a time-based measuring unit like "week" or "month."]

Response scale 3:

a) *Yes,* b) *No*

[**Item Evaluation:** Acceptable in terms of clarity but information may be lost with a forced binary choice. May lead to missing data for those who wish to give a more refined response.]

Response scale 4:

a) *More than last year,* b) *About the same as last year,* c) *Less than last year*

[**Item Evaluation:** Weak. Choices not ideal unless measuring a *change* in attitudinal behavior.

BOX 7.6 Closed-Ended Items for Self-Report Tools: Optional Responses

Type of response desired	
Endorsement	*Endorsement options are useful for measuring strength of opinions, beliefs, attitudes, and perceptions. Common response scales:* • Definitely true, True, Don't know, False, Definitely false • Strongly agree, Agree, Uncertain, Disagree, Strongly disagree • Yes, Not sure, No
Frequency	*Frequency-based options apply best when measuring degrees to which a behavior, action, or practice occurs or is evident. For example:* • Always, Most of the time, Sometimes, Rarely, Never • All the time, Most of the time, Some of the time, Occasionally, Very occasionally, Never
Intensity	*Intensity-based response scales are useful for measuring strength of a feeling about something or for describing the severity of a need, condition, or painful situation. For example:* • Absent, Very mild, Mild, Moderate, Severe, Very severe • To a great extent, To a moderate extent, To some extent, Very little, Not at all • Very low, Low, High, Very high
Comparison	*Comparison response scales apply best for measuring perceptions about a change of situation or condition. For example:* • More than last year, About the same as last year, Less than last year

Acceptable when the item also presents the past year as a comparison point.]

Response scale 5:

a) *Strongly agree,* b) *Agree,* c) *Disagree,* d) *Strongly disagree*

[**Item Evaluation:** Weak choices. Degrees of agreement or endorsement add vagueness and do not logically match behavior-based items. Regular attendees may vacillate between SA or A, while irregular ones may do the same with SD and D. The absence of a midpoint option, "Uncertain," could also yield unreliable data.]

Response scale 6:

To a great extent, a) To a moderate extent, b) To some extent, c) Very little d) Not at all

[**Item Evaluation:** Another weak set of choices. "Extent" or "degree" of an action is not the best logical or semantic match to the item stem. "Extent" is also unsuitable for measuring behavior-based indicators.]

The number of response choices for closed-ended items (2-, 3-, or multipoint) should be given due thought. For populations that do not have the attention span, time, capacity, or the inclination to respond to demanding item structures, a simplified 3-point scale may be the most appropriate, such as a) *Yes*, b) *Not sure*, c) *No.*

A Likert scale *without* the "Uncertain" option is often viewed as more effective as it forces a choice. Although sometimes desirable, a forced two-option scale should be chosen carefully. The approach may precipitate problems for respondents who wish to make their choice conditionally or have a position that requires finer gradations. Measurement issues, for instance, are well documented for the Myers–Briggs Type Indicator (Gardner & Martinko, 1996; Pittenger, 2005). Applied in occupational contexts, this widely used instrument is a self-reported personality measure with binary, forced-choice items that require just one answer. As the opening section of this chapter suggested, the use of a "Don't know," "Not applicable," or "Cannot respond" option could yield more valid information in circumstances where segments of the population may not know about or have a position on the topic.

Elsewhere, however, a binary choice may be the most fitting response option for the question stimulus. See the next item example:

Item: *Did you (the client) consent to participate in counseling? Circle one response.*

Response scale 1: *1-2-3-4-5-6-7-8-9*

Response scale 2: a) *No,* b) *Yes*

Given that this is fact-based item, a binary response option ("Yes/No") would suffice and is the only logical fit. The 9-point rating scale shown is not only inapplicable, it is also problematic as the numerals have no descriptors to indicate what each denotes.

Rating scales for closed-ended items could go up to 10 or even 12 or more scale points. The literature suggests *five to seven* response options as ideal for most structured self-report items (Babbie, 1998, 2020; Fink, 1995). The goal should be to have each item discriminate among the *true differences* of persons on the variable of interest—a validity issue. From a classical test theory perspective, more scale points would potentially add higher levels of **variability** to response distributions—a desirable property in construct measures (Bandalos, 2018; Crocker & Algina, 2006; Price, 2018). However, if the number of scale points fails to map the typical item response distributions we could expect, random error variability may cloud the results—a reliability issue.

As the examples showed, points on the response scale need to be anchored with appropriately worded descriptors that are semantically consistent with the item stem. These descriptors should indicate logically what the degrees of difference are on an increasing gradient. For young children, pictorial icons (e.g., smiley faces) have been employed as effective descriptors on 3- or 4-point scales. Consider the next poorly matched item-to-response scale intended to measure feelings:

Poor stem-to-response wording match	Stimulus: *How do you feel about your relationship with your counselor?*
	Responses: a. *Unhappy* b. *Satisfied* c. *Sad*

This heterogeneous mix of descriptors is problematic, reflecting perhaps different aspects of "feeling" to some—happiness versus satisfaction. A more semantically consistent set of options on an increasing scale gradient might be: a) Happy; b) Neither happy nor unhappy; c) Unhappy. The use of the vague and broad words like *feel* invites responses from different perspectives and reference points (more on this in Section 7.6). Lastly, the response scale is biased given that two of three options are negatively oriented words—a) and c).

7.5.6 Choosing between Open- and Closed-Ended Item Formats

As evident, open-ended interview item formats are sometimes necessary in self-reported assessments. Five guiding considerations to inform that choice are occasions when:

- respondents are likely to vary so greatly on the subject of interest that a highly structured item response format will result in a loss of information.
- the measurement process is still exploratory and not enough is known about the constructs and/or the population to design structured-response items effectively.
- we seek to follow up on previously obtained answers to closed-ended items with open-ended question probes (Figure 7.3).
- the respondents are unable to respond to a structured-response tool due to special needs or other barriers.
- time and resources are available to permit proper application of open-ended assessments, including administration, scoring, data compilation, and analysis.

7.5.7 Instrument Assembly: Standardizing the Assessment Conditions, Scoring, and Instructions for Self-Report Tools

A finished self-report tool must be complete and easy-to-apply for both participants and users, yielding the highest quality of data possible that meets the primary users' needs. The recommendations that follow are consistent with ethical research and professional practice standards in assessment and evaluation generally, and applicable across fields. Readers may wish to further consult the Ethical Guiding Principles of the American Evaluation Association (AEA, 2018, at *www.eval.org*; see also AERA et al., 2014; Yarbrough et al., 2011). These and similar resources will provide a useful base for guiding the design, assembly, and use of various instruments employed for a wide array of purposes.

To complete the assembly of a self-report instrument, we need to give attention to the following areas:

- A brief statement of the purpose for the tool
- Clear and easy-to-comprehend general directions for all respondents, interviewees, examiners, and assessment users/administrators, as applicable
- Special instructions for subsections of the tool, as applicable
- A user-friendly design and layout of the tool
- Guidelines for administering the instrument, as necessary
- Guidelines for a scoring procedure, interpretation, and use of results
- Assurance of confidentiality and/or anonymity for respondents and other users, as applicable

Declaring the assessment purpose for an instrument openly is necessary. Outside improving the likelihood of a higher response rate, transparency of purpose earns the trust of respondents and other assessment users. The statement need be no more than two to five sentences long and should ideally include a note of appreciation. For example:

> **Purpose:** This survey is for research purposes only. Do *not* enter your name or personal information. Please be as honest as possible. The results will be kept *completely confidential*. You can learn more about the study and obtain a copy of the report here [add website]. Thank you for your participation.

When subsections of the instrument change, such as shifting from open-ended to closed-ended questions, or between item sets with different response scales, special directions are necessary to alert respondents to make the transitions smoothly. The overall survey or interview presentation format must be inviting, readable, printed in sufficiently large font size for the screen or on paper, as the case might be.

Assurance of confidentiality and anonymity, as appropriate to the application, are critical for compliance with ethical standards, as well as securing the trust and full participation of the respondents.

As shown in highly abbreviated form with the Thurstone scale in Box 7.2, directions are necessary to guide respondents on how to complete the assessment exactly as designed. Depending on the instruments, instructions are necessary for interviewers, examiners, or other users involved to standardize the conditions for assessment delivery and administration, scoring, score interpretation, and proper uses of the tool, or for making allowable accommodations for those who might need it. The standardization guidelines may apply to any videos, printed materials, other supporting materials for the instrument. Interviewer orientation and training protocols may be necessary for self-report assessments intended for high-stakes decisions, such as certifying professionals.

QUICK RECAP: To build useful self-report tools, the specific steps of the domain sampling method are adapted. As with other modalities, item-writing, instrument design and assembly, and design-related actions should be informed by the particulars of the assessment user context. Apt choices in item structures, wording, and response scales increase the likelihood of meaningful, rather than invalid, whimsical, and unreliable, responses. A vast number of item functioning issues can be addressed by following established guidelines and, when possible, pilot-testing the items.

Reflection Break 7.4: Objectives 3–6

- Describe *three steps* you would take differently to design a useful self-report tool for a *cognitive construct* versus a *noncognitive construct*. What are some measurement benefits of using this approach?
- What is the difference between a *maximum performance response* versus a *typical response* for items on a self-report tool? Give examples.
- Describe factors you would consider to match the choice of a self-report modality (interview or survey) to the backgrounds of your desired *population*.
- Describe factors you would consider to match the choice of a specific self-report modality (interview or survey) to your desired *construct*.
- List the main components of a well-assembled self-report tool and explain why each is important.

7.6 Ten More Guidelines for Writing Closed-Ended Survey Items

Even when self-report items appear to match the indicator and domain specifications closely, as we saw, good writing skills and word choices are essential for good item design or selection. Ten guidelines follow next for *closed-ended item writing*, with demonstrations of common issues. Refer back to the items in Figures 7.2 and 7.3 again, as needed.

1. **Write or select concretely stated, succinct items that provide a common reference framework for all respondents.** A concrete item is clear because it provides a well-defined and shared reference framework that all respondents can use to generate the response. To write concretely situated items, we could provide a timeframe, location, common episode, or particular experience. Consider the three items next (A–C), intended to measure beliefs about the effectiveness of a counselor accompanied with a standard Likert response scale.

- Item A: *My counselor considers my feelings.*
- Item B: *In the past month, my counselor considered my feelings.*
- Item C: *In the past month, my counselor helped me deal with my negative thoughts.*

  Item Evaluation:
- Item C is the best item of the three. It is situated within a concrete timeframe. Rather than a vague reference to feelings, it refers to a specific type of counseling experience, "dealing with negative thoughts." It is also short and on point. Compared

to A and B, it will likely yield the most useful information on a respondent's beliefs about their counselor's performance.]

2. Use either a complete sentence or direct question format in each item stem. The item stem is sometimes presented as an incomplete sentence. On many occasions with literate and educated participants, this would be adequate. In others, a more desirable format is a direct question or complete sentence that communicates the main idea to the respondent clearly and fully. Item-writers should exercise judgment in deciding which strategy facilitates a clear and reader-friendly communication, staying faithful to the indicator being measured. For example, to measure a person's beliefs about the counselor–client relationship, the *question format* next may be the best one, as shown below:

A. **Incomplete statement stem:** *My working relationship with my counselor is:*
   a) Satisfactory
   b) Neither Satisfactory nor Unsatisfactory
   c) Unsatisfactory

B. **Question stem:** *To what extent do you have a satisfactory working relationship with your counselor?*

C. **Complete sentence stem:** *Indicate the extent to which you have a satisfactory working relationship with your counselor.*

   Response scale for B–C:
   a) To a great extent
   b) To a moderate extent
   c) Barely
   d) Not at all

3. Avoid writing highly verbose items, and the use of complex vocabulary, technical language, and jargon. Consider this next item to measure perceived levels of concern about partner abuse among college students.

Academic jargon in an item:

Year-specific perceived norms of partner abuse in dating relationships of college freshman students are a cause for concern.

Likert response scale: SA-A-U-D-SD

This item has 18 words and appears to be excerpted in part from an academic book or technical paper. Overly wordy items, and use of technical language like "year-specific perceived norms," may carry little meaning for typical respondents. If used at all, technical terms and jargon should be defined in user-friendly terms. A better item would use fewer words, a more personalized sentence structure, direct language, and a reading and vocabulary level appropriate for the population, as follows.

A jargon-free, shorter item:

I worry when I hear that undergraduate students physically assault their dates.

4. Avoid the use of abbreviations and acronyms in items, unless defined. For those unfamiliar, an item using acronyms, such as UNICEF or WHO (to refer to the United Nations Children's Educational Fund and World Health Organization, respectively), could obstruct readability and comprehension levels.

Item with an undefined acronym:

I am glad that the WHO supports health counseling for college students.

Response scale: SA-A-U-D-SD

As a rule, we should spell out all acronyms in a dedicated section of the tool to prevent confusions. All abbreviated terms should be defined simply and clearly.

5. Avoid double-, triple-, or multi-barreled items. Self-report items that contain more than one idea in the statement or question are multi-barreled. For example, the item "My counselor helps me deal with my anger and anxiety" is double-barreled in focusing on two separate behavioral issues. Individuals who vary in their experience on one or the other issue would be unable to respond accurately. Such an item is better when split into two separate items.

6. Avoid leading questions. An item that is leading strongly suggests a socially desirable answer to the respondent. When the goal is to capture the actual and typical response, the item wording should not point to what the "appropriate" response might be. Consider the following item to measure opinions about requiring mental health counseling:

A leading item:

As gun violence is rising in public schools, every student should receive counseling services.

Response scale: SA-A-U-D-SD

The clause "as gun violence is rising in public schools" is leading. To measure opinions, the item stimulus is better presented as "Counseling services should be available for public school students."

7. **Avoid loaded questions.** An item is "loaded" when it incorporates presupposed assumptions that may or may not be true for all individuals, such as the following:

A loaded item stem:

How often do you get angry with your husband about issues in your household?

This item assumes that all respondents are (1) married with a "husband," (2) living in the same household with their husband, and (3) probably female. One or more of these assumptions may not be true for certain members of the population. The use of traditional labeling of a life partner could raise other issues. Reviewing the items and instructions carefully could clear up these ambiguities, but as a rule, loaded items should be avoided.

Alternatively, the items could be presented after screening out the subgroups of interest. An item to screen persons based on self-identified gender may look like this:

Please indicate your gender identity.

a) Male
b) Female
c) Other (fill in) ____________

If you answered b), please complete the next two questions.

8. **Balance the number of positively and negatively worded item response options equally.** A heavier loading with more positively worded response options creates a built-in bias in an item that may also be leading. An equally balanced set of options would give equal chances to each and not suggest any direction for respondents.

An item with a 50% built-in positive bias	**Item stimulus:** *How happy do you feel about your marital relationship?*
	Responses: a) Very happy [positive] b) Happy [positive] c) Indifferent [neutral] d) Unhappy [negative]

9. **Mix in a small number of negatively worded or reverse-oriented items randomly in the subscales, scales, or overall instrument.** A *few* negatively oriented items in a tool are useful in preventing response sets or thoughtless, disengaged responses, as previous examples showed. However, factor analytic research suggests that negatively worded items tend to measure a "negative semantic factor" instead of the targeted constructs (see, e.g., DiStephano & Motl, 2006). Hence, including negatively oriented items sparsely, and evaluating how such items perform empirically *before* including them in the instrument, may be the most prudent approach. If negative words are used in items, they should be italicized, bolded, or underlined to draw the readers' attention. Double negatives should be avoided regardless, as they tend to add confusion and are problematic grammatically. For example, "I <u>do not</u> support students receiving <u>no</u> counseling in public schools" may leave respondents unsure as to whether they should agree or disagree.

10. **Screen items for the appearance of bias toward diverse or minority groups.** This final guideline applies to all self-report items, both closed-ended and open-ended alike. The self-report assessment must *appear to be free of biases* toward any minorities during the initial item screening, review, and instrument compilation process. For this step, majority and minority participants in the population—whether based on age, ethnicity, gender, special needs, culture, or other background factors—must first be identified. Careful reviews of the instrument and items must verify that

the language, pictorials, references, or other parts of the tool will not bar access, or otherwise demean or portray particular individuals or subgroups in a negative light. This process may be carried out by the assessment designers themselves or by external reviewers for higher-stakes tools.

QUICK RECAP: Table 7.1 provides a checklist to guide preliminary reviews of different types of self-report items and tools during the assessment design or selection process, including the 10 item-writing guidelines provided for closed-ended items. These are commonsense tactics that could help reduce errors rooted in the item or response wording, sentence construction, scale structures, or presentation formats. Biases can be inadvertently and easily incorporated item stems and response choices. However, most such problems can be rectified through carefully performed reviews before assembling an instrument in final form.

Reflection Break 7.5: Objectives 3–6

- From existing self-report tools used in your field or organization, identify *closed-ended items* that fall in each of these categories.
  - Items having rating scales with too few or too many points than necessary
  - Items with no descriptors or poor descriptors for rating scale points
  - Items that have wording, language, or structural issues
  - Item stems that are too long or too short
  - Items that fail to communicate the question clearly
  - Items that are not concretely situated
  - Items that are leading <u>or</u> loaded
  - Items with other kinds of issues, such as negative wording, jargon, acronyms, biases, complex vocabulary, and the like (identify the specific issue you see)
- For each item, indicate how you would address the issue.

7.7 A Case Study: Designing Self-Report Tools with the Process Model

To end the chapter, we turn to an application of the Process Model focusing on a complementary set of assessments designed for mental health screening purposes, a survey-based and an interview-based tool. The title of the original instrumentation was *Subjective Perceptions of Unhealthy Intimate Relationships* (Bogart, 2003). That design is slightly modified here for illustration purposes with permission of the author (Bogart, personal communication, June 15, 2021). See Boxes 7.7 and 7.8 and Tables 7.2 and 7.3. Terms pertinent to applying a user-centerd design process are presented in italics as we proceed.

7.7.1 The Setting

The assessment designer in this case was a psychologist at the student services division of a large urban university located in the Northeast. At the time, there was a compelling, data-based rationale for undertaking the project at that institution, with possible applications in other higher education institutions in the region. Violence and abuse in intimate relationships were on the rise in many college campuses, affecting younger and older adults alike. Research studies showed that in adult dating, cohabitating, or marital partnership situations, the intimate relationship status of individuals was associated with one or more kinds of abuse—physical, verbal, emotional, or other serious forms of partner neglect (see, e.g., Wiersma, Cleveland, Herrera, & Fischer, 2010).

For potential victims, initial screening is the first step toward identifying a need for further assistance. Intake assessments of student-clients are standard practice at university clinics; the new two-part screening assessment was added to existing intake protocols at the institution where the author worked (Bogart, 2003).

7.7.2 Phases of the Process Model

7.7.2.1 Phase I: Specifying the Assessment User Context

To begin the design process, the *What?*, *Who?*, and *Why?* questions were addressed, situated in mental health service settings at university clinics (Figure 7.1). The main construct was identified as noncognitive in

TABLE 7.1. A Checklist for Designing Self-Report Tools

Checklist for overall tool

1. Does the overall assessment and items show a match with:
   - the content and behaviors in the indicators and overall construct domains?
   - the demographic and socioecological context specifications of the intended population?
   - the assessment purposes, including the specific inferences and uses planned with scores?
2. Are the directions clear? Are the directions sufficient?
3. Are the assessment conditions and materials clearly outlined?
4. Are the scoring procedures clearly described?
5. Are there enough items by domain and subdomain to generate reliable scores?
6. Are the overall layout and presentation user-friendly?
7. Does the assessment *appear to be* free of the following?
   - Readability bias
   - Inflammatory bias
   - Stereotypical bias
   - Materials- or conditions-related biases

Checklist for closed-ended survey items

1. Are item statements or questions clearly written?
2. Is the language in items concrete?
3. Are wordy items absent?
4. Do the answer options fit the stem of the item?
5. Are double- or triple-barreled items absent?
6. Are there sufficient response categories to capture the variability of expected responses?
7. Are there any "leading" questions?
8. Are there any "loaded" questions?
9. Is the number of points on the response scale reasonable? Does each response point have a clear descriptor?
10. Are negative words, if used, in italics or underscored (e.g., not)? Are double negatives avoided?
11. Are negatively oriented items used sparingly and with judgment?
12. Are items free of:
    - jargon (e.g., use of technical terms)?
    - abbreviations (e.g., ADD for attention-deficit disorder)?
    - biased language or content (e.g., boys are more violent than girls)?

Added checklist for interview-based items

1. Is there a script to accompany interview questions? Is the script sufficiently clear?
2. Is the script interviewer-friendly?
3. Are there adequate directions for each step of the interview?
4. Do instructions for interviewers/recorders clarify:
   - the time allowed for each prompt?
   - the probes allowed for each prompt?
   - when to skip items?
   - pause periods (e.g., between item prompt and probes)?
   - how to deal with unexpected responses (e.g., rambling)?
   - the methods for recording, scoring, and coding responses?

nature, dealing with so-called subjective perceptions of an unhealthy relationship with intimate partners (*What?*). The population comprised all students age 18 or older enrolled at the local university and other universities in that state who were involved in intimate relationships and who had reached out to the university clinics for health care needs (*Who?*). A review of demographic distributions in student databases enabled the designer to align the instrument design specifications (detailed next) with students' diversity profiles and backgrounds. The *population unit*, for assessment administration and making inferences from the results, was the individual student-client.

The broad *assessment purpose* of the two-part screening procedure was specified as mental health screening in university-based clinical settings (*Why?*). The *specific uses* were to screen student-clients involved in intimate relationships for signs of distress due to exposure to abuse, assault, or neglect by partners. The assessment was expected to inform decisions on the immediate next steps necessary, such as more in-depth diagnostic testing and provision of targeted support or treatment for those in critical need. To allow for more trustworthy *inferences* about any "red flags," the scores from both parts were to be interpreted together.

The initially identified *primary users* of the assessment results were (1) the counseling and clinical psychologists at the university clinic, including the designer; (2) administrators and support staff of the student services divisions of the university; and (3) the student-clients themselves. For "red-flagged" clients, the *secondary users* of the assessment results included other medical and clinical professionals involved in any subsequent interventions or support.

7.7.2.2 Phase II: Specifying the Assessment Operations

DOMAIN AND SUBDOMAINS

An excerpt of the domain, with selected behavioral *indicators* on emotional abuse only, is shown in Box 7.7. The general indicator of the domain was broken down in terms of *four subdomains* dealing with emotional, physical, and verbal abuse, and other harmful forms of negligent behavior. The assessment designer drew on relevant psychological literature, clinical assessment resources, and practice guidelines to specify the domain (see the excerpt in Box 7.7). To set item-writing parameters, the designer applied the functional taxonomy for assessing noncognitive constructs, focusing on measuring clients' *feelings* and *beliefs* about self-perceived behaviors of intimate partners, given their best recollections.

ASSESSMENT MODALITIES SELECTED.

By definition, screening involves short and quick assessments (Chapter 2; AERA et al., 2014). Initially, both parts of the screening assessment were designed to be administered to every client: a 10- to 12-minute *paper-and-pencil survey* (Part 1), followed by a 15- to 20-minute one-on-one *verbal interview* (Part 2), the latter conducted by credentialed psychologists or counselors. Given that diverse student-clients were expected to share private and sensitive details about their intimate relationships, two different avenues of response afforded greater flexibility for making accommodations. Combining two modes also afforded better domain coverage, assuring higher levels of content-based validity. With a greater number of items overall, the reliability of scores was expected to increase. The two-part assessment was to be kept short enough so that the entire process could be completed in 30 minutes for individual clients.

MODIFIED "PARALLEL FORMS" DESIGN

Strictly speaking, parallel forms of an instrument must be equivalent in every aspect, including the item formats, the distribution of items by content and taxonomic categories, as well as the statistical and psychometric properties of the scores (AERA et al., 2014; Bandalos, 2018; Price, 2018). In this case, a modified set of design specifications were prepared for creating *parallel forms* consisting of closed-ended items (Parts 1 and 2). Both forms were built with Likert-scaled or modified Likert-type items linked to the same subdomain indicators, with similar percentages of items distributed to match the four kinds of abuse specified in the domain (Box 7.7). Part 1 focused on measuring participant *feelings* about partner behaviors; Part 2 measured participant *beliefs* about partner behaviors with fewer closed-ended items, alongside six to eight open-ended *item probes*.

BOX 7.7 Domain Specifications for Measuring Subjective Perceptions of Unhealthy Intimate Relationships

General Indicator

Adults involved in intimate relationships report experiences of abuse or harmful neglect by their spouse/partner based on their recollections within the past 6 months.

Taxonomic levels

- *Beliefs*
- *Feelings*

Specific Indicators

- Recalls experiences of *emotional abuse* by partners
- Recalls experiences of *physical abuse*, including sexual abuse and assault by partners
- Recalls experiences of *verbal abuse* by partners
- Reports experiences of *harmful neglect* by partners

Subindicators of Emotional Abuse [Excerpted]

Subject indicates that partner:

1.1. Uses guilt or other forms of coercion to get desired reaction from subject
1.2 Displays extreme mood swings (highs and lows) when with subject
1.3 Gives subject the "silent treatment" (ignores partner) for periods of time
1.4 Isolates subject from family and/or friends
1.5 Restricts subject's use of phone or other forms of communication with others
1.6 Tracks subject's whereabouts
1.7 Shows irrational reactions to subject's behavior
1.8 Blames subject for things that go wrong, regardless of whether the subject is responsible

References [Excerpted]:

1. Burge, S. K. (1998). How do you define abuse? *Family Medicine, 7*(1), 3132.
2. Eisenstat, B. D. (1999). Examples of abusive behavior. *New England Journal of Medicine, 341*(12), 886–892 (Table 1).

Source: Adapted with permission from Bogart (2021) and Chatterji and Freda (2003). © Madhabi Chatterji.

ITEM DESIGN SPECIFICATIONS

Items were written or selected in accordance with established item-writing rules. To control for avoidance, the designer selected a 4-point *forced-choice* Likert rating scale on Part 1, with the "Uncertain" option removed. Part 2 used a modified a 4-point frequency-based scale to indicate client-perceived levels of specific behaviors of partners. On each form, the designer included three to four affirmatively worded items that were randomly distributed; these were *reverse-scored*. The readability and vocabulary were deliberately kept at a high school level (Tables 7.1–7.3).

Part 2 was designed for the purposes of confirming details of specific types and episodes of abuse. These included client-reported facts about why, who, when, where, and how often the episodes occurred (see Items a–e in Table 7.3).

Specifications of Assessment Conditions and Materials. Both tools were administered in print form in one visit, after obtaining voluntary consent and client permissions. Clients were allocated a quiet and private office space for completing the assessment, with the assigned psychologist/counselor nearby for assistance as necessary, and for administering Part 2; no other persons were present.

Scoring Specifications. For the closed-ended item sections on both Parts 1 and 2, the designer specified a scoring procedure yielding a summated total score for

TABLE 7.2. Survey-Based Screening Assessment: Subjective Perceptions of Unhealthy Relationships

Purpose: This self-assessment will be used for *screening purposes only*. Your answers will be kept completely confidential. There are no right or wrong answers. Please be as honest as you can in your responses. After you finish, a counselor will discuss the next steps with you.

Directions: The statements below describe your feelings about your partner's behaviors *in the past 6 months*. Place a check to indicate if you Strongly Agree (SA), Agree (A), Disagree (D), or Strongly disagree (SD) with each statement. Choose only one response to each statement.

Thank you for your participation.

	Response choices**			
In the past six (6) months, I *felt:*	SA	A	D	SD
1. *afraid* I would do things that would make my partner angry.				
2. *anxious* about how my partner would react to things I did.				
3. *safe* when I was with my partner.*				
4. *a need to make excuses* to others about my partner's behavior.				
5. *confident I could trust my partner* with my personal items.*				
6. *afraid* my partner would be unhappy no matter what I did.				
7. *worried my partner would prevent me* from doing what I wanted.				
8. *anxious* that I must have done something wrong whenever my partner was angry.				
9. *happy* that I was a valued partner in the relationship.*				
10. *afraid to end the relationship*, although it was a bad situation.				
[*Excerpted from original tool*]				

Note. *Indicates reverse-oriented items; **point allocations: SA = 3 points, A = 2 points, D = 1 point, SD = 0 points; points reversed for reverse-oriented items. Adapted with permission from Bogart (2021) and Chatterji and Freda (2003).

TABLE 7.3. Interview-Based Screening Tool: Measuring Subjective Perceptions of Unhealthy Relationships

Items	Response choices**			
In the past 6 months, *how often* did your partner:	Very often	Often	Sometimes	Never
1. *embarrass you* in front of others?	______	______	______	______
2. *compliment you* for something you did well?*	______	______	______	______
3. *blame you* for making them angry?	______	______	______	______
4. *treat you roughly*, like grab, pinch, shove, or hit you?	______	______	______	______
5. *encourage you* to spend time with friends and family?*	______	______	______	______
6. *check up on you* to make sure you were exactly where you said you would be?	______	______	______	______
7. *say things that made you feel incapable* of making a decision on your own?	______	______	______	______
8. *pressure you to do things sexually* that you do not want to do?	______	______	______	______
9. *take money without your knowledge* and not pay you back?	______	______	______	______
10. *blame you* for something that did not do?	______	______	______	______
11. *support you* in your professional life?*	______	______	______	______
12. *express displeasure* with the way you look?	______	______	______	______

Directions to interviewers and script for item probes:

In Items 1, 3, 6, 7–10, and 12, for probing, choose <u>any two items</u> on which the client gave a Sometimes, Often, or Very often answer.

- *You chose* ______ *to Item* ______ (insert answers). *How many times did this happen?*
- *Tell me more about what happened exactly on the latest occasion. Could you give me some details—what was going on at the time? When did it happen? Where? Who else was present? Why did it happen? What do you think caused it? Were you alone?*
- *In the latest episode, how did you respond? For example, did you share how you felt with your partner?*
- *What else did they do that seemed wrong or hurtful (or supportive and caring) to you?*

From the reverse-oriented items, Items 2, 5, and 11, choose <u>any one item</u> for probing. Repeat the bulleted steps above.

Note. *Indicates reverse-oriented items; **point allocations: Very often = 3 points, Often = 2 points, Sometimes = 1 point, Never = 0 points; points reversed for reverse-oriented items.

Adapted with permission from Bogart (2021) and Chatterji and Freda (2003).

each client (see Box 7.3 for reference). Recorded interview notes were coded for matches with a preprepared list of terms signifying indicators of partner abuse drawn from the literature. These included words such as "silent treatment," "yell," "hit," "secret," "bruise," "cried," "scared," "push," "pain," "trust."

Initially, drafted tools were pilot-tested. The data distributions helped the designer set cut points on the quantitative scale for identifying clients with the highest service needs. All final decisions following client screening were made using the combined results of the survey and interview process.

7.7.2.3 Phase III: Design the Instrument

INITIAL VERSIONS OF TOOLS—PARTS 1 AND 2

See Tables 7.2 and 7.3 and Box 7.8 again. The designer assembled early drafts of 30–50 items for a preliminary content validation by experts. Of these, the items that matched to the domain specifications and complied with item-writing guidelines were selected for inclusion in the instruments.

Table 7.2 shows an excerpt of Part 1 of the tool. The form included 24 items in all, with three reverse-oriented items.

BOX 7.8 Interview Script and Instructions: Measuring Subjective Perceptions of Unhealthy Relationships

- Greet client.
  Obtain voluntary consent and permission.
  Explain any paperwork on obtaining consent and permission.
  Make client comfortable.
  State, before starting, *The assessment can be stopped whenever you want. May we begin?*

- State assessment purpose.
  Please read aloud to interviewee, if needed, or adapt to the situation: *This is a "relationship screening assessment" with a short survey and an interview. The results will be used for screening purposes only; that is, we will only use the results to evaluate if there are needs for further assessments, a follow-up consultation, or no need for any of these. This interview or the survey is not for diagnosing any health issues or providing services or treatments. Are you comfortable with this purpose?*

- Provide directions for the interview.

  Begin only when interviewee is ready.

  This interview will take 15 to 20 minutes in all. All your answers will be kept ***completely confidential.*** *Please be honest in your responses. Shall we start?*

  This interview has ***two*** *parts.*
  In Section A, I will read aloud ***12 short questions****, one by one, about your partner's behavior toward you over the past 6 months. Tell me what you remember. Here is an example.* [Read aloud Item 2 with the response options.]
  For each question, please choose only ***one*** *answer that best describes your partner's behavior as you remember it: a) Very often, b) Often, c) Sometimes, or d) Never. I will put an X in the column that matches your response.*

- Provide directions for open-ended questions.
- Begin open-ended interview only when interviewee is ready.

State, *In Section B, I will ask a* ***few*** *follow-up questions. Describe your experiences in your own words. I will note down your answers as you are speaking and read my notes back so that you can correct any omissions or mistakes I may have made. Comfortable? Ready to start?*

Added Instructions:
Allow a 1- to 1½-minute pause between each question, as necessary, to allow interviewee to provide complete answers.

Skip item or stop the interview process if client resists, is upset, rambles, or gives far-fetched, impossible, and/or contradictory responses.

For Part 2, a semi-standardized script and interview protocol were constructed to provide guidance to interviewers. As this protocol was self-explanatory, there were minimal needs for staff orientation or training (Box 7.8). The interview included 12 closed-ended items and 8 item probes (Table 7.3).

7.7.2.4 Phase IV: Validate the Items, Instrument, and Measures

The designer conducted (1) a content validation and critical review of all the assessment materials by three external experts; (2) **cognitive interviews** of a small group of student-clients and interviewers after the pilot testing was over; and (3) a pilot test of the assessment procedure with 20 student-clients.

CONTENT VALIDATION OF INITIAL ITEMS AND TOOLS BY EXTERNAL EXPERTS

This critical review informed the revisions that followed (Polit, Beck, & Owen, 2007). The validation was performed by two clinical and counseling psychologists from the student services division, and a faculty-researcher in measurement from another university who were not involved in the instrument design process.

Bearing in mind the confidential, sensitive, and potentially high-stakes nature of the screening procedure for individual clients, the guiding questions for the content validation were comprehensive.

- *Domain coverage.* Are the domain's indicators consistent with the most up-to-date research literature on intimate partner abuse and related mental health issues? Are all the important indicators represented in the domain and subdomains?
- *Content relevance and content representativeness.* Do items on both instruments match the indicators? Are items distributed appropriately to cover each subdomain?
- *Item clarity, succinctness, and directness.* Is the wording/language in the items, instructions, and assessment materials clear? Is the communication direct (not confusing)? Are any items too long or wordy? Are the presentation and layout of items and forms clean and easy-to-read?
- *Usefulness.* Are both parts of the screening assessment likely to yield information that is beneficial to the student-clients and primary users of the tools? Could the assessment or information gathered in any way harm or have a negative consequence on clients, their families, or the university clinic?
- *Usability.* Are interview instructions, scoring, and interview protocols easy to use? Is the language in items and assessment forms interviewer- and student-friendly? Can the process (Parts 1 and 2) be completed in the allocated time?
- *Reliability.* Are there sufficient items to produce reliable scores from each part of the assessment?
- *Appearance of bias.* Do any parts of the screening assessment appear to be unfairly biased, inaccessible, or inflammatory toward diverse or minority individuals and subgroups?

Cognitive Interviewing of Respondents. A *cognitive interview* is a qualitative interview to examine how individual respondents mentally processed the information as they interacted with specific items and the assessment; effective cognitive interviews help validate the extent to which the designer's intentions are borne out in the participants' response processes (Carbone, Campbell, & Honess-Morreale, 2002). In this project, the designer used a **focus group interview** for this purpose (Rabiee, 2004). She asked a small group of five clients and their interviewers a brief set of open-ended questions. Specifically, they were asked to share why they chose particular responses to items, how they interpreted different items, how comfortable they felt responding, and any concerns or barriers they experienced during the two-part screening assessment. Insights gained led to added revisions to both parts of the assessment.

Decision Criteria for Identifying Client Needs. The results obtained from testing the first 20 clients at the clinic helped improve the administration procedures and tighten scoring criteria and other guidelines. They further helped set "standards" as *cut-score points* on the scale for identifying client need levels. The designer completed this step in consultation with the three external experts, setting score-based criteria for three client groups (see, e.g., Cizek, 2013; more on this topic in Chapter 9): *high needs* (those with the highest score range, reflecting long-term and clear patterns of abuse and neglect); *moderate to low needs* (those with scores in the middle range, reflecting mild or occasional abuse and/or neglect); and *no needs* (those reporting negligible or no signs of abuse and neglect by partners).

7.7.2.5 Phase V: Evaluate Readiness of Tool for Use

REVISIONS AND DECISIONS FOLLOWING INITIAL VALIDATION

Following the initial validation, several items were revised/rewritten or removed altogether due to flaws. The lengths of the survey and interview were altered to better balance the number of items by subdomain. Other procedures, directions, and the interview script were similarly refined. The cognitive interview indicated that the two-part screening was unduly time-consuming when administered to every client. The procedure was changed to a two-stage assessment, where only the subset of clients "red-flagged" in Part 1 were to be administered in Part 2.

IMPLEMENTING THE REVISED ASSESSMENT

The modified "final" versions of the tools, not shown here, were considered ready for use for screening purposes at the university clinic (Phase V). As more clients were screened, a database was gradually built. This ongoing data-collection effort allowed further validation and psychometric evaluations to continue (Phase IV).

QUICK RECAP: Flowing directly from the specified context of use (Phase I), this case study demonstrated the how-to steps within the framework of a user-centered approach. The case illustrated the actions and thought processes of the designer in Phases II, II, and IV of the Process Model, that followed. The self-report modality is vulnerable to unique types of errors; the case study showed how to circumvent or mitigate some of the major issues during the design process.

Reflection Break 7.6: Objectives 4–6

- What are the *benefits* of taking the design approach shown in the case study for the *primary users* of the assessment?
- Create a new "parallel form" of (1) a *survey-based assessment* or (2) an *interview-based assessment* based on the domain specifications provided in Box 7.7.
- Critique the quality of self-report items shown in Tables 7.2 and 7.3 based on guidelines discussed in Sections 7.5 and 7.6. Select any five items from each tool to revise. Explain why they need revisions.
- Create some new "reverse-oriented" items using indicators in the domain shown in Box 7.7. Self-critique the items based on guidelines in this chapter.

7.8 Summary

This chapter discussed measurement principles and theory applicable for creating well-designed self-report assessments. This assessment modality is best applied on occasions when direct questioning of respondents is the most appropriate or only means for learning more about the constructs of interest. The tools can be built with various item types, with historical designs for scaling psychological constructs offering useful ideas to build on.

The chapter reviewed the literature on the numerous measurement challenges with self-reported data. It discussed several methods, established standards and guidelines, with examples of well- and poorly constructed items and tools.

As in Chapters 5 and 6, this chapter presented a real-world case study in applying the Process Model (Phases I–V), focusing on survey-based or interview-based instruments. The case delineated the steps of the design process, as well as the habits of thinking and decision making that accompany the implementation of each phase.

SECTION III

VALIDATION AND USE OF ASSESSMENTS

CHAPTER 8

Analyzing Data from Assessments
A Statistics Refresher

8.1 Chapter Overview

8.1.1 Introduction

Chapter 8 offers a refresher in basic statistics as a precursor to Chapters 9–11. Figure 8.1 shows where the chapter fits with the rest of the book and the Process Model, falling largely under empirical validation methods in Phase IV, A and B. Competence on the topics in Chapter 8 is necessary when reading or preparing "Methods" and "Instrumentation" sections of dissertations, journal articles, and technical measurement reports; the material is applicable in a number of academic and professional fields.

Readers should consider the chapter a *basic* introduction to statistical methods, as relevant to selected applications of classical test theory (CTT) and, to some extent, item response theory (IRT). For more in-depth treatments, readers should consult added textbooks and advanced resources on statistics, psychometrics, and research methods (e.g., Aron & Elliot, 2012; Bandalos, 2018; Best & Kahn, 2016; Price, 2018; see also online statistical software manuals, such as Statistical Package for Social Sciences [SPSS] at *www.statistics-solutions.com/spss-statistics-help*).

Departing from the previous chapters, Chapter 8 is intended as a *self-teaching guide*. It has eight main sections corresponding with the objectives that follow. Two small datasets are used for computations embedded in so-called Demonstration boxes. Formulas with interpretive guidelines are given alongside each topic. Key Concept boxes replace Quick Recaps. Practice Breaks replace the Reflection Breaks in other chapters.

8.1.2 Chapter Objectives

After reading this chapter and completing the accompanying exercises, the reader should be able to:

1. Distinguish among nominal, ordinal, interval, or ratio scales (levels of measurement), and discretely or continuously distributed variables.
2. Tabulate, organize, and graph data obtained from tests/assessments in rank-ordered distributions, simple (ungrouped) frequency distributions, and grouped frequency distributions.
3. Compute and interpret commonly used measures of central tendency and variability for given datasets: mean, median, mode, variance, standard deviation, range.
4. Describe mathematical properties of the *standard normal distribution* and its applications in measurement problems.

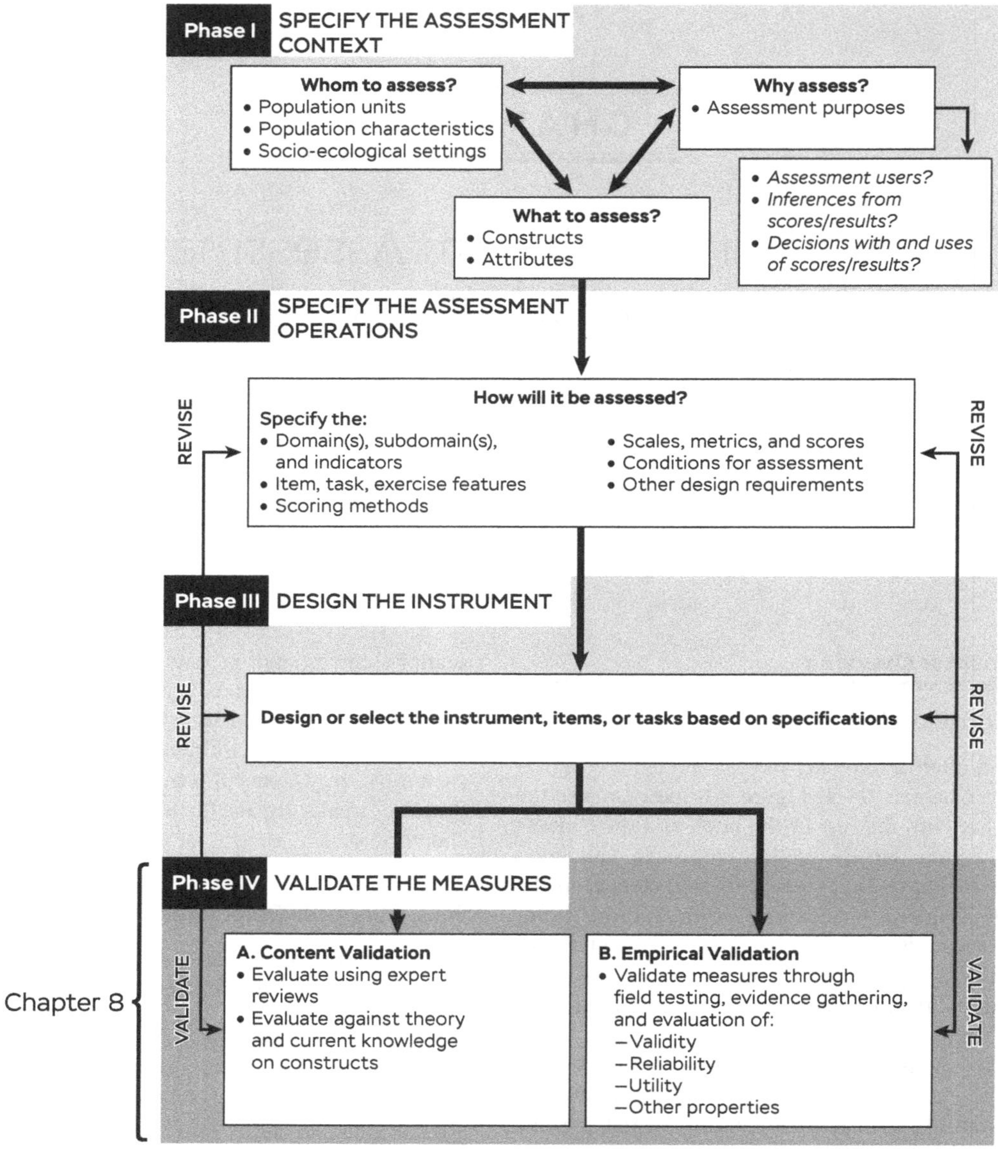

FIGURE 8.1. Connecting Chapter 8 to the Process Model and the rest of the book.

5 Compute and interpret standard scores and percentile ranks in normal and non-normal distributions.

6 Apply bivariate correlation coefficients for continuous variables meaningfully (Pearson's r).

7 Show awareness of the applications of various correlational statistics and advanced analytic methods in measurement problems, including multiple regression, factor analytic methods, and IRT techniques.

8.2 Preparing for Data Analysis

Tests *do* produce scores, and scores *are* numbers. So, if we are to think about and use test scores, we must be prepared to think with and work with numbers.
—ROBERT M. THORNDIKE (1997, p. 24, original emphasis)

8.2.1 Preparing the Dataset

Once the measures are produced from an assessment instrument, the first step is to prepare a dataset that can be analyzed. Figure 8.2 illustrates a hypothetical dataset from a self-report assessment. The responses for Item_1–Item_n are entered in a person-by-item data matrix. These data would have no right or wrong answers and could be obtained from 5-point Likert-type items (Chapter 7). The item-level data are in columns, with the responses for each person in separate rows. Had Items 1–4 represented a scale, we could generate summed *total raw scores* (X) from those ratings, as shown.

With similar data from a cognitive test with 20 items, the item-level data would appear as 1's and 0's or as ratings denoting correctness of answers. In this latter case, the raw score for different individuals would be the sum of the total number of *correctly answered* items according to preset scoring criteria, such as an answer key yielding 1's and 0's (Chapters 5 and 6).

Unless everyone has exactly same item responses, the total raw score X would present as a **variable**. Notice in Figure 8.2 that the item-level responses differ in value from person to person, and hence, each item is a variable, too. For analytic steps that follow, the typical dataset would be **multivariate**, holding data from several items and construct measures, including any background item data produced by an instrument. A majority of analytic procedures in Chapter 8 utilizes the raw data at the total score or subscale score level; in Chapters 9–11, item-level data will be necessary for certain computations, such as for computing statistics for item analysis, reliability, or specific types of scale derivation.

Before data analysis can begin, all datasets must be "cleaned." This process involves ensuring that the response data are entered correctly in the right cells and evaluating the extent to which data are missing for different persons or items. There is a vast literature on treating "missing data" to inform decisions on how best to fill any observed gaps (see, e.g., Sterne et al., 2009). The goal should be to either impute the missing data with a suitable mathematical algorithm *or* to delete individual item or person data with a list-wise or pair-wise procedure while holding intact most of the dataset. The procedural options for this step lie outside the scope of this discussion, but are available in standard statistical software packages (see, e.g., SPSS at *www.statisticssolutions.com/spss-statistics-help*). We should remember, however, that a dataset with too much missing data is undesirable even when much of it may be imputable in a statistically defensible manner.

	Item_1	Item_2	Item_3	Item_4 ... Item_n	Score
Person_1	2	2	5	4	13
Person_2	1	4	3	3	11
Person_3	2	3	3	3	11
Person_4		5	1	4	13
Person_5	2	2	2	2	12
...					
Person_p					

FIGURE 8.2. A "person-by-item" data matrix.

8.2.2 Levels of Measurement

Next, we need to identify the level of measurement of the numeric data obtained from the items, subscales, or total scales. This step informs the interpretations possible and the selection of the most appropriate analytic methods to follow. Refer back to the levels of measurement introduced in Chapter 1, namely—**nominal**, **ordinal**, **interval**, and **ratio** scales (Stevens, 1946) and the operations, examples, and definitions of each in

Table 1.2 for each. Another quick review of each type of scale follows again in Table 8.1.

Recall that assessment designers could choose to scale given constructs on any level of measurement, depending on user interests and information needs. For instance, classroom teachers often create tests to measure student achievement levels, where the original test scores may range from, say, 1 to 100; typically, such test scores are treated as *interval*-level data. Subsequently, however, the teachers could group the same scores in marking categories, for example, with 90–100 (A), 80–89 (B), 70–79 (C), and 69 and below (F), for assigning student grades. In this second application, the categorical numerals are ordered and would now be on an *ordinal* scale.

Use of the term *numeral* is deliberate here, as the data at the lower levels of measurement in Stevens's scheme (i.e., the nominal or ordinal scale) do not carry the properties of a real number line. Hence, the 0 for measuring *sex* in Table 8.1 is not a true zero indicating a total absence of the attribute, but rather denotes the membership of a person in a different category from the 1. On an ordinal scale, in contrast, a 0 denotes the lowest category value relative to a 1, 2, 3, or higher numeral; as each value increases in order, we infer that there is more of the underlying attribute being measured but cannot tell how much more in exact terms.

Stevens's (1946) scale typology included an *invariance* requirement that prescribed how the numerals from each type of scale could (or should) be manipulated mathematically, given their properties. Here, *invariance* implies that the essential properties of the numerals would remain intact even after analytic treatments. While statisticians tend to treat all numbers similarly regardless of their origins, meanings, or properties—akin to numerals on football jerseys (see, e.g., Lord, 1953)—Stevens (1946, 1968) held that the numerals on measurement scales should depict the underlying properties of the targeted constructs. His scale classification system continues to be widely employed in the social and behavioral sciences; in this book, we use it as a general guide.

If we apply Stevens's (1946) invariance requirements strictly, some added statistical assumptions could be imposed about how the measured variables would be distributed. Distributional assumptions usually come into play when computing and applying different statistics. For example, individuals scaled on the interval and ratio levels would be expected to have *parametric* distributions, with a known shape, param-

TABLE 8.1. Four Levels of Measurement: A Quick Review

Scale type	Example	Interpretations
Nominal scale	Scaling people on *sex*, where *0* = Males *1* = Females	Numerals denote a qualitatively different class or category in which individuals are placed.
Ordinal scale	Scaling *formal education level*, where: *0* = None *1* = Completed primary school *2* = Completed secondary school *3* = Completed 2-year college *4* = Completed 4-year college or more	Numerals denote ordered categories in which individuals are placed. Values have a property of increasing order, but units are not necessarily equal in size. Individuals assigned 0 have less of the attribute than those with 1; both 1 and 2 have less of the attribute than those with 3, and so on.
Interval scale	Scaling *attitude toward community service* using the total scores from a multi-item survey.	This is a linear scale with an arbitrary 0 as a starting point, after which values increase in equal-sized units. Individuals with a score of 12 have 6 more units of the attribute than those with 6. But 12 is *not* twice that of 6, due to the arbitrary zero point.
Ratio scale	Scaling *height* with a meter rule in children and youth.	This is a linear scale with a true zero and equidistant units. Individuals with a score of 4 have twice as much of the measured attribute as those with 2.

eters, and properties. The familiar bell curve, the **normal distribution**, has an expected parametric distribution. In comparison, with nominal- or ordinal-level data, the distribution shapes and properties are often relatively unknown; the latter are viewed as *nonparametric* distributions with less restrictive assumptions. More on data distributions to follow shortly.

There is recurring debate as to whether tests and assessments in the social and behavioral sciences could yield anything beyond ordinal data. With most multi-item measures of latent constructs, whether cognitive abilities or affective characteristics, we strive to achieve at least interval-level properties. Most researchers and practitioners are willing to assume continuous, interval-level properties of the raw scores, while others may choose to mathematically transform the data to achieve interval-level properties for particular statistical procedures.

8.2.3 Continuous and Discontinuous Variables

Prior to beginning data analysis, it is also necessary to determine whether the measured variable is distributed in a *continuous* or *discrete* manner. Common observations will indicate that some variables, such as height, weight, intelligence, and achievement, naturally occur in a form that permits scaling on a linear continuum with every possible fractional amount possible in between units. For example, we can meaningfully express the measured heights of different persons as 5.5, 5.56, or 5.567 feet. Similarly, distances can be measured as 10 meters (m), 10.2 m, 10.25 m, or 10.2559 m. Both these are examples of continuously distributed variables, appropriately measured with ratio scales. Interval scaling also lends itself to measuring continuous variables.

Discontinuous or discrete variables, such as *sex* in Table 8.1, are those that are naturally distributed or vary in a way that increases in whole unit increments, with intermediate values impossible, unknown or not meaningful. In the 0/1 scaling shown for *sex*, values of 0.5, 0.58, or 1.50 would make no sense as the two categories are discrete. Similarly, think of the variable *family size,* operationally defined based on counts of people living together in a household. *Family size* could increase as 1, 2, 3, . . . , or more, but the increments are meaningful only in whole-person counts; it makes little sense to say 2.52 persons. Discretely distributed variables are usually scaled on nominal or ordinal scales. This treatment makes the data suitable for various types of categorical data analysis.

8.3 Organizing the Data

Appropriate methods of data organization assist in depicting generally where a group of individuals stand on the measured constructs. They are also necessary for computing various **descriptive statistics**, which are statistical indices used to describe the groups on measured variables. There are three major methods for tabulating and arranging datasets. These arrangements could apply to item-level data, raw test scores, and mathematically transformed or derived construct measures. They are:

1. Rank-ordered distributions
2. Simple (or ungrouped) frequency distributions
3. Grouped frequency distributions

Each method has its advantages and disadvantages in particular situations. To illustrate each of these procedures, suppose that we administer a 10-item achievement test to a sample of 20 sixth graders. The number of individuals tested, N, is 20. The raw scores are represented with X. Each individual in the group tested would have a score, yielding X_1, X_2, X_3, . . . , X_{20}. A score of 10 denotes that the student answered 10 of 10 items correctly. Assuming we have interval-scaled, continuous data, Demonstration 8.1 next shows the tal-

DEMONSTRATION 8.1. Organizing a Dataset

	0	1	2	3	4	5	6	7	8	9	10
			X_1								X_{20}
People tested:			/	/	//	//	///	/		////	/
							//			///	

0—1—2—3—4—5—6—7—8—9—10

Achievement Scale

X_1, raw score for student 1 = 2
X_{20}, raw score for student 20 = 10
N, number of individuals tested = 20

lied scores distributed along the underlying scale continuum. Recall that "achievement" is a generic label for performance measures tied to curricula in schooling or professional training contexts (Chapter 5).

8.3.1 Rank-Ordered Distribution

In the **rank-ordered distribution**, we would simply place the scores in an ascending array from the lowest to the highest, as shown next in Demonstration 8.2. Once displayed in a rank-ordered arrangement, we can discern the patterns suggesting how the group is distributed on the variable.

An advantage of the rank-ordered arrangement is that it gives us instant information on several characteristics of the group. The **frequency (*f*)** of each score is the number of times a given score appears in a distribution. We see immediately that a raw score of 6 has a frequency of 5, denoting that five students obtained that score. A raw score of 2 has a frequency of 1. We also get an idea of the **mode (Mo)**, defined as the most frequently occurring score in a data distribution. The Mo in this distribution is 9, with a frequency of 7. The Mo is a rough "average" and an easy-to-obtain measure of **central tendency** for a group. Finally, we also see the **range (*R*)** of the score distribution, which is the difference between the highest and lowest score. In this case, the R is 8. The R denotes the degree of spread of the scores and is a measure of the **variability** of a distribution.

A practical disadvantage in using the rank-ordered arrangement becomes apparent when we have very large sample sizes. Similarly, when the measurement scale is long (say, with 100 or more operative points), the rank-ordered arrangement becomes difficult to depict visually on a page. One can envision the rank-ordered layout of a large dataset of, say, $N > 150$, becoming cumbersome to tabulate and analyze when spread out over multiple pages.

DEMONSTRATION 8.2. Rank-Ordered Distribution of Test Scores

X	
10	
9	
9	
9	
9	
9	
9	
9	Range $(R) = X_{maximum} - X_{minimum}$
7	
6	Frequency (f) of raw score of 6 = 5
6	
6	Mode (Mo) = most frequently occurring raw score in a distribution
6	Mo = 9
6	
5	
5	
4	
4	
3	
2	
$N = 20$	

KEY CONCEPT

★ *Rank-ordered distributions* involve arranging scores on a measured construct from the lowest to the highest value.

8.3.2 Simple or Ungrouped Frequency Distribution

More commonly, we might organize and tabulate the data in a **simple frequency distribution**. A simple or **ungrouped frequency distribution** results from simply tallying how many individuals received a different score (see Demonstration 8.3).

Demonstration 8.3 shows a simple frequency table. As the scores are treated as a continuous, interval-level variable, each scale unit is represented as an "interval" ranging from half a unit below a score to half a unit above the score. For example, for a score of 5, the **score interval** extends from half a unit below (4.5, the lower limit of the interval) to half a unit above a score (5.5, the upper limit of the interval). A score of 6 is defined by an interval extending from 5.5, the lower limit, to 6.5, the upper limit of the score. We see here that the score interval for 9, extending from 8.5 to 9.5, has a

DEMONSTRATION 8.3. Simple or Ungrouped Frequency Distribution

(Scale) $\underline{X}$	(People) Tallies	(Frequency) $\underline{f}$
10	/	1
9	𝍸 //	7
8		0
7	/	1
6	𝍸	5
5	//	2
4	//	2
3	/	1
2	/	1
		$N = 20$

A Score Interval of 6 on a Continuous Scale

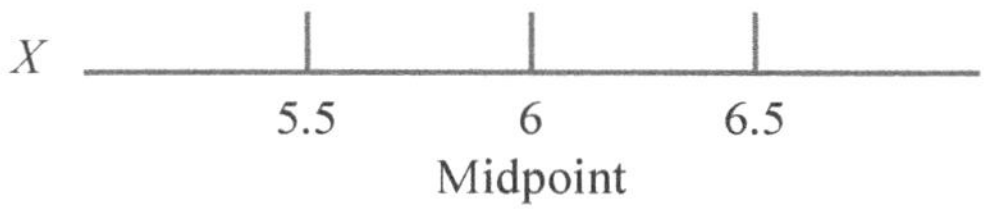

frequency of 7; while the score interval of 8, extending from 7.5 to 8.5, has a frequency of 0. Why? No one in the tested group obtained a score of 8.

The advantage of the simple frequency distribution lies in a more compact presentation of data without loss of any of the information from the rank-ordered arrangement. We still know the frequencies of each score; we can immediately identify the modal score interval of 9; and we can see that the R is 8.

From a theoretical standpoint, a continuous scale is unlimited. However, when arranging the data in frequency distributions, we typically depict only the operative part of the scale, or the range of intervals within which individuals actually obtain scores. By convention, it is acceptable to leave score intervals such as 8 out of the arrangement when their frequency is zero. Alternatively, we can include them in the arrangement, as shown in Demonstration 8.3. Computationally, this decision will not make a difference for the statistics we will calculate. Inclusion of all the scores is favored to obtain a more complete picture of how the group's scores are distributed, as the graphs to follow will illustrate.

KEY CONCEPTS

★ A *simple frequency distribution* involves arranging a group of scores to show how many individual scores fall within each interval on the continuous scale.

★ Each score in a *simple frequency distribution* is not a discrete point, but a *score interval* with a theoretical upper and lower limit.

8.3.3 Grouped Frequency Distribution

A third alternative in data organization is the **grouped frequency distribution**. In a grouped frequency arrangement, the interval includes two or more consecutive scale units and is called a **class interval**. See Demonstrations 8.4A and 8.4B next. In Demonstration 8.4A, the class interval size is set at 3 and includes three units on the scale defined by the exact upper and lower limits. Given the rather small R and N in the dataset, a class interval size of 3 is reasonable. Frequencies are tallied within the class intervals of the specified size. Using the exact upper and lower limits and a class interval size of 3, we see that the first interval in the dataset extends from 0.5 to 3.5, with 2 as the midpoint. That class interval has a frequency of 2, representing the two individuals' scores that fall within that range.

DEMONSTRATION 8.4A. Grouped Frequency Distribution

(Scale) $\underline{X}$	(People) Tallies	(Frequency) $\underline{f}$
10–12	/	1
7–9	𝍸 ///	8
4–6	𝍸 ////	9
1–3	//	2
		$N = 20$

A Class Interval on a Continuous Scale
(Class Interval Size = 3)

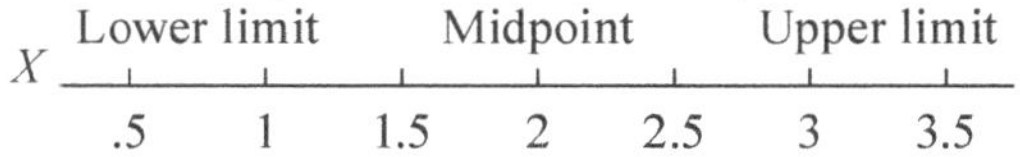

DEMONSTRATION 8.4B. Determining the Class Interval Size for a Grouped Frequency Distribution

X	f
95–99	4
90–94	0
85–89	3
80–84	10
75–79	11
70–74	5
65–69	2
60–64	1
55–59	8
50–54	8
45–49	2
$N =$	54

Range = 98 – 46 = 52
Desired number of classes = 10
Class interval size = 52 ÷ 10 = 5.2

Class Interval Size = 5 (rounded)

By convention, the class interval sizes for a grouped frequency distribution are more typically 5, 10, 15, and 20. Demonstration 8.4B applies these interval conventions with an example of a 100-point test administered to a group of 54 students, where the scores range from 46 to 98. To determine the class interval size suitable for a similarly large dataset, we would typically use the calculated R and a specification for the *number of classes* we desire for presenting the data. The typically accepted number of classes is 10 to 20 for complete visual displays limited to a printed page or computer screen. Since R is 52 in the illustrative dataset, if we desire 10 classes in the distribution, our class interval size would be 5 based on the following calculation:

$R = 98 - 46 = 52$

Interval size = 52/10 = 5.2 (rounded to 5)

If we find that the R in the distribution is too small, using a grouped distribution will not be advantageous over the ungrouped approach.

We might pay a price for the convenience of a more compact arrangement of a grouped frequency distribution. Notice that in grouping the scale points into class intervals in Demonstration 8.4A, some information is lost or distorted. For example, the exact R of the actual data is masked, as is the exact Mo of the distribution. The *modal interval* appears as 4–6, although the actual Mo of 9 is now located in the next class interval of 7–9. The exact frequencies of individual scores are also lost.

KEY CONCEPTS

★ A *grouped frequency distribution* involves arranging a set of scores in class intervals of a given size, showing how many individual scores fall within each interval.

★ A *class interval* consists of consecutive scale values with an upper and lower limit. The *class interval size* in a grouped frequency distribution is usually 5 or 10.

8.4 Measures of Central Tendency

The statistical term for "average" is a measure of central tendency. This section will present three statistical averages: the already encountered mode (Mo), along with the **mean (M)** and the **median (Mdn)**. In the sections that follow, computational formulas and examples will assume the use of a simple or ungrouped frequency distribution, with variations of formulas applicable to a rank-ordered or grouped frequency tables also provided on occasion. To follow the computations, read the frequency tables horizontally by row. Occasionally, formulas will call for summing of a vertical column of tabulated numbers.

8.4.1 Mode

The mode (Mo) is the score with the highest frequency in a given data distribution. See Demonstrations 8.2 and 8.3 again, alongside Demonstration 8.5 next. As shown, the Mo becomes evident once the data are organized in either a rank-ordered or simple frequency distribution. Note that there may be *more than one* Mo in a given distribution. In such cases, both the Mo values are reported separated by a comma. Distributions with two Mo values are called **bimodal**; those with more are

DEMONSTRATION 8.5. Bimodal Distribution

X	Tallies	f
12	/	1
11	~~////~~ ///	8
10	///	3
8	//	2
7	/	4
5	//	2
4	~~////~~ ///	8
3	//	2
		$N = 30$

Mo = 4,11

called **multimodal**. The bimodal distribution shown in Demonstration 8.5 suggests that there are two distinct groups on the measured variable, one with very high scores and the other with relatively low scores.

The number of modes carries implications for **assessment uses**; see Figure 8.1. For example, to a classroom teacher, a bimodal distribution would suggest that there are two distinct subgroups showing clearly different levels of performance on the tested domains. Accordingly, subsequent instructional decisions could be varied for students clustered around a score of 4 versus those around 11. In a service profession, bimodal or multimodal distributions from a needs assessment survey, for example, would suggest varying service needs for distinct subgroups of clients. For researchers investigating the effects of an experimental intervention, two or more modes on the outcome measure would suggest very different impacts of the new treatment on subsets of the investigated group.

8.4.1.1 Formulas

There are no mathematical calculations nor formulas necessary for the Mo.

8.4.1.2 Steps in Computation

Organize and tabulate the data in a rank-ordered or simple frequency table. The Mo can be quickly derived by inspection of the data distribution.

8.4.1.3 Interpretations and Uses

The Mo is easy to understand, and it is a quick method for evaluating a group's overall performance. The main disadvantage of this index of central tendency is that it is vulnerable to sampling errors and tends to be unstable in samples drawn from a given population.

KEY CONCEPTS

- ★ The *mode* is the most frequently occurring score in a data distribution.
- ★ Data distributions could be *unimodal, bimodal,* or *multimodal*, each with different interpretations and uses.

8.4.2 Mean

The mean (M), also called the *arithmetic mean* of a set of test scores, is obtained by taking their sum and dividing by the total number of persons in the group (N). See Demonstrations 8.6A and 8.6B. The

DEMONSTRATION 8.6A. Calculation of the Arithmetic Mean in a Simple Frequency Distribution

X	f	fX (Step 1)		How Derived
10	1	10	⇒	10 × 1 = 10 (Step 1)
9	7	63	⇒	9 × 7 = 63
8	0	0		
7	1	7		
6	5	30		
5	2	10		
4	2	8		
3	1	3		
2	1	2		
	$N = 20$	$\Sigma fX = 133$	⇒	(10 + 63 + 0 + 7 + 30 + 10 + 8 + 3 + 2) (Step 2)

$$\bar{X} = \frac{\Sigma fX}{N}, \text{ or } \bar{X} = 133 \div 20 = 6.65 \checkmark \text{ (Step 3)}$$

Note. To apply the above formula twith a *grouped frequency distribution*, simply use the *midpoint of each class interval* as the X value.

DEMONSTRATION 8.6B. Mean Calculation in a Rank-Ordered Distribution

X	
10	
9	
9	
9	
9	
9	
9	
9	
7	Step 2 = $\overline{X} = \frac{\Sigma X}{N}$
6	
6	$N = 20$
6	$\Sigma X = 133 \div 20 = 6.65$ ✓
6	
6	
5	
5	
4	
4	
3	
2	
Step 1: $\Sigma X = 133$	

algebraic sum of the deviations (distances) of all the scores from their M in a distribution, weighted by their corresponding frequencies, is always equal to 0. Thus, the mean is sometimes referred to as the center of gravity of a distribution. For the **population**, the statistical symbol for the mean is μ. For a selected subset of the population, the **sample**, the statistical notation is $\overline{X}$.

8.4.2.1 Formulas

Two formulas for calculating the arithmetic mean follow; these apply for (1) a simple frequency distribution and (2) a rank-ordered arrangement, respectively. Both yield the same result, but the steps vary slightly because they assume different arrangements of the dataset.

1. The formula for a simple frequency distribution is

$$\overline{X} = \frac{\Sigma fX}{N}$$

where fX = the f(requency) times each raw score, X
ΣfX = the sum of the product of f and X for all scores
N = the number of cases (or individuals) in the group.

2. The formula for a rank-ordered distribution is

$$\overline{X} = \frac{\Sigma X}{N}$$

where ΣX = the sum of all raw scores
N = the number of scores (or individuals) in the group.

8.4.2.2 Steps in Computation

To compute the M in a simple frequency distribution using Formula 1, follow the steps next.

1. Set up a fX column in the frequency table. Compute the product, f times X, for each score value that has a frequency greater than 0.
2. Make a sum of the fX column. This should give you ΣfX, the numerator in the formula for the arithmetic mean.
3. Divide the ΣfX by the N. The N is the sum of the frequency column, and is the denominator in the formula.

8.4.2.3 Interpretation

Unlike the Mo, the M is the most stable measure of central tendency; that is, the M on a measured variable is likely to remain the same in different samples drawn from the same population. Several descriptive statistics use the M as the reference point, such as the **variance** and **standard deviation**, two measures of variability that we will consider soon. In research studies involving multiple group comparisons, statistical hypothesis tests like the t-test and F-test need the M as a starting descriptive statistic for groups investigated.

A disadvantage of the M is that it is sensitive to outlying scores in the distribution. Outliers are values that are extremely low or high compared to the majority of scores in a group. Because the M is computed by taking into account every score in the distribution weighted by its frequency, it is influenced by outlying scores. If the outlying score is a very low value, the M will be lower than the average for the vast majority of the group. It will be higher when the outlying scores are extremely high values.

A "trimmed" mean is more representative of a data distribution that has outliers. To obtain a trimmed M, we delete the outlying scores and recompute the M for the remaining scores. Choosing an alternate measure of central tendency, as with the **median** discussed next, is another option for dealing with outliers.

KEY CONCEPT

★The arithmetic *mean* of a set of values is their sum divided by their number.

8.4.3 Median

The median (Mdn) is the midpoint of a distribution of scores. Another name for the median is the *50th percentile.*

8.4.3.1 Formulas

There are two formulas, depending on the data organization:

1. When data are organized in a simple frequency distribution, the computational formula is

$$\text{Mdn} = \text{L}_{\text{MI}} + \left[\frac{i\left(\frac{N}{2} - \text{Cum}f_{\text{below MI}}\right)}{f_{\text{in MI}}}\right]$$

   where MI = middle interval or score interval within which the median is located
   L_{MI} = lower limit of the middle interval
   $N/2$ = half of the total number of scores (individuals) in the group
   $\text{Cum}f_{\text{below MI}}$ = cumulative frequency in the interval below MI
   $f_{\text{in MI}}$ = frequency in the middle interval
   i = size of the interval (in a simple frequency distribution, this number is always 1)

2. When scores are organized in a rank-ordered distribution, with no tied score values (each score occurs only once), the median is simply the middle value that divides the N into equal halves. If the N is odd (say, $N = 7$), the Mdn is the score located in the middle with three ordered scores on either side. For example, the median below is 4.

   X: 1 2 3 <u>4</u> 5 6 7

   When the number of cases is even ($N = 6$), the median is the midpoint, or arithmetic mean of the two middle scores (3 and 4).

   X: 1 2 3 | <u>4</u> 5 6

   3.5

   Mdn = (3 + 4)/2 = 3.5

8.4.3.2 Steps in Computation

More typically, we would have a larger dataset than $N = 20$. There, we would need a simple frequency table arrangement to apply the Mdn formula. See Demonstration 8.7. The steps are shown with the sixth-grade dataset.

1. Set up a cumulative frequency (Cum f) column by obtaining a running total of the frequencies in the f column for each interval, going from bottom upward:

   $$\text{Cum}\,f = f \text{ in given interval} + \text{Cum}\,f \text{ in previous interval}$$

   The running total is the cumulative frequency; it should reach a value equal to N when you reach the topmost interval.
2. Find $N/2$. This is half of the total number of scores. The $N/2$ term is key to the definition of the Mdn.
3. Find the middle interval (MI). The MI is the interval within which the Mdn is located. You will find MI in the Cum f column by going from bottom upward until you find the *first interval* where the cumulative frequency value equals $N/2$ or a value just higher than $N/2$. In Demonstration 8.7,

$N/2$ = 10. There is no interval with exactly 10 people, but the MI has a cumulative total of 11, including the 10 we need.

4. Mark the lower limit of the MI. This value is the L_{MI} in the formula.
5. Go to the Cum f column again. Highlight or identify the Cum f value found in the interval *just below* the middle interval. This is the Cum $f_{\text{below MI}}$
6. Now, go to the f column. Identify the f-value found inside the middle interval (MI). This is the Cum $f_{\text{in MI}}$.
7. Substitute the values in the formula below and solve.

$$\text{Mdn} = L_{MI} + \left[\frac{i\left(\frac{N}{2} - \text{Cum}f_{\text{below MI}}\right)}{f_{\text{in MI}}} \right]$$

DEMONSTRATION 8.7. Computing the Median

$N/2 = 20/2 = 10$ (Step 1)

	X	*f*	*Cum fX*(Step 1)		How Derived
	10	1	20	⇒	1 + 19 = 20 (Step 2)
	9	7	19	⇒	cum f = cum f in previous interval or 7 + 12 = 19
	8	0	12		
	7	1	12		
6.5					
Middle Interval	6	5	*11*	(Step 3)	
5.5					
(Step 4)	5	2	*6*	(Step 5)	
	4	2	4		
	3	1	2	⇒	cum f = cum f in previous interval or 1 + 1 = 2
	2	1	1		
		N = 20			

$$\text{Mdn} = L_{MI} + \left[\frac{i\left(\frac{N}{2} - \text{Cum}f_{\text{below MI}}\right)}{f_{\text{in MI}}} \right] \quad \text{(Step 6)}$$

$N/2 = 10$
$L_{MI} = 5.5$
$\text{Cum} f_{\text{below MI}} = 6$
$f_{\text{in MI}} = 5$
$i = 1$

Mdn = 5.5 + [1 × (10 – 6) ÷ 5] = *6.3*

Note. To apply the above formula with a grouped frequency distribution, replace $i = 1$, with the actual size of the class interval in the distribution, for example, $i = 3$, or $i = 5$. The remaining calculations will be unchanged.

8.4.3.3 Interpretations and Uses

The Mdn is called the *50th percentile* because it is the point in the distribution above and below which exactly half (50%) of the total number of scores fall. Unlike the M, the Mdn is not influenced by the magnitude of outlying scores on either side, but simply by their counts. Thus, even when there are extremely high or low scores that may be outlying, the computed value of the Mdn will reflect the midpoint of the tested group. For this reason, the Mdn is the preferred measure of central tendency in distributions with outliers. The Mdn is also a relatively stable measure of central tendency. Although it does not have the precision and sampling stability of the M, it is more stable than the Mo.

By definition, **percentiles** are points in a distribution below which certain percentages of the total group (N) fall. As the Mdn is a point in a distribution below which 50% of the group lies, it is the 50th percentile. The *25th percentile* is the point below which a quarter of the group falls and is also called the first quartile. Similarly, the *75th percentile* is the point below which three-quarters of the group tested falls and is the third quartile.

KEY CONCEPT

★ The *median* of a set of scores is the point on the scale below which exactly 50% of the scores in a distribution fall. The median is the *50th percentile*.

It is easy to see that other **percentiles** can be derived by modifying the $N/2$ term in the formula for the median to reflect the proportion that corresponds to the desired percentile. For the 25th percentile, the term should be $N/4$, and for the 75th percentile it is $3/4N$, as shown in the formulas below. Computing the 25th percentile in a simple frequency distribution would occur as before with the demonstration dataset.

$$\text{25th Percentile} = \mathrm{L}_{\text{Interval with first quartile}} + \left[i \frac{\left(\dfrac{N}{4} - \mathrm{Cum}\, f_{\text{below first quartile}} \right)}{f_{\text{in interval with first quartile}}} \right]$$

Computing the 75th percentile in a simple frequency distribution:

$$\text{75th Percentile} = \mathrm{L}_{\text{Interval with third quartile}} + \left[i \frac{\left(\dfrac{3N}{4} - \mathrm{Cum}\, f_{\text{below third quartile}} \right)}{f_{\text{in interval with third quartile}}} \right]$$

8.5 Measures of Variability

A measure of central tendency is an important first step in understanding a group's distribution on a variable. But, for obtaining a complete picture, one also needs to evaluate the group's **variability** on the measure with a statistic that describes the dispersion of the scores. Score distributions with exactly the same M might have a very different "spread." More homogeneous distributions on a variable will tend to cluster closely around the most "typical" score, while dissimilar measures will show a wider, more heterogeneous spread around the average. This section presents two commonly used statistical indices of variability: **range** and **standard deviation**. A third index—the **variance**—is addressed along the way.

8.5.1 Range

As we saw, close scrutiny of a frequency distribution gives away its range once the two extreme scores are located. The R denotes the number of scale units between the highest and lowest score in the distribution. It is the difference between the lowest and highest scores in a distribution.

8.5.1.1 Formulas

The R, as indicated earlier, is calculated by the formula

$$R = X_{\max} - X_{\min}$$

where R = range
$X_{\max}$ = the highest obtained score
$X_{\min}$ = the lowest obtained score.

Sometimes, the **inclusive range** is used, which denotes

the total number of different scores represented *within* the range:

$$R' = X_{max} - X_{min} + 1$$

Of the two indices, most researchers prefer to use the simpler index, R.

8.5.1.2 Steps in Computation

Computation of the R has already been illustrated in the demonstration dataset. It is

$$\text{Range } (R) = X_{max} - X_{min}$$
$$R = 10 - 2 = 8$$

8.5.1.3 Interpretations and Uses

The greatest advantage of the R is its ease of computation and interpretation. Its greatest disadvantage is its sampling instability. Because it relies only on the two extreme scores in a dataset, the R is prone to fluctuate from sample to sample.

KEY CONCEPT

★ The range R is the difference between the lowest and highest scores in a distribution.

8.5.2 Variance and Standard Deviation

The **standard deviation** s is the principal descriptive measure of the spread of scores in a distribution; it is derived from the **variance** s^2. In the population, the corresponding statistical notations are σ and σ^2. Both indices are calculated by using the arithmetic mean as the central point of reference. The term *deviation* stands for the distance of any given score, X, from the arithmetic mean of the distribution. Two definitions follow:

1. The mean-squared deviation is called the variance s^2.
2. The standard deviation s is the positive square root of the mean-squared deviation of a set of scores from the arithmetic mean. It is calculated from the variance.

8.5.2.1 Formulas

The formula for obtaining the standard deviation s, starting with a simple frequency distribution, is

$$s = \sqrt{\frac{\Sigma fx^2}{N}}$$

where $x = X - \overline{X}$, or the deviation of each raw score from the mean
x^2 stands for the squared deviation scores
fx^2 represents the product of the frequency f times the squared deviation scores (needed because scores may have frequencies >1)
$(\Sigma fx^2)/N$ represents the mean-squared deviation (variance or the sum of squared deviations divided by their number)

The formula in Demonstration 8.8, next, is for the *deviation score method* for computing s and is consistent with the conceptual definition of the index.

Another formula for a raw score method follows. Although this book will not demonstrate it, the raw score formula can be derived mathematically from the deviation score formula for s. It is

$$s = \sqrt{\frac{\Sigma fX^2}{N} - \overline{X}^2}$$

8.5.2.2 Steps in Computation

See the deviation score method in Demonstration 8.8. To start, the dataset is organized in a simple frequency table; the M is 6.65 here. The standard deviation s is calculated by first obtaining the deviation scores x for all the raw scores in the dataset; for a score of 10, it is $10 - 6.65 = 3.35$. Each deviation score is then squared; for a X of 10, the x is 3.35 and x^2 is 11.22, as shown. Each x^2 is multiplied by that score's frequency and averaged by taking their sum and dividing by N. This yields the variance s^2 or the mean-squared deviation. The final step is to take a positive square root of the variance. In Demonstration 8.8, s^2 is $106/20 = 5.30$; s is 2.30.

In sequence, the steps are as follows:

1. Find the deviation score for each raw score using $x = X - M$ and set up an x column.
2. Square the deviation scores for each raw score

DEMONSTRATION 8.8. Calculating the Standard Deviation

X	f	x (Step 1)	x^2 (Step 2)	x^2 (Step 3)
10	1	3.35 (10 – 6.65 = 3.35)	11.22 (3.35 × 3.35 = 11.22)	11.22 (1 × 11.22)
9	7	2.35	5.52	38.64
8	0	1.35	1.82	0.00
7	1	0.35	0.12	0.12
6	5	–0.65	0.42	2.10
5	2	–1.65	2.72	5.44
4	2	–2.65	7.02	14.04
3	1	–3.65	13.32	13.32
2	1	–4.65	21.62	21.62
	$N = 20$			$\Sigma fx^2 = 106.5$

$$s = \sqrt{\frac{\Sigma fx^2}{N}} \text{ or } \sqrt{\frac{(106.5)}{20}} = 2.30 \checkmark \text{ (Steps 4 and 5)}$$

to obtain an x^2 column. (Note that if you were to sum the deviation scores taking into account their frequencies, their sum would be zero. This happens because of the way the arithmetic mean is defined. We square the x values to bypass this problem.)

3. Multiply the x^2-values with the f-values in the frequency column to set up a fx^2column.
4. Sum the values in the fx^2 column and divide by N to obtain the variance s^2:

$$\frac{\Sigma fx^2}{N}$$

Find the positive square root of the variance to obtain the standard deviation s:

$$s = \sqrt{\frac{\Sigma fx^2}{N}}$$

In a *rank-ordered* distribution, the f column would be absent; hence, the same basic procedure would apply without Step 3. The formula would be

$$s = \sqrt{\frac{\Sigma x^2}{N}}$$

The same steps would apply in a grouped frequency distribution, except that in Step 1, we would use the *midpoint of each class interval* to find the deviation from the mean.

8.5.2.3 Interpretations and Uses

Conceptually, both the variance and standard deviation in a distribution describe how far, on average, the scores stray away from the mean. The deviation score method utilizes the distances of every score from the mean in the formula. A higher value of s or s^2 indicates a wider, more heterogeneous spread on the measured variable. A lower value indicates the reverse. Both statistics demand the inclusion of every score in the distribution and display greater sampling stability than R.

The standard deviation has widespread use as a descriptive statistic and for constructing a family of *derived score scales* called **standard scores** (Section 8.7). The variance metric is similarly necessary for numerous statistical computations, including the analysis of variance (ANOVA). ANOVAs are applied in experimental research for conducting multiple group comparisons accompanied with tests of statistical significance, falling under methods of *Inferential Statistics* that are not discussed in this chapter.

KEY CONCEPTS

★ The *standard deviation* s is the square root of the sum of the squared deviations of a set of scores from their mean.

★ The *variance* is the mean-squared deviation of a set of scores from their mean.

8.6 Graphical Displays of Data

Graphing of frequency distributions facilitates visual interpretations of a group's performance on measured constructs and variables. We could also compare empirically obtained distributions with mathematical models, one of which is the bell-shaped **standard normal distribution**. Three common procedures involve displays in the form of a frequency polygon, the histogram, and the ogive. All graphs should vbe clearly titled with appropriate labels for the axes. We examine all three display methods and then consider the properties of the normal curve.

8.6.1 Frequency Polygon

In a **frequency polygon**, the horizontal x-axis is represented by the scores on the scale; the vertical y-axis is represented by the frequencies f. The frequencies are plotted at the midpoints of the intervals. Here, we will use the raw scores X for the hypothetical sixth-grade dataset.

8.6.1.1 Steps in Constructing a Frequency Polygon

Figure 8.3 shows a completed graph with the same dataset (Demonstrations 8.1–8.8).

1. Organize the data in a simple frequency table. A grouped frequency distribution could also be used.
2. Set up the horizontal x-axis of the graph with its origin at 0 and with equal-sized units for the score scale X. End the x-axis a couple of units *beyond* the observed maximum and minimum scores. In Figure 8.3, the origin is at 0, each unit equals 1 score unit on the continuous interval scale for X, and the x-axis extends to 11th score interval, or up to 11.5.
3. Set up the vertical y-axis also starting at 0 with equal-sized units representing the frequencies. The y-axis units should extend beyond the highest frequency. In Figure 8.1, the y-axis units are equal to 1 and also extend up to 11, four counts above the highest frequency of 7 in the distribution.
4. Plot and connect the *midpoints* of each score interval against the frequency at that interval by drawing a continuous line, as shown (see Demonstration 8.3). For a grouped frequency distribution, we would use the midpoints of each class interval instead.
5. Anchor the polygon to the baseline by extending the line to the midpoints of the two extreme intervals at each end, next to the maximum and minimum scores.

If the range of scores is very high, say, with scores of 22–95, $R = 73$, it might be better to opt for the grouped frequency distribution with class intervals of a suitable size. With an R of 73, we could establish class intervals of size 10, with the two extreme intervals being 20.5–25.5 (midpoint = 23), and 95.5–100.5 (midpoint = 98). The procedures are similar for both arrangements. With the given dataset of 20 cases and $R = 7$, starting

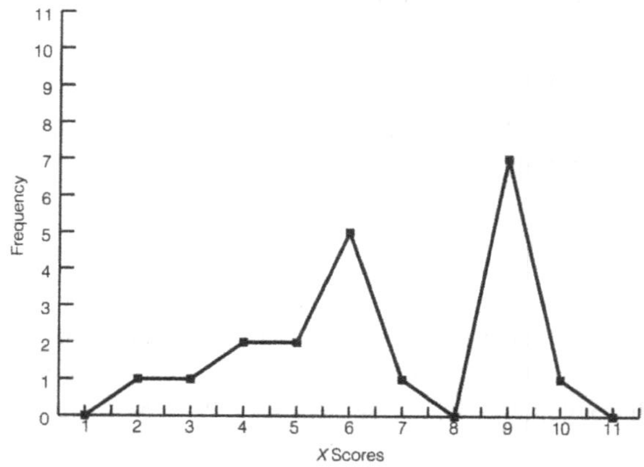

FIGURE 8.3. A frequency polygon.

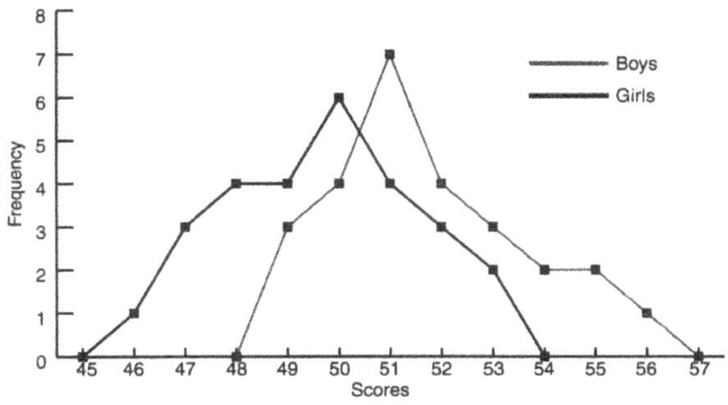

FIGURE 8.4. Comparing frequency polygons of boys (right) and girls (left).

with a simple frequency distribution is reasonable and appropriate.

In Figure 8.4, there are two frequency polygons comparing score distributions for sixth-grade boys (N = 27) and girls (N = 26) on an arithmetic test. Should the dataset have scores starting at a higher point on the scale, say, at 46, we could still display the data as shown. To be more accurate, we could also begin with the 0 at the origin, include the first couple of units, then break the scale with two vertical slashes, and restart the scale with units close to the region where people scored, say, 44.

If the N is small, the unit size for frequencies on the y-axis can be set at 1. If the N is large, say, 100 or more, then it may be more practical to use a unit size of 10 units, with points increasing by 10, 20, 30, 40, and so on.

8.6.1.2 Interpretations and Uses

The frequency polygon is a line graph that characterizes the shape of the data distribution visually. It is built from the data organized in a frequency table. The distributions can be described in terms of modality, variability, and symmetry.

In Figure 8.3, the distribution is unimodal. The Mo of the distribution is depicted by the highest point, or the peak of the polygon. Although 9 is the Mo, we see that 6 is another score with a high frequency. The spread of the distribution is quite wide, suggesting heterogeneity. As there were only 10 test items, the variability is limited by the extreme intervals on the scale, referred to as the upper *ceiling* and lower *floor* of the test, respectively. The R is visually evident in the graph.

The distribution suggests some asymmetry. Technically, a distribution is symmetrical if the M and Mdn have equal or close to equal values. The scores of 2 and 3 can be called outliers, with a vast majority of the scores (70% exactly) hovering around scores of 6–10. The outliers contribute to the lack of symmetry.

When two groups with near-equal N's are given the same test, the frequency polygon is useful in making comparisons between groups. Comparisons are meaningful when the unit sizes on x- and y-axes for both distributions also match. Figure 8.4 shows two comparable polygons for boys and girls. The boys have a slightly higher Mo than the girls and are distributed on a somewhat higher region of the scale than girls. In terms of the R, the maximum and minimum scores vary, but the distributions seem to have similar dispersions.

8.6.2 Histogram

The **histogram** is a bar graph of data from a frequency table. See Figure 8.5.

As in a frequency polygon, to construct a histogram, the horizontal x-axis is represented by the scores on the scale; the vertical y-axis is represented by the frequen-

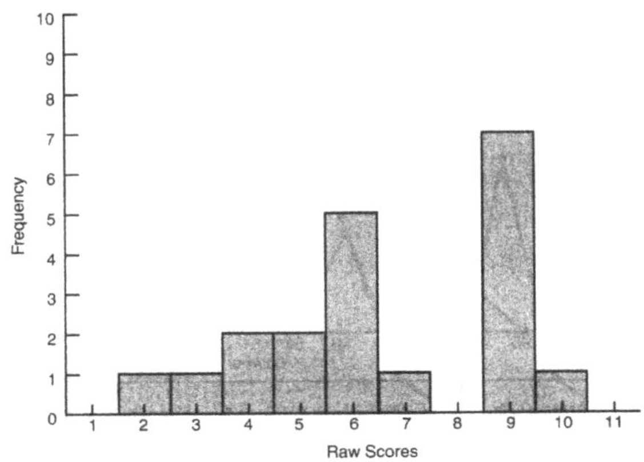

FIGURE 8.5. A histogram.

cies. However, in a histogram, the frequencies are plotted as bars that extend over the exact upper and lower limits of each interval on the *x*-axis, with the midpoints at the center of each bar.

8.6.2.1 Steps in Constructing a Histogram

A histogram of the demonstration dataset is shown in Figure 8.5, constructed with the following steps:

1. Organize the data in a simple or grouped frequency table.
2. Set up the *x*-axis for the graph with its origin at 0 and equal-sized units representing the score scale.
3. Set up the vertical *y*-axis starting with a 0, with frequencies increasing in equal-sized units and extending beyond the *N* by a couple of units.
4. Plot a bar for each score interval or class interval against the frequencies from the data in the frequency table, using the *exact* lower and upper limits of the intervals. For a score of 5, the width of the bar extends from 4.5 to 5.5; the midpoint of the bar is at 5.

8.6.2.2 Interpretations and Uses

The histogram is simply an alternate way to depict the data in a frequency table. It yields much the same visual information as a frequency polygon. Again, the overall performance of a group could be interpreted using modality, variability, and symmetry. Visual comparisons of the performance of two more groups, however, is not as easy with histograms as it is with the frequency polygons. Overlapping bars are difficult to read, and some of the information may be clouded or lost.

8.6.3 Ogive

An **ogive** is a graph based on cumulative proportions of frequencies relative to the *N*, as found at each interval of a frequency distribution. It is an S-shaped graph. Recall the Cumulative *f* column used for computation of the median. Ogives rely on the same statistic. To create an ogive, frequency distributions are graphed using cumulative percentages of the frequencies in the *y*-axis against upper limits of intervals on the *x*-axis.

8.6.3.1 Steps in Constructing an Ogive

See Demonstration 8.9 and Figure 8.6. To construct an ogive, we add two columns to the frequency table for an ungrouped or grouped score distribution: the Cumulative Frequency (Cum *f*) column and the Cumulative Percent (Cum %) column. The Cum % column is set up by dividing the Cum *f* value at each interval by *N*, as shown. The ogive is constructed with each score interval and the corresponding Cum % value.

1. Set up a frequency table with a Cum *f* and Cum % column.
2. Set up the *x*-axis for the graph with its origin at 0 and equal-sized units representing the score scale.
3. Set up the vertical *y*-axis with percentages starting with 0 at the origin. The %'s increase in equal units of 10 from 0 through 100.
4. Plot the *upper limits of each interval* on the *x*-axis against the Cum % on the *y*-axis.
5. Connect the points with a line.

8.6.3.2 Interpretations and Uses

Ogives have several uses. They are useful for comparing the performance of two or more groups that have

DEMONSTRATION 8.9. Frequency Distribution with Cumulative Frequency and Cumulative % Columns

X	*f*	Cum *f*	Cum %	How Cum % is derived
10	1	20	100	⇒ 20/20 × 100 = 100
9	7	19	95	⇒ 19/20 × 100 = 95
8	0	12	60	
7	1	12	60	
6	5	11	55	
5	2	6	30	
4	2	4	20	⇒ 4/20 × 100 = 20
3	1	2	10	
2	1	1	5	

N = 20

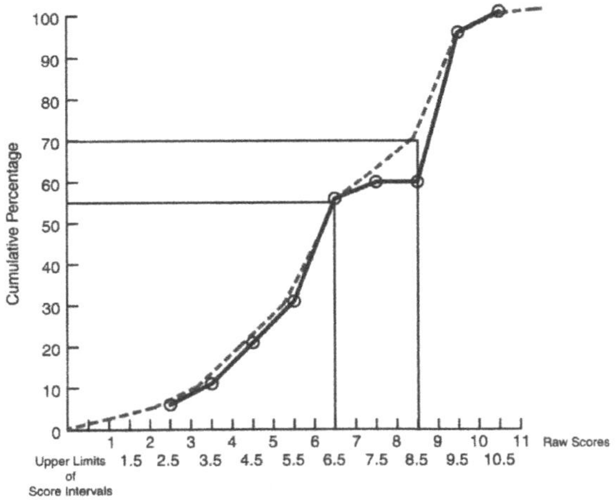

FIGURE 8.6. An ogive: A cumulative percentage graph.

different N's but are measured on the same scale. If multiple measurements are made on the same group of individuals over time using the same instrument, the rightward movement of the ogives from Time 1, to Time 2, to Time *t* will illustrate the changes of the group on the measured construct. Ogives can also be used for deriving *approximate* percentile ranks (PRs) corresponding to upper limits of particular score intervals.

See Figure 8.6 again. In this illustration, percentile ranks are derived for score intervals of 6 and 8. The ogive has been smoothed in the dotted line shown in the graph. *Smoothing* is a procedure that helps make a line graph more continuous when points are jagged due to gaps in the data. In such cases, a best prediction of the points is made based on the rest of the data points and inserted to obtain a smoothed graph. Graphs from opinion polls are often smoothed with a procedure called 90-day weighted, moving averages.

As we see in the ogive shown, the score of 6 has a PR of 55, obtained by drawing a straight line from the axes to the point. A PR of 55 indicates that individuals obtaining scores at that interval were ranked above 55% of the rest of the group. Similarly, a score of 9 has an approximate PR of 95, meaning that the persons located at that score point surpassed 95% of the group. Using the ogive, we could also approximate the PR for a score of 8, although no one in the group received that particular score. Percentile ranks obtained in this manner are *approximations* because the percentages correspond with the upper limits of intervals, rather than the actual percentile location within an interval. Precise computational procedures for PRs follow in a later section.

KEY CONCEPTS

★ A *frequency polygon* is a line graph depicting the frequencies of each score at the midpoints of each interval in a distribution.

★ A *histogram* is a bar graph depicting the frequencies of each score in a distribution; the bars are built with the exact upper and lower limits of the score intervals.

★ An *ogive* is a graph depicting the cumulative percentage frequency at each score interval of a distribution.

Practice Break: Objectives 1–3

Examine the test scores for a class (Dataset 1) provided below. Set up a simple frequency table. Calculate all the descriptive statistics you will need to answer the questions that follow.

Dataset 1: 13, 21, 20, 17, 16, 15, 14, 20, 17, 16, 15, 20, 15, 15, 20, 20, 15, 13, 11, 10

- Find the *mean*, *median*, *mode*, *range*, and *standard deviation.*
- Define each statistic and interpret it with reference to the dataset.
- Plot the scores in a *frequency polygon.* Describe the shape of the distribution with respect to its modality, symmetry, and variability.
- Suppose an instructor obtained the above distribution after a *pretest.* What do the descriptive statistics and the shape of the distribution tell you about the students? Identify two classroom decisions that could be made with the results. Explain.
- Identify constructs that could be measured at each of the *ratio*, *interval*, *ordinal*, and *nominal* levels. Justify your choice of the level of measurement.
- In the classroom context, give examples of variables that have a *continuous* versus a *discrete* distribution.

8.7 The Standard Normal Distribution and Its Applications

8.7.1 Properties of the Standard Normal Curve

The standard normal distribution, shown in Figure 8.7, is a bilaterally symmetrical, bell-shaped curve based on a mathematical probability function that describes the expected distribution of a continuous, random normal variable. It has a fixed mean (μ) of 0 and a standard deviation (σ) of 1.0 for a population and is also called the *z-distribution* or the Gaussian distribution. Several measured human characteristics approximate the shape of the normal distribution, including measures of cognitive abilities, attitudes, height, and weight. Hence, the mathematical model has proven useful in interpreting real-world distributions that are normal, near normal, or non-normal in shape. In the measurement and testing field, the standard normal distribution has been applied widely for deriving various *norm-referenced scores*, including the *normalized z-score* and its derivatives, and **normalized percentile ranks**.

What are some of its useful properties? The base of the normal curve is represented in continuous standard deviation units σ, ranging from $+\infty$ to $-\infty$ (infinity). The distribution has a total area of 1.0, representing 100% of the region under the curve. The normal probability function makes it possible to predict the height of the normal curve for any σ-value at its base. We could also predict the percentages of the area under the curve that lie between given σ-units on the baseline. The height of the normal curve at any point reflects the probability of the corresponding σ-value at the base. The important properties can be summarized as follows:

1. The standard normal distribution is unimodal.
2. The mean, median, and mode lie at the same point and have equal values.
3. The distribution is bilaterally symmetrical; the left side of the bell curve is a mirror image of the right.
4. Although, in theory, the units at the base range from $+\infty$ to $-\infty$, 99.9% of the area under the curve lies between –3.0 and +3.0 σ-units.
5. The areas between given σ-units of the normal curve correspond to probabilities of expected values of a random variable.
6. The two "tails" of the distribution approach but never touch or intersect with the baseline.

Of the area under the curve, as Figure 8.7 shows, 34.13% lies between the mean and 1.0 standard deviation unit; 13.59% lies between 1.0 and 2.0 standard deviation units; and about 2.14% lies between 2.0 and 3.0 standard deviation units. The corresponding areas on the left are replicated exactly on the right. Moving from the left to right, one could calculate cumulative percentages of the total area between given units, as shown. The mean is located at the 50th percentile (which is the median by definition); at that point, the cumulative percentage of the area under the curve between –3.0 σ-units (left tail) and 0.0 σ-units (midpoint) is 50%.

Note also the correspondences with a frequency polygon that we might construct with real data. In a frequency polygon that is near normal or "normalized" to take the shape of a standard normal distribution, the areas under the curve would correspond with *percent of individuals* with scores or measures in those regions; the height at a given point would reflect the frequency of that score value. These parallels open up other useful applications that now follow.

KEY CONCEPT

★ The *standard normal distribution* is a bell-shaped curve based on the normal probability function.

8.7.2 Comparing Distribution Shapes with the Standard Normal Curve

Skewness is an indicator of non-normality (see Figures 8.8 and 8.9). If we superimpose an imaginary standard normal curve over a real data distribution, we could identify the degree of its non-normality by comparison. A distribution is *positively skewed* when a vast majority of persons are concentrated at the lower end of the score scale, with the "tail" of the curve overlapping the part of the normal distribution with positive σ-values on the baseline. In a positively skewed distribution, there will be relatively few scores located *above* the mean of the distribution or in the right tail area. In a *negatively skewed* distribution, a reverse picture is obtained with fewer persons located *below* the mean. The left tail of the curve is over the part of the

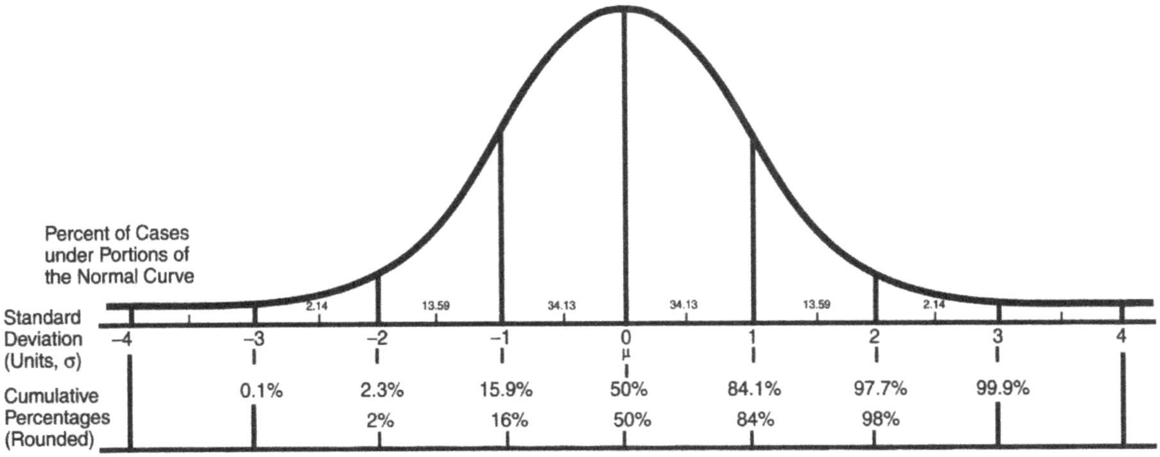

FIGURE 8.7. The standard normal distribution.

normal distribution where the σ-values on the baseline are negative.

Skewness can be calculated as the difference between the mean and mode of a distribution in standard deviation units. Because of the low sampling stability of the mode, another formula for skewness uses the difference between the mean and median (not shown):

$$\text{Skewness} = \frac{(\mu - \text{Mo})}{\sigma}$$

In skewed distributions that are unimodal, the mean, median, and mode usually have predictable locations on the score scale (see Figure 8.8A,B). In a negatively skewed distribution, the mean tends to be pulled toward the tail, especially when there are outliers at the lower end. Hence, the calculated mean will have the lowest value, followed by the median and mode. The opposite pattern is found in positively skewed distributions, where the mean tends to be pulled toward the high end of the scale, especially by outlying scores. Hence, the mean would now have the highest value, with the mode at the lowest value and the median in between.

Kurtosis is another measure of non-normality in a distribution and refers to how flat or peaked a distribution is in comparison with the normal curve (Figure

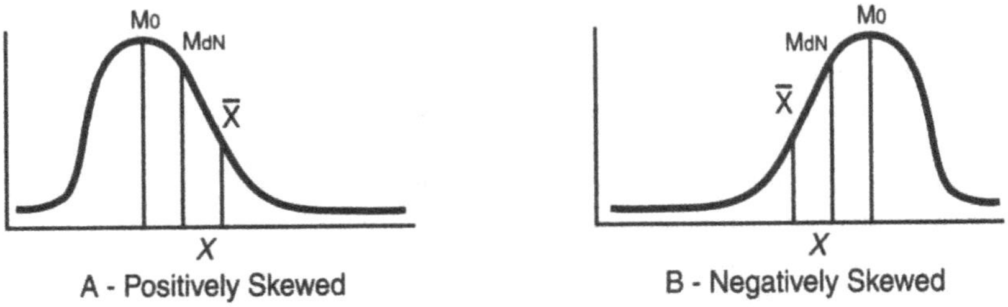

FIGURE 8.8. Positively (A) and negatively (B) skewed data distributions with relative locations of measures of central tendency.

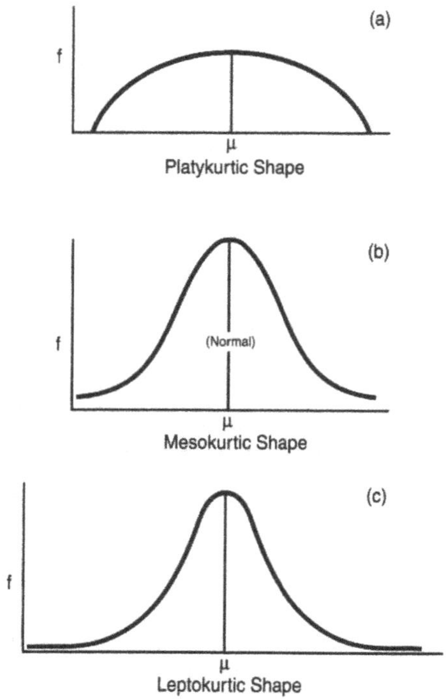

FIGURE 8.9. Distributions with different degrees of kurtosis.

8.9). If a distribution is narrow and sharply peaked relative to a normal distribution, it is called a *leptokurtic* distribution. When a distribution is flat and spread out, resembling a plateau, it is described as *platykurtic.* The bell-shaped normal distribution lies somewhere in between and is described as *mesokurtic* in shape.

8.7.3 Measures of Relative Position

A **measure of relative position** is useful for interpreting measurements in a comparative manner, providing a means for ranking individuals in a distribution. The reference distribution is the group to which a score is compared. In most informal, local, or small-scale assessment projects, it is the tested group itself. In large-scale, commercial, or standardized test design contexts, the reference group is a separate **norm group** of carefully selected respondents who ideally meet certain population specifications. We will consider two frequently used measures of relative position: (1) standard scores or, specifically, *z*-scores and (2) percentile ranks.

8.7.3.1 *z*-Scores

THE *Z*-SCORE FORMULA

The most basic form of a standard score is the *z-score.* The *z*-score is the raw score expressed in standard deviation units, and the conversion yields a continuous, equal-interval scale. For an individual score on a given variable *X*, the *z*-score would be computed with the formula

$$z_X = (\overline{X} - \text{mean}_x) \div \text{standard deviation}_x$$

For another variable, *Y*, the z_y would be as follows, starting with the raw scores on *Y*.

$$z_Y = (Y - \text{mean}_y) \div \text{standard deviation}_y$$

COMPUTATION OF *Z*-SCORES

Computation of the *z*-score is shown in Demonstration 8.10. We see the scores for six students (A–F) from two assessments: reading (*X*) and mathematics (*Y*); the distributions are not shown in their entirety. Given the mean and standard deviation of each of the *X* and *Y* distributions, respectively, the *z*-score calculations for each requires two simple steps, shown in Demonstration 8.10.

INTERPRETATION OF *Z*-SCORES

The *z*-score tells us how far a given score deviates from the mean of the distribution, expressed in standard deviation units. Depending on whether the score is located above or below the mean, the *z*-scores can be positive or negative. A value of +1.0 indicates that the student's raw score is located exactly 1 standard deviation *above the mean* of the distribution. See Student A's performance on *X* and Student B's on *Y.* When the *z*-score is 0.0, as with Student B on *X*, the student's score coincides exactly with the mean of the distribution.

Keeping in mind the different means and standard deviations of the two distributions, one can still make comparisons of performance on two different tests

DEMONSTRATION 8.10. Computation of *z*-Scores for *X* and *Y*

1. Find the deviation of each score from the mean of the distribution ($x = X - \text{mean}_x$).
2. Divide the deviation score by the standard deviation of the distribution ($z = x/s$).

Student	X	z_x	Y	z_y	How Derived for $z_{\hat{y}}$
A	9	+1.0	24	+3.0	⇒ (24 – 12) = 12 (Step 1) 12/4 = +3.0 (Step 2)
B	7	0.0	16	+1.0	
C	5	–1.0	12	0.0	
D	2	–2.5	8	–1.0	
E	10	+1.5	19	+1.75	
F	12	+2.5	22	+2.5	

$\text{Mean}_x = 7$, $s_x = 2$

$\text{Mean}_y = 12$, $s_{\hat{y}} = 4$

using a common z-scale. Thus, we can say that Student B's performance ($z = 0$) on Test X is average relative to the rest of the group; however, the same student is 1 standard deviation *above the mean* on Test Y ($z = +1.0$). Student F's comparative performance, on the other hand, is 2.5 standard deviation units *above the mean* of both the X and Y distributions.

Note that z-scores have a one-to-one and straight-line relationship with raw scores; hence, the shape of the distribution remains unchanged after the conversion. If the original raw score distribution is skewed, the same shape will be replicated in a frequency polygon with the z-scores we derive. If the original distribution is normal, the z-scores will retain that normal shape. When we use z-scores to derive percentile ranks (next, another widely applied measure of relative position), the characteristics and shape of the distribution will matter.

8.7.3.2 Percentile Ranks

The percentile rank or PR, referenced several times in this chapter and book, indicates the proportion of scores that a given individual's score surpasses in a distribution, expressed as a percentage. The distribution to which the score is compared is called the *comparison group* (or the *reference group*). When designing standardized tests for facilitating norm-referenced score interpretations, the comparison group is referred to as the *norm group*.

To recap, if a student with a score of 10 is located *above 35%* of the comparison group, that student would have a PR of 35. The score of 10 would correspond with the 35th percentile. While PRs represent the cumulative percentage of persons falling below a given score, the percentile indicates the specific point in the distribution where that score is located. Refer back to PRs in the context of ogives (cumulative percent graphs) and the normal curve.

Note the correspondence of z-scores and σ-units in the standard normal distribution in Figure 8.7. Figure 8.10 shows a hypothetical empirical distribution of a normally distributed variable X. When a measured variable distributes normally, we could use this information to predict the PRs that correspond with particular z-scores. Most statistics textbooks or online statistical resources provide statistical tables for the normal curve for determining PRs for every z-value that lies

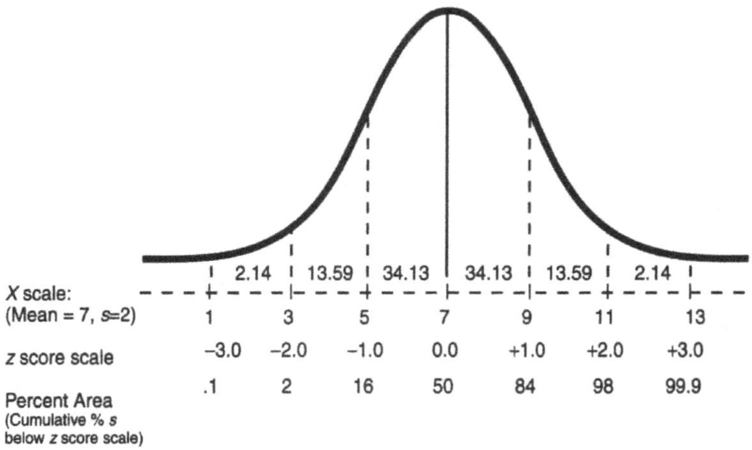

FIGURE 8.10. Mapping *z*-scores against percentile ranks for a normally distributed variable, *X*.

between −3.0 and +3.0. See Demonstration 8.11 next. Given the normal probability function, the areas under the theoretical distribution have a predictable relationship with the σ-units on the base.

Relationship of *z*-units and PRs in the standard normal distribution:

z	PR	
−3.0	0.1	(rounded 0)
−2.0	2.3	(rounded 2)
−1.0	15.9	(rounded 16)
0.0	50.0	(rounded 50)
+1.0	84.1	(rounded 84)
+2.0	97.7	(rounded 98)
+3.0	99.9	(rounded 100)

When the shape of empirical distributions is nonnormal, we need to apply a formula that does not assume normality of the score distribution. See Demonstration 8.12, and note the formula using the cumulative frequencies at each interval of the empirical distribution:

$$\text{PR} = 100\left[\frac{\frac{f(X - \text{Lower limit of interval of X})}{\text{interval size, } i} + \text{Cum} f_{\text{in interval below}}}{N}\right]$$

DEMONSTRATION 8.11. Deriving PRs in a Normal Distribution

Student	X	z_X	PR	How derived
L	9	+1.0	84	Read cumulative % below *z*-score in graph
M	7	0.0	50	
N	5	−1.0	16	

(Mean = 7, s = 2)

Step 1: Convert raw scores to *z*-scores.

Step 3: Read the PR directly from the abscissa of the graph of a normal curve by obtaining the cumulative percent of scores lying below a *z*-score.

Example: The cumulative percent of scores lying below a z of +1.0 is 84%; hence, the PR of a person who obtains a *z*-score of +1.0 in a normal distribution is 84.

DEMONSTRATION 8.12. Determining Percentile Ranks in a Non-Normal Distribution

X	f	Cum f	Cum %
10	1	20	100
9	7	19	95
8	0	12	60
7	1	12	60
6	5	11	55
5	2	6	30
4	2	4	20
3	1	2	10
2	1	1	5

$N = 20$

What is the PR for a raw score of 6?

PR = 100[6 – 5.5) ÷ 1 × (5) + (6)] ÷ 20
100 [.5/1 × 5 + 6] ÷ 20
100 × 8.5 ÷ 20 = *42.5*

KEY CONCEPTS

★ *Measures of relative position* help compare a person's score with the scores of a comparison group, also called the norm group for standardized tests.

★ A *standard score* indicates the distance of a score from the mean of the distribution in standard deviation units. The *z-score* is the basic standard score.

★ A *percentile rank* indicates where a person's score is placed based on the percentage of scores that it surpasses in the comparison group.

★ The *standard score* and *percentile ranks* are commonly used derived scores for *norm referencing* purposes.

8.8 Correlation Coefficients and Their Applications

In in both CTT and IRT applications, two useful and closely related statistical concepts are *correlation* and *prediction*. The degree to which different variables relate to one another in given populatons is often of general interest to researchers and practitioners in a number of fields. Correlations also serve as the basic building block for obtaining several different validity and reliability coefficients, discussed in greater depth in Chapters 10 and 11.

8.8.1 Types of Correlation Coefficients

Correlation coefficients are descriptive statistics that portray the extent to which two or more variables are associated. To express the relationships with data at different levels of measurement, we need to compute and interpret specific types of **correlation coefficients.** Some of these are listed in Table 8.2. When two variables are correlated, the resulting relationship yields a **bivariate correlation**. If more than two variables are involved, we obtain a **multiple correlation**.

Correlations are group-specific. That is, while we could calculate these statistics for any sets of variables in any group, like students, teachers, patients, counselors, administrators, parents, clients, or the general public, the correlation coefficients may not replicate in the same way in different populations or subpopulations.

Here are some research questions answerable with correlational statistics:

- To what extent is attendance rate (X, Variable 1) related to measured achievement levels (Y, Variable 2) in high school students?
- To what degree do daily physical activity levels (X, Variable 1) predict weight measures (Y, Variable 2) in young adults?
- To what extent is time spent at work (X, Variable 1) associated with worker productivity levels (Y, Variable 2)?

For investigating properties of new or adopted construct measures during the validation phases (Figure 8.1), the following types of questions would require correlational analyses:

TABLE 8.2. Bivariate Correlation Coefficients: Recommended Levels of Measurement

		Level of measurement	
Correlation coefficient	Symbol	Variable 1	Variable 2
Pearson product-moment correlation	r	Interval or ratio	Interval or ratio
Spearman rank-order correlation	ρ or r_s	Ordinal	Ordinal
Kendall's tau	τ	Ordinal	Ordinal
Point-biserial correlation	r_{pb}	Nominal	Interval
Phi	Φ	Nominal	Nominal
Contingency coefficient	C	Nominal	Nominal
Tetrachoric	r^t	Transformed nominal	Transformed nominal
Biserial	r_{bis}	Interval	Transformed nominal

- **Predictive validity:** To what degree do the measures from a new recruitment test (X) predict future performance (Y) of workers in an organization?
- **Test–retest reliability:** To what extent do the measures taken at Time 1 (X) correlate with measures taken with the same test at Time 2 (Y) in typical workers, indicating stability within a two-week period?

As indicated, the type of correlation coefficient most applicable for a given situation depends on the level of measurement of the variables. Table 8.2 delineates some general guidelines for selecting bivariate correlation coefficients based on their scaling properties. Of these, the computational procedure and interpretation of the **product–moment correlation** r, are illustrated next.

Correlation coefficients describe variable relationships in two ways and are interpreted similarly. First, they shed light on the *strength* of the relationship, based on the size or magnitude of the correlation coefficient. Second, they indicate the *direction* of the relationship: Is the correlation positive, negative, or nondirectional? Correlation coefficients typically range in value from –1.0 to +1.0. Both these extremes reflect perfect relationships. The middle value of 0 represents that no relationship exists between the variables. An exception is the *phi* coefficient, which ranges from 0 to +1.0. Positive correlations indicate that individuals with high values (scores) on one variable also tend to have high values on the other, and vice versa. Negative correlations denote that those who receive high scores in one variable tend to obtain low scores on the other, and vice versa.

8.8.2 The Product–Moment Correlation (r)

Pearson's r indicates the degree to which the same individuals occupy the same relative position in the distributions of each of the two variables, expressed in terms of their distance from the mean in standard deviation units. Both variables must be measured on interval or ratio scales.

8.8.2.1 Formula

The "conceptual" formula for the Pearson's r for two variables, X and Y, is given by the z-score method next. See Demonstration 8.13.

$$r = \frac{\Sigma z_x z_y}{N}$$

where $z_x = (X - \overline{X})/s_x$, or the deviation of each raw score from the mean of X, expressed in standard deviation units of the X distribution (also called "z-scores for X")

$z_y = (Y - \overline{Y})/s_y$, or the deviation of each raw score from the mean of Y, expressed in standard deviation units of the Y distribution ("z-scores for Y")

$z_x z_y$ = the cross product of the z-scores for X and Y

$(\Sigma z_x z_y)/N$ represents the sum of the cross products of z-scores divided by the number of individuals measured.

The corresponding "raw score" formula, which is a derivative of the z-score method, is as follows:

$$r = \frac{\Sigma XY - \frac{(\Sigma X)(\Sigma Y)}{N}}{\sqrt{\left[\Sigma X^2 - \frac{(\Sigma X)^2}{N}\right]\left[\Sigma Y^2 - \frac{(\Sigma Y)^2}{N}\right]}}$$

As evident from the preceding, the z-scores provide a method for assigning "ranks" to individuals within a distribution using its arithmetic mean and standard deviation. When the z-scores on both measured variables are in perfect agreement for every individual in the group, the computed r-value is 1.0.

Step 1: Compute z-scores for all the X scores in the distribution using $z_x = (X - \overline{X})/s_x$.

In example, where $X = 2$, $z_x = (2 - 9)/4 = -1.75$

Step 2: Compute z-scores for all the Y scores in the distribution using $z_y = (Y - \overline{Y})/s_y$.

In example, where $Y = 4$, $z_y = (4 - 16)/7 = -1.71$

Step 3: Set up a cross products column, $z_x z_y$, by multiplying z_x values with z_y values.

In example, where for student A, the $z_x = -1.75$ and $z_y = -1.71$, the $z_x z_y = (-1.75)(-1.71) = +2.99$

Step 4: Sum the values in the $z_x z_y$ column to obtain $\Sigma z_x z_y$.

In example, [(+2.99) + (+1.43) + (.65) + (–.07) + (.14) + (.22) + (–1.43) + (2.99)] = 6.92

Step 5: Solve using the formula $r = \frac{\Sigma z_x z_y}{N}$

In example, 6.92/8 = .865

DEMONSTRATION 8.13. Computation of Pearson's *r*

Given: $\overline{X} = 9$, $s_x = 4$
$\overline{Y} = 16$, $s_y = 7$
$N = 8$

People	X	z_x (Step 1)	Y	z_y (Step 2)	$z_x z_y$ (Step 3)
A	2	–1.75	4	–1.71	+2.99
B	4	–1.25	8	–1.14	+1.43
C	6	–0.75	10	–0.86	+0.65
D	8	–0.25	18	+0.29	–0.07
E	10	+0.25	20	+0.57	+0.14
F	12	+0.75	18	+0.29	+0.22
G	14	+1.25	8	–1.14	–1.43
H	16	+1.75	28	+1.71	+2.99
$N = 8$					$\Sigma z_x z_y = 6.92$ (Step 4)

$r = \frac{\Sigma z_x z_y}{N} = 6.92/8 = .865$ ✓ (Step 5)

8.8.2.2 Interpretation

See the data for Students A and H in Demonstration 8.13. Student A has z-scores of –1.75 on X and –1.71 on the Y distribution (low performance on both tests); while not in exact agreement, these values are very close, indicating the student performed well below average on both tests. Student H shows similar results on both variables, with +1.75 and +1.71 (very high performance on both tests). On close examination, we find the same pattern for every student in the group, more or less. The agreement levels in the paired z-values of each student yield the high correlation coefficient of .87 (as rounded) that we observe.

8.8.2.3 Limitations of *r*

There are two limitations that we should bear in mind. The calculation of Pearson's r assumes that the two variables have a *linear* relationship. Pearson's r works best when the distributions of both variables are unimodal and relatively symmetrical, although not necessarily normal. Second, r also assumes that the distributions of both variables have an adequate variance. If the range on either variable is restricted, the statistic will underestimate the actual relationship between the two variables. Prior to computing r in a sample, we should ensure that there is sufficient variability on both variables, as can be reasonably expected in the population.

8.8.3 Bivariate Scatterplots

Relationships between pairs of variables can also be depicted visually without the computations, with bivariate **scatterplots**, also called scattergrams. Figure 8.11 illustrates scatterplots that vary with respect to the strength and direction of the correlation coefficient, r. To construct a scatterplot, set up the x-axis with score intervals on the first variable (X), starting with 0 at the origin. Set up the *y-axis* in the same way for the second variable (Y). Then, plot the coordinate points of the two variables for each individual in the group.

Examine carefully the scatterplot for the data presented in Figure 8.11A. One could draw an ellipse around the plotted points and a diagonal line passing through the center of the ellipse. The narrower the ellipse, the more concentrated the points are toward the central line, and the stronger the correlation between the two variables. When the correlation has an absolute value of 1.0, all the points fall exactly on the straight line (Figure 8.11B).

The direction of the scatter suggests whether the relationship is positive or negative. When the points move upward from left to right in a straight line, the relationship is linear and positive. In the group displayed, as values on X go up, values on Y go up as well; and when X-values go down, the Y-values are correspondingly low. This pattern remains consistent in all the individuals. If we find that the points in a scatterplot move downward from right to left, a negative relationship is indicated. When there is a random scatter of points that cannot be represented with a straight line in either direction, the correlation is 0.

Note that a scatterplot will also reveal if the relationship is *curvilinear* (Figure 8.11E), instead of linear. The relationship between age (X) and physical strength (Y) of persons is likely to yield a curvilinear relationship. As age increases, physical strength increases in most individuals; however, after a certain age, as age increases, we tend to become physically weaker. A curvilinear relationship indicates that the relationship between the two variables is positive up to a point but reverses to negative thereafter. Pearson's r is not an appropriate statistic for measuring nonlinear relationships.

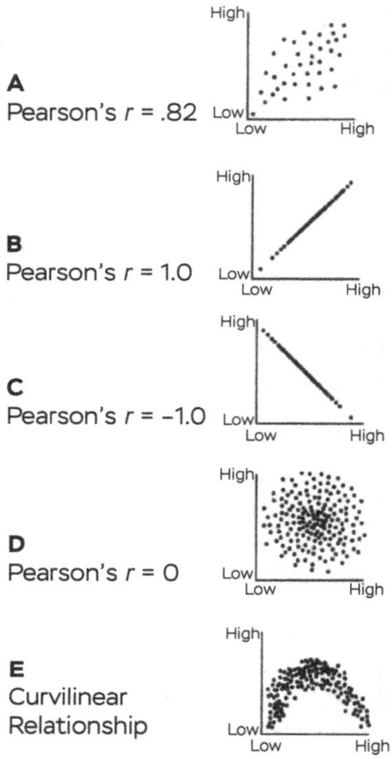

FIGURE 8.11. Bivariate scatterplots showing different directions and strengths between two variables.

8.8.4 Caveats for Correlations

Evaluations of correlations require a command of the existing literature on the measured variables (or related variables). They should be interpreted with reference to the relationships expected in given populations. Correlations are affected by the units of analysis (e.g., are we measuring persons or groups?) and their variance on the measured variable; groups tend to have a much narrower spread than individuals on given variables. The measurement scales for each variable also matter.

What is a reasonable range for a "high" correlation for most constructs in the social and behavioral sciences? Some *very general* rules of thumb are provided next with the caveat that the magnitude of correlation coefficients should be interpreted in context, taking all the above factors into consideration:

.80–1.0	High correlation
.40–.60	Moderate correlation
.20 or less	Low to very low correlation

An aid to interpreting r is the **coefficient of determination** r^2. While r-values cannot be interpreted directly as percentages, if we squared them, the corresponding r^2 is interpretable as the *percent of variance in* X *accounted for by* Y. Once converted to r^2, negative correlations are interpreted in the same way as positive correlations. The greater the r^2-value, the stronger the relationship.

r	r^2	Interpretation
.82	.67	67% of the variability in the X distribution is explained by the Y scores.
.50	.25	25% of the variability in the X distribution is explained by the Y scores.
–.22	.05	About 5% of the variability in the X distribution is explained by the Y scores.

In interpreting r-values, we should also remind ourselves that correlation is *not* the same as causation. Correlation coefficients simply tell us that the variables are associated.

For example, if the salary earned by sports coaches (Variable A) is found to be highly and positively correlated with the performance of players (Variable B), we cannot automatically conclude that higher-paid coaches are *the cause* for better-performing players (or that better players lead to higher-paid coaches). Often there are other variables that influence both variables, causing them to correlate. It could be that the more experienced coaches (Variable C) earn higher salaries (Variable A) and also prepare better players (Variable B).

Direct causal inferences are not warranted based solely on correlational statistics, unless there are additional experimental or statistical controls built into the research design.

There may also be situations where multiple variables together cause two variables to correlate. A bivariate correlation coefficient will not shed light on the influence of these other factors or reveal any information on which of the causal explanations is most plausible.

Finally, when we read published reports with correlational statistics, we might encounter probability information such as the following (shown for r):

$$r_{xy} = .38, p < .05$$

The $p < .05$ refers to the **statistical significance** of the r-value obtained ($r_{xy} = .38$). The X and Y measurements were made in a sample of individuals drawn from a larger population. The p stands for the probability that the population r is 0 in a so-called null hypothesis test. Literally, such a finding would mean that the chances of the population correlation being 0 were found to be less than 5%. Most researchers would consider that result to be "statistically significant" for rejecting the null hypothesis, deeming the 5% error in the decision to be tolerable.

For evaluating its implications for practice or theory, the results on statistical significance tests must be evaluated in concert with the size and direction of the r. Note that the p has nothing to do with the magnitude or direction of r. When the sample size is large, we could obtain a very small r_{xy} of .09 with $p < .05$, a statistically significant result. However, as the r_{XY} of .09 translates to an r^2_{xy} of only about .01 (suggesting little or no overlap in the variables), the statistical significance at 5% here has little **practical significance**.

8.9 Related Statistical Techniques

Several statistical concepts and terms in forthcoming chapters build on the material presented in Chapter 8. Three concepts are introduced in highly abbreviated form to end the chapter: regression, factor analysis, and IRT models (AERA et al., 2014). More follow in Chapters 9–11.

Regression methods are useful in predictive validity studies, as well as in investigations of group-specific prediction biases, among other investigations of construct validity. Chapter 3 offered an illustrative case study showing how prediction biases could manifest in results of college entrance exams for males versus females. Regression procedures utilize the observed correlation between one or more "predictor" variables with a desired "criterion" measure, represented as linear equations, to make future predictions. Think of a two-variable relationship in a scatterplot, as given in Figure 8.11A. A statistical regression analysis attempts to derive a "line of best fit" mathematically that represents the degree of overlap between the two variables. A linear equation can then be used to predict any value on the criterion from given predictor measures.

Factor analyses are a family of multivariate techniques useful in examining and validating the hypothesized internal structure of measures. Starting with correlations of item response data generated by assessments from a matrix like that in Figure 8.2, we can evaluate the extent to which the variance in the response data obtained from the items is explained by mathematically derived factors that correspond with theory. Factors derived are also called latent dimensions. There are different methods for performing **exploratory factor analysis (EFA)** and **confirmatory factor analysis (CFA)**. If a satisfactory factor structure is determined with one or more of these methods, we have validation of the theoretical model on which the assessment was built. From Figure 8.1, the domain specifications usually suggest hypotheses to test the theoretically expected internal structure of an assessment tool.

Finally, **item response theory (IRT)** models are a variety of mathematical models that represent the expected functional relationship between the responses to an item, the item's characteristics (e.g., its difficulty), and the respondent's standing on the overall construct measure scaled unidimensionally. Item characteristic curves (ICCs) generated by IRT models provide the probability of a certain response to an item based on the mathematical function and show the item's relationship to the overall construct measures visually. Most IRT models are mathematically stringent, requiring that items on an assessment measure a single dominant construct with items ordered in terms of their strength or difficulty on a linear scale. Hence, IRT models are useful in **unidimensional** scale construction and for verifying the dimensionality of scale structures according to that intended design. When the item response data fit the IRT model, we obtain unidimensional scales. ICCs are useful for item evaluation purposes, such as detecting measurement biases in items. IRT procedures are also used for setting standards for making criterion-referenced performance interpretations (further discussed in Chapter 9).

Practice Break: Objectives 4–7

- See Dataset 1 again (below) to answer the four bulleted items):
  13, 21, 20, 17, 16, 15, 14, 20, 17, 16, 15, 20, 15, 15, 20, 20, 15, 13, 11, 10
  - Plot the distribution of student's test scores in Dataset 1 this time as a *histogram* and an *ogive*. Which graphing technique was more useful for deriving a measure of relative position? Why?
  - Define the terms *skewness* and *kurtosis*. Describe the shape of the distribution in Dataset 1 with respect to its skewness and kurtosis.
  - Identify the similarities and differences between the distribution in Dataset 1 and the *standard normal distribution*.
  - What are the *z-scores* and *percentile ranks* for students who received scores of 13 and 20? What method did you use to calculate the PRs and why?
- A student obtained a score of 600 on a standardized verbal assessment. What is their *percentile rank* in a "normalized" distribution with a mean of 500 and a standard deviation of 100? What is their *z-score*? Explain the steps of your procedures. Interpret each measure of relative position.
- In a *correlational study* relating college performance to class attendance, a researcher found an $r = .78$, $p < .02$. Make a statement describing what they can conclude about the strength, direction, statistical significance, and practical significance of the correlation.
- The Wechsler Adult Intelligence Scale (WAIS) scores are normally distributed with a mean of 100 and a standard deviation of 16. John Doe and Jane Doe obtained the following WAIS scores. Find their percentile ranks. What percent of cases lie between John's and Jane's scores?
  - John Doe = 116
  - Jane Doe = 84

- What is the most likely Pearson correlation between the following two sets of scores? Interpret their correlation with respect to strength and direction.

Student	*X*	*Y*
A	16	25
B	14	23
C	18	21
D	10	19
E	11	17

- Briefly describe assessment reports or other research studies where you have seen any of the procedures described in this chapter. Which ones were applied and for what purposes? Interpret the statistics in a meaningful way using information from this chapter.

8.10 Summary

Chapter 8 discussed a number of descriptive statistics and methods for examining distributional properties of items, scales and scores from assessment tools. The measurement scale and the variable's distribution properties should guide decisions on specific analytic procedures. Appropriate data organization techniques are necessary for the computation of different statistics, which help in gaining information on variable distributions. Graphing of frequency distributions facilitates visual interpretation of a group's performance.

Shapes of distributions can be described with reference to the properties of the standard normal distribution, namely, in terms of their variability, symmetry, modality, skewness, and kurtosis. The chapter demonstrated methods for deriving measures of relative position in normal and non-normal distributions, specifically for standard scores and percentile ranks.

Relationships among measured constructs could be evaluated with bivariate scatterplots and a number of different correlation coefficients. Deviation scores, variance and correlation coefficients, among others, serve as the foundational concepts for several statistical procedures used for psychometric scaling and validation research, including regression, factor analysis and IRT-based methods that we touched upon.

CHAPTER 9

Improving the Inferential Utility of Assessment Results

Methods and Limitations

9.1 Chapter Overview

9.1.1 Introduction

Building on Chapter 8, this chapter presents the basic theory, statistical procedures, interpretive guidelines, and common uses of selected types of *derived scores* and *transformed measures*, drawing largely from classical test theory (CTT). Most of the techniques were developed by testing agencies, researchers, or practitioners for large-scale, standardized test design purposes in education or psychology, or for more restricted instrument uses in specialized fields. As needed, readers should seek out added psychometrics textbooks and statistical resources to supplement the information given here (see, e.g., Bandalos, 2018; Crocker & Algina, 2006; Price, 2018).

Figure 9.1 illustrates where the Chapter 9 topics fit within the process model and rest of the book. Derived score scales and transformed scores need to be purposefully designed as a part of the assessment operations in Phases II and III, guided by the projected inferences, assessment uses, and overall user context in Phase I. Validation in Phase IV is addressed in Chapters 10 and 11, and should be performed to ensure the overall quality of derived scores and scales (Phase I).

9.1.2 Chapter Objectives

1. Identify the basic properties of derived scores and scales for making *norm-referenced* interpretations, along with their applications, design procedures, advantages and disadvantages.
2. Identify the basic properties of derived scores and scales for making *criterion-referenced* interpretations, along with their applications, design procedures, advantages and disadvantages.
3. Identify the basic properties of derived scores and scales for making *ipsative* interpretations, along with their applications, advantages and disadvantages.
4. Describe common applications of *composite scores* with attention to their derivation, properties, and limitations in specific scenarios.
5. Describe common applications of *grouped scores* or other forms of aggregated assessment data in specific scenarios.
6. Show awareness of the purposes of "linked" or "equated" score metrics and common methods of linking scales in different scenarios.

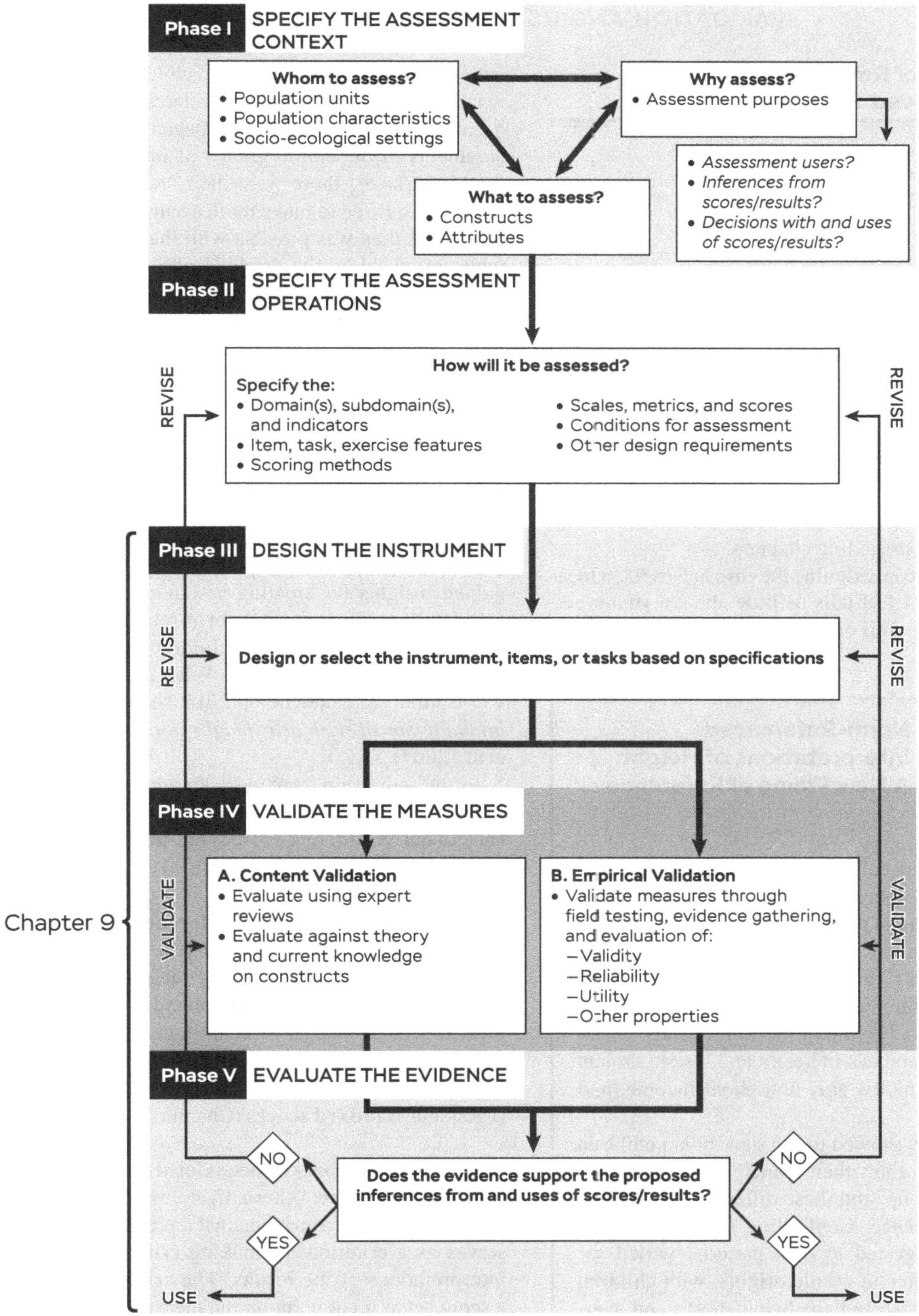

FIGURE 9.1. Connecting Chapter 9 with the Process Model and the rest of the book.

9.2 Frames of Reference and Derived Scores

The way we derive meaning from a test score depends on the context or frame of reference in which we wish to interpret it.

—ROBERT M. THORNDIKE (1997, pp. 52–53)

To begin Chapter 9, recall the distinction made between *raw scores*—the scores or information produced in original form directly from a test or assessment instrument—and a *derived score*, which refers to any transformed scores and scales obtained from the raw assessment data. Derived scores add inferential value to the information produced from assessments by adding a frame of reference, thereby making the results more useful for an intended research or practice-related purpose. Readers will recall references to many examples in the preceding chapters.

For a quick recap, examine the case in Box 9.1; a measured height of 4 feet tells us little about a young person's well-being until one compares it with the heights and weights of other similar-aged children or youth. But what would be the *best* frame of reference? In this study, a team of biological researchers began with height measurements of the ethnic groups of interest to them in the Netherlands; these were their "raw scores." However, they desired to make more accurate health-related inferences than was possible with the universal norms tables provided by the World Health Organization. To do so, they compared the height measures with that of children and youth growing up in the *same* region over time. This provided them with a better-situated frame of reference; they were able to derive more accurate percentile ranks from the raw measures of height.

Health researchers know today that height and weight together serve as important indicators of a person's physical and psychological well-being. Furthermore, height is also known to be related to age, ethnic origins, cultures, and the socioeconomic backgrounds of different peoples. Through the study, the researchers gained insights for creating new regional norms that could enhance their desired norm-referenced interpretations of the health status of children and youth growing up in the Netherlands (de Wilde, van Dommelen, van Buuren, & Middelkoop 2014; see also *www.who.int/childgrowth/standards/height_for_age/en*; de Onis et al., 2007).

In the same vein, starting with any given raw measures, we could utilize *three* possible frames of reference to derive different score types for adding inferential value to the results (see Table 9.1). These are:

1. **Norms as the frame of reference:** As in the case study in Box 9.1, we could compare an individual's raw scores with those of a carefully selected *norm group* where every member is administered the same assessment tool under the same conditions. Two commonly found derived scores for making norm-referenced interpretations, readers will recall, are **percentile ranks (PRs)** and **standard scores** (Chapter 8).

2. **Criterion scores or behavioral standards as the frame of reference:** Alternatively, we could compare an individual's measures against a preset standard that serves as a criterion for making criterion-referenced interpretations of the results. The criterion is usually a score set as a cut point on the measurement scale, or a series of ordered cut scores, for placing individuals in separate categories like Level 1, Level 2, and so on.

BOX 9.1 Norm-Referenced Interpretations of Height: A New Frame of Reference

Case Study

De Wilde and colleagues (2014) measured and compared the heights of Asian Indian children and young adults growing up in the Netherlands against height and weight standards given by the World Health Organization (WHO). They studied a large sample of over 3,000 children and youth ages 0–20 years in the Netherlands, charting their differences in height and weight broken down by ethnicity, age, household income, and affluence.

The results showed that Asian Indian children were shorter than their Dutch counterparts in every age group, and these differences increased after adolescence. Controlling for age, the differences suggested growth patterns varied for groups of different ethnic origins, with children of affluent Asian Indians being shorter, on average, than children of affluent Dutch.

Elsewhere, it could be a previously set profile of behavioral indicators that meets the definition of a condition or an expected level of performance. Note that use of the term *criterion* here is different from *criterion measures* we might use for measuring future outcomes in predictive validity studies.

3. **Self as the frame of reference:** Lastly, one could compare a person's measures with their *own* prior performances or behaviors over time in domain-specific areas. Known also as *ipsative* measurements in education, self-referenced interpretations of assessment results permit growth-based inferences. Ipsative interpretations are necessary when evaluating changes on measured constructs in students, disabled individuals, or patients, following specific treatments or interventions in health care or education contexts.

Table 9.1 shows examples of these three classes of derived scores with their respective frames of reference; in order, Sections 9.3 through 9.6 that follow detail their common applications, design requirements, advantages and limitations. For ease of communication, the generic terms *test* and *test score* are used; however, the concepts and procedures are applicable across different assessment tools and modalities.

9.3 Using Norms as the Frame of Reference

When designing instruments intended for norm referencing (norm-referenced tests [NRTs]), we need a distribution of scores to serve as the primary referent and database for deriving the new scores and scales. For specific illustrations of steps of these procedures, this section refers to the Universal Nonverbal Intelligence Test—Second Edition (UNIT-2; Friedlander Moore, McCallum & Bracken, 2017), a commercially distributed standardized test, and a hypothetical classroom test shown in Figure 9.2, as we proceed.

9.3.1 The *z*-Score: A Building Block

See Figure 9.2. A basic building block for a family of standard scores we find in different NRTs is the *z-score*. We begin this section with a quick review of the properties of the *z*-score. Suppose that a student obtained a score of 25 on an arithmetic quiz at school, where the class mean (M) was 15 with a standard deviation (s) of 10. That raw score of 25 would yield a $z = +1.0$ as follows:

$$
\begin{aligned}
z &= (X - M)/s \\
&= (25 - 15)/10 = +1.0
\end{aligned}
$$

Given its formula, a *z*-score represents the calculated linear distance of any raw score from the mean of the distribution, expressed in standard deviation units. We would interpret the score of +1.0 and all positive *z*-score values in Figure 9.2 as "above average" in the class's distribution of scores. The class in this scenario serves as its own norm group. As a measure of relative position in a distribution of scores, the *z*-score scale is useful in distinguishing among individuals who are average, above average, or below average given the mean and standard deviation of the norm group.

TABLE 9.1. Three Frames of Reference for Deriving Scores

Frame of reference	Type of derived scores	Intended inferences	Examples
1. Norms, based on a distribution of test scores	Norm-referenced scores	Rank or placement of a person's score in the norm group	• Percentile ranks • *z*-scores • Standard scores
2. An absolute standard or criterion score(s) on a domain-referenced test	Criterion-referenced scores or domain-referenced score categories	Determinations of the proficiency or severity levels in specified domains	• Pass versus fail categorizations • Severity levels of a diseased condition
3. Self as referent, using prior assessment results on the same persons	Ipsative (self-referenced) change scores over time	Ipsative interpretations of change over time	• Gain scores • Graphed growth trajectories • Time-series graphs

Recall that the *z-score scale* is an equal-interval scale with a one-to-one relationship with the raw scores (Chapter 8). Distributions of z-scores take the shape of the original distribution of scores in a group—whether normal, near normal, or non-normal. This shape influences their properties.

9.3.2 Common Applications of Norm-Referenced Scores

Norm-referenced scores are used for a number of research or practice-related purposes in both educational and noneducational contexts. Interestingly, most of these applications require *cut points* to be set in the score distribution, such as a z-score of +2.0 or a percentile rank of 90. Typical uses include:

- Selection and/or placement of students in gifted, enrichment, or special education programs based on cut points set on the NRT score scale
- Selection of individuals for competitive college admissions and scholarships, or for merit pay, rewards, or sanctions in the workplace, also with cut points set in an NRT score distribution
- Diagnosis and/or treatment of mental disabilities or serious health conditions in persons, using cut points on NRT scales denoting the severity of the pathological condition
- Selection, hiring, and recruitment decisions using cut scores on job-related test score scales, especially in fixed-quota occupational settings
- Instructional decisions as in Figure 9.2, both formative and summative, using distributions of classroom test scores as the comparison group.

Taking up the last, teachers often make a number of NRT score uses with easy-to-apply methods that can be replicated elsewhere. Assigning end-of-year report card marks using distribution of percentile ranks or z-scores from a classroom test is a typical **summative use**. The colloquial expression "curving the grades" refers to norm-referenced methods for assigning marks. The method relies entirely on the shape and properties of the test score distribution to which the remaining scores are compared, and the background characteristics of the other test-takers.

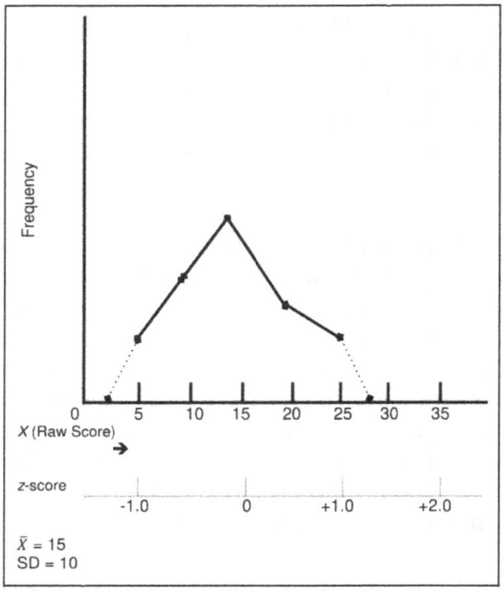

FIGURE 9.2. A distribution of raw scores and z-scores for a class.

As an example, see Figure 9.3 illustrating an ogive-based, norm-referenced marking scheme. It employs cumulative percentile ranges on final examination scores with the top 20% of students in the score distribution receiving A marks (PRs of 80 and above), the next 20% receiving B marks (PRs of 60–79.9), and so forth. Figure 9.3 makes clear why the characteristics of the comparison group matter when making norm-referenced interpretations and uses of test scores. We see that the *range* of scores is rather narrow with the class as a whole performing poorly on the test. Regardless, students ranked in the top 40% are awarded A and B marks because of their relatively higher location in *that* distribution. In a norm-referenced grading scheme, the mark does not reflect the students' proficiency level on the tested domains per se, but only their rank or placement relative to that of the class's score distribution. This could be a limitation in some user contexts.

A contrasting **formative use** of NRT results would be one where a teacher might select students with z-scores ≤ -0.5 on a classroom test for providing added educational supports. Public education systems fre-

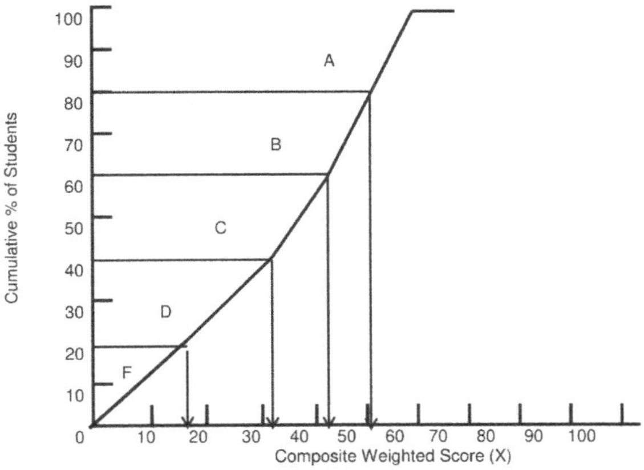

FIGURE 9.3. Ogive-based system for assigning marks.

quently use cut points on standardized NRT score distributions for identifying students in need of special instructional assistance, such as supporting students with limited English skills via English language learner (ELL) programs (Valentino & Reardon, 2015).

9.3.3 Design Requirements for Norm-Referenced Tests

To derive and interpret norm-referenced scores accurately, the tests must be carefully constructed so as to ensure certain properties. There are *four* main design requirements for well-functioning NRTs: (1) a focus on general domains, (2) high variance and reliability of test scores, (3) quality and characteristics of the norming sample, and (4) rigor in the procedures for norming and score derivation. In addition, validation of NRT scores is always necessary (more on this in Chapters 10 and 11). Refer back to Figures 9.2 and 9.3 and Table 9.1 again and see Tables 9.2 and 9.3 as we continue.

9.3.3.1 A Focus on General Construct Domains

NRTs are best designed to measure general domains, as the priority is placed on obtaining reliable, comparative placements of individuals in the distribution of *total scores* representing that overall domain. To assure construct validity, the general domain must be conceptualized in a defensible manner and grounded in some theoretical base of knowledge (Chapter 4).

For example, the UNIT-2 (Friedlander Moore et al., 2017; McCallum & Bracken, 2018) is an NRT purported to measure *general intelligence*. The UNIT-2 includes three subtests that focus on different cognitive ability dimensions (memory, fluid reasoning, and symbolic and nonsymbolic forms of quantitative reasoning), but these subconstructs are all linked theoretically to an underlying general cognitive ability. According to one of its authors, the test "is first and foremost a strong measure of *g*" (McCallum, 2003, p. 1, Abstract). The *g* refers to a broad, general ability factor based on Charles Spearman's 1904 theory of general intelligence (Deary, 2001). The *g*-factor continues to have currency in interpreting results of modern mental ability tests and is theorized to dominate intellectual capacities of human beings.

In the same vein, standardized educational achievement tests intended for norm referencing should also aim to measure broad, general domains, yielding the most reliable scores for the total test. For a recently designed NRT that displays these properties, examine the English language arts (ELA) or math assessments developed for grade school students by the Smarter Balanced Assessment Consortium or SBAC (National Center for Research on Evaluation, Standards, and Student Testing [CRESST], 2017). For each grade level, the total test scores of the SBAC reflect achievement in a specified, general domain based on the Common Core content standards.

9.3.3.2 Variance and Reliability of Test Scores

Well-functioning NRTs are designed to spread out the test-takers widely on the total score distributions. Higher variability, such as a distribution with *z*-scores ranging from –3.0 to +3.0, enables more accurate and reliable sorting and placement of candidates in the distribution. To do so, NRT designers may deliberately incorporate items with wide-ranging difficulty levels for the tested population. Reliability estimation methods for NRTs based on CTT techniques also require high variance in test scores. When high-stakes uses are planned with the results, the relative placements of scores of NRTs should be highly reliable within tolerable margins of error (Crocker & Algina, 2006).

Returning to the UNIT-2 as an example (Friedlander Moore et al., 2017), the developers deliberately "normalized" the standard score distribution derived from the raw scores to achieve a wider z-score range from –3.0 to +3.0 that they desired. More details on the normalization procedures follow in a later section. The reliability estimates reported for the overall test scores are in the order of .90 (rounded), generally considered to fall in the high range.

9.3.3.3 Quality and Characteristics of the Norm Group

Three criteria for determining the quality and suitability of the norms are their recency, relevance, and representativeness (AERA et al., 2014). Depending on the test's purposes, the norms established could consist of national, local, or more specialized samples of test-takers. Developers usually undertake **standardization studies** with a carefully selected "norming sample" to ensure the quality of the norms and norm-referenced scores for the populations specified for the test.

We should ask three questions for assuring the quality of norms when designing or adopting NRTs:

- *Norm group recency.* Were the comparison group's data collected recently enough to allow meaningful comparisons with current groups of examinees?
- *Norm group relevance.* Did individuals in the norm group have similar experiences to the prospective test-takers, facilitating relevant and meaningful score comparisons on the constructs measured?
- *Norm group representativeness.* Are the members of the norm group similar to the prospective test-takers on major sociodemographic, contextual, and background variables?

For the illustrative classroom test (Figure 9.2), these three requirements would be met *if* the students being compared:

1. took the same test at about the same time, possibly during the same school semester or term (*recency*);
2. were in the same grade, and exposed to similar curricular experiences in comparable schooling environments (*relevance*); and
3. were of the same age, with similar distributions on major background characteristics (*representativeness*).

Standardization requires that designers of NRTs collect data from an appropriately selected norming sample. Guided by the assessment design specifications, this sample is administered the test following all the standardized protocols applicable, such as controlled directions, use of media, timing constraints, scoring criteria, or any accommodations for disabled, linguistically or otherwise diverse test-takers. Examiners and proctors must be trained or appropriately qualified to administer the test. The results are then compiled into a database from which the required norm-referenced scores and scales are derived.

Norm groups for most standardized NRTs are carefully stratified with respect to region, socioeconomic status, urban–rural–suburban location, ethnicity, and age of subjects (see Table 9.2 for an example). The age range of the norming sample should concur with that of the intended population for the NRT and be sufficiently large to be representative of other key background variables. To enable prospective NRT users/adopters to evaluate its quality, the standardization procedures should be documented in technical manuals or other publications disseminated by the test developers (AERA et al., 2014).

Table 9.2 shows an excerpted table from the technical materials of the UNIT-2 (Friedlander Moore et al., 2017). Here, the test publishers provide a breakdown of the standardization sample of 2,100 examinees taken from North America, from 5 to 18 years old. Comparisons with U.S. census data breakdowns on the selected background variables are shown at the bottom. Such information allows future test users and adopters to evaluate the national representativeness of the data.

Notice that every age group listed in Table 9.2 is crossed with data on sex and parental education levels—these are background variables selected by the developers for optimizing score interpretations. Elsewhere in the examiner's manual, the developers provide a number of added tables with breakdowns on stratification variables they used, including race, sex, and disability status of the individuals. The foot-

TABLE 9.2. Composition of the UNIT-2 Standardization Sample: Percentages by Age, Sex, and Parent Education

	Female				Male				Total			
Parent's education level → / Age in years ↓	<HS	HS	Some college	≥4 years college	<HS	HS	Some college	≥4 years college	<HS	HS	Some college	≥4 years college
5:0–5:11	6.9	12.6	14.3	16.6	4.0	16.0	17.1	12.6	10.9	28.6	31.4	29.1
6:0–6:11	6.9	16.6	16.0	10.9	5.7	13.7	14.3	16.0	12.6	30.3	30.3	26.9
7:0–7:11	7.4	15.4	15.4	11.4	6.3	12.0	16.6	15.4	13.7	27.4	32.0	26.9
8:0–8:11	6.9	13.1	19.4	9.7	6.3	16.0	12.0	16.6	13.1	29.1	31.4	26.3
9:0–9:11	10.3	13.1	15.4	11.4	3.4	17.1	14.9	14.3	13.7	30.3	30.3	25.7
10:0–10:11	5.7	14.3	15.4	13.7	6.9	16.0	15.4	12.6	12.6	30.3	30.9	26.3
11:0–11:11	10.9	14.9	11.4	12.0	5.7	14.3	17.7	13.1	16.6	29.1	29.1	25.1
12:0–12:11	5.7	16.6	16.6	11.4	7.4	13.7	12.0	16.6	13.1	30.3	28.5	28.0
13:0–13:11	8.6	13.1	12.0	16.6	6.3	14.3	18.3	10.9	14.9	27.4	30.3	27.3
14:0–14:11	6.3	14.3	15.4	13.7	9.7	15.4	9.7	15.4	16.0	29.7	25.1	29.1
15:0–15:11	8.6	13.7	12.6	15.4	6.9	19.4	8.6	14.9	15.4	33.1	21.1	30.3
16:0–16:11	5.1	16.0	13.1	16.0	9.7	12.0	17.1	10.9	14.9	28.0	30.3	26.9
UNIT norming sample	7.4	14.5	14.8	13.2	6.5	15.0	14.5	14.1	14.0	29.5	29.2	27.3
U.S. population*	6.9	14.6	14.9	13.8	6.9	14.6	14.9	13.8	13.7	29.1	29.7	27.5

Note. $N = 2{,}100$; for each age group, $n = 175$. Population percentages for each sex were adjusted to ensure equal representation of male and female participants. Parent education is classified as Less than high school (<HS), High school graduate or equivalent (HS), Some college or technical school, Four or more years of college (≥4 Years college). Due to rounding, values may not always sum exactly to the totals.

*U.S. Population data are from *Current Population Survey, March 1995*, by U.S. Bureau of the Census, 1995, Washington, DC: Author.

note here indicates that the U.S. census data are from 1995. To meet the national *representativeness* criterion today, test users and adopters should evaluate the norming sample breakdowns against the most current U.S. census data on those variables.

To enable comparative determinations of the performances of all future test-takers, NRT developers prepare **norms tables**. A norms table displays each raw score in the original distribution, with the corresponding derived scores presented in columns; see Table 9.3 for an illustration. Test scores of all future test-takers are referenced back to these norms tables for interpretation purposes. Consistency and adherence to standardized protocols during norming facilitate construct-relevant, norm-referenced score comparisons afterward.

Norms tables for NRTs can become outdated over time, diminishing in their relevance and representativeness for given assessment user contexts. Although there is no fixed rule, renorming after a 5-year period and no later than 10 years is the recommended practice (AERA et al., 2014; Russell, 2010). The UNIT was originally normed and published in 1997; the second edition was renormed and published in 2015, about 10 years later (Friedlander Moore et al., 2017).

For high-stakes NRTs, norms should be updated every 5–7 years. With standardized achievement tests used in education systems for high-stakes, accountability purposes, new norms may be necessary whenever there are major shifts in scholastic curricula, population demographics, and/or reform policies under which particular assessments are adopted and used. To assure the relevance of the norms, the reformed curricula and instructional programs must be implemented *before* the norming and standardization process begins (see the case studies in Chapter 2).

TABLE 9.3. Normalized *z*-Scores and Percentile Ranks with Raw Scores and Linear *z*-Scores in a Norms Table

Raw score	Percentile	Normalized *z*-score	Linear[a] *z*-score
36	98	2.05	2.43
33	96	1.75	1.64
32	94	1.55	1.38
31	90	1.28	1.12
30	88	1.18	0.86
29	84	0.99	0.59
28	72	0.58	0.33
27	54	0.10	0.07
26	32	−0.47	−0.20
25	16	−0.99	−0.46
24	10	−1.28	−0.72
22	8	−1.41	−1.25
21	6	−1.55	−1.51
15	4	−1.75	−3.09
14	2	−2.05	−3.36

[a]*z*-Values based on the actual distribution and using the equation: $z = \frac{X - M}{SD}$ where $M = 26.75$ and SD = 3.80.

9.3.3.4 Rigor of the Norming and Score Derivation Procedures

Finally, how thoroughly we execute the steps of the norming and score derivation procedures determines the quality of the NRT. Although individual projects may vary, there are five main steps. Each one is listed next, supported with descriptions of the procedures reported for the UNIT-2 (see Friedlander Moore et al., 2017, UNIT-2 Examiner's Manual, Chap. 3, pp. 32–35);

- **Step 1:** Administer the test according to standardized protocols to a selected norming sample and check the integrity of the data collected.

  To ensure quality of the UNIT normative data, the project staff followed a stringent quality control procedure. Every submitted record and response booklet was checked against a 33-point checklist.

- **Step 2:** Ensure representativeness of the normative database against the specified population of potential test-takers on major sociodemographic and contextual variables.

  The UNIT standardization was designed so that the sample conformed with the contemporary U.S. population on important demographic variables. The sample was randomly selected within the demographically determined strata.

- **Step 3:** Follow the design specifications to score the items in the norming sample and generate raw score distributions for all subtests and total test.

  After the UNIT normative data were collected and analyzed, raw scores were determined for each subtest, for each examinee.

- **Step 4:** Derive the norm-referenced scores to create norms tables with all derived scores listed in columns for the overall test and all subtests that apply.

  Subtest total raw scores were converted to percentile ranks for each full year age group. For each age group, percentile ranks were then converted to z-scores; these were then converted to subtest scaled scores with a mean of 10 and a standard deviation of 3 (range = 1–19, or +/–3 SD).

- **Step 5:** Examine the shape of the score distributions and normalize the distributions, as appropriate, to enhance score interpretability and utility of the derived scores for the designated uses of the NRT.

  [The] normalized scaled scores were then smoothed in each age group and across each age group. For the intermediate age levels within an age group, subtest scaled scores were interpolated from the smoothed norms. The result was a smoothed distribution of scores that reflects the intellectual growth patterns of children and adolescents assessed.

Note that the terms *norming* and *normalizing* in NRT design, described for the UNIT-2 in Step 5 above, are not the same thing.

Even when the norming sample is very large (N = 2,100 on the UNIT-2), the raw score distribution may be non-normal to different degrees. Hence, standardized test developers often choose to **normalize** the score distributions. Normalizing involves stretching or scrunching the original *z*-score values forcibly to match the *z*-values of the **standard normal distribution.** This procedure is justifiable when the measured construct naturally distributes in a near normal fashion. Once normalized, the percentile ranks, *z*-scores, and other forms of derived scores have a shape and properties that mimic the standard normal curve, with the z-scores (σ-units on the base) and percent areas under the curve, related in fixed ways. This procedure offers distinctive interpretive advantages (Chapter 8).

Table 9.3 demonstrates how the normalization procedure may be carried out starting with the originally obtained "linear" z-scores; as indicated earlier, it also illustrates what a typical "norms table" might look like. The descriptive statistics from any raw score distribution is first employed to derive the linear z-scores (here, mean = 26.75 and standard deviation = 3.8). Using a statistical table of the standard normal distribution, these linear z-scores are mapped against normalized PRs, as shown. In the last step, using the same statistical table, the normalized PRs are mapped against the corresponding normalized z-scores of the standard normal distribution. The normal curve table is available online, or in most statistics textbooks (see, e.g., Larson & Farber, 2004)

Smoothing, also described for the UNIT-2 in Step 5 above, is necessary when the empirical data from the norming sample do not provide all the z-score points in the theoretical normal distribution. To "smooth" the graph, some data points are interpolated or extrapolated to give it a continuous shape.

9.3.4 Computation Procedures of Different Norm-Referenced Scores

Different standardized test-makers have proposed the use of different derived scores, mostly in normalized form. Examine Figures 9.4 and 9.5 next as we review the procedures for deriving norm-referenced scores of the following types:

- Normalized percentile ranks
- Normalized standard scores
- Normalized stanines
- Grade-equivalent and age-equivalent scores

9.3.4.1 Normalized Percentile Ranks

DEFINITION

Normalized percentile ranks (NPRs) denote the percent of examinees/respondents in the norm group's distribution who scored below a given raw score in that distribution. Percentiles and NPRs have ordinal scale properties, distributing as shown in Figure 9.4, consistent with the standard normal distribution.

DERIVATION

See Figure 9.4 and Table 9.3. NPRs corresponding with specific σ-units (z-scores) can be read from statistical tables on the normal curve, as demonstrated earlier. From Chapter 8, we also know the mathematical formula for a PR for any raw score, X. Applicable in either normalized or non-normalized frequency distributions of scores, it is

$$\text{PR} = 100\left[\frac{\frac{f(X - \text{Lower limit of interval of X})}{\text{interval size, } i} + \text{Cum} f_{\text{in interval below}}}{N}\right]$$

where X = raw score for which PR needs to be calculated
f = frequency
i = size of class or score interval (in a simple frequency distribution, this value is always 1)
Cum f = cumulative frequency
N = total number of cases

INTERPRETATION

For Person A with a reported NPR of 48 on a standardized NRT, the interpretation is that Person A's raw score places them above 48% of similar test-takers in the norm group.

9.3.4.2 Normalized Standard Scores

DEFINITION

Most commercial developers of NRTs normalize their z-scores first and then derive standard score distributions (NSSs) that are on an equal-interval scale, as shown in Table 9.3 and Figure 9.4. All NSSs describe the distance of any raw score from the mean of the norming sample in standard deviation units. These z-units correspond with fixed NPRs in the normal distribution.

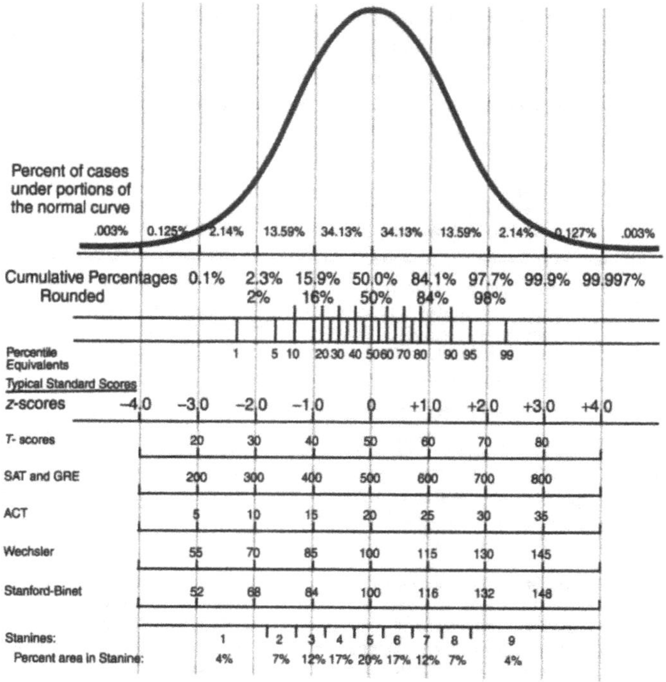

FIGURE 9.4. Normalized distributions of standard scores, percentile ranks, and stanines.

DERIVATION

The starting point for obtaining a normalized NSS is always the *z-score*, calculated with the formula

$$z = (X - M_{\text{norm group}}) \div SD_{\text{norm group}}$$

To convert the normalized *z*-score to a given NSS, we use two constants in the conversion formula for the M and S, as shown below. Various test developers have designated different values for the S and M constants in their conversion formulas:

$$\text{NSS} = z(\text{S}) + \text{M}$$

For example, see Step 4 again for the UNIT-2 description given in the previous subsection. These test developers used values of M = 10 and S = 3 to obtain their desired range of 1–19 on their NSS scale, extending from +/–3.0 standard deviation units in a normalized distribution. For an examinee with a normalized *z*-score of +1.0 on the UNIT-2, the converted SS is 13, computed as follows:

$$\text{UNIT-2, NSS} = 1.0\ (3) + 10 = 13$$

Now see Figure 9.4 that shows the NSS scales of several well-known standardized tests, each with different constants replacing the values of M and S: the T-score (M = 50, S = 10); Scholastic Assessment Test and Graduate Record Examination (SAT and GRE; M = 500, S = 100); Stanford–Binet (S-B; M = 100, S = 15); and Wechsler Adult Intelligence Scale (WAIS; M = 100, S = 15) being some examples.

Why are there so many different constants employed for deriving these different NSS scales? As with the UNIT-2, each NSS is rooted in the scale properties that each test developer desired for the specific user contexts they had in mind. The negative and decimal values of the z-score scale are not user-friendly. To remove these, different NSS conversions were conceptualized by different test developers.

As another example, the T-score scale is employed by a number of test-makers in psychology and education. To detect clinical levels of adolescent psychopathology, Reynolds (2004) used the normalized T-score scale with cut points to determine five levels of severity of the psychological condition. The two clinical categories are the "moderate clinical symptom" range of $70T$ to $79T$ and the "severe clinical symptom" range of $80T$ and above. Utility and meaningfulness of the NSS scale for the specific user context are the main drivers of such differences in decisions.

The normal curve equivalent (NCE, not shown), is another historic NSS scale developed by the U.S. Department of Education in 1976 for monitoring student performance in federally funded public school programs. Many state and federal departments of education continue to utilize NCEs for educational evaluation and accountability purposes (Gewertz, 2017; Morgan, 2016). The converted and normalized NCE scale is derived from z-scores using the constants of M = 50 and S = 21.06 to yield a scale that corresponds with the normalized PR range of from 1 to 99. This scale is considered more useful for showing annual changes in student achievement (Mertler, 2002).

INTERPRETATION

An NSS is interpreted exactly like the z-score, with predictable NPRs readable directly from the normal curve table. To illustrate with the T, we would use this formula: $T = z(10) + 50$. For a Person A with a z-score of 1.0, the T is calculated to be 60, as follows:

$$T = 1.0(10) + 50 = 60$$

The T of 60 indicates that the student is placed 1 standard deviation unit above the mean of the national norm group. Given a normalized distribution, for a T-score of 60, the PR is 84 (Figure 9.4). Similarly, we can read off the PRs corresponding to various SS values, as follows, in Figure 9.4: z of –1.0 (T = 40, PR = 16); z of 0 (T = 50, PR of 50); z of +1.0 (T = 60, PR of 84); and so forth. The PR for every intermediate value of z is available from published normal curve tables online or in statistics textbooks.

9.3.4.3 Normalized Stanine

DEFINITION

Figure 9.5 shows a normalized stanine (NS) distribution. The word "stanine" is rooted in the contraction *standard nine*. It refers to the nine bands at the bottom. If we divide the σ-units (z-units) at the base of a normal distribution into nine parts, we would create ordered bands called *stanines*. Stanines yield an ordinal scale, with scores ranging from 1 (lowest) to 9 (highest). Psychometric legend has it that stanines were developed as a space-saving mechanism for reporting test results. The single-digit scores were preferred as they fit in one column on data entry cards fed into early computers for scoring and analysis.

DERIVATION

No calculations are necessary. Fixed z-units set the boundaries for each stanine. For example, as Figure 9.5 shows, z-units of –1.75 to –1.25 define a stanine of 2.

The stanine scale is constructed in a normal distribution starting from the mean as the center point and by marking off a quarter of a standard deviation unit on either side. This defines the middle stanine of 5. Next, if we mark off similar bands on either side of the fifth stanine, each exactly half a standard deviation unit in width until we reach the two extreme bands of 1 and 9, we will have created a stanine scale. The two extreme bands are undefined. Note that each NS band has a fixed percentage of measured individuals or examinees within.

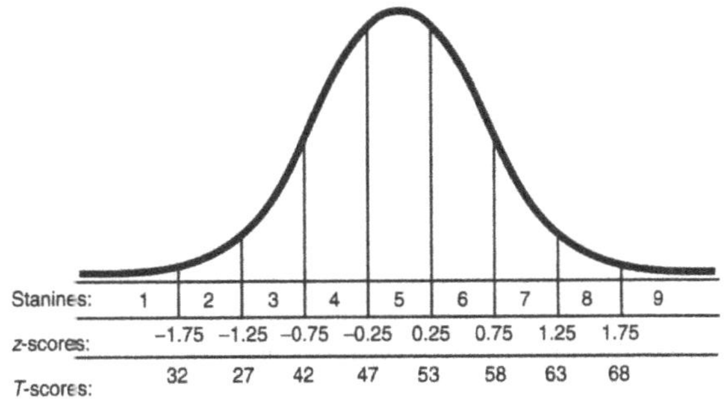

FIGURE 9.5. Normalized stanine distribution.

INTERPRETATION

Stanines of 1, 2, and 3 are considered below average; values of 4, 5, and 6 are considered average; while values of 7, 8, and 9 indicate above average performance. If Person A's NS is 5, it would correspond with a NPR range of 47 – 53, falling in the middle range of scores. We would correctly interpret that performance as average relative to the norm group in the tested domain. An advantage of stanines is that they are more reliable than the NPR or NSS at a given point. The stanine score bands tend to absorb random measurement errors.

9.3.4.4 Grade- and Age-Equivalent Scores

All the norm-referenced scores presented so far compared an individual's score with those of a cross-sectional norming sample, collected at a given time. In contrast, the grade-equivalent (GE) and age-equivalent (AE) scales are built with multiyear, developmentally ordered norming samples. By design, AE and GE scores are intended for mapping *changes* as individuals develop in given construct domains, say, from one grade level to the next, or from age 5 to 7 years, in verbal skills.

AE score scales accompany most intelligence tests; for example, the UNIT-2 Examiner's Manual discusses age-equivalent scores. GEs apply to grade school students; these scales are reported for many standardized achievement tests intended for making growth-based, norm-referenced inferences. Although IRT-based *vertically linked scales* are devised today for measuring student achievement from grade to grade with NRTs (Student, 2022), the AE and GE are growth-based scales by design and offer some advantages.

GE scores are reported as two-digit, decimalized numbers like 3.9. With 10 months in a typical school year, GE scores range from 3.0 to 3.9 for grade 3. Correspondingly, the AE scale accounts for 12 months in the calendar year for age, with decimals ranging from 0 to 11.

DERIVATION

Figure 9.6 illustrates the procedures for GE scale development. To build a GE scale, assessment designers start with a multilevel test, or a series of leveled tests in a domain, such as reading comprehension tests for grades 2, 3, and 4. The multilevel test (or each separate grade-level test) is administered either in the fall or spring term of a school year, to a multigrade norming sample, usually for three successive grades. From the norm group data at each grade level, the *median* score is identified. The GE scale is constructed around these empirically obtained medians. The medians serve as the anchoring points for creating the remaining segments of the developmental GE scale.

See the horizontal axis of Figure 9.6, which shows how the scale would be built if the norming were performed in the fifth month of the school year. The empirical median points of 1.5, 2.5, 3.5, and 4.5 are marked for the four grades in the norming sample. The intermediate point values in between the medians are interpolated; points beyond those empirical medians are extrapolated. In Figure 9.6, points falling in between 1.5 and 2.5 are interpolated, while a GE score of 1.0 is extrapolated downward from the empirical 1.5 point. The difference between GEs of 1.5 and 2.5 is much greater than the difference between GEs of 3.5 and 4.5, showing the ordinal properties of the GE scale.

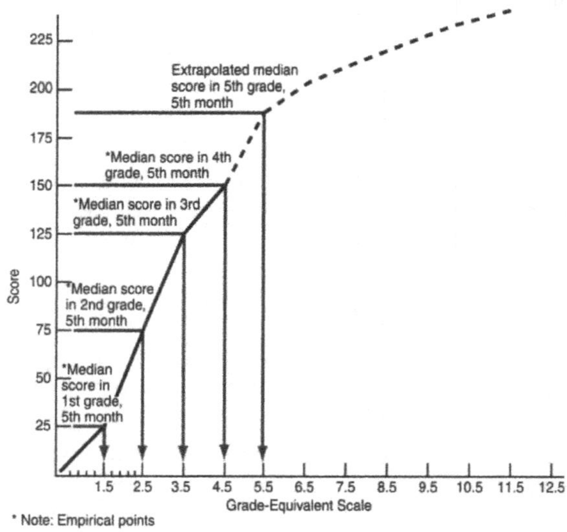

FIGURE 9.6. Deriving grade-equivalent scores: An illustration.

INTERPRETATIONS

A GE score of 2.5 denotes that the student's performance is equivalent to the *average performance* of a second grader in the fifth month of the school year in the measured domain. A number like 3.9 on the AE scale would denote *average development* on the measured construct for a child of 3 years and 9 months of age.

The empirically based points of the GE and AE scales permit the most valid interpretations of expected "gains" across the levels. The interpolated and extrapolated regions tend to become overinterpreted and could easily mislead laypersons and professionals alike. If a first grader receives a GE score of 6.4, for example, a common misinterpretation is that the child is reading at the sixth-grade level. In reality, the students in the norming sample neither received a sixth-grade curriculum, nor took a sixth-grade test; the GE score is just a rough estimate for a first grader's relative reading level compared to grade-level peers on a grade-level test. Hence, the most conservative and accurate interpretation would be that the child is reading well above the median score for that grade level. As with all norm-referenced scores, interpretations of curriculum mastery cannot be made with a GE score.

QUICK RECAP: NRT scores offer advantages but have limitations in specific scenarios. The characteristics of the norming sample, along with the standardization and scale development procedures, determine the properties of specific NRT scores and scales. With the exception of AE and GE scales, most derived scores for NRTs begin with linear *z*-scores. Designers should try to adhere to the main technical requirements and conduct validation studies, as necessary, in specific user contexts. To adopt NRTs for a local need, users should carefully review the scale and score derivation procedures.

Reflection Break 9.1: Objective 1

- What are the *pros* and *cons* of using *norms* as a frame of reference for interpreting a "raw" construct measure? Why are NRTs popular in so many application contexts, despite the *cons*?
- On a standardized NRT used for college admissions, a test-taker got 80% of the items correct and a percentile rank (NPR) of 70. Given that the NPR fell below the cut-point of 84, the individual was not admitted. Interpret each score separately and explain the discrepancy in the two scores.
- Describe the steps that you would follow to design an NRT for a specified purpose in your work sphere. Which technical properties would you prioritize? Explain.
- Provide two reasons why NRT developers *normalize* the raw score distributions. Give an example of an assessment design situation where it would *not* be advisable to normalize the raw scores. Explain.
- Describe the derivation procedures and correct interpretations of (1) normalized standard scores, (2) normalized stanines, (3) normalized percentile ranks, and (4) grade-equivalent scores.
- Is the following statement true? *We will always find the highest 4% of the examinees in a stanine band of 9 in a normal distribution.* Explain.

9.4 Using Criterion Scores or Standards as the Frame of Reference

9.4.1 Criteria, Performance Standards, and Domains

Review the middle panel of Table 9.1 and Figure 9.7 now, and consider this quote:

"An 'A' in English means only that some adult thought the student's work was excellent. Compared to what . . . ? As determined by what criteria? [With] reference to what subject area? (Wiggins, 1989, p. 42). An alternative to designing NRTs, and perhaps the more common approach in educational contexts, is to design a criterion-referenced test (CRT).

For CRT design, the expected criterion behaviors tied to a construct domain are set beforehand; this serves as an absolute standard or benchmark, against which we interpret a given person's performance or condition. The criterion enables us to generate *categorical scores*, such as Pass (Score = 1) versus Fail (Score = 0). As Figure 9.7 shows, the categories are

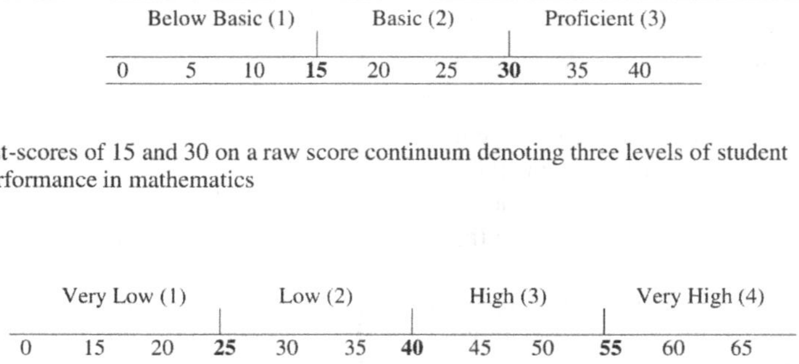

A. Cut-scores of 15 and 30 on a raw score continuum denoting three levels of student performance in mathematics

B. Cut-scores of 25, 40, and 55 to distinguish among four levels on a Depression scale

FIGURE 9.7. Deriving ordinal score categories for criterion-referenced performance interpretations.

the "derived scores." Typically, the categories carry ordinal scale properties. The criteria set are a series of cut scores, and each successive category denotes a progressively higher level on the measured construct. However, if the underlying scale is an interval or ratio scale, the category criteria can also be set at equal intervals.

To generate a multidimensional profile of scores, cut scores may sometimes be set on each indicator in a specified behavioral domain or subdomain, with a rating such as 4 as the minimum passing standard on a 5-point rating scale (Chapter 6 offers examples). When educational and skill-based proficiency domains are assessed, the criteria set are also called **performance standards**. Depending on the situation, the criterion may reflect a **minimum competency standard** or a **standard of excellence**.

In notable contrast to cut scores employed on NRT scales, the standard here is set in advance, *regardless* of the distribution of test scores. The primary referents for score interpretation purposes are the performance standard, or a series of standards, along with the specified domain.

Importantly, a *dual* frame of reference is necessary for interpreting scores meaningfully in the criterion-referenced approach—both the domain and the cut scores are important. Unless the specified domain of indicators is simultaneously considered, the categorical placements shed only partial light on the caliber of a performance or an underlying condition. For example, a severity rating of 5 denoting an "unhealthy" status yields limited information, unless we also consider the domain of symptomatic indicators for a health-related disorder. To interpret the category score comprehensively, we must refer it directly back to the domain of behaviors, symptoms, or indicators that operationally define the construct.

The term **domain-referenced assessment** is historically connected to CRT design in education (AERA et al., 2014; Berk, 1984b; Crocker & Algina, 2006; Glaser, 1994). For example, the depth and breadth of demonstrated mastery in different areas of a curricular domain in education are only partly revealed by a Pass score. The profile of content and cognitive behaviors in indicators, and the category score, together help in making sound criterion-refenced interpretations of the performance level.

9.4.2 Common Uses of Criterion-Referenced Tests

The most typical CRT applications include:

- Formative decision making in classroom teaching and training contexts
- Summative exit testing of students at different levels of education

- Minimum competency assessments at all levels of education
- Certification testing of professionals in different fields
- Diagnostic testing for identifying given health conditions, disorders, or diseases
- Classifying individuals by levels of need in special education or therapeutic contexts for providing differentiated or individualized supports

For a concrete example of the last, see the Gross Motor Function Classification System (GMFCS) shown in Table 9.4. The GMFCS is a criterion-referenced assessment system used in the movement sciences and occupational therapy settings. It is used to classify children affected with cerebral palsy who have compromised levels of physical mobility. (Harvey, Rosenbaum, Graham, & Palisano, 2009). As the descriptors in Table 9.2 illustrate, domain-referenced indicators operationalize each level of physical mobility, complemented with indicators in manual ability and communication skills. Together, these aid professionals in differentiating patients at Levels I–V, requiring variable types and degrees of therapeutic support. The system recognizes five criterion levels of mobility in children based on their physical capacities, ranging from individuals who are immobile and wheelchair-bound (the lowest, Level V), to those who can walk without limitations (the highest, Level I).

Domain-referenced CRTs are particularly useful for various formative instructional uses in classroom learning environments, and for providing coaching and feedback in professional development, sports training, and other adult training contexts. State certification examinations for professionals before they enter the workplace frequently rely on CRTs as well (e.g., certification of teachers or physicians in different specialties in medicine). The performance standards for summative uses could be set by other educators, health care professionals, therapists, internal or external professional agencies.

9.4.3 Design Requirements for Criterion-Referenced Score Interpretations

Unlike NRTs that measure broad, general domains, well-performing CRTs require more detailed domain breakdowns and design specifications. To maximize

TABLE 9.4. Criterion-Referenced Category Scores with a Behavior-Based Assessment

Score level	Classification systems		
	GMFCS	MACS	CFCS
I	Walks without limitations.	Handles objects easily and successfully.	Sends and receives information with familiar and unfamiliar partners effectively and efficiently.
II	Walks with limitations.	Handles most objects but with somewhat reduced quality and/or speed of achievement.	Sends and receives information with familiar and unfamiliar partners but may need extra time.
III	Walks using a hand-held mobility device.	Handles objects with difficulty; needs help to prepare.	Sends and receives information with familiar partners effectively, but not with unfamiliar partners.
IV	Self-mobility with limitations; may use powered mobility.	Handles a limited selection of easily managed objects in adapted situations.	Inconsistently sends and/or receives information even with familiar partners.
V	Transported in a manual wheelchair.	Does not handle objects and has severely limited ability to perform even simple actions.	Seldom effectively sends and receives information even with familiar partners.

Note. GMFCS, Gross Motor Function Classification System; MACS, Manual Ability Classification System; CFCS, Communication Function Classification System. Reprinted with permission from Hidecker et al. (2011). © John Wiley & Sons.

sound criterion-referenced score interpretations, *five* technical qualities should be prioritized during test design: (1) well-specified domains, subdomains, and indicators; (2) domain-referenced item or task sampling; (3) high reliability of all relevant domain, subdomain, and test component scores; (4) defensible cut scores and performance standards; and (5) reliability at cut points set for decision making. Each is explained next.

1. **Well-specified and detailed domains:** Detailed domain, subdomain, and indicator specifications allow for modular, domain-referenced assessment design procedures that, in turn, facilitate more fine-grained interpretations and uses of the CRT results. The domains and subdomains must be adequately broken down. When defined with clear indicators that link directly with the items and tasks, the resulting score categories and score profiles can be better aligned, thus enabling more valid interpretations and uses of results.

2. **Domain-referenced item sampling:** Tied to the first requirement, careful sampling of items by domain, subdomains, and indicators allows for better domain coverage and standard setting (next). To facilitate "content-valid" inferences, the items and tasks must show adequate levels of content relevance and content representativeness vis-à-vis the domain.

3. **High reliability of scores by domain, subdomain, or modular test components:** CRTs should yield highly reliable scores by domain, subdomain, or subcomponents of the test that users desire to interpret and use. To obtain the requisite reliability levels, larger numbers of items/tasks for each modular component of a CRT may be necessary. This property is unlike that of NRTs, where reliability is necessary mainly for the total scores from which the norm-referenced scores and scales are derived.

4. **Defensible cut scores and performance standards:** The criteria and standards set for CRT categorizations should not be arbitrary, but domain-referenced and suited to the populations. For high-stakes, summative decisions, these cut scores should be informed by judgments of carefully selected experts who are knowledgeable about the construct domains *and* the population to be tested.

5. **Reliability of decisions at cut points:** The cutoff points used for classification of examinees or respondents into categories must be reliable (see Figure 9.7). Candidate classifications should be replicable, assuring high levels of decision consistency. For high-stakes uses, the margins of error around cut points should be tolerable for the CRT users. This requirement applies for users of NRT scales where cut scores may be employed.

9.4.4 Standard-Setting Procedures for CRTs

There are a number of established procedures to arrive at accurate, fair, and defensible cut scores on measured scale continua for differentiating levels of a condition or performance. Most standard-setting procedures were developed in the 1970s–1990s, an era marked by widespread use of large-scale competency tests in the United States (Cizek, 2013; Hambleton & Pitoniak, 2006). These methods offer useful and adaptable ideas for both research- and practice-based CRT applications today.

Methods of standard setting with CRTs are largely *judgment-based*, and some involve lengthy procedures. A main purpose is to arrive at rational procedures to differentiate between two or more states or performance levels. In contrast to cut scores in NRTs, the standard-setting process is carried out in a *norm-free* mode; no standardization samples are necessary, nor any *z*-score distributions. However, validation of the judgment-based criteria is necessary with empirical data from examinees, especially when the testing stakes are high. This chapter recommends the use of a combination of expert judgments and reviews of empirical evidence from the populations tested.

How we define and select an "expert" judge is key to implementing standard-setting methods effectively. In the Common Core educational reform context, the SBAC initially selected judges with curricular and teaching expertise in the domains of interest and grade levels to be tested. To secure broad stakeholder buy-in in a politically charged reform setting, they also sought online feedback later from various other constituents, including teachers at large, parents, members of the larger community, and the state legislature (CRESST, 2017). For admitting students into a competitive high school fine arts program, for instance, we might select a panel of qualified art teachers with the most teaching experience with students at that level.

A summary of the main steps in standard-setting procedures follows:

- **Step 1:** Convene, orient, or train a panel of carefully selected experts on the process.
- **Step 2:** Review the content and domain specifications of an assessment, along with the tasks and items, with panelists. It helps to train the panel on how to match items or tasks to domains, domain indicators, and item-scoring methods.
- **Step 3:** Educate the panel on the number of score categories and decision-maker needs. Present details of existing research, decision-making examples, and policy contexts where CRT results will be used.
- **Step 4:** Familiarize panelists with a range of actual responses to items/assessment and other data from the population to be tested.
- **Step 5:** Apply a selected standard-setting procedure with the panel to arrive at different levels of performance or cutoff points in scaled responses.
- **Step 6:** Draft descriptive labels or statements to represent each level or category of response, based on a review of the response data, such as highly proficient, proficient, and not proficient. (Refer back to the section on scoring rubrics in Chapter 6.)
- **Step 7:** Develop a final consensus, with or without use of data and computational summaries, to complete the standard-setting procedure. Arrive at the final categories defining the score levels and descriptors.

The better techniques tend to combine the expertise of panelists along with empirical data from populations of focus. Combining methods is sometimes referred to as "compromise" methods (Hambleton & Pitoniak, 2006). This usage, however, does not imply that quality considerations should be compromised in any way.

Different standard-setting methods are distinguished based on the types of assessment artifacts and empirical data that judges review, such as (Hambleton & Pitoniak, 2006):

- The overall item pool in a domain
- Content of individual items, tasks, or item clusters by domain
- Empirical data on item or score distributions from examinees
- Hybrid approaches that combine one or more of the above

Note that the term *standard* in a CRT design context is different from a *content standard* in curriculum design (connoting a broadly stated, expected learning outcome, like the Common Core State Standards in mathematics; see Chapter 2). To enable prospective users to use CRT results appropriately, evidence of validity, reliability, and utility of the performance standards must be documented (AERA et al., 2014). Each is now discussed.

9.4.4.1 Standards or Criteria Based on the Overall Item Pool

In the first method for standard setting, we ask expert judges to carefully review the overall domain, the content of all the assessment items or tasks in the pool, and have them answer questions (see below) on cutoff points that would represent either minimum or excellent levels of performance or a state/condition in the population. This procedure was devised originally for structured-response tests but can be adapted to other assessment modalities, as shown.

To set a minimum competency standard on a multiple-choice test, a question might be.

> What percent of the items would be answered correctly by examinees who are *minimally competent* or borderline in terms of skill mastery in this domain?

If multilevel cut points are required, a series of such questions may be presented.

> What percent of the items tapping this domain would be answered correctly by examinees who are:
> - *Highly competent*?
> - *Competent*?

- *Minimally competent*?
- *Not competent at all*?

For a behavior-based assessment like the GMFCS (Table 9.4), the questions are modified as follows:

> Taking into consideration the population and domain of motor functioning skills, what level would denote the *lowest level of functionality*? What would be the defining behaviors at that level? What behaviors would define the *next higher functionality level* in the same group? What would be the defining behaviors at the *next* level?

The responses from experts would then be averaged to obtain the final cut points for score levels.

9.4.4.2 Standards Based on Individual Items, Tasks, or Classes of Items

THE ANGOFF AND MODIFIED ANGOFF PROCEDURES

In Angoff's (1971) procedure for multiple-choice tests, judges conducted an item review before answering questions like this:

> What is the probability that an examinee with *minimum competence* in the domain will answer this item correctly?

The sum of the projected probabilities (expected percent of examinees who will answer correctly) for all items on a test yields a minimum passing score from a given judge. The range of passing scores obtained from the judging panel is considered, and judges are asked to arrive at a consensus on the final passing score.

For performance assessments with scoring rubrics and rating scales, the original Angoff procedure has been altered. In a modified Angoff procedure, the judges are typically given at least two opportunities to project probabilities for the minimum "passing" rating on tasks. Ratings are collected in each round as a part of the deliberation process. After the first round of judgments is completed, judges may review data on the actual proportions of typical examinees found to perform at particular levels. The passing score is derived by averaging the responses across all judges, rather than by consensus. In practice, the second round of ratings is given more importance because by then the judges' ratings show less variability in their opinions.

THE EBEL AND MODIFIED EBEL PROCEDURE

In a similar procedure, Ebel and Frisbie (1972) used a table to classify items by their degree of difficulty (from easy to difficult) and their level of relevance (from essential to questionable) to set a minimum passing score. Each cell in the table was weighted by the number of items it held. As before, the judges were asked: What percent of the items *in each cell* would an examinee with minimum competence in the domain answer correctly? In contrast to the Angoff procedure, the minimum passing score is identified by summing probabilities (projected percentages) of items in the cells. For each cell in the table, agreement is reached by consensus among the judges. Then, the sum of the percentages across all cells yields the minimum passing score for the test.

Ebel's "relevance" dimension was criticized on the grounds that tests should not be designed to include items that are of questionable relevance. Others pointed out that judges (who are usually practitioners) might have difficulty separating the relevance dimension from the difficulty dimension, because the two dimensions tend to be correlated.

See Table 9.5 for an adaptation of the Ebel method to address the above concerns. This approach uses a table of test specifications that we would produce during Phase II when applying the Process Model (Figure 9.1). Utilizing information we routinely enter into the columns, rows, and cells of a table of test specifications—namely, the number of items by the *taxonomic levels* and *content areas/topics* to be tested—we would apply Ebel's questions for each cell. In Table 9.5, the taxonomic level crossed by main topics replaces Ebel's difficulty and relevance dimensions, respectively (after Chatterji, 2003; Chapters 4 and 5).

Once the items are organized and tabulated, experts are asked to identify the probability (%) that a minimally qualified examinee would answer the items in each cell correctly. For each cell, we would obtain a consensus-based *or* average percentage, projected by all judges. The sum of these projected percentages

TABLE 9.5. Setting Standards: A Minimum Passing Score for a 24-Item Multiple-Choice Test

Domain	Cognitive levels			Marginal total
	Factual knowledge	Application	Higher-order thinking	
Competencies				
State definitions	**10 *(80%)			10
Use formulas		**8 *(60%)		8
Evaluate conclusions			**6 *(30%)	6
Marginal total	10	8	6	24

Weight for each item = 1

Minimum passing score on test = 10 (.80) + 8 (.60) + 6 (.30) = 8 + 4.8 + 1.8 = 14.6 out of 24

Minimum percent score = 61%

**No. of items allocated to each cell of table of specifications.

*Percent of items that should be answered correctly by minimally competent examinees, as determined by consensus among expert teachers.

would yield the minimum passing score, as shown in the table note. The illustration assumes that all items have an equal weighting of 1 point. The two-step formula for setting a standard is:

1. *Minimum passing score* (Min X) =

   (Projected % items to be correctly answered per cell × no. of items per cell)

2. *Minimum percent correct score* (Min %) =

   Min X ÷ Total no. of items on test

In the event that items in some cells were weighted more than 1 point, we would multiply the weighting factor (e.g., × 2, × 3, as applicable) to the number of items in the cell to arrive at the weighted passing score. The performance standard can be refined by allowing participating judges to also look at data on percentages of examinees who are actually able to answer the items correctly by cell.

HOLISTIC STANDARD SETTING FOR PERFORMANCE ASSESSMENTS

A lot of the work on setting standards occurred with writing assessments that translate easily to other performance assessment modes. In this method, judges are provided with sample tasks, the rating scale (rubric), and samples of examinee performances to review. The samples could be a range of typical answers or recorded behaviors on video or audiotape. Once the judges are thoroughly familiar with the assessment tasks and the rubric, they identify "benchmark" papers or performances at particular rating levels. This decision may be arrived at through iterative discussions and consensus seeking (Chapter 4 discussed some group consensus methods). Multiple cutoff points may be set at progressively higher levels on a rating scale.

9.4.4.3 Standards Based on Empirical Score Distributions

Comparing the subjectively proposed cut scores from judges against real data distributions helps in validating the initial judgments, as well as refining or adjusting the cutoffs. To employ these methods effectively, the composition of the group used for standard setting should mimic the intended CRT populations on relevant socioecological and background factors.

CONTRASTING GROUPS METHOD FOR SETTING STANDARDS

See Figures 9.8 and 9.9. In this procedure, data distributions obtained from two distinct groups help derive an appropriate cut score, such as instructed (IG) versus uninstructed groups (UG) in educational settings. Others may be diagnosed versus undiagnosed persons, experts versus novices in a field, and so on. To begin, two groups that are known to be different with respect to the measured construct domain(s) are selected and administered the CRT under similar conditions. Test scores are plotted in frequency polygons, and the score at the *intersection point* is selected as the cut score. See the point at which the two distributions overlap in Figure 9.8.

Alternatively, we could also compare ogives (cumulative percentage graphs) for two distinct tested groups for standard-setting purposes. In Figure 9.9, a score interval of 150 (149.5–150.5), lying between the medians of the two distributions of 130 and 170, may be selected as a cutoff. Again, informed judges should review the data distributions to make a final decision on an appropriate cut score. The assumptions about one group being clearly more knowledgeable or having higher levels of a pathological condition must be borne out with data. Cut score(s) may be difficult to ascertain when the distributions overlap too much and are not clearly separated on the measure.

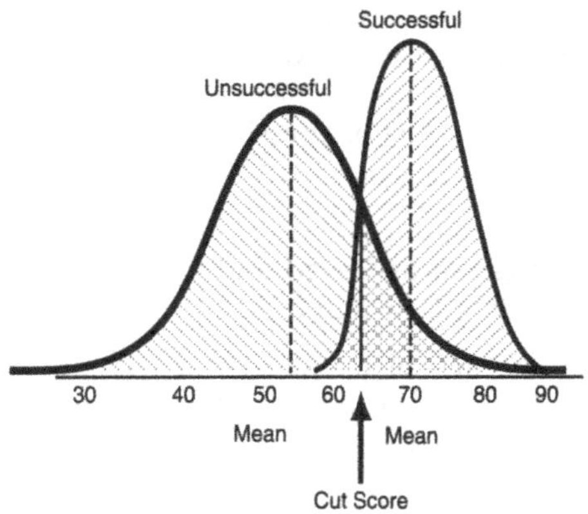

FIGURE 9.8. Contrasting groups method for setting standards.

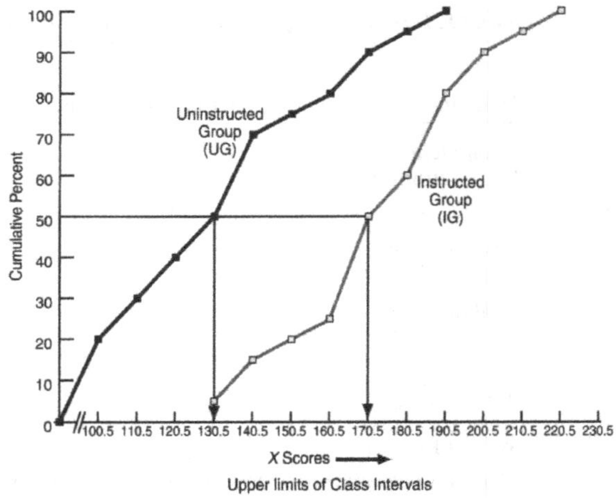

FIGURE 9.9. Using ogives of contrasting groups for setting standards.

BOOKMARKING METHOD

The bookmarking method is based on IRT scaling models and routinely applied by standardized test-makers of achievement tests. Judges are involved, as before, to make the final decisions on the performance standards (see Figure 9.10).

This method requires administration of the assessment to a typical group of test-takers as a prerequisite. Using the item response data from the testing, the items are ordered by their estimated difficulty levels on an *item map* using logit (log odds) units along the common linear scale. The item map separates the easier items from the more difficult (see the mostly recall-level items at the bottom with the higher-order thinking items at the top). The distribution of individuals on the scale is shown to the left. On such a map, judges would place a "bookmark" showing items that minimally competent examinees should be able to answer correctly. In Figure 9.10, the items ordered by difficulty are shown using taxonomic labels as added descriptors. One concept recall item (Item 7) is located above the bookmark, as it is estimated to be at a higher difficulty level than expected in logit units (after Wyer & Chatterji, 2013).

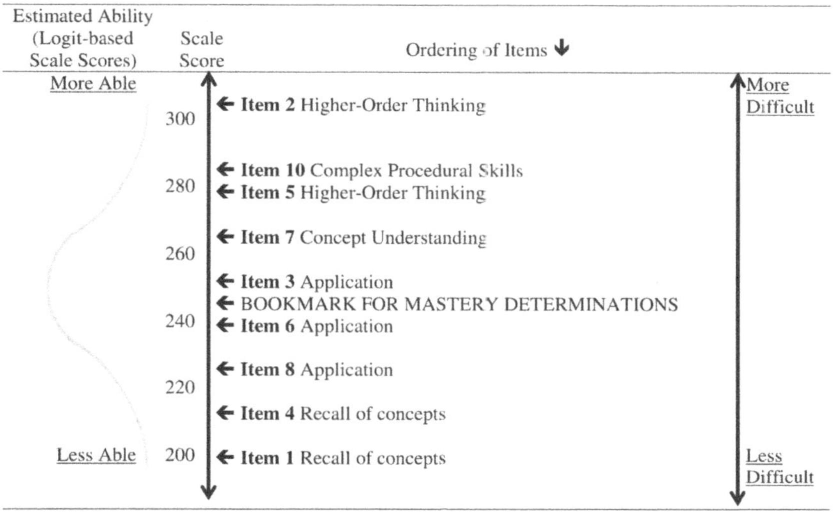

FIGURE 9.10. The bookmarking method for setting standards: An illustration.

HYBRID METHODS

Some standard-setting techniques are "hybrids" of one or more approaches described. These have proven useful in various large-scale assessment programs over time. In these, judgments of panelists may come into play at the start, during the interim review processes, or toward the end of the procedure. Two methods are the dominant profile method and the judgment policy capturing method (see AERA et al., 2014; Hambleton & Pitoniak, 2006).

QUICK RECAP: CRTs intended for enhancing criterion- and domain-referenced interpretations of the results have five main design requirements. There are several alternative procedures for standard setting. Of these, methods that combine the use of expert judgments and reviews of empirical test data distributions offer several advantages over either one used alone. We should examine the validity, reliability, and utility of standards set to ensure that the cut scores are reasonable for the contexts of assessment use.

Reflection Break 9.2: Objective 2

- Identify the *benefits* of following a domain-referenced CRT design approach for a specified use and user context in (1) the workplace, (2) education, (3) health, or (4) another field. Describe the context. What could be some *limitations* of using CRTs?
- Provide examples of assessments in your field that meet the design criteria given for a well-performing CRT.
- Would you recommend that a CRT *or* NRT design approach to test for licensing automobile drivers in a region? Assume that the driver population consists of adults of age 18+? Justify your answer.
- Compare the different methods of standard setting by listing one advantage and one disadvantage of each. Which would you recommend for certifying professionals in your own field? Explain why.

9.5 Using Self as the Frame of Reference

9.5.1 Ipsative Assessments of Change

The third frame of reference for deriving scores is presented in the bottom panel of Table 9.1. Here, measures taken at one point in time for a person are compared against the same individual's earlier measures, usually on the same construct measure. The ipsative assessment approach is motivated by a need to make a growth-based interpretation, or track a person's or entity's change, on a measured domain. As such, conceptually, the assessment's scale should enable the derivation of *growth scores* or *gain scores*. The term ipsative originates from the Latin term *ipse*, meaning "of the self" (*www.dictionary.reference.com*).

In K–12 education, ipsative assessment is valued especially when assessing growth in children with learning difficulties or other forms of disabilities. Whereas students may experience peer pressure from the competitive elements of the NRT approach or feel discouraged by failing to meet the performance expectations in the CRT approach, the ipsative approach tends to foster a continuous improvement and "growth mindset" that is intrinsically more motivating. Ipsative measurement could also be applied to monitor an organizational entity's change over time with aggregated data collected at two or more time points on valued constructs; this approach in common for studying change in organizations undergoing reforms. However, it is fraught with several technical challenges (see the next subsection).

As an aside, readers should note that the word "ipsative" has a different meaning in psychology. This section will not discuss psychological ipsative applications, but a brief description follows. Psychologists distinguish among two types of assessments for measuring personality and attitudinal constructs in the workplace: *ipsative* and *normative*. Normative assessment is essentially the NRT approach described in Section 9.3. Ipsative measurement in psychology employs *forced-choice items*. The two contrasting item formats on a personality assessment for managers in a workplace, shown next, illustrates ipsative measurement with forced-choice items.

Normative assessment with a Likert-type item

> *I rely on my own judgments to make decisions at work. (Response options:* Strongly agree, Agree, Uncertain, Disagree, Strongly disagree)

Ipsative assessment with a forced-choice item pair

- *When I make decisions at work, I rely on my own judgment.*
- *When I make decisions at work, I collaborate with others.*

Instead of indicating a level of agreement with a series of attitudinal statements (which can be falsified), in a forced-choice format, respondents must select which item of the two *equally desirable* options applies to them most. In the item examples above, both independent and collaborative decision making are equally desirable behaviors in managerial decision making. This method was designed to control for socially desirable or faked responses.

9.5.2 Derived Scores in Ipsative Assessments of Change

A common "ipsative score" for self-referenced change measurement is a **difference score**, also called a **gain score**. This method of measuring change involves just two measurements of a given individual or group of individuals. One assessment administration may occur before an instructional or treatment intervention (prescores), with the second performed afterward (postscores). The gain could be expressed in either raw score or *z*-score units for individuals. For groups, the difference in standard deviation units is shown next:

$$\text{Gain in raw score units}_{\text{(Individual)}} = (\text{Postscores}_{\text{(Individual)}} - \text{Prescores}_{\text{(Individual)}})$$

$$\text{Gain score in standard deviation units}_{\text{(Group)}} = (\text{Mean postscores}_{\text{(Group)}} - \text{Mean prescores}_{\text{(Group)}}) / \text{Standard deviation prescores}_{\text{(Group)}}$$

An alternative to gain scores is to interpret the growth trajectories of individuals or groups using advanced statistical approaches called **growth curve models**, elsewhere referred to as value-added models (VAMs) (Raudenbush & Jean, 2012). The statistics of VAMs are beyond the scope of this book, but some of the ideas may be useful descriptively. For example, we could plot growth graphically in line graphs for individuals in small groups, displaying progress over time with descriptive statistics like the mean and standard deviation.

See Figure 9.11A and B next. It is possible to plot growth of individuals in a line graph where the y-axis (vertical axis) is used for the test scores and the x-axis (horizontal axis) for the time points or occasions of measurement, as shown. When a number of individual growth trajectories are plotted, we may find that there is variability in the slope of each line, points at which the lines start, as well as the spread of score points in the group on each measurement occasion. This spread at a given time point is measurable with a standard deviation, shown for five individuals. To study the changes in a group over time, the points of origin of the lines, the average scores at time points, and the spread at each time point of measurement could be computed and interpreted together. For example, a person starting higher may show less gain overall with a flatter slope than a person starting at a lower point.

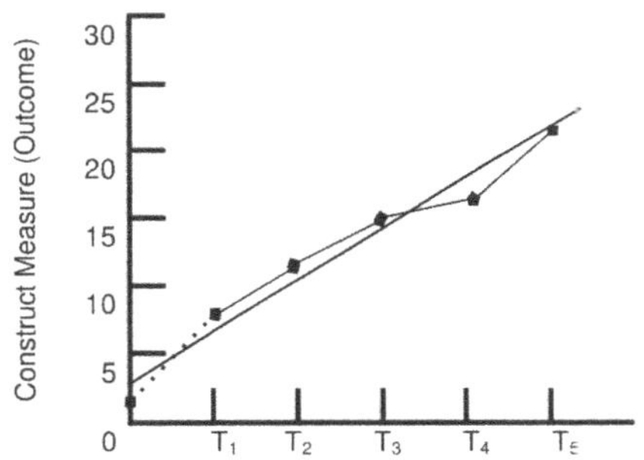

$T_1 - T_5$: Time points

A. Change in one individual over 5 time points with the "Line of Best Fit" overlapping actual measurements

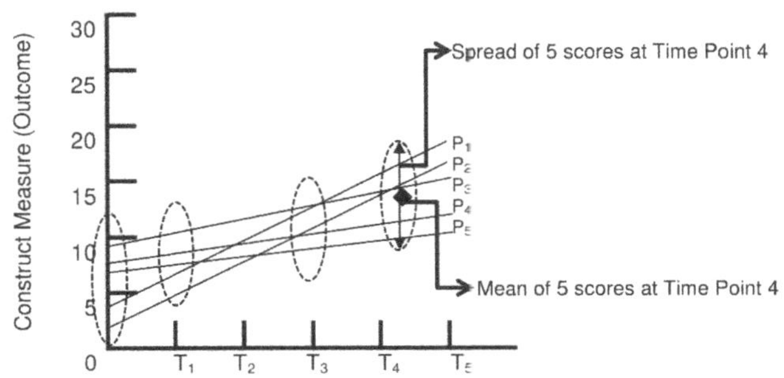

B. Linear Trends in 5 Individuals, P_1-P_5

FIGURE 9.11. Mapping growth trajectories for an individual (A) and small group (B) with ipsative assessment.

9.5.3 Uses of Ipsative Assessments

Self as a referent is common in many measurements we take in everyday life, such as when monitoring changes in body weight over time. The approach is easily applied with physical measures of height and weight, and is used widely in sports, physical education, and computer games as well.

Ipsative assessment has gained advocates in higher education recently as well, with some who promote it over traditional assessments with NRTs (and even CRTs) as it enables individualized monitoring of progress with feedback (Martinez-Arboleda, 2021). As indicated, the approach has been practiced in special education and clinical contexts, especially with individuals with exceptional needs or disabilities (Hughes, 2017; Penn & Wells, 2018). With grouped student test scores at the classroom, school, or school system level, ipsative approaches have also been used for tracking school improvement trends (New Hampshire Department of Education, 2018). But the latter application relies on vertical scaling methods with NRTs that have their own technical limitations (AERA, 2015).

9.5.4 Design Requirements for Ipsative Assessment

To register measured changes with validity, reliability, and utility, the assessment instrument must have certain properties. Constructs like height and weight that are measurable on linear scales (ratio scales, typically) are well suited for making self-referenced interpretations of growth. Other constructs need to be conceptualized and scaled in developmental terms. This could be challenging.

With behavioral constructs (Table 9.4), once the domains are defined in concrete observable terms, we would need to map an evidence-based developmental trajectory on the indicators that is typical for the population of focus. Given this, we could depict individual changes descriptively on the indicators over multiple time points with well-designed, domain-referenced rubrics. Checklists and line graphs can prove useful in such applications, as suggested (Figure 9.11A,B).

Pre- to posttreatment *gain scores* are also useful when valid and reliable outcome measures are available on a developmental scale. The AE or GE scales may be useful for this purpose, with their built-in limitations borne in mind. Time-series analysis is another way to visually depict growth on developmentally scaled construct measures. To complement the quantitative descriptions of change, qualitative and anecdotal note taking can be helpful for special needs or disabled populations.

NRTs that are built with cross-sectional norming samples for a given age or grade level are *not* appropriate for ipsative interpretations. By design, NRTs are fundamentally incompatible with the growth-based premises of ipsative assessment. Although IRT-based and other methods have been developed to vertically "link" achievement construct measures from NRTs across grade levels, these "growth" scaling techniques have several limitations (Section 9.7; AERA, 2015; Dorans, Pommerich, & Holland, 2007; Student, 2022). Many "grouped" achievement indexes, like the Student Growth Percentile, are used for monitoring school improvement with NRT data tracked over a given number of years. These applications are similarly controversial (Sireci, Wells, & Keller, 2016). Vertical scales are discussed in Section 9.7.

In sum, the main challenge of ipsative assessments has to do with designing a single scale continuum that can longitudinally map the *same* construct as it evolves developmentally in given persons or groups. From a validation standpoint, the challenge lies in establishing **construct invariance**—that is, holding the construct definition and score meanings constant, even as individuals or groups change on the construct.

At least *five* technical issues should be borne in mind. These are some questions we should ask:

1. **Properties of the "growth" scale, validity, reliability, and utility issues:** To what extent does the score scale yield valid information on an individual's or a group's change over time on the construct? To what extent is this growth depicted reliably? Is the growth-based information transparent and easy-to-understand for the test-takers and other assessment users?
2. **Floor and ceiling effects:** Might the maximum and minimum scores possible on a test, as established by test-makers (called the *floor* and *ceiling* of a test), artificially limit the measurement and

tracking of true change on the construct domain? How can we remove the effects of "regression toward the mean" in individuals who have extreme scores on the test score metric on the first measurement?

3. **Numbers of, and time points for, measurements:** How many measurements will best depict growth—2, 3, 5 or more? What are the best time points for taking those measurements?
4. **Confounders:** How can we remove the effects of outside confounders that may detract from obtaining valid measurements of true change on the constructs of interest, such as practice effects due to exposure to the same test items in the first and second measurements?
5. **Individual differences:** For evaluating change in groups, how can we take into account interindividual and intraindividual differences in growth patterns on the construct measure of interest?

The psychometric issue of regression toward the mean is related to floor and ceiling effects on a test when used to study change in a group over two time points. The problem occurs with individuals who obtain *extreme scores* in the pretesting phase. When we measure the same individuals twice on the same testing instrument, those who get the highest and lowest scores in the first testing will tend to obtain scores toward the middle of the distribution the second time. That is, the highest performers will always *drop* or regress toward the mean, and appear to lose ground due to the ceiling on the test's metric (the maximum score possible is fixed). The lowest performers who were located at the floor of the test on the first measurement, in contrast, will appear to *gain* by regressing upward toward the mean on the second measurement. This is a predictable result due to the combination of a floor and ceiling effect and unreliable scores. The problem can be partially mitigated by taking multiple measurements instead of two.

The matter of unreliable scores at each time point remains an issue. All tools yield measures that are unreliable to some degree; hence, they will also yield unreliable *gain scores*. Random errors of measurement attenuate the true levels of change; these issues must be taken into account during interpretation of ipsative measures.

For all these reasons, change measurement has long had its critics. Despite attempts, ipsative methods are not easily applied with ambiguous and hard-to-measure constructs (McDermott, Fantuzzo, Glutting, Watkins, & Baggaley, 1992). Several measurement, statistical, and research design issues need to be addressed beforehand, and limitations understood.

QUICK RECAP: Self-referenced interpretation of growth on given constructs is an appealing but technically complex concept. A prerequisite is a developmentally scaled construct measure with adequate validity, reliability, and utility levels for the desired ipsative interpretations and uses that users desire. Yet, ipsative methods are often necessary in clinical, rehabilitation, and special education contexts. Change monitoring with descriptive statistics, visual line graphs, domain-referenced rubrics, and anecdotal records can be useful for these purposes. Gain scores and time-series analyses on constructs scaled on interval or ratio scales could facilitate ipsative inferences.

Reflection Break 9.3: Objective 3

- Provide an example of ipsative measurement application in a field of your choice. What is the construct? What is the instrument? What type of ipsative "derived score" or scaling method is used for tracking? Who is tracked (individuals or groups)?
- See the preceding question. Which design requirements would you consider to be uppermost in designing the tool? How would you address the issue of *floor* and *ceiling* on the scale?
- Which of these NRT score scales would be better for ipsative measurements? (1) *T*-scores *or* (2) grade-equivalent scores? Justify your answer.
- See the GMFCS system in Table 9.4. Describe *two* added design procedures you would implement to enhance the ipsative interpretations of children's changes over multiple years. Justify your answer.

9.6 Composite Scores

9.6.1 Types of Composite Scores

Many assessment applications require that we derive a **composite score** with data from one or more assessments to serve a specific user need. A composite in measurement and testing refers to a single score that combines the scores of two or more different subtests of a given assessment instrument. In the simplest case, we would simply add the scores from the subtests to build a composite score for the total test—the UNIT-2 *total raw score* is an example of a composite built by adding the raw scores of three subtests.

In other examples, grade point averages and individual grades in school marking systems (GPA based on A–F grades) are also composite scores. GPAs are derived from students' assessment results on a number of tests and school assignments gathered over a period of time. Elsewhere, the data from different instruments, added data sources, and indicators may be statistically combined to generate a multi-indicator composite for serving a particular purpose. Weights are sometimes applied so that some data sources count for more than others in a "weighted composite."

Once a composite is created, it has a "character" and distribution properties of its own. Review this quote from Mark Twain in the Preface to *The Adventures of Tom Sawyer and Huckleberry Finn* (1876/1996): "Tom Sawyer . . . is a combination of the characteristics of three boys whom I knew, and therefore belongs to the composite order of architecture. . . ." Just as with Mark Twain's character composition of Tom Sawyer, the original information is not recognizable in the composite score. For high-stakes uses, composite scores should be transparent, fair, and supported with the requisite evidence of validity, reliability, and utility. In ideal scenarios, the properties of composites are examined and validated so that they can be interpreted and used appropriately.

Let us consider next two examples of composite scores with two units of analysis, organization versus the individual. To illustrate particular procedures, we will revisit the second example again.

9.6.1.1 A Diversity and Inclusion Index for Ranking Corporate Organizations

The Thomson Reuters' Diversity and Inclusion (D&I) Index is a composite measure that applies to organizations as the population units. It was developed to rank-order global corporations and companies on their D&I commitments and activities, for the purposes of informing investors and clients on their quality. The D&I Index incorporates multiple metrics, categorized under four "pillars," the broad domains: workforce diversity, inclusion, people development, and news controversy. Companies are assigned an overall score obtained as the average of the four pillar scores. A recent news release announced the top 100 most diverse and inclusive organizations on the D&I Index, indicating that the index ratings are informed by Thomson Reuters environmental, social, and governance data, designed to "transparently and objectively measure the relative performance of more than 7,000 companies and provide clients with differentiated insight" (Thomson Reuters, 2018, see *https://thomsonreutors.com*). Individual *organizations* serve as the units for interpreting the D&I Index, which may then be used for further research or decision-making purposes.

9.6.1.2 GPAs and School Marks for Individual Students

The GPA and marks (mentioned before) awarded at school are also composite scores. These apply to individual *students* as the population units, in contrast to the D&I Index. Depending on the subject areas and level of the students, instructors could use a variety of tests and data sources for allocating marks. In practice, we see a wide range, from weekly quizzes, midterm tests, final examinations, products and performances, to records of student attendance, classroom participation, effort, and conduct. These choices and their weighting impact validity, connoting what the composite score eventually represents, and inferences that are reasonable.

9.6.2 Four Issues to Resolve: Constructing Composite Scores

In given contexts of use, four design-related questions need to be addressed before we can build the composite score. These decisions should be guided by primary users' and stakeholder values, as well as technical criteria.

- **Issue 1: What constructs and indicators should define the composite?** Ideally, a composite should be meaningful to its primary users and based on a well-rationalized and coherent set of assessments, data sources, and indicators. Amalgamating very disparate data sources into a single composite must be justified and communicated clearly to the primary users of the information.

With GPAs and marking systems, for instance, the academic (cognitive) and nonacademic (noncognitive) areas to be graded must be clearly identified and communicated to the primary users and stakeholders, in this case, students, parents, school administrators, and teachers themselves. Behavioral areas, like attendance and effort, should be graded separately from the marks for academic subjects like science, math, and reading. This is necessary to uphold the meaningfulness (validity), clarity, and transparency (utility) of the grades. It is always better to assign and communicate the separate grades for broad construct-relevant areas before combining the results in the form of a GPA. A single composite GPA would mask details and may miscommunicate the level of performance to students and other users in individual areas.

• **Issue 2: What is the population unit for inference making?** The population unit is the "unit of analysis" to whom the composite scores will apply. Clarity on the population units helps us maintain the integrity of the conceptualization, computation procedures, and interpretation of the composite.

For instance, individual students are the primary units for composites used to assign A–F marks and GPAs. In contrast, the organization is the unit of analysis for the D&I Index, which is developed, interpreted, and used to compare several thousand organizations globally. Although the data on the four pillars of the D&I may be collected from employees, departments, or divisions, the composite score is derived at the highest level of an organizational entity, which is then used for the rankings and communication with shareholders and clients. It is at that upper level that the D&I Index must demonstrate the highest levels of validity, reliability, and utility.

• **Issue 3: Which instruments will be used for each construct or indicator that feeds into the composite? How many assessments in all should contribute to the composite, and are they individually of good quality?** The number of different data-gathering tools and assessment methods that we use to build a composite must be selected judicially. Individually, they should yield high-quality data on their own before inclusion in a composite.

For instance: Should the A–F marks be based on results of end-of-term assessments only, or should they utilize the results of added assessments, homework, and classwork exercises as well? How many formal tests should be included that are designed to have the highest levels of content-based validity? Likewise: Should the D&I Index be based on employee surveys or other "hard data" indicators, too, such as statistics on ethnic minority representation in organizations? These types of questions must be resolved beforehand.

• **Issue 4: How should the different assessments be "weighted" in the composite?** The number and kinds of data sources on which to base a composite score, along with the importance allocated (in terms of weights) to the different elements, are value-based judgments of designers and stakeholders. This decision cannot be a purely technical or statistical one. The weighting plan and mathematical procedures used to create the composite scores should also be transparent to all stakeholders and users, especially when high-stakes actions are taken with the results, such as global visibility of the D&I score of a corporation.

Marking system configurations, as we know, can vary greatly from teacher to teacher. Some teachers might decide to have scores from three unit tests and one paper, all weighted equally in a mark. Others might choose to have a portfolio-based assessment carrying 33% weight, with midterm and end-of-term test scores carrying the remaining 67% of the grade. Stakeholders must accept the weights in the marking systems to be reasonable and fair.

• **Issue 5: Will the composite scores be used for making norm-referenced or criterion-referenced interpretations and uses?** The computation procedures differ for composites intended to serve norm-referencing versus criterion-referencing purposes. This decision should, again, be guided by stakeholder values and the users' information needs. When stakeholders wish to select the best performers in a large group, the choice of a comparative ranking system is indicated. The composite should be criterion-referenced when the reverse is true; for example, when users place more value on how well the entity performed on the domains of interest in an absolute sense.

Currently, the Thomson Reuters D&I Index is a norm-referenced, ranking system for organizations. There are large numbers of entities in the pool, and the aim is to highlight the topmost exemplars. If the stakeholders choose to alter course by setting an expectation that *all* organizations should aim to meet a certain D&I performance profile on the four pillars, a criterion-referenced system might be preferred.

9.6.3 Alternate Methods for Deriving Composites

Once the five issues are resolved, a composite can be derived and applied. Two approaches are demonstrated next for deriving composites with a norm-referenced and a criterion-referenced method, respectively. Although the example is of a composite for report card marks, the computational steps in the illustrations are generalizable to other applications like the D&I Index.

9.6.3.1 Deriving a Composite Using *T*-Scores

Let us say that on Issues 1–5 above, we have a classroom scenario defined by the following parameters. For a norm-referenced marking system that relies on three data sources, with scores from an exam, a speech, and a paper, we could derive a weighted composite *T*-score in five steps.

Constructs and indicators

Achievement in a school semester

Cognitive domain (subject area: English literature)

Population units for inference making

Individual students

Number of instruments and data sources

Three assessments (exam, paper, speech)

Weights allocated to each data source

25% (exam), 50% (paper), 25% (speech)

Desired interpretations and uses

Norm-referenced interpretations of performance using a composite in a classroom context

- **Step 1:** *Compute z-scores and study distributions of scores on each assessment for students in the class.* The first step would be to score each assessment and calculate the descriptive statistics for the distributions of scores in the class. Suppose the following results were obtained for Student A and the class as a whole:

1. *Exam*

   Mean $_{class}$ = 17, s = 2.45 (maximum possible score = 20)

   Student A's raw score = 13

   Student A's z-score (exam) = –1.63
2. *Speech*

   Mean $_{class}$ = 12.2, s = 2.48 (maximum possible score = 15)

   Student A's raw score = 8

   Student A's z-score (speech)= –1.69
3. *Paper*

   Mean $_{class}$ = 78, s = 14.6 (maximum possible score = 100)

   Student A's raw score = 53

   Student A's z-score (paper) = –1.71

- **Step 2:** *Calculate T-scores for each student.* Obtain *T*-scores for every student on each assessment (the relevant unit of analysis here), using descriptive statistics of the respective score distributions, as shown.

Student A's score on the exam = 13, z = –1.63

T = 10(–1.63) + 50 = 33.7

Student A's score on the speech = 8, z = –1.69

T = 10(–1.69) + 50 = 33.1

Student A's score on the paper = 8, z = –1.69

T = 10(–1.69) + 50 = 33.1

- **Step 3:** *Apply the weights to the T-score for each assessment or data source.* Multiply the numeric weight allocated previously (by the teacher) to each student's *T*-score on each assessment to obtain *weighted T-scores* on each. For Student A:

Weighted *T*-score on exam: 33.7 × .25 = 8.43

Weighted *T*-score on speech: 33.1 × .25 = 8.28

Weighted *T*-score on paper: 33.1 × .50 = 16.45

• **Step 4:** *Sum the weighted T-scores from each assessment to obtain a composite score for each student.* For Student A, the weighted composite *T*-score = 8.43 + 8.28 + 16.45 = **33.16.**

• **Step 5:** *Assign the mark based on the class's distribution of composite scores.* Study the distribution of composite scores for the class and set the desired cut points for Grades A–F on a scale continuum. Standard setting here would be based on teacher judgments. For example, see the scheme below:

Student A's assigned mark = **D** based on a weighted composite *T*-score of *33.16*.

Standards for a *T*-score Based Marking System:

Composite *T*-Score Ranges	Mark
60 and above	A
50–59	B
40–49	C
30–39	D
29 and below	F

9.6.3.2 Deriving a Composite Using Percentage Scores

In the CRT method for the same scenario and parameters, we would apply *previously set criteria* on a weighted composite scale to determine the marks. Distributional statistics like the mean or standard deviation are not employed. The computational steps follow in five steps.

• **Step 1:** *Set the standards for criterion-referencing the marks.* Start by setting cut points on a weighted composite score scale of 0–100 for the A–F marking categories, such as

90–100 = A, 80–89 = B, 70–79 = C,
60–69 = D, and <60 = F

• **Step 2:** *Convert the scores of each student on each of the three assessments onto a common scale, 1–100.* For each student (population unit), calculate the percentage score out of the maximum possible score on each assessment. This will create a common standardized scale of 0–100 for all students on all the assessments.

For example, Student A receives: 13/20 or 65% score out of the maximum on the exam, 8/15 or 53.3% on the speech, and so on.

• **Step 3:** *Apply the weights to each assessment for each student.* For each student, multiply each score from the different assessments by the allocated weight.

For example, using the same numeric weights in the scenario, Student A receives 65% × 0.25 = 16.25 weighted points on the exam.

• **Step 4:** *Create a weighted composite by summing the weighted percentage score for each student across all assessments.*

For example, using the same weights, Student A receives 56.06 points:

Weighted composite = 16.25 (exam) + 13.33 (speech) + 26.5 (paper) = **56.08**

• **Step 5:** *Apply the criterion-referenced marking scheme with the weighted composite scores.*

For example,

Student A's grade = **F**

Both the illustrations shown are of summative classroom uses for the composites derived. The norm-referenced scheme offers a kinder depiction of Student A's performance on the three assessments than the criterion-referenced one.

Derivation of the GPA composite would require an added layer of computations. Again, the formulas or procedures should be clearly communicated and defended to stakeholders. In the typical case, grade points awarded are A = 4 points, B = 3 points, C = 2 points, D = 1 point, and F = 0 points. The GPA could be computed as a cumulative average or a cumulative total of all the grades earned over every course completed by individual students, in an academic year or a degree program. Commonly, an unweighted average is used, yielding GPAs on a scale of 1 to 4.

QUICK RECAP: Composite indices combine information from multiple measuring instruments and data sources and could be designed for different population units (students, groups, organizations). When used, they should be appropriately rationalized, transparent, meaningful, and user-friendly. Computational steps for deriving composite indices vary depending on whether users desire norm-referenced or criterion-refenced systems. Both were demonstrated with school marks; the procedural steps are transferable to other applications. When composites are used for visible high-stakes applications, validation is necessary.

Reflection Break 9.4: Objective 4

- Derive a composite index of your own for use in a setting of your choice.
  - What are the constructs, the instruments/measures, and data sources? How did you decide on the five issues outlined in the subsection?
  - What is the main inference you will make from the composite? What is it to be used for? At what unit of analysis? Who are the primary users?
  - How did you compute the index? Outline the steps.
  - Why is the index best suited for the users and user context?
- Consider this scenario. The Connecticut State Department of Education (CSDE; 2019) derived a composite called the Accountability Index, intended for grading high schools based on their annual performance. The composite is built with 12 indicators, for example, average test scores of students, student absenteeism rate, student graduation rate, and the like. Each school receives a mathematical score on each indicator, which is then weighted to derive a composite index on which schools are ranked.
  - Identify the unit of analysis for the CSDE composite.
  - List *three* procedures you would recommend so that the composite is meaningful, transparent, fair, and user-friendly. Justify your recommendations.
  - The CSDE includes several high schools dedicated to serving only students with disabilities. Is the composite reasonable for ranking such a school against the rest? Explain how you would advise the CSDE to evaluate specialized schools.

9.7 Grouped Scores, Equated Scales, and Linked Tests

This section of Chapter 9 introduces three specialized psychometric concepts: grouped scores, equated scores, and linked scores. Awareness of these concepts, including their underlying rationales and limitations, is helpful in deterring misuses or misinterpretations of assessment results. Details of the statistical techniques, variously based on classical test theory (CTT) or item response theory (IRT), lie outside the scope of this book.

9.7.1 Grouped Scores

Sometimes, assessment scores from individual units may need to be averaged or aggregated statistically in larger groups for facilitating interpretations and uses at more than one level of an organization, or at the uppermost levels of an organizational system. These are called *group scores* (Mazzeo, Lazer, & Zieky, 2006). A mean achievement test score, derived from test scores of all enrolled students at a school, is an example of a *grouped score*. (Note that a grouped score is different from a composite score.)

In such cases, both the individual level scores and grouped scores may be interpreted and used, with each carrying a different connotation. For example, when students' achievement test scores are used, the individual-level measures convey a single student's level of *achievement* in the tested curricular domain. At the upper organizational levels, the grouped scores from the same test may be treated as an indicator of *educational quality* for a school or school system.

Similarly, we might administer a job satisfaction survey to individual employees of an organization, as well as to different departments and teams within those departments. Here, we would have grouped scores for the teams nested within departments, each representing a different unit of analysis. At the individual level, the survey measures might simply stand for *job satisfaction* levels of individual employees; however, the grouped job satisfaction scores for teams and departments might be interpreted differently based on business management theory, for example, as an indicator of the *organizational climate*.

In both of the above examples, the evidence from grouped scores at different levels of the system is generally used for program evaluation purposes, such as to evaluate the organization's overall functioning and performance.

During validation, it is important to remember that score meanings often alter after aggregation or averaging the individual-level data from a given instrument. Hence, guided by the user context, each score-based inference must be supported with validity evidence for the intended *population units*, or at the *levels of an organizational entity* that are prioritized for making inferences. In program-based studies, issues of nestedness should be considered in the choice of statistics and research design.

9.7.2 Test Equating

Test equating is a procedure used by standardized test developers when multiple test forms or test modalities are necessary to measure a given domain, and the scores generated from the various test forms or testing modes for given persons are not exactly the same. The score and scales must therefore be mathematically adjusted to establish equivalence of the test forms (Bandalos, 2018; Kolen & Hendrikson, 2013).

Let's start with an example in college admissions. Think of two students who take the same standardized entrance test before applying to colleges. Although they take the same test on the same date and time, they find that their test forms shared very few common items! In truth, they took two different but *parallel test forms*, containing items sampled from the same domain. Despite the common test and item design specifications, in fact, there may be minor discrepancies in the tests and test scores produced by parallel forms. This raises the question: Were the two test forms comparable, equivalent, and interchangeable?

Parallel test forms should be assembled such that each form matches the same content and statistical specifications for a given construct domain (AERA et al., 2014). Albeit "parallel" in theory, in practice, it may be that Form A is slightly more difficult than Form B for typical examinees, or vice versa. See the scores below for four test-takers.

Persons	Form A Score	Form B Score
Allen	55	56
Bea	60	61
Carlos	42	43
Dela	64	65

Here, we see that every person gets 1 score point more on Form B than on Form A, suggesting that Form B is easier. To mathematically equate Form A scores with those on Form B, we could add a constant of +1 to each Form A score. Equating functions are derived and calculated with a similar logic but using more complex CTT- or IRT-based statistical formulas. The goal is to have comparable and interchangeable scores, regardless of which test form or testing format an individual examinee is given.

When thousands of examinees take a standardized entrance assessment in given years (like the GRE or SAT), parallel test forms help keep the overall item pool secure by preventing potential item exposure and leakage of test information, and occasional cheating on high-stakes tests. All these problems could arise if only one test form were used. Over repeated administrations of the same test, parallel test forms are necessary to ensure the validity and integrity of the testing, and test scores are maintained by keeping items secure (AERA et al., 2014; Bandalos, 2018; Kolen & Brennan, 2013).

9.7.3 Linking Scales

The goal when linking two or more tests or scales is to place individual scores from *different tests* on a common numeric scale. For example, in theory, we could create a common z-score scale ranging from +/–3.0 for a math test and a reading test for a given group of students. Here, note that the content and construct definitions of the linked tests are *not* the same—in fact, they are significantly different. But, using the separate means and standard deviations of the distribution of scores on the math and reading tests for a common group of students, we could establish a common numeric z-score scale. If we do so, we would have "linked" the two tests. But interpretations of the common scale scores would have to be done cautiously, as the z-scores in each subject are not only different with respect to the content tested, but also the distributional properties. Average or above average performance would *not* be interchangeable in meaning in the two distributions!

Regardless, using the same logic, standardized test-makers may link two different tests that are at the *same* level as with the z-score example above. This is called **horizontal linking** (or **horizontal scaling**). Think of linking two college entrance examinations, like the SAT and the ACT, that are popular in different regions of the United States. As students typically take only one of the tests, horizontal linking studies are expected to allow the prediction of the ACT scores from the SAT scores, and vice versa. Horizontal linking should only be performed with tests at the same level that intend to measure the *same* general domain. Ideally, the group of students should also be the same.

Elsewhere, test developers may statistically link multilevel reading tests designed for different grade levels, say, from grades 3 to 10, to generate a common longitudinal scale that is increasingly higher. This linking procedure is called **vertical linking** (or **vertical scaling**). Vertically linked tests yield longitudinal "scaled scores" intended for facilitating inferences of student growth over time.

Both CTT- and IRT-based techniques are available for test-linking studies (Kolen & Brenan, 2014). In the usual case, test developers rely on an "anchor" test, built with a small sample of common items shared by the two tests to conduct the linking procedures. When an anchor test is very short (e.g., include just one to four items instead of, say, 10), there could be large measurement errors in the regions of the common scale where the tests are joined.

As indicated, interpreting what linked scales mean in specific user contexts is challenging unless one delves into the details of the shared items of anchor tests, research designs, student samples, and mathematical procedures used. Because of the substantive differences in (1) content domains or grade-level curricula, (2) background differences in test-takers who took the different tests, (3) built-in limitations of the anchoring test, or (4) unmet assumptions of the statistical methods/formulas, the linked scales produced must be interpreted with great caution. Their uses must be defensible.

Measurement researchers have consistently warned users of the limitations of vertical scaling, for example, when evaluating school or teacher performance with VAMs in high-stakes educational accountability contexts (AERA, 2015; Lockwood et al., 2007). Despite the warnings, there were recent proposals to use vertically linked test score scales for such purposes (New Hampshire Department of Education, 2018).

QUICK RECAP: Grouped scores, test equating, and test-linking procedures are highly specialized methods. Each was developed to support particular evaluative uses of data obtained from tests and assessments. Each entails very different psychometric, statistical, and research design procedures. Whether used in individual, group, or organizational contexts, their undergirding logic and limitations should be carefully heeded.

Reflection Break 9.5: Objectives 4–6

- Define the term *grouped score*. How is it different from a *composite*? Describe an application of grouped scores used at more than one level. Identify the construct(s) measured and the units of analysis. Did the score meanings change for different units?
- Distinguish between test equating, vertical linking, and horizontal linking. When would you expect each to be applied?
- Would you recommend using vertically scaled achievement test scores for tracking changes in students enrolled in *special education programs* (e.g., students with learning disabilities) in a school? Why or why not? Explain.

9.8 Summary

Chapter 9 described a number of procedures for deriving measures from raw scores, each with different frames of reference, and guided by different inferential needs and uses. The topics addressed were norm referencing, criterion referencing, ipsative assessments of growth, composites, grouped scores, test equating, and test-linking methods. There is a distinct rationale for each of the methods discussed. The different methods offer advantages and disadvantages in given instrument design or use scenarios. Some are technically complex. Execution of others may be lengthy and painstaking, requiring resources. The choice of method should be made with careful judgment.

For each type of derived score and derivation method, the chapter presented the detailed steps for meeting the basic design requirements and best practice guidelines. The different derived scores or transformed scales have different psychometric properties. To correctly interpret these, we must understand the derivation methods, underlying rationale, and limitations of the methods.

When applying the Process Model, we should execute the selected score derivation or transformation procedures in Phases II–III (see Figure 9.1). A prerequisite is that we specify the assessment use and user context clearly in Phase I to guide our design choices and procedures. It may be difficult and sometimes impossible for designers to shift course once a commitment is made to design an assessment to optimize a particular inferential need and use; for example, the logic and steps for designing an NRT versus a CRT are considerably different. Careful validation can help avoid untoward consequences and contingencies (more on this in Chapters 10 and 11).

CHAPTER 10

A Unified Approach to Construct Validity and Validation

Theory to Evidence

10.1 Chapter Overview

10.1.1 Introduction

Chapter 10 discusses the background theory and evidence we need to establish the construct validity of measures, endorsing a "unitary" approach to instrument design and validation (after AERA et al., 1999, p. 11). Building on the introductory information in Chapter 1, this chapter elaborates on the different kinds of evidence necessary to produce measures of high quality, including evidence of validity, reliability, and utility as different facets of the unitary approach to construct validation. The discussion is mainly from a classical test theory (CTT) perspective. Chapter 10 sets the stage for Chapter 11, which focuses on empirical validation methods. For more advanced or different treatments of the topics, see books by Bandalos (2018), Crocker and Algina (2006), and Price (2018), among other resources.

Figure 10.1 shows that validation would occur in an integrated manner in Phase IV, A and B, of the Process Model. This process is guided by the specified contexts of instrument use (Phase I) and sets iterative cycles in motion for revising the tools, as needed, to arrive at optimally functioning measures.

10.1.2 Chapter Objectives

After reading this chapter and completing the accompanying exercises, the reader should be able to:

1. Compare and contrast the predictive, trinitarian, and unitarian views of validity from a historical perspective.
2. Elaborate on the theoretical concepts of construct validity and validation from a unitary perspective.
3. Identify the main clusters of *validity evidence* necessary in given assessment user contexts, with a rationale for each.
4. Identify the main types of *reliability evidence* necessary in given assessment user contexts, with a rationale for each.
5. Identify common types of *utility evidence* required in given assessment user contexts, with a rationale for each.
6. Develop *unified validation plans* under the framework of the Process Model, to investigate overall construct validity of measures.

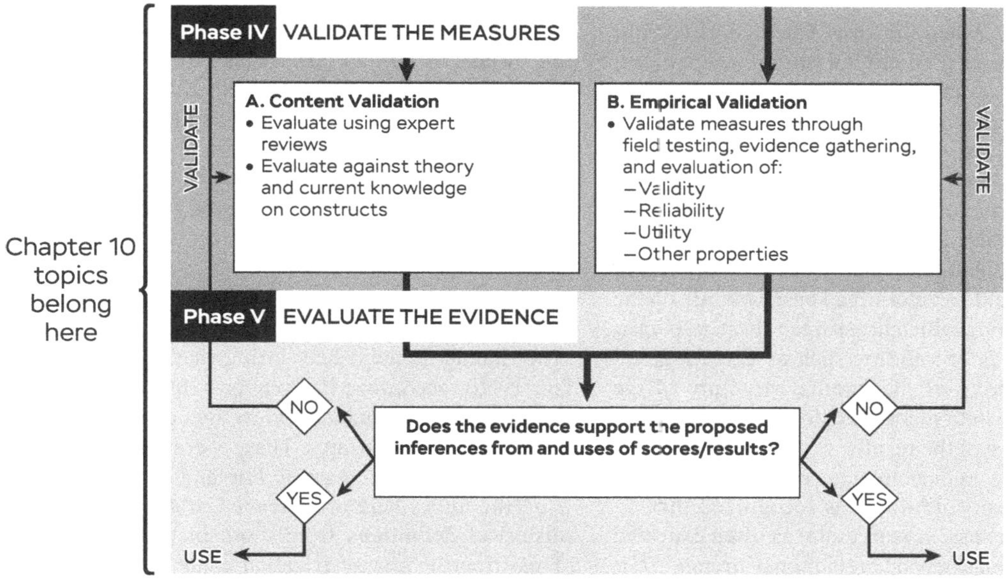

FIGURE 10.1. Connecting Chapter 10 to the Process Model and the rest of the book.

10.2 Construct Validity: An Evolving Concept

"I know who I was when I got up this morning, but I think I must have been changed several times since then."

"What do you mean by that?" said the Caterpillar, sternly. "Explain yourself!"

"I can't explain myself, I'm afraid, Sir," said Alice, "because I am not myself, you see."

—Lewis Carroll (1865/2011, Chap. 5)

Much like Alice's changing persona in Wonderland in Lewis Carroll's famous tale, theoretical ideas and definitions of validity have undergone several shifts over the decades (Baker, 2013). Ongoing challenges in applied measurement practices instigated much of the collective rethinking that occurred on the concept since the 1950s. For a "then and now" comparison leading up to the present, a quick survey of the mindsets of selected measurement scholars, including published positions of professional organizations, follows. See Table 10.1. As we consider what validity means in theory and practice today, think of *construct measures* in the broadest possible sense, extending from raw scores to various forms of derived scores, composites, and transformed measures discussed in Chapters 8 and 9.

10.2.1 An Old Idea: Predictive Validity as the Whole of Validity

Until the 1960s, discussions on validity centered largely on **predictive validity**, defined as empirically collected evidence showing the degree to which a given test's scores predict the measures of a future criterion in a defined group of respondents. In a predictor–criterion relationship, the word "criterion" refers to the outcome or dependent variable measured at some later point and is usually identified by the primary users of an assessment. From examples in Chapters 3 and 8, recall that predictive validity is commonly evaluated with bivariate **correlation coefficients** using the distributions of the desired construct measures.

Espousing a predictive perspective to validity would mean that we would rely almost entirely on predictive validity evidence for making determinations of the quality of an assessment and its measures. This is a reasonable stance when the chief function of the test (and its results) is in predicting a future criterion performance of the test-takers.

For example, suppose an organization designed a general ability test to select the best candidates for their firm. Here, the examinees' ability scores would serve as the *predictor* measures; the *criterion* measures could be their productivity levels, measured a year after recruitment. The quality of the ability test in this scenario would be determined based mainly on the predictive validity coefficient between these two variables. Other kinds of validity, such as content-based validity, the validity of the internal structure of the test, and so on, would matter less to the test designers and primary users of the results.

The predictive perspective to validity dominated measurement theory until it was recognized that, in practice, the same assessment tool was often expected to perform functions beyond prediction (Cureton, 1951; Ebel, 1961). When this was the case, the added inferences and uses of the measures needed support with appropriate forms of validity evidence; for instance, suppose the recruiters in the above scenario also desired to know the proficiency levels of the recruits in job-specific cognitive skills. Now, evidence of **content-based validity** of the test scores would be minimally necessary for those valued domains. No matter, during that period, the predictive purposes of tests tended to eclipse all others. In effect, predictive validity became the "whole of validity" (Brennan, 2006, p. 3).

The singular emphasis on predictive validity led to both controversies and practical challenges in applied contexts. A primary barrier dealt with locating suitable criterion measures for particular instruments that would themselves yield sufficiently valid and reliable data.

10.2.2 A Trinitarian View of Validity

The Standards published during that period (APA et al., 1966), according to Brennan (2006), presented a revisionist and expanded view by identifying *three* main aspects of validity. These were labeled as *content validity*, *predictive validity*, and *construct validity*—the italics here are intended to distinguish these historical definitions from those of the modern era. This tripartite characterization came to be called the trinitarian conception of validity (Brennan, 2006, p. 3; Kane, 2006).

To contrast the trinitarian view with the prior predictive perspective of validity, see Table 10.1 again. As evident, the notion of validity came to be thought of differently for different types of assessment tools: content validity was deemed necessary for achievement tests, predictive validity for assessments intended for prediction, and construct validity for psychologi-

TABLE 10.1. Evolving Perspectives on Validity

	Key principles	Typical methods
Predictive perspective	Predictive validity is the "whole of validity," prioritizing predictive purposes of all tests and assessments	Obtaining predictive validity coefficients in specified persons, groups, or entities
Trinitarian perspective	Three types of validity: • Content validity • Predictive validity • Construct validity	Reviewing of a test's content, applied mainly for achievement test design purposes Obtaining predictive validity coefficients applied for tests intended for prediction purposes Applying correlational and factor analysis methods for psychological test design purposes
Unitarian perspective	Construct validity is "all of validity" Unified evaluation of relevant kinds of evidence to: • Confirm the properties of construct measures • Justify the planned inferences and uses of the construct measures.	Evidence-based evaluations of the measures to support their meanings against construct theory and justify the desired inferences and uses of the chosen measures

cal assessments. On the surface, it appeared that the dominant purposes for an assessment tool influenced exactly what kind of validity investigation would be undertaken and the evidence that was to be valued for each. At the same time, the notion of "construct validity" seemed reserved mainly for assessments of psychological constructs, such as personality assessments and attitude inventories. There was a logical inconsistency in the trinitarian conception of validity, suggesting that *not* all assessments measured constructs!

Robert Ebel (1961) criticized the piecemeal trinitarian view of validity due to the confusion it created among researchers, measurement practitioners, and assessment users alike. Each type of validity evidence yielded starkly different kinds of information on the construct measures, yet was inadequate by itself. The approach led to bewilderment as to which kind of validity counted for specific instruments, especially if a given tool was used for more than one purpose. In a sarcastic title to an influential paper published by the American Psychologist, Ebel asked: "Must all tests be valid?" However, he was not urging for an abandonment of the concept of validity altogether, but rather, to forgo the confusing notion of three, instrument-specific kinds of validity. In his opinion, the focus needed to shift to the overall "meaningfulness" of the construct measures tied to the assessment's purposes (Ebel, 1961, pp. 640–647). That essential line of thinking was repeated by R. L. Thorndike a decade later, who said: "[T]o be able to decide when and where a test should be used, whether for research or for practical inferences about a person, one needs an understanding of what the test score means, of what it signifies for the individual" (1971, pp. 13–14).

10.2.3 The Unitarian View of Validity

The unitarian view of construct validity and validation holds that "all of validity is construct validity" (Brennan, 2006, p. 2). This view was endorsed in the Standards published successively in 1985, 1999, and 2014, where validity is defined as (AERA et al., 2014, p. 11): "the degree to which evidence and theory support the interpretations of test scores for the proposed uses of tests." With some variations, this basic view was articulated in an earlier seminal work by Cronbach and Meehl (1955), and endorsed later by Messick (1989), Kane (2006), and many others—further discussed in Section 10.4.

A practical translation of the above ideas is that the evidence we need to claim construct validity of measures is dictated by the specific inferences and uses that we plan with those measures. The operative words to remember in the 2014 Standards' definition are *theory*, *interpretations*, *uses*, and *evidence*. What do these terms, central to the unitary view of validity, mean? Situated in an applied example, a breakdown follows.

10.2.3.1 Theory, Inferences, and Uses

Every assessment tool aims to measure one or more "theoretical" constructs, whether it is an achievement test, a personality assessment, or an anxiety scale. Furthermore, the measures that each tool produces are intended for making particular score-based interpretations (inferences) about those constructs in some specified individuals or groups (units of the population) and for taking specific types of actions in the contexts where we use the tool. Hence, it stands to reason that we validate those *inferences* about the constructs measured guided by the underlying construct theories and couched in the situations where we (the primary users) plan to use the tool. See the Process Model in Figure 10.1.

Suppose we wish to validate measures of anxiety obtained with a survey-based instrument. Suppose also that the tool was purposefully designed for diagnosing clinical levels of anxiety in adults in health care settings. When investigating construct validity, we must ask: To what extent do the survey's scores permit *meaningful inferences* about clinical anxiety levels in adults, given the existing knowledge and theory about human anxiety? Second: Do the survey's scores have the properties to support the *diagnostic decisions* that clinicians plan to take in health care settings? The primary users of the assessment's results in the scenario would be the clinicians, as well as the adult patients/clients and their families.

10.2.3.2 Evidence

In the clinical example, the word "unitary" implies that *all* the evidence we need to support the intended interpretations and uses of the anxiety scores must be collected and evaluated together. This should certainly include evidence on content-based validity, guided by questions like, *Are clinical levels of anxiety operation-*

alized according to the latest science and theory about the construct? Simultaneously, however, we would also need evidence to confirm the reliability of the scores and of any diagnostic classifications that may follow. Finally, added evidence of utility of the assessment procedures would validate that the instrument is easy to apply in practice settings and beneficial to both the clinicians and their patient-clients, for the purposes that they prioritize and value. In the unitarian view, all of this evidence must be evaluated *as a whole* situated in the contexts where the survey is used.

Recall from Chapters 1 and 2 that, depending on the user contexts and projected stakes tied to the assessment's results, **validation** could be performed informally or on a limited scale; elsewhere, it would require formal studies and sometimes longer-term research programs (Angoff, 1988; Cronbach, 1971, 1988; see Henry, Lipsey, & Rossi, 2019, for a definition of *evaluation research*). Because clinical decisions are relatively high stakes, validation of the anxiety measures would likely require comprehensive evidence-gathering efforts.

Implicitly, the unitarian approach assumes that an assessment tool may be useful for a range of different purposes, serving the interests of different assessment users and user paths. For each different user context, however, a *different mix of evidence* could be necessary to claim adequate levels of construct validity of the measures.

QUICK RECAP: Historically, three major conceptions of validity dominated the testing and measurement field: the predictive, trinitarian, and unitarian. The unitarian perspective dominates today and is endorsed by the latest Standards. To claim construct validity, the body of evidence we gather during validation must be linked to the underpinning construct theories and justify the proposed inferences and uses of the measures situated in given user contexts. The Process Model (Figure 10.1) adopts the main premises of the unitarian perspective.

Reflection Break 10.1: Objective 1

- Explain the similarities and differences in the concepts of *construct validity* and *construct validation* from the (1) predictive, (2) trinitarian, and (3) unitarian perspectives. Give examples of assessment design or selection cases where one or the other approach seems dominant. Explain.
- Identify the principles of the unitarian approach that are especially meaningful to you. Explain how you would apply these for an instrument design/selection project of your own. In what ways could following the Process Model enhance your project's goals?

10.3 The Unitarian View of Validation: Moving from Theory to Application

The foundational tenets of the unitarian view of validity and validation were formalized over time with ideas from several measurement theorists. Box 10.1 offers a summary of four major ideas that this book adopts to guide measurement practices.

10.3.1 Four Tenets to Applying a Unitarian View of Construct Validation

1. Validation is a form of scientific inquiry. A construct validation mindset should be no different from one we would adopt for conducting any scientific study, placing the constructs at the center of the inquiry process. Borrowing from Cronbach and Meehl

BOX 10.1 Unitarian View of Construct Validation: Four Tenets

1. Validation is a form of scientific inquiry.
2. Validation is a theory-guided effort in search for construct meanings.
3. Validation calls for integrating and evaluating relevant kinds of evidence in the contexts where the construct measures are to be interpreted and used.
4. Validation includes investigations of the social consequences of the uses of high-stakes assessments on individuals and other concerned entities.

(1955): "The investigation of a test's construct validity is not essentially different from the general scientific procedures for developing and confirming theories" (pp. 301–303). All tests and assessment instruments tap into constructs about which we might have prior hunches or theories. Therefore, it is sensible to investigate the properties of the construct measures with a systematic, theory-guided, and hypothesis-driven approach.

2. **Validation research involves a quest for construct meanings.** To derive theoretically grounded systems of meanings for new construct measures, again it was Cronbach and Meehl (1955) who posited that a "construct is defined implicitly by a network of associations or propositions. . . ." (pp. 302–303). They called this network of expected variable associations a **nomological network**. In operation, Cronbach and Meehl were saying that all new construct measures about which we have little knowledge could be situated within a network of theoretically related variables that we *did* know more about. That network of hypothetical relationships could then be tested empirically. The intervariable correlations would provide insights into what the new construct measures mean.

Review Figure 10.2 for a concrete example, excerpted from an earlier study (Benson, 2005). The central construct investigated is *test anxiety*, representing the negative emotions individuals might experience during test taking. It is operationalized by the researcher with two subconstructs: worry and emotionality, as shown. These two *focal construct measures* were then situated within a network of other variables with which they were expected to correlate, namely, academic self-concept, motive to avoid failure, and achievement. The directional arrows show the pathways and relationships expected among the selected variables and the focal constructs. For example, if the test anxiety measures were valid and true to theory, they would correlate *negatively* with academic self-concept and achievement. Similarly, with the connecting paths, the test anxiety measures were hypothesized to play an *intervening* role in the relationship between self-concept and measured achievement levels. The researcher tested the proposed *nomological network* with empirical data from a sample of school-going students, mostly confirming the hypothesized relationships (Benson, 2005).

3. **Validation calls for integrating and evaluating relevant kinds of evidence situated in the specified user contexts.** Several authors have spoken to this validity tenet in different ways, starting with Cronbach and Meehl (1955, p. 302), who said: "Many types of evidence are relevant to construct validity . . . content validity, inter-item correlations, intertest correlations, predictive validity coefficients and stability of

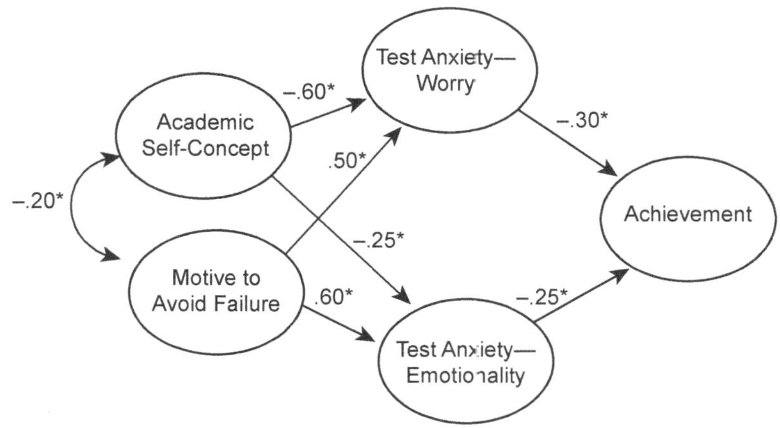

FIGURE 10.2. A nomological network to validate measures of test anxiety: An illustrative case. Reprinted with permission from Benson (2005). © John Wiley & Sons.

test scores." Likewise, Robert Ebel (1961) argued for gathering and unifying *six* different kinds of evidence when examining the validity of an assessment intended for norm-referenced score interpretations and uses. With the example of a mental test, Ebel delineated the types of evidence essential for establishing validity as (1) "operational definition of the measurement procedure"; (2) "relationships of scores to other measures"; (3) "appropriate norms"; (4) "reliability"; (5) "convenience of the test in use"; and (6) "the importance of the inferences that can be made from the test scores" (p. 647). As may be evident, he was calling for the integration of evidence on the validity, reliability, and utility of the measures, as defined in this book.

Later, Messick (1989, pp. 56–58; see the quote in Chapter 1) endorsed a similar integrative definition of validity. Also taking a comprehensive, evaluative approach to validating measures, he emphasized the need to combine empirical evidence with the theoretical rationales underlying a test, to adequately justify the score-based inferences and actions we plan to take with the test's scores, in predefined contexts.

Subsequently, Kane (2006, 2013a, 2013b) proposed an *argument-based approach* for conducting unified validation studies, taking *every* score-based interpretation and use deliberately into consideration when multiple uses, users, and stakeholders are likely. Kane's approach translates to addressing two pragmatic questions during validation, as follows:

- *Testing the interpretive argument.* Is the argument for the intended interpretations and uses of construct measures complete, coherent, and plausible?
- *Testing the validity argument.* Given the proposed uses of construct measures, are the claims regarding their properties warranted with evidence?

That is, he recommended that we begin by evaluating the reasonableness of the *interpretive arguments* about what the construct measures are supposed to mean when the instrument is put to use in specific ways. Then, we should test the *validity arguments* by verifying those claims with empirical evidence.

4. **Validation includes investigations of the social consequences of using an assessment and its construct measures on concerned stakeholders.** Finally, evaluating the potential consequences of assessment uses should be a pertinent validation issue for investigation, especially in high-stakes contexts. Designers of all tests and assessments typically expect the measurement tools to contribute positively to specific societal functions and organizational missions, with positive impacts on the persons, groups, and entities assessed. For instance, workplace competency assessments are designed to ensure that the professionals and workers in an organization uphold high standards of practice. In most situations where assessment adopters and users employ the tests appropriately, we can expect positive consequences of testing for all the stakeholders.

Yet, validity issues could arise due to misuse of tools, or misinterpretations of the measures in original or modified form. In any given user context, misinterpreting or overinterpreting the results of a test or assessment, or using the same for specific actions *without* the necessary validity evidence in hand, is labeled as a *misuse*. In many instances, the negative consequences of inappropriate test uses have raised issues of equity, fairness, or social justice for one or more stakeholder groups, including individuals who are assessed in high-stakes decision-making contexts (see the cases in Chapter 2; Chatterji, 2013a, 2013b).

There is, therefore, a need to validate the extent to which the desired positive consequences of using an instrument appropriately are realized in all or most settings. Any potential adverse impacts of actions taken with an assessment's results for individuals and groups should also be investigated and ruled out, especially in high-stakes scenarios. To ameliorate potential long-term societal issues, stakeholders should be alerted of any negative results of testing promptly. Messick (1989) referred to this aspect of construct validation as the "consequential basis of test [score] interpretation" (p. 58). Several publications have since abbreviated the expression to **consequential validity** (see, e.g., Feuer, 2013), a usage adopted in this book. The latest Standards call for studies on the consequences of test use for all published instruments (AERA et al., 2014).

10.3.2 Opposing Viewpoints on Construct Validity

While the unitarian conception is dominant today, some continue to subscribe to older or alternate views of validity. A recent textbook on psychometric methods breaks down validity under the three categories of *criterion validity*, *content validity*, and *construct validity* (Price, 2018), corresponding closely with the traditional trinitarian perspective. Other contrarian perspectives discount the need for validating the *uses* of construct measures at all, arguing that validity is a built-in property of a test or measuring instrument (Borsboom & Mellenberg, 2007; Borsboom, Mellenberg, & Van Heerden, 2004). Yet others believe that attention to "uses" of assessment results has posed barriers to theoretical, empirical, and practical advancements in measurement. There is a fear that validation could become a never-ending process once users and all possible uses of assessments are factored into validation procedures (Cizek, 2012).

To elaborate briefly, the first perspective (Borsboom et al., 2004) holds that "[v]alidity is a property of tests: A valid test can convey the effect of variation in the attribute one intends to measure. . . . A test is valid if a variation in the attribute causes a variation in the test scores" (p. 1067). In this view, if the latent constructs measured by an assessment are found to cause variations in the item responses, subscale scores, or other scores, we have evidence of validity. And, that is *all* the validity evidence we need. In this view, to claim that a "test is valid," we would rely largely on correlational evidence on its internal structure.

Arguing in a similar vein, the second opposing view (Cizek, 2012) concurs: "Validity is the degree to which scores on an appropriately administered instrument support inferences about variation in the characteristic that the instrument was developed to measure" (pp. 35–36). This author's definition of validation is also restricted to studying variations in the scores that are attributable to variations in the purported constructs. It discards the need to investigate the validity of various *uses* of assessment results, or the social consequences of proper or improper assessment uses. Validation within a user-centered assessment design framework, as presented in this book, is incompatible with both these contrarian perspectives.

QUICK RECAP: The unitarian approach to validation requires that we investigate the meanings that construct measures convey in given situations and justify the measure-based inferences for user-specified uses of the assessments. The proposed measure-based inferences and uses must be defended with scientifically gathered evidence. In high-stakes scenarios, it asks for investigations of the consequences of assessment use. Alternate positions on validity discount the relevance and necessity of validating assessment uses.

Reflection Break 10.2: Objective 2

- Recap the *four* main tenets of the unitarian approach to construct validation. Describe how you would apply each during instrument design or adoption with the Process Model.
- Make arguments to *support* **or** *refute* the positions of one or more authors referenced in this section. Situate the arguments with an assessment example from your experience.
- In your own words, describe the concept of a *nomological network*. Is it a reasonable way to better understand what the constructs measured by a tool mean?
- What is test *misuse*? Explain with an example. How could validation help correct this?

10.4 Main Clusters and Types of Validity Evidence

From a methodological perspective, the goal of construct validation studies is to identify the influences of internal and external factors that could interfere with pure measurement of the constructs of interest. We begin with attention to systematic errors, their sources, and the major types of valid evidence we could secure to examine these interferences. In the following sections, we draw on the theoretical distinction between *systematic* and *random* sources of measurement error for differentiating between validity and reliability (after Stanley, 1971).

10.4.1 Sources of Systematic Error

To start with a quick reminder and a case study, systematic interferences undermine the meaningfulness of construct measures (Chapters 1–3). For example, unknowingly, we might include item content that is biased toward a given subgroup of examinees. Think of a language comprehension test that incorporates too many items to which only boys can relate—such as items dealing with analytics in baseball, a sport that girls do not play. Here, the girls may receive lower scores, predictably and repeatedly, due to their lack of exposure to that sport. This outcome is not due to their inferior language understanding abilities, but rather the gender-biased item content. When this interference affects the test score interpretations each time we use that test's results, it is a systematic error. Predictably and systematically, the factor lowers the validity of the score-based inferences about the language abilities of the girls, and to the same degree.

Systematic errors could result from a variety of sources. Consider Box 10.2 for a real-world assessment scenario in a refugee migration setting. Should a particular subgroup of refugees in this particular assessment context obtain systematically lower (or higher) scores for reasons unrelated to their psychological functioning levels, there would be validity concerns. In this situation, the major sources of systematic error are identified to deal with:

1. Construct-irrelevant item content in the daily life skills domain
2. Construct underrepresentation by the omission of items that *should* define the domains
3. Invalid composite scores built with limited or inappropriate subscale scores
4. Language interferences, due to item translation or communication issues
5. Cultural interferences and potential gender biases, due to untenable assumptions about the living circumstances, customs, beliefs, and sociodemographic profiles of segments of the surveyed populations

10.4.2 Three Clusters of Validity Evidence

Validation studies are intended to interrogate different sources of systematic error, as in Box 10.2, by gathering and evaluating different kinds of **validity evidence** appropriate to the assessment context. See the accompanying Tables 10.2–10.4 and Boxes 10.3–10.5. This section describes *three* broad Evidence Clusters I–III, with specific kinds under each listed as A–J. Note that

BOX 10.2 Validity and Systematic Errors: A New Application of an Existing Instrument

Case Study

A team of psychological researchers designed a self-report screening assessment—*Instrument A*—to measure general psychological functioning levels of English-speaking adults. The tool comprised five subscales, measuring physical functioning, interpersonal relationships, social acceptability, daily skills, and applied skills. It yielded five subscale scores and a global composite score. After field-testing the tool with English-speaking adult populations in a number of Western nations, the researchers found satisfactory evidence of validity and reliability.

During the Arab Spring in 2012–2016, a refugee crisis developed in Jordan. At a camp, a team of international health care providers selected *Instrument A* to screen incoming refugees on their psychological functioning needs. The clinicians modified the survey into a shorter interview and translated the items into Arabic.

Issues during Assessment Use:

- In the daily life skills domain, the items were not relevant to daily life in a refugee camp setting.
- There were too few items that were relevant to the experiences of refugees in some scales (e.g., social acceptability).
- Due to dialectic differences in the Arabic language, there were barriers to interviewee understandings of the items. Refugees were mostly from Tunisia.
- Some parts of the instrument were translated poorly or incorrectly, altering the construct definitions.
- Some items assumed equal roles and activities for men and women. These items were inconsistent with the cultural traditions of many refugees, who could not respond comfortably or honestly.

the tables are not exhaustive lists of validation questions to guide the studies, or possible systematic errors under each; they are intended to initiate thinking toward preparing *unified validation plans* (Section 10.7).

In large part, the Evidence Clusters I–III (A–J) conform with the latest Standards, which recognize *five* categories of validity evidence described in Chapter 1 (AERA et al., 2014, pp. 13–22), namely, evidence based on test content, response processes, internal structure, relations of the construct measures with other variables, and the consequences of testing. Added evidence categories under Clusters I–III are intended to support the instrument design process and justify the uses of various derived scores and scales under a unified framework.

10.4.2.1 Validity Evidence: Cluster I

The first cluster in Table 10.2 includes three types of evidence, namely, content-based validity, validity of response processes, and validity of item properties (A–C). This body of evidence alerts designers as to the specific weaknesses and strengths of the initially drafted items and assessment tools, informing the next iterations of the design process. The end goal is to assemble a "final" version of the instrument after poorly functioning parts are revised or deleted.

BEST TIME TO COLLECT THE EVIDENCE

Evidence under Cluster I should be collected in the *early stages* of the design process for a new instrument, or immediately after we select items or an existing instrument for use in a new or different setting. These studies are often small-scale empirical try-outs or pilot tests of the entire or relevant portions of the assessments.

*A. **Content-Based Validity Evidence.*** See the "Typical validation questions" in the top panel of Table 10.2. Content-based validity should be established to some degree for all assessments, including teacher-made classroom tests and instruments intended for informal uses. As discussed elsewhere in the book, the procedure relies on logically performed, critical reviews of the domains, item content, and the overall instrument. Content validation could be performed by the assessment designers themselves, or by qualified peers and external experts.

Procedurally, content-based validity is established by asking reviewers to systematically review and verify that the assessment's items and operations are sufficiently aligned with the assessment's purposes, constructs and construct theories, and population profiles. The domains, items, presentation mode, response formats, scoring systems, and administration media

TABLE 10.2. Types of Validity Evidence: Cluster I

Validity evidence and definition	Typical validation questions	Sources of systematic error
A: Content-based validity Evidence of content relevance and content representativeness of the domains, items, and overall assessment operations	To what extent is the content of items, domains, and assessment operations . . . • . . . representative of the construct? • . . . match the theoretical definition of the construct? • . . . well matched to the population and assessment purposes?	Mismatches of the assessment's content with construct theory Poor item sampling Mismatched assessment content for the population or the purposes of assessment
B: Validity of response processes Evidence that the responses reflect the intended cognitive, affective, or behavioral processes of respondents	When responding to items and the assessment . . . • . . . are respondents engaging in the intended thought processes or other processual behaviors relevant to the construct(s)?	Poorly conceived items or assessment operations Oversight of "process indicators"
C: Validity based on item properties Evidence that the statistical properties of item-level data are consistent with the assessment design specifications	To what degree . . . • . . . do the item-level statistics suggest properties consistent with the designer's intents?	Item construction issues Item selection issues

could all be reviewed. Two major guiding criteria are *content relevance* and *content representativeness* of the items and overall assessment tool. This book provided several checklists in Chapters 4–7 to facilitate content evaluations.

Formal content validation procedures may involve surveys or interviews of experts, yielding both quantitative ratings and qualitative comments. Expert agreement levels may be evaluated statistically with content validation indices (CVIs; see Lynn, 1986; Pollitt et al., 2007; see also Chapter 11 for further discussion).

Locating appropriately qualified researchers or practitioners with expertise relevant to the construct domains and populations is key to executing effective content validation studies. For example, teachers might ask peer teachers who are subject-area specialists to content-validate their classroom assessments; psychologists with appropriate specializations could review assessments of psychological constructs; banking professionals could conduct content reviews of a test of finance or banking concepts. In standardized test design settings, measurement experts are also often invited to ensure that appropriate design procedures and item construction techniques were followed.

CONTENT-BASED VALIDITY VERSUS FACE VALIDITY

We should be clear about the distinctions between content-based validity and face validity, as the two are often confused in common usage (Gravetter & Farzano, 2012; Holden, 2010). **Face validity** refers to surface features of an instrument that make it acceptable to *lay audiences* of test-takers and other assessment users, such as parents of student examinees. On the surface, to laypeople, it looks as if the instrument is authentic and credible, measuring what it professes to measure. Studies of face validity rarely or never include experts, although some data may be collected. The Standards (AERA et al., 2014) do not include, or even mention, face validity as necessary for assessment design or validation purposes. However, the notion continues to have some valence with assessments in psychology and the health fields, where lay respondents may need to be convinced of the authenticity of the assessment procedures.

B. Validity of Response Processes. See the "Typical validation question" in the middle panel in Table 10.2. This category of evidence deals with validating the *cognitive processes* that individuals utilize when responding to tasks or items on assessments against some prior hypotheses of the designers. Think of process indicators when specifying cognitive domains (Chapters 4 and 5). Many assessments rest on theoretical assumptions about *how* respondents will approach a task or the specific mental processes that they will employ to solve a problem, such as reasoning or trial-and-error processes. With performance assessments, designers may make assumptions about the cognitive, decision-making processes that examiners will engage in when assigning ratings to respondents or examinees. Yet others may make assumptions about affective processes, emotions, or behaviors that respondents will engage in, leading to a particular mindset or attitude toward something.

The best means for examining the **validity of the response processes** is evidence collected "in the moment." That is, the data must be procured as the respondents engage with the tasks and items, or shortly thereafter, so that individuals are better able to recollect and reflect on their thought processes. Qualitative research methods offer useful approaches. A method called **cognitive interviewing** is useful for engaging participants in guided meta-cognitive and reflective exercises with probing techniques (Cacioppo, Petty, & Feng Kao,1984; Carbone, Campbell, & Honess-Morreale, 2002; see Chapter 11 for more on the methods). Keywords and phrases in their verbal communications lend insights into the construct relevance of the response processes employed during task execution.

C. Validity Based on Item Properties. See the "Typical validation question" in the bottom panel of Table 10.2. Evidence on the statistical properties of items is gathered with a range of **item analysis** methods, treated in greater depth in Chapter 11. Item analysis procedures require field testing and empirical tryouts of the items with typical samples of examinees or respondents. These techniques are useful for reviewing the distributional and statistical properties of item response data against the assessment designer's specifications, and in diagnosing possible causes for item malfunctioning. Any flaws detected are addressed before the final versions of assessment tools are compiled. Results could lead to item deletions, revisions, or rewriting. Some item statistics are also useful in item bias studies.

Different statistics help validate different item design expectations, as guided by the stated purposes of an assessment tool. For instance, item analysis methods differ for tests aiming to support criterion-referenced versus norm-referenced score interpretations. Similarly, entirely different statistics are useful for self-report items developed with domain-sampling methods. Three statistics are discussed next.

ITEM DIFFICULTY AND DISCRIMINATION STATISTICS

When testing cognitive domains, two useful item analysis statistics are the **item difficulty index**, the *p*-value, and **item discrimination index**, the *D*-value. Invented for multiple-choice and structured-response items, these statistics are adaptable for numerically rated cognitive tasks.

Item difficulty is calculated based on the proportions (%) of examinees who select the correct answer to a multiple-choice item. The *p*-values range from 0 to 1, indicating 0 to 100% of persons selecting the correct answer. For example, a *p*-value of .40 indicates that 40% of the examinees identified the correct answer. Higher *p*-values denote easier items (e.g., >.80); low *p*-values indicate more difficult items (<.30). In the typical test design scenario, cognitively demanding items measuring higher-order skills would be expected to show lower *p*-values than items tapping lower-order skills, like concept recall.

The *D*-value is the *difference* in proportions of examinees belonging to the lower and higher subgroups of the test score distribution who select the right answer. For this, we need to calculate the *p*-values for the top performers and bottom performers in the overall test score distribution. For example, for an item with a *p*-value of .40, the *D* could also turn out to be .40, as follows:

Highest-scoring 1/3 of examinees, Item *p*-value = .60 (60% selected the right answer)

Lowest-scoring 1/3 of examinees, Item *p*-value = .20 (20% selected the right answer)

Mean Item *p*-value for both groups = (.60 + .20)/2 = .40

Item *D*-value = .60 – .20 = .40

Interpretation: This is a difficult item overall, but useful in discriminating between persons located at higher and lower regions of the test score distribution.

Although relatively difficult, the item above would have the separation and sorting properties consistent with norm-referenced test design specifications (Chapter 9). For making item improvements or to decide that an item is acceptable, careful deliberation must follow after item statistics are obtained.

ITEM HOMOGENEITY STATISTICS

To test the assumptions of domain sampling theory, **item homogeneity** indices are other useful statistics. Recall that by design, domain-referenced items should all be homogeneous, measuring the same underlying construct. Each item's response data should therefore add to the variance of the total score distribution, with each item correlating positively with the total scores.

A homogeneity statistic called the *item-to-total score correlation* gauges this covariance. After deleting the item under investigation from the total score computation, it tells us the extent to which the item's responses are correlated with those adjusted total scores. Descriptive statistics such as item-level means, standard deviations, variances, and inter-item correlations yield additional information on an item's distributional and statistical properties. These statistics are applicable for all structured-response items, such as self-report items of noncognitive constructs, as well as for cognitive test items.

10.4.2.2 Validity Evidence: Cluster II

The second evidence cluster shown in Table 10.3 deals with two main categories of correlational evidence of validity (D–E). Correlational evidence could focus on the *internal structure* of an assessment, speaking to its latent factor structure or dimensional properties based on item-level responses. Alternatively, the evidence could show the relationships of the focal construct measures with *external variables*, similar to the logic of a nomological network in Figure 10.2. The following correlational validity indices are presented here: convergent validity, discriminant validity, predictive validity, concurrent validity, and validity of group differences. Examinations of systematic group biases are variations of these.

TABLE 10.3. Types of Validity Evidence: Cluster II

Type of validity evidence	Typical validation questions	Sources of systematic error
D: Validity evidence of internal structure Evidence confirming that the variance and covariance in item responses is explained by the expected "latent" factors or dimensions	To what extent . . . • . . . do mathematically derived factors match the theoretically proposed structure? • . . . do the factors intercorrelate, as hypothesized? • . . . is the assessment's scoring system consistent with validated internal structure? • . . . are the item response data consistent with a unidimensional mathematical model?	Item-level issues Item-level language interferences Item organization issues by domain or subdomain
E: Correlational validity evidence with external variables Evidence showing that the construct measures correlate, as suggested by theory or logic, with selected external variables • Convergent validity • Discriminant validity • Predictive validity • Concurrent validity • Validity based on group differences • Lack of systematic group biases	To what extent . . . • . . . do the construct measures converge with, or diverge from, selected external measures, as expected? • . . . do measures predict future performance on selected criterion variables, as expected? • . . . do the construct measures overlap sufficiently with other measures to permit substitutions? • . . . are there significant between-group differences on the construct measures, as expected? • . . . are there *no* systematic biases evident in the measures for any individuals or specific groups?	Degree of interferences from external variables

BEST TIME TO COLLECT THE EVIDENCE

Cluster II data should ideally be gathered *after* early versions of instruments are refined, that is, after completing some preliminary content validation and item analysis studies. All these procedures should be hypotheses-guided and informed by reasoned logic and theory. Refer back to Chapter 8 to review computation and interpretation procedures for correlation coefficients in general.

D. Validity of Internal Structure. Validation of the internal structure of assessments is often pursued with a family of specialized mathematical techniques called **factor analysis** (Gorsuch, 2014). These procedures rely on inter-item correlations or inter-item covariance matrices. Various factor analytic tools have evolved for this purpose. Validation of the internal structure yields evidence of the construct meanings and helps in devising scoring schemes linked to the validated structures. Consider a simplified example shown in Box 10.3.

Suppose, for developing the writing assessment in Box 10.3, the designers started with theoretical notions of what strong writing skills represented, such as clarity in communication, logical thought processes, and so on. Guided by that theory, they designed a 20-item assessment organized into five subdomains as shown, each intended to yield a separate score. They theorized about the interrelationships among the different subskill areas as well, expecting a higher correlation of the scores from the first two subdomains (I and II) than with the other three (III–V), and so on. All of these design-related assumptions suggested a hypothetical "latent" structure of the writing construct. This structure was then tested and validated with factor analysis.

In Box 10.3, the design of the assessment suggests a multidimensional internal structure, with five latent abilities expected to explain overall writing performance ability. Here, factor analysis methods could help verify the extent to which the variance of the item-level data, organized by subdomain, is explained by different mathematically derived factors, as hypothesized. Are the responses to each item set explained by a distinguishable factor, as expected? Are these latent factors intercorrelated, as expected? To justify the interpretability of each score, we would need evidence to support the proposed multipart internal structure.

BOX 10.3 Proposed Internal Structure of a Writing Skills Assessment: Subdomains, Items, and Scoring Scheme

Subdomains (item no.'s.)	Scoring scheme
I *Clarity of communication* (Items 1–5)	Score 1
II *Logical thought processes* (Items 6–9)	Score 2
III *Organization* (Items 10–12)	Score 3
IV *Correct use of grammar and language conventions* (Items 13–16)	Score 4
V *Correct use of punctuation* (Items 17–20)	Score 5
Writing skills domain (Items 1–20)	Total score

Different factor analytic methods are useful for exploring the properties of latent constructs with unknown structures in an open-ended manner, or for confirming a proposed, fixed internal structure of assessments. The methods are particularly well suited to assessments built with domain-sampling methods. For validating the scale structure of tests purported to measure unidimensional linear constructs, item response theory (IRT) models offer alternative (and sometimes better-suited) mathematical procedures.

E. Validity Based on Correlations with External Variables. The second type of validity evidence under Cluster II in Table 10.3 deals with verifying claims that an assessment's scores will correlate with, or predict performance on, other external measures and variables. The external variables could either be continuous or categorical grouping variables. The statistical procedures we use are usually correlation and regression, or variants of these techniques.

CONVERGENT AND DISCRIMINANT VALIDITY EVIDENCE

By definition, **convergent validity** studies yield concurrently gathered correlations on two or more instruments. The results confirm that instruments purporting to measure the *same* or *similar* constructs yield measures that intercorrelate positively to the degree expected. Conversely, results of **discriminant validity** studies verify that instruments intentionally measuring *different* constructs at the same time yield measures that do not correlate at all or correlate to a much lesser degree. Sometimes, measures may even be expected to correlate negatively, based on existing theory or past research.

Box 10.4 provides an illustration with tabulated correlations of subtest scores of an achievement test intended to measure verbal versus mathematics domains. In theory, the scores from the different verbal subtests should show strong convergent validity with each other, with strengths and directions of correlations consistent with the literature. Similarly, we should expect stronger convergence and higher correlations of the mathematics subtest scores. In contrast, we would expect the verbal subtest scores to show *much weaker* correlations with the scores of the mathematics subtests, giving evidence of discriminant validity.

These expectations are verified by Pearson's correlation coefficients in Box 10.4. See the values of .75 and 65 of paired mathematics subtests; a strong overlap in the underlying constructs is revealed in the high convergent validity coefficients. Why not an $r = 1$ for measures of the same construct? Recall that test scores are unreliable to some degree, due to random interferences. Furthermore, as math assessments are usually presented with some verbal instructions and question prompts, the degree of overlap shown is reasonable. Interpretations of two highlighted correlations from the table follow.

Pearson's $r =$ **.73**

Interpretation: This is a high correlation compared to the others shown. By calculating r^2, we find that the coefficient of determination is .53, indicating 53% overlapping variance in the two measures. This is an acceptable *convergent validity coefficient* for the reading subtests and likely supported by the literature.

BOX 10.4 Convergent and Discriminant Validity Evidence: Pearson Correlation Coefficients

Correlation Matrix

Subtest 1	2	3	4	5	6	Test no. and description
1.0	*.73*	.77	.49	.42	.61	1. Reading comprehension
	1.00	.69	**.38**	**.35**	.59	2. Vocabulary
		1.00	.39	.40	.58	3. Language skills
			1.00	*.75*	.60	4. Number concepts
				1.00	.65	5. Math computation
					1.00	6. Math problem solving

Note. *.73* Convergent validity evidence for two verbal tests; *.75* convergent validity evidence for two mathematics tests; **.35** discriminant validity evidence for a mathematics test and vocabulary test; **.38** discriminant validity evidence for a mathematics test and vocabulary test.

Pearson's $r = .35$

Interpretation: This is a relatively low correlation. The coefficient of determination is low at .12, indicating only a 12% overlapping variance in the two measures. This much lower but still positive correlation provides satisfactory *discriminant validity evidence* for two different construct measures, a math computation and a verbal vocabulary test.

Taken together, the convergent and discriminant validity evidence suggests that the mathematics and verbal assessments are measuring sufficiently different constructs, as intended, but cohere together in small amounts, as expected by the literature on similar measures.

PREDICTIVE VALIDITY EVIDENCE

Predictive validity evidence was discussed at length already, as defined in Section 10.2 and Table 10.1. These data require a longitudinal data-collection design. The data collected on the predictor and criterion measures must be *separated in time* for given groups of persons or entities. Interpretations are similar to other correlation coefficients.

CONCURRENT VALIDITY EVIDENCE

By tradition, a **concurrent validity** study is motivated by a desire to substitute an earlier version of a test with the new version and involves a correlation of the scores obtained from each *at the same time*. The term *criterion-related validity* is sometimes applied to refer to predictive validity and concurrent validity together. In terms of empirical design, convergent validity and concurrent validity studies are the same with data on both variables collected at the same time; in purpose, they are slightly different.

For example, the authors of the Vineland Adaptive Behavior Scales (VABS) gathered and reported concurrent validity evidence to convince their test adopters that the new version of the VABS yielded much the same information as the old test. For this, they had to show high correlation coefficients of scores from the two versions with concurrently gathered data on the same respondent group.

VALIDITY EVIDENCE OF GROUP DIFFERENCES

For some assessments, designers may want to demonstrate that the construct measures can reveal the theoretically expected differences between two or more *groups*. For example, to validate measures of a curriculum-based achievement test, a designer might examine if the average test scores of instructed versus uninstructed groups of examinees are significantly different in statistical terms. This finding would justify claims that the achievement test scores are sensitive to curriculum exposure and hence valid.

Box 10.5 shows another example. Here, the assessment purported to measure a construct that was expected to develop with age, with corresponding score increases. To validate the properties of the "developmental" measure, the study examined the differences in mean scores of children grouped by age (birth year). As compared to the youngest children, the validation hypothesis on group differences was confirmed in all the age groups, except for the group born in 1985. When added contextual factors applicable to each group were considered to interpret the results, it was found that this group included a high number of students with learning disabilities.

Group-based comparative studies require careful selection of individuals concerning the grouping attribute. Both univariate and multivariate group comparisons may be useful, accompanied by appropriate descriptive and inferential statistics. The grouping characteristic could be any relevant categorical variable, such as the respondents' neighborhood, institution, education level, age, race, or sex.

EVIDENCE ON THE LACK OF SYSTEMATIC MEASUREMENT BIASES IN GROUPS

By comparing the performance of selected minority and majority subgroups of the *same ability* on given items or construct measures, we could detect the presence of systematic measurement biases. Subgroup biases in measurement were illustrated and discussed briefly in Chapter 3. Issues investigated could include item biases in ethnic minority versus majority subgroups of examinees on achievement tests or prediction biases for male and female applicant groups on college entrance examinations. Although groups are compared, the logic guiding studies of measurement bias is reversed. That is, we look for systematic biases in the assessment results to rule out, correct, or mitigate the detected issues. This type of validity evidence is necessary for all high-stakes tests. Illustrations of item bias studies follow in Chapter 11.

10.4.2.3 Validity Evidence: Cluster III

The third cluster in Table 10.4 includes evidence necessary for validating various forms of derived or modified scores and securing consequential validity evidence (F–J). The following specific score types are treated separately: norm-referenced scores, criterion-referenced scores, composites, and grouped scores.

BOX 10.5 Validity Evidence of Group Differences by Age

Mean Scores on a Developmental Ability Test

	1986 (youngest)		1985		1984		1983		1982 and earlier	
Birth year	Mean	SD	Mean	SD	Mean	SD	Mean	SD	Mean	SD
Ability score	25.20	8.57	24.34	9.68	31.57	8.26	30.15	10.07	26.30	5.77
Group difference score (SD units)			**<u>–0.09</u>**		**+0.74**		**+0.58**		**+0.13**	

Note. SD, standard deviation units (rounded to 100th place). Group difference scores are shown in SD units compared to the youngest group. For example, for birth year 1984, Difference score = (31.57 – 25.20)/8.57 = +0.74.

For illustrations of each, the section refers to recently proposed uses of state-adopted standardized test data for educational accountability purposes (Gewertz, 2017). Issues with linked and equated test scores were discussed at length in Chapter 9; these are not revisited here. Before embarking on Cluster III validation efforts, the need for each form of validity evidence should be carefully evaluated. The same derived score investigations would not apply to every assessment design or use scenario.

BEST TIME TO COLLECT THE EVIDENCE

This evidence should be gathered *as applicable* to the proposed uses of each derived score type, and an extension of validity studies under Cluster II. For instance, in scenarios where users plan to use criterion-referenced test scores for placement actions with examinees, consider the evidence listed under G in Table 10.4.

F. Validity Evidence for Norm-Referenced Score Interpretations. Refer again to Chapter 9 on design criteria for norm-referenced tests and scores. Validating norm-referenced scores requires evidence of the quality and appropriateness of the norms, the standardization, and the score derivation procedures. These derived scores must be reliable, transparent, and easy for potential assessment users to understand, interpret, and use correctly. To further ensure meaningfulness, it may be necessary to ensure that the derived scores correlate with appropriate external variables, as expected (see the evidence listed under F in Table 10.4).

G. Validity Evidence for Criterion-Referenced Score Interpretations. Again, see Chapter 9. For validating inferences from criterion-referenced scores, ensuring the quality of the domains, indicators, and domain-referenced scores is a first requirement. The usability of the categorical scores and their correlation with external variables will further affirm the validity of the measures. Outside the reliability of domain and subdomain scores, we should also verify the consistency of any classification decisions using the cut score points. Standard-setting procedures for categorical placements of respondents must also be checked for soundness (see the evidence listed under G in Table 10.4).

H. Validity of Composite Scores. While not common, composite scores and their uses should be supported with appropriate kinds of construct validity evidence in practice settings. For a high-stakes example of a weighted multi-indicator index designed under the Every Student Succeeds Act (ESSA) for public school and school system evaluations, consider the composite scores developed by some states. To design school ranking systems for educational accountability purposes, these states statistically combined students' test score data with other school-level indicators of quality (e.g., number of board-certified teachers), attaching different weights to each (Gewertz, 2017). The evidence under H in Table 10.4 is listed to facilitate validation studies of such composite indexes.

With any multi-indicator index, questions could arise about both their validity and reliability for the intended inferences and uses. Transparency and usability of the composites for the intended primary users and other stakeholders also play an important role when high-stakes actions are desired. The defensibility of different indicators, the weights assigned to each, the statistical formulas for deriving composite indices, should all be examined and validated objectively (Chatterji, 2019).

I. Validity of Grouped Scores. Grouped scores from tests rarely distribute similarly to individual-level scores. Hence, separate validations are often necessary, particularly for summative decision-making purposes (Chatterji, 2019). How the scores of individuals are grouped may differ mathematically; these differences should be considered during validation. For educational accountability reports produced annually under ESSA (Gewertz, 2017), for example again, several states had proposed using aggregated percentages of students at different performance levels (Levels 1–4) on their adopted standardized test. In other studies, grouped mean scores by region are derived and used for evaluating the overall performance of regional education systems, such as for tests under the National Assessment of Educational Progress program (NAEP; see *The Nation's Report Card* at *https://nces.ed.gov/nationsreportcard*). The evidence listed under I in Table 10.4 applies to such validation studies.

J. Evidence of Consequential Validity. Lastly, the two questions listed under J in Table 10.4 could begin

TABLE 10.4. Types of Validity Evidence: Cluster III

Type of validity evidence	Typical validation questions	Sources of systematic error
F: Validity evidence for norm-referenced score interpretations Evidence showing the quality of norms, norms tables, and norm-referenced scores	To what extent . . . • . . . are the norms recent, relevant, and representative of the intended populations? • . . . were the norm-referenced scores derived using appropriate procedures? • . . . are the norm-referenced scores reliable, transparent, and user-friendly? • . . . do the norm-referenced scores correlate with performance in expected areas?	Irrelevant or outdated norms Nonrepresentative norms Improperly derived norm-referenced scores Misinterpretations or misuses of norm-referenced scores
G: Validity evidence for criterion-referenced score interpretations Evidence showing the quality of domain-referenced scores, cut scores, and standards	To what extent . . . • . . . are criterion-referenced scores meaningful with respect to the domains? • . . . are placements using cut scores reliable, transparent, and user-friendly? • . . . do the categorical scores correlate with performance in expected areas? • . . . were the criterion-referenced scores derived using appropriate procedures?	Poorly specified domains Poorly designed domain-referenced items or test Improperly set performance standards and cut points Misinterpretation or misuses of criterion-referenced scores
H: Evidence on the validity of composite scores Evidence showing the meaningfulness, reliability, and quality of composite scores	To what extent . . . • . . . are the data sources that define composite theoretically and logically meaningful and transparent? • . . . are the individual data sources valid and reliable? • . . . do the composite scores correlate with external variables, as expected? • . . . do the composite scores distribute as expected in the population units? • . . . are the composite scores reliable?	Poorly conceived composites Procedural or mathematical issues in deriving composites Nontransparent composites Misinterpretation or misuses of composites
I: Evidence on the validity of grouped scores Evidence showing the meaningfulness, reliability, and quality of grouped scores	To what extent . . . • . . . are the grouped scores reliable? • . . . do the grouped scores correlate with external variables, as expected? • . . . do the grouped scores distribute as expected in the population units?	Poorly conceived grouped scores Procedural or mathematical issues in deriving aggregates Misinterpretation, overinterpretation, or misuses of composites
J: Evidence on the consequences of assessment use Evidence showing that uses of construct measures have the expected positive impacts, without undue adverse consequences	To what extent . . . • . . . are the expected positive outcomes of using the assessment's results achieved for individuals, groups, or other entities? • . . . are there any unintended or harmful effects of using the assessment's results on individuals, groups, or other entities in the short or long term?	Unjustified actions with, or misuses of, assessment results Oversight of undesirable consequences for individuals, groups, or entities assessed

the evidence gathering for examining consequential validity. With recent COVID-19 testing, we have seen potent examples of positive health policy changes ensuing from the documented consequences of timely usage of COVID "home" tests. Although not called consequential validity studies, these epidemiological studies showed the positive effects of the *test–trace–quarantine* strategy for society at large in combating the disease (Kerr et al., 2021). Instead of widespread school and workplace closures, the test–trace–quarantine interventions altered the course of the disease prevention efforts, validating an expected positive consequence of using the at-home tests.

For all high-stakes uses of assessment results in fields linked to the social and behavioral sciences, similarly, we need to gather the *essential evidence* necessary to evaluate the expected consequences of testing. On occasion, there might be a "test–treatment" package as with the COVID-19 test that needs to be evaluated. These investigations could be conducted in the short or long term. Issues that might arise at the individual level, such as with examinees themselves, or at the group, organizational, or societal levels, should all be studied, including any differential impacts on specific ethnic or social groups.

QUICK RECAP: Three main clusters of validity evidence, labeled under A–J, should be considered during validation. Cluster I enables preliminary evaluations of tools and construct measures; Cluster II is necessary after the "final" instruments are ready; Cluster III is necessary for specific types of derived scores, or for consequential validity studies. Each type of evidence investigates particular sources of systematic error and should be thoughtfully rationalized for given instrument design or adoption situations.

Reflection Break 10.3: Objectives 2, 3, and 6

- See the case in Box 10.2. Identify the types of validity evidence you would seek if you were adopting Instrument A for use in that refugee camp setting. Provide a rationale for why each is *essential* and *relevant* to the assessment use context.
- Explain the difference between *content-based validity* and *face validity*. Which would you prioritize in your own assessment design scenario? Explain.
- Define the concept of *systematic errors* as threats to validity. Explain with an example.
- Think of an instrument design or adoption project. Select the types of *evidence* under Clusters I and II that you would prioritize, with a rationale for each. Would you need any under Cluster III? Explain.

10.5 Random Errors of Measurement and Types of Reliability Evidence

Reliability refers to the degree of consistency or reproducibility of an assessment's results under different conditions, given that construct measures will always have some random error. Even under the best of assessment conditions, random events could affect the reliability of the measures in various ways, such as (1) distractions in the assessment environment; (2) sudden occurrences, such as illness or fatigue of examinees during assessment; (3) changes in observer or examiner behaviors; or (4) sudden conditions that affect the item or assessment delivery systems (e.g., sudden computer malfunctions), and so on. Unlike systematic errors, random errors are unpredictable. In given testing scenarios, the test scores could either increase or decrease due to their influences.

10.5.1 Some Reliability Theory: True Score and Error Score Distributions

In classical test theory, the conceptualization of reliability rests on three assumptions associated with the notion of random errors of measurement in test scores and construct measures (Bandalos, 2018; Crocker & Algina, 2006; Stanley, 1971; *test scores* hereafter). First, we assume that each tested individual has a fixed amount of the measured characteristic, referred to as the "true score" for that person, *T*. Second, we hold that there will always be some degree of random error associated with the test score of a person, referred to as *E*. Third, we assume that a person's raw score, called the *observed score X*, is made up of two additive components: the *true score* and *error score*, as follows:

$$X = T + E$$

Examine Figure 10.3. The standard normal distribution shown mimics the distribution of any random variable. In this case, it is the hypothetical distribution of X for a person over repeated measurements on the same test. The curve shows the degree to which a person's observed score is likely to vary from its mean, the T, due to the influences of random error. Because of the random component in the test scores, if we were to make, say, 100 or more observations of the same person on a given test, the observed scores would distribute normally, as shown. The mean of this distribution would be equal to the person's true score on the measured characteristic, T.

The standard deviation of this normal distribution is called the standard error of measurement (SEM). The SEM is one indicator of test score reliability that can be estimated using the assumptions of normal curve theory. Using the areas under the normal distribution and an estimate of the SEM, as shown in Figure 10.3, it is possible to say that there is a 68% chance a person's T would lie between +/– 1.0 SEM. Or, that there is a 95% chance that one's T would lie between +/– 2.0 SEM, and so on.

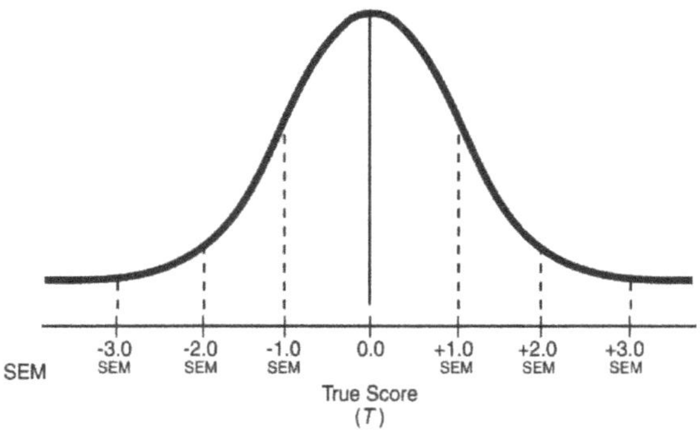

Hypothetical Distribution of a Person's *X* Scores Resulting from Numerous Repeated Measurements

$X = T + E$

There is a 68% chance that a person's *T* would lie between ± 1 SEM units.

There is a 95% chance that a person's *T* would lie between ± 1.96 SEM units (rounded to ± 2 SEM).

There is a 99% chance that a person's *T* would lie between ± 2.58 SEM units.

FIGURE 10.3. Normal distribution of errors of measurement.

Based on the T-, X-, and E-scores, there would be *three* respective distributions for each person in a given testing situation. Generalizing to multiple tested individuals, the variability estimates of these distributions would yield, respectively: the true score variance, observed score variance, and error score variance. Although the T-scores are unknown in any given test score distribution, the *variance of T-scores* can be obtained indirectly by subtracting the estimated random error variance from the observed score variance, using normal theory assumptions.

Two indices of score reliability, derived from the abbreviated presentation from classical test theory above, are the **standard error of measurement (SEM)** and the **reliability coefficient** $r_{XX'}$. The SEM is a measure of the expected variability in observed scores, X, that is due to the random error component E. The reliability coefficient reflects the extent to which variance in observed scores, X, reflects true score variance rather than error variance.

Mathematically, the reliability coefficient is the square of the correlation between observed scores and true scores and should be represented in pure form as r_{XT}^2. However, we do not commonly see the r_{XT}^2 notation for the reliability coefficient. Rather, the symbol is $r_{XX'}$. The derivation of the reliability coefficient, $r_{XX'}$ from the r_{XT}^2, requires an assumption of **parallel forms** of a test. Assuming that two tests are *strictly parallel*, the r_{XT}^2 formula can be shown to be the same mathematically as $r_{XX'}$.

Recall next the ideas from domain sampling theory discussed in Chapter 4. The $r_{XX'}$ refers to the correlation between the observed scores of two strictly parallel forms composed of items sampled randomly from a defined universe of all possible items. When test forms are strictly parallel, a given group of examinees will have the same true scores, and the error variance of both distributions will be equal. Using these assumptions, the reliability coefficient $r_{XX'}$ can be equated mathematically to the r_{XT}^2. It is the $r_{XX'}$ statistic that we find commonly reported in research, technical manuals of tests, and other measurement publications. It is the one we apply going forward. For more on the mathematical derivation procedures, see Crocker and Algina (2006).

10.5.2 Interpreting Reliability Coefficients

See Table 10.5 for four main types of reliability coefficients that we will consider. When investigating reliability empirically, we think about the $r_{XX'}$ as showing the correlation of the test scores from two strictly parallel forms of a test, sampled from the same domain or content universe. This yields a *parallel forms reliability coefficient*. For the other reliability coefficients, one extends this theoretical idea from parallel test forms built with equivalent item samples taken from a given universe, to "parallel" assessment conditions, "parallel" raters, or "parallel" occasions of assessment taken from a universe containing all possible items, conditions, raters, or testing occasions. Each reliability coefficient, described further in the next section, provides an estimate of the random sampling error we would encounter when we correlate data from items, raters, occasions, or conditions of testing sampled from those universes.

For any group of examinees, the reliability coefficient denotes the proportion of the variance in the observed scores, X, that is explained by the true scores, T. If the obtained $r_{XX'}$ is .98, we conclude that the influence of random errors is only (1 – .98) = .02 or 2%. Or, conversely, it indicates that 98% of the variability in observed scores is accounted for by the true scores of the respondents. Similarly, if a $r_{XX'}$ = .70 is reported, it indicates that 70% of the variability in the observed scores is accounted for by the true scores of respondents.

As a rule, the closer the reliability coefficient is to 1, the better the reliability level; reliability coefficients approaching or higher than .90 are considered very strong for most assessment purposes. Although there are no fixed rules of thumb for every possible situation, a reliability estimate that falls too far below .70 is considered unacceptable.

10.5.3 The Relationship between SEM and $r_{XX'}$

The reliability coefficient $r_{XX'}$ and the SEM are inversely related. Hence, when the reported SEM is high, the $r_{XX'}$ value will be low. Conversely, when the SEM is low, the $r_{XX'}$ value will be high. The relationship is mathematically represented as follows, with population parameters:

$$\sigma_e = \sigma_X \sqrt{1 - \rho_{XX'}}$$

The version of the formula given next applies to examinee samples:

$$s_X \sqrt{1 - r_{XX}}$$

SEM = the standard error of measurement
s_X = the standard deviation of the observed scores
r_{XX} = the reliability coefficient

Review the demonstration in Box 10.6. Here, two SEMs are calculated starting with two illustrative reliability coefficients of .60 and .95. They apply to two test score distributions with the same standard deviation of 5. As we see, the calculated SEM is three times greater when the reliability coefficient is lower at .60.

BOX 10.6 Relationship between Standard Error of Measurement and the Reliability Coefficient

Case 1

$r_{xx'} = .60$

$s_x = 5.0$

$$\begin{aligned} \text{SEM} &= 5.0\sqrt{(1-.60)} \\ &= 5.0\sqrt{.40} \\ &= 3.162 \checkmark\checkmark \end{aligned}$$

Case 2

$r_{xx'} = .95$

$s_x = 5.0$

$$\begin{aligned} \text{SEM} &= 5.0\sqrt{(1-.95)} \\ &= 5.0\sqrt{.05} \\ &= 1.118 \checkmark\checkmark \end{aligned}$$

10.5.4 Types of Reliability Evidence

In this chapter, we focus on four reliability coefficients that are most commonly reported and applied, as Table 10.5 shows. Each has a different purpose; that is, each coefficient attempts to evaluate the influences of random error from a different source when measuring the *same* construct domains in the *same* group of individuals. These are **test–retest reliability** for estimating random error influences related to two or more occasions of testing; **parallel forms reliability** for estimating errors related to responding to one or another parallel test form; **internal consistency reliability** for estimating the degree to which individuals respond consistently to all the items meant to measure the same construct domains; and **interrater reliability** for estimating random variances introduced through examiner, observer, or rater behaviors.

Table 10.5 suggests when to apply each reliability coefficient. Each is interpreted differently. We would need different research designs and data-collection procedures, which are addressed in Chapter 11. Conceptually, however, they all derive from the theoretical notion of sampling "parallel" items, forms, raters, occasions, or testing conditions randomly from an infinitely large domain or universe. Up to a limit, the larger the sample size of items or conditions sampled for an assessment, the higher will be the empirical reliability estimates.

For all assessment instruments, it is advisable to examine the internal consistency reliability. When resources permit, test–retest reliability levels of the scores that users will interpret are also desirable. A parallel forms reliability coefficient is necessary only for tests of the same construct domains designed with parallel forms or modalities, say, Forms A and B. That coefficient would indicate how unreliable the scores would likely be if examinees were to respond to Form A versus Form B. For performance assessments and tasks involving human raters or observers, interrater reliability coefficients should be estimated.

When examining reliability information reported in research articles or technical manuals of published instruments, we should heed the following:

- Different methods for obtaining reliability coefficients will yield different results. Hence, each must be interpreted as guided by its purpose. When more than one applies to an assessment situation, they should all be treated separately but evaluated together.
- The reliability coefficients are all correlation coefficients. These are group-dependent statistics, and the results may change depending on the composition of the groups used for estimation purposes and the variability of the test scores in that group. A narrow range of test scores could underestimate the reliability coefficients.
- Up to a limit, the greater the number of items, behaviors, or products sampled for building an assessment tool, the better the reliability estimates will likely be for the test scores produced.

TABLE 10.5. Different Types of Reliability Coefficients

Type	Purpose is to evaluate . . .	Applies to . . .
1. Test–retest reliability coefficient	The stability of measures in the same persons over short time periods of 10 days to 2 weeks	All assessments
2. Parallel forms reliability coefficient	The consistency of measures from two equivalent test forms with items from the same domain	Assessments with parallel forms or modalities
3. Internal consistency reliability coefficients	The degree of within-person consistency of responses to items sampled from the same domain	All assessments
4. Interrater reliability coefficient	The degree of consistency of ratings or scores given by different observers or raters to the same persons on the same tasks	All constructed- response or performance assessments

- Objectively scored assessments (e.g., multiple-choice tests) tend to be more reliable than more subjectively scored assessments (e.g., behavior- or portfolio-based assessments).
- The SEM estimates for examinees or respondents at different levels of a measured construct can vary, with SEM being higher at the extreme ends of a normal distribution of scores. Note that standardized test-makers generally report an *average* SEM estimate for all test-takers in their standardization or field-testing samples.

Table 10.6 shows that the validation demands would be dictated by the stakes tied to the decisions in any given user scenario. Taking Tables 10.3–10.6 together, we see that evidence on validity and evidence on reliability are *not* the same thing. We need both. If the assessment design process ensures the high validity of measures, chances are that we will also have high reliability. The reverse, however, is not necessarily true. That is, we could have high reliability in the results, but cannot be certain that the test scores are also valid without added evidence. It could be that we are assessing something unrelated to what we intended, but the assessment is yielding highly consistent results each time we use the tool.

TABLE 10.6. Validation Demands and Stakes Tied to the Decision

More convincing evidence is needed when . . .	
• Decisions are final. • Decisions are irreversible. • Decisions have lasting consequences for individuals, groups, or institutions. • Decisions are based on constructs that are not well understood. • Decisions depend heavily on results of one assessment tool.	*Examples of high-stakes or summative actions:* • Diagnosis of a serious health condition • Granting selective awards, college admissions, certification of professionals • Accreditation or accountability decisions for entities or persons
More limited evidence is sufficient when . . .	
• Decisions are reversible. • Decisions have less important impacts on individuals or entities. • Decisions have temporary effects for individuals or entities. • Decisions can be confirmed with other data and assessments.	*Examples of low-stakes or formative actions:* • Reteaching a lesson in school • Improving an intervention strategy • Improving processes, products, or services • Research and information gathering

QUICK RECAP: The concept of reliability is associated with random errors of measurement. The two main indices of reliability, derived based on classical test theory assumptions, are standard error of measurement and reliability coefficient. Reliability levels can be estimated using four different reliability coefficients in Table 10.6. Each examines a different source of random error and should be interpreted accordingly.

Reflection Break 10.4: Objectives 2, 4, and 6

- Define the following reliability concepts: true score, observed score, standard error of measurement, and reliability coefficient.
- In what ways are the evidence categories *different* for evaluating *reliability* versus *validity*? Explain.
- See the Case in Box 10.2 and refer to Table 10.5. Assuming you were adopting Instrument A in that setting, identify the types of *reliability evidence* you would seek. Provide a rationale for why your selection is *essential* and *relevant* to the context.

10.6 Utility of Measures, Assessments, and Assessment Systems

10.6.1 Two Components of Utility

The concept of **utility** is central to a user-centered design process (see Chapter 1). The concept has two components:

1. *Usefulness* refers to the intended benefits of using the assessments and the assessment's results as designed, for the primary users and relevant stakeholders of an instrument, including the test-takers or respondents, and any involved researchers, professionals, or the lay public.
2. *Usability* of the assessments, the raw scores and

any derived construct measures, applies mainly to the primary assessment users and refers to the practicality, transparency, and ease of use of these products.

For published and commercially distributed instruments, the notion of usability applies to any supplemental technologies, assessment materials or manuals, data systems, or reports that accompany the assessments and assessment systems. With all assessments, it is necessary to weigh validity and reliability factors against both aspects of utility.

Usefulness, as defined above, overlaps a good deal with the idea of consequential validity. See the evidence listed under J for Cluster III and the validation questions in Table 10.4. The intended benefits *are* a major part of the expected positive consequences of using a given assessment and its results. Recollect that potential users include the members of the tested populations, the decision-makers who take action with the results, and stakeholders in the larger assessment context who could be indirectly affected by the assessment applications.

Usability, the second part, again deals with feasibility and the practical aspects of applying the instruments. Time and resources available for conducting assessments are almost always in competition with other responsibilities. From a typical user's perspective, usability is perhaps the more important quality of an assessment or testing program, when compared to validity and reliability.

10.6.2 Factors That Influence Assessment Utility

See Box 10.7. Considered as a whole, the utility of assessments is determined by multiple factors, of which 10 are listed in the box. For self-designed or self-selected assessments, as mentioned, utility levels would be governed by time and resource demands associated with assembling, administering, interpreting, and using the data obtained from particular assessments according to the specifications. For standardized assessments, utility is affected by several added factors, including the accessibility, transparency, and built-in complexities of the print-, media- or technology-based materials, such as the items, assessment platforms, score types, and reports.

BOX 10.7 Utility Criteria for Assessments and Construct Measures

- Documentable benefits for respondents and primary users, in the short and long term
- Practicality of administration requirements
- Time, resources, and human and material costs
- Ease and efficiency of scoring procedures
- Ease in interpreting results correctly (applies to raw scores, derived scores and composites, and reports)
- User-perceived transparency
- User-perceived fairness
- User access to information
- Clear communication of built-in limitations of assessment and construct measures
- Timeliness of release of results to primary users

10.6.2.1 Administration Conditions

We should design or select assessments to optimize administration conditions for the primary users. Ease of administration deals with the simplicity and directness of the instructions, the length of time needed to administer the assessment, the completeness or availability of supporting materials needed for appropriate assessment administration, and the ease with which the procedures can be conducted. An assessment tool with high utility in administration conditions is one that relatively untrained or inexperienced individuals can apply with little or no obvious issues. A long cumbersome assessment, needing complicated materials and instructions, should be avoided as it could adversely affect both the validity and reliability of the results.

10.6.2.2 Time, Resources, Human, and Material Costs

Factors that increase the time demands, human and material costs, and other requirements for assessment resources must be borne in mind during assessment design or selection. The use of multiple-choice tests or surveys via online delivery systems today is more cost-efficient, with an instantaneous and wide reach.

For instance, performance assessment uses make high demands on instructional time in educational settings. Training of observers and scorers can also be burdensome and costly to sustain over time. When assessments require expensive equipment or expendable supplies that need replenishment, usability will be affected.

10.6.2.3 Scoring Procedures

One of the most burdensome, and often tedious, chores associated with assessment is scoring. As a rule, we should prefer assessment designs that offer both ease and speed of scoring without sacrificing the accuracy of scores. The assessment results must be defensible to test-takers and other users if questioned.

To the extent possible, assessments should be designed with provisions made for maximizing scoring utility. Developments such as computerized scoring, stencil keys, separate answer sheets, and improved directions for scoring significantly contribute to raising the utility of both structured response and essay tests today. The need for human scorers or judges in performance assessment applications, however, could present challenges to users.

10.6.2.4 Ease of Score Interpretation, Transparency, and Timeliness of Results

How easily and accurately the assessment's results can be interpreted and therefore used appropriately in particular user contexts, is of paramount importance. Clear and transparent communication is key. In any given assessment context, the success or failure of an assessment is a direct function of the interpretative accuracy and timely use of the assessment's results by the primary users. For assessments, the human user groups could include both professionals and nonprofessionals, such as classroom students, public participants in research studies, or members of organizations. Data on the *user-perceived* levels of ease of use, user-friendliness, and transparency of the assessments and reports, in such instances, can help improve utility during the design process.

In multilevel organizations where assessments are used, users at each level might have different information needs, with each interested in different kinds of test reports and test scores. For each, the test scores and any derived construct measures should be clear, transparent, and unambiguously presented. To prevent misuse, human users should be clear about the specific limitations of the tools and assessment results—the do's and don'ts when interpreting scores must be explicit.

10.6.3 Investigating Utility Issues

In theory, user-centered design should be informed throughout with *user feedback* in the areas just discussed. A user-centered design philosophy, prevalent in many technology and engineering fields today, places the users' capacities, limitations, needs, and desires at the center of the design process from beginning to end. These design principles are adopted in the Process Model in Figure 10.1 for designing assessments, which calls for iterative cycles of data gathering to improve the quality of tools and construct measures placing users first.

Typical methods for gathering data could include user surveys; direct observations of users in action at sites as they engage with the assessment materials; data reviews and data analytics with logged user information on computer-based or online assessment systems; human emotion studies; and analyses of "user flow," for example, examining whether the ideal flow of required assessment activities is achieved during application of the tools (Norman, 2013; Still & Crane, 2017).

As mentioned, several utility concerns surrounding the usefulness of assessments intersect with consequential validity issues and user perceptions of fairness (Table 10.4 under Evidence Cluster III; see Chatterji, 2013a, 2013b). Consequential validity studies on the short- and long-term benefits of assessment uses could be evaluated with causal path diagrams called *logic models.* These research designs are also referred to as *program theory-guided evaluations* (Henry et al., 2019).

By tradition, standardized and commercial testing programs in education and psychology rarely place assessment utility on a par with the validity, reliability, or scaling properties of tests. Potential assessment user groups are infrequently, if ever, included during the design process. Most human adopters and users of assessments, however, must work within their own personal and professional limitations and practical constraints. Hence, oversights of usefulness and usability are inadvisable, and sometimes undermine the larger goals of assessment programs.

QUICK RECAP: Utility has two parts, dealing with the *usefulness* (benefits for user groups) and *usability* (ease of use and practicality) of assessments and construct measures for various human user groups. Involving users actively in the design processes could help address the factors affecting utility levels of tests and measures. Gathering user feedback and studies of consequential validity could mitigate or avert possible negative outcomes of assessment uses for different individuals or user groups.

Reflection Break 10.5: Objectives 2, 4, and 6

- See the case in Box 10.2 again. If you selected and were adapting Instrument A in that setting, which design factors would you prioritize to maximize *utility*? Explain.
- With an example, describe some ways in which the *validity* or *reliability* of construct measures can be undermined when we ignore or overlook utility issues.
- Do you agree that *consequential validity* and *usefulness* could be examined with the same questions and evidence? Explain.
- Create a utility checklist to improve the quality of assessments for *primary users* in an assessment project or scenario.

10.7 Unified Validation Plans

10.7.1 Validation Specifications

We now return to Figure 10.1, at the top of the chapter, that offers an evidence-based procedural framework for evaluating construct validity guided by unitarian principles. The body of evidence in Phase IV, A and B, combines validity, reliability, and utility comprehensively, but it should be *limited by* the prespecified context of assessment use. To narrow the body of evidence sought, we need to specify the inferences and uses that users intend with the construct measures in Phase I (*Why?*). In Phases I and II (*How?*), existing theory and knowledge should come into play when we operationalize the constructs. These steps, consistent with the unitarian view of validity, will assist in framing appropriate validation questions.

Added "user-centered" requirements unique to the Process Model are important:

- Identifying the *primary users* of the assessments and their desired purposes for the assessment (*Why?*)
- Specifying the population, the population units, and their socioecological contexts (*Who?*)
- Clarifying the specific score types and construct measures to be validated (*What?*)

As the measure-based inferences would apply to only the population units we specify, we must be clear—Are these units the individual respondents, groups, or organizational entities, or more than one? We also need to be clear about *which* construct measures will be validated—Do the *score types* include the raw scores, derived scores, grouped or composite scores, or more than one? Field testing of the instruments and gathering and evaluating appropriate kinds of evidence would apply to these *validation specifications*.

Second: *How much validity evidence is enough?* Table 10.6 provides guidelines for tightening validation goals to secure and evaluate the most relevant and essential evidence. Review these against Tables 10.2–10.5 and Box 10.7. Some evidence is minimally necessary even for informal applications of a new or adopted instrument (e.g., content-based validity, internal consistency reliability, and basic usability). Added evidence categories should be selected with judgment. How much, and which types, would depend on the assessment purposes, stakes tied to decisions, and resources available to carry out the work. More convincing evidence is necessary for irreversible, high-stakes decisions; less will suffice for decisions that have lower stakes with reversible consequences for respondents, researchers, or stakeholders. On occasion, a complete redesign of a tool may be necessary when the measures fail to perform as intended in a new context.

10.7.2 A Unified Validation Plan

To create a unified validation plan, we need to address the following needs:

- *Validation questions.* State the questions to guide the evidence-gathering and evaluation procedures.
- *Type of evidence,* Identify the categories of validity, reliability, and utility evidence necessary to claim the overall construct validity of the measures to be used.
- *Rationale.* State why the evidence is essential to justify the inferences for those particular uses of the measures.

For a concrete application, consider this scenario next in tandem with Table 10.7:

> A global technology corporation employs a mental ability test to select the top 16% of candidates every year from its job applicant pool. The corporate leaders wish to interpret and use the normalized standard scores (z-scores) produced by the subtests and overall test for this purpose. The cut point for identifying candidates is a z-score = +1 on the overall test score distribution. Once recruited, candidates are matched to specialized jobs around the world based on strengths they showed on the raw scores of different subtests.

What are the major parameters to consider in order to devise a plan? Here, the *primary users* in the scenario are the applicants themselves and the corporate leaders, with the latter making the recruitment decisions. The *score types* to be interpreted and used are the normalized z-score for recruitment decisions and raw subtest score profiles for matching recruits with jobs. Candidate selection using the standard scores is a high-stakes decision that could affect both the candidates and organization. Relatively, using subtest score profiles after recruitment for job matches carries lower stakes. The sociodemographic and ecological profile of the population units, the individual candidates here, is relevant for validating the measures. Lastly, we know that the leaders intend to make both predictive and content-based inferences from the standard scores and raw scores.

Given the above, review the proposed validation plan in Table 10.7. Each type of evidence is selected and rationalized. Refer back to Tables 10.3–10.6 and Box 10.5 for details on each evidence category. In every instance where instruments are adopted or designed, however, it is necessary to weigh the time and resources available to execute the proposed validation plan appropriately.

TABLE 10.7. Unified Validation Plan

Validation questions	Evidence	Rationale
To what extent do the standard scores predict future job performance of applicants?	Predictive validity	Ensures the validity of inferences on the examinees' potential to succeed in the workplace and supports the high-stakes selection decisions.
To what extent do the items in the subtests cover skills that match the jobs in our organization?	Content-based validity	Ensures subtest scores match the key indicators of domains of job performance.
What is the quality of the standard scores, given the norms and norming procedures reported by the designers?	Quality of norm-referenced scores	Ensures validity of comparative inferences and decisions made with norm-referenced scores.
What levels of reliability are reported for the total test and subtest scores that will be interpreted and used?	Test–retest reliability	Ensures the scores are replicable over short time periods, with tolerable margins of error.
Is the assessment easy to use, cost-effective, and practical? Are the scores understandable to decision-makers and examinees?	Usability	Ensures utility of the assessment and results for the primary users.

A closer review might reveal gaps in the validation table shown, which could be revised with stakeholder feedback. For example, we might ask: Why is there no study on the reliability of the selection decisions? What about evidence of consequential validity, confirming the benefits of recruitment, or negating any possible adverse consequences? Why is there no examination of possible measurement biases, given the global diversity levels in the population? These are legitimate validation questions that could be added and evaluated.

QUICK RECAP: For any given user scenario, unified construct validation plans address the most important validity, reliability, and utility concerns that might be raised. Plans can be improved with stakeholder participation. The focus should be on the *relevant* score types and population units. The actions hinging on the assessment's results should dictate the essential categories of evidence included in the plan.

Reflection Break 10.6: Objective 6

For an assessment situation of your choice, develop a unified validation plan. Delineate the questions, evidence, and rationale to address validity, reliability, and utility concerns together.

10.8 Summary

This chapter discussed validation theory and different kinds of evidence necessary to claim validity, reliability, and utility of construct measures holistically, situated in assessment user contexts. It recommended a unitarian approach to construct validation, with scientifically rigorous studies that are also practical.

Depending on the user contexts, validation could focus on the raw scores, derived scores, grouped scores, composite scores, or other score types. The proposed uses could involve either low-stakes or high-stakes decisions. One or more population units may be the focus of the desired inferences. For each of these, a different combination of evidence might be necessary.

The chapter organized validity evidence (A–J) under three major clusters. It identified four main classes of reliability evidence and two broad classes of utility evidence. These evidence categories are not interchangeable. Before beginning validation, we should use judgment to make situation-specific selections.

To keep validation efforts manageable, the essential types of evidence must be carefully rationalized. Multipurposing existing assessments beyond their originally intended functions, oversight of built-in limitations, and major gaps in the existing evidence will increase the validation burden in new user contexts. Guided by the Process Model, the chapter provided an example of a unified validation plan.

CHAPTER 11

Empirical Methods of Validation

11.1 Chapter Overview

11.1.1 Introduction

Chapter 11 focuses on *selected* methods of validation guided by the unitarian framework and is intended to build skills in conducting empirical validation studies and critically reviewing published technical information on tests and assessments. The chapter extends concepts introduced in Chapters 8–10 and is lengthier than others. Readers are encouraged to reread different sections and, as necessary, take advantage of the hands-on practice and reflection exercises. Refer to more advanced textbooks and journal articles to broaden backgrounds on particular topics (see citations in the introductions to Chapters 8–10).

Figure 11.1 shows where Chapter 11 topics fit with the rest of the book and the Process Model. Validation occurs in Phase IV, with evidence evaluations following in Phase V. Redesigning and refinements continue until the instrument and construct measures meet the specifications set forth in Phases I and II (see Figure 1.4).

11.1.2 Chapter Objectives

After reading this chapter and completing the accompanying exercises, the reader should be able to:

1. Implement a *unified validation plan* guided by a user-centered rationale, validation questions, specific types of evidence, and appropriate empirical methods.
2. Gather, analyze, and interpret selected kinds of *validity evidence*, namely, evidence on item functioning, content-based validity, validity of response processes, validity of the internal structure, convergent and discriminant validity, and predictive validity.
3. Gather and interpret selected kinds of evidence on *perceived fairness* and *measurement bias.*
4. Gather, analyze, and interpret selected types of *reliability evidence*, namely, internal consistency reliability, test–retest reliability, parallel forms reliability and interrater reliability, reliability of cut scores, and domain scores.
5. Gather, analyze, and interpret *selected types* of utility evidence.
6. Evaluate the evidence holistically in predefined contexts of assessment design, adoption, and/or use.

11.2 Planning Empirical Validation Studies

Validation always requires empirical investigations, with the nature of the measure and the form of validity dictating the needed form of evidence.

—JUM C. NUNNALLY AND IRA H. BERNSTEIN (1994, p. 84)

Empirical investigations lie at the heart of a unified validation exercise. The term *empirical* refers to information obtained through verifiable observations or experiences, as opposed to theory or pure logic. In all instrument design or adoption situations, the evidence

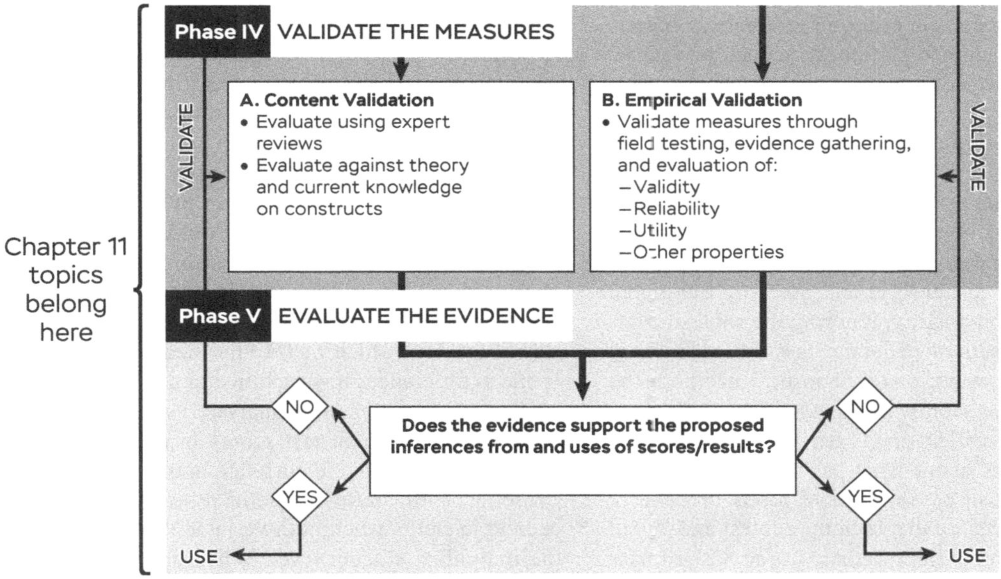

FIGURE 11.1. Connecting Chapter 11 to the Process Model and the rest of the book.

gathering, analyses, and evaluations should be guided by a well-conceived **validation plan**.

To set the stage, we begin with a review of the validation planning process, building on the initial components of a plan introduced in Chapter 10. We then examine a published validation study of an existing self-report survey, the Pittsburgh Sleep Quality Index (PSQI). That work suggests how the planning and empirical aspects of a unified validation effort could be approached (Beaudreau et al., 2012). Sections 11.3–11.9 that follow next, elaborate on the empirical methods identified in the chapter's objectives. In Section 11.10, we revisit the PSQI validation study again to evaluate the evidence in light of the methods discussed.

11.2.1 A Quick Look-Back: Validation Planning with a Unitary Framework

When applying a unified validation approach, the assessment user context is key. The goal is to collect only the requisite amounts and kinds of empirical evidence to justify the measure-based inferences and uses desired by the primary users of a tool. The selected validity, reliability, and/or utility evidence must be obtained systematically, integrated, and then evaluated meaningfully in the specified user contexts. Both quantitative and qualitative research methods could be useful for this purpose (Figure 11.4; Chapter 1; see also AERA et al., 1999, 2014).

11.2.2 Before Validation: Four Issues to Resolve

As a part of the validation planning, and before we begin the investigations, it is necessary to clarify four issues with regard to the focal construct measures that we wish to validate. Refer to Phase I in Figure 11.1, as we review these essentials.

1. **Clarity about the construct(s) we desire to measure and the score types that must be validated:** Along with the major constructs of interest to the assessment users (specified in Phase I), we need to identify the different "score types" to be validated. These could be, for instance, (1) the raw scores for a total test or scale, (2) the raw scores for any subscales that could apply, and/or (3) one or more derived scores. Remember that derived scores could include specific kinds

of norm-referenced or criterion-referenced scores, weighted or unweighted composite scores, or various mathematically scaled or transformed scores (Chapters 8 and 9).

Suppose we designed a competency assessment for certifying psychologists in a higher education context, and the assessment yielded five separate *subtest scores* and a *global score*, the latter obtained by summing the subtest scores for a person. As the educator-designers, we could decide to interpret and use only the global scores for decision making, ignoring the subtest information. Other users of the same assessment, such as prospective employers, could choose to use both the subtest and global scores. In this scenario, both score types should be validated guided by the underlying construct theories about what each different score is supposed to measure. Appropriate kinds of validity evidence would ensure that both the subtest and global scores are accurately interpretable in the desired user contexts.

2. Clarity about the specific uses and also the primary users of the assessment results: The "uses" deal with specific actions to be taken with assessment-based information. The primary users and the specific uses they plan with the scores are essential and corollary pieces of information. To keep the validation process efficient and manageable, it helps to limit the focus to the *highest-priority* uses projected for an assessment tool.

In small-scale or local projects, the primary users of the assessment results could be the designers, researchers, or professional practitioners themselves. With more complex undertakings, relevant users could fall into several user groups, such as other researchers, organizational leaders and workers, teachers, employers, policymakers, examinees, students, patients, or clients and their families. Identifying only the *main* assessment users or user paths keeps the validation procedures within reasonable boundaries. Chapter 2 identified eight typical **user paths**.

3. Clarity on the levels and units of analysis where the assessment results will be interpreted: Related to the two previous issues, the population units (e.g., individuals, groups, or organizational units)—elsewhere called the *units of analysis*—must also be clear during validation planning. The validity evidence we gather and analyze must be appropriate for the units to which the desired score-based inferences and uses would apply. In the professional certification example, the individual psychologists-in-training are the population units.

As we identify the relevant units of analysis, we should be alert to any differences in interpretive implications at the different levels. Ample research today suggests that the empirical relationship among any two measured constructs can vary significantly in size and sometimes direction, depending on the units of analysis and levels at which we take the measurements. This is due to differences in variability, or dispersions of the measures at a given unit of analysis. For instance, standardized achievement test scores in grade K–12 settings are documented to correlate in the order of about .30 to .40 with commonly defined measures of socioeconomic status when both variables are measured at the individual student level. When aggregated at the school or school district levels, these same variables correlate in the range of .60 to .70 (see American Psychological Association, 2007; Reardon, 2016; Sirin, 2005).

Furthermore, the measure-based interpretations often change in different population units (Chapter 2). For example, school-level test score aggregates typically serve as proxy measures indicating the quality of the schools, whereas test scores of individual students indicate their levels of achievement in a given curricular domain in an academic year. It is important to bear these differences in mind during validation planning.

4. Clarity on the stakes tied to assessment uses and their potential consequences: Finally, clarity on the stakes tied to the planned score-based decisions also assists in framing the validation plans and specifying the evidence necessary. Every assessment use carries with it some "stakes" tied to the results, varying from very low and relatively inconsequential, to very high and consequential. Implicit in every assessment use is also the assumption—subject to verification—that applying the instruments and measures will benefit the tested individuals, groups, and organizations involved, or improve some societal conditions (Chapters 1 and 2).

It is prudent to limit the body of validity evidence to the most necessary kinds; the stakes to be tied to the assessment results could inform these choices. Any possible adverse consequences of testing should also be considered concurrently (Messick, 1989). This clarity is especially necessary for the higher-stakes assessment uses. In particular, we should seek compelling evidence that potentially *negative* outcomes of assessment uses are minimal and resolvable in the intended decision-making contexts.

Certification testing in the opening example involves high-stakes uses of test scores, with occupation-related consequences that could manifest in the short or long term. Assuming there could be disabled individuals or diverse minority groups in the tested population, it is important to evaluate systematically whether there were any differential outcomes with undesirable social consequences for some subgroups of examinees or related stakeholders.

11.2.3 An Illustrative Validation Study: The Pittsburgh Sleep Quality Index Survey

Now, consider an actual validation study to which we will apply the preceding four criteria. Validation studies on particular instruments all have implicit, if not declared, validation plans. In the following study, the focal measures are different scores from the Pittsburgh Sleep Quality Index (PSQI), an instrument developed earlier by Buysse, Reynolds, Monk, Berman, and Kupfer (1989). A new team of researchers revalidated the PSQI measures subsequently, with a focus on racially diverse subpopulations of women (Beaudreau et al., 2012). This work, as we will see, reflects several elements of a unitarian approach. This section first describes that published validation study in some depth and then discusses what a guiding validation plan for the effort might have looked like. Readers are encouraged to read the original work by the authors for added details.

11.2.3.1 The PSQI Case Description

WHAT WAS THE STUDY'S PURPOSE?

Research shows that sleep disorders and disturbances become more prevalent as adults age. The authors' purpose was to revalidate the PSQI scores for making sleep-related clinical inferences in elderly Black and White women of age 70+ years living in community dwellings. For the study, the authors analyzed a preexisting dataset from a national osteoporosis study. The revalidation was necessary at the time, according to Beaudreau et al. (2012), because past research on the PSQI had focused mostly on middle-aged adults and males. Specifically, the authors aimed to fill gaps in the existing evidence base on the validity and reliability of the PSQI scores in older Black women living in community dwellings. In addition, they desired to examine normative, descriptive data on important sleep-related, demographic, and health indicators in Black women as compared with their same-aged White counterparts.

WHAT WAS THE ORIGINALLY DESIGNED PSQI TOOL AND WHAT WERE ITS STATED PURPOSES?

The PSQI is a 19-item self-report survey for adults (Buysse et al., 1989). Respondents rate the quality of sleep on selected indicators based on their subjective perceptions and recall. Each item is self-rated on a 4-point Likert-type scale, indicating the frequency of sleep-specific behaviors or experiences (0 = Not at all, 3 = Three or more times a week). While the tool was originally designed for use by psychiatrists and clinicians with adults in the United States in mind, it has been used widely since in both the United States and overseas settings.

In theory, the PSQI global score is intended to denote subjective perceptions of overall sleep quality, with each of the seven subscale scores reflecting, in order: subjective sleep quality, sleep latency, sleep duration, habitual sleep efficiency, sleep disturbances, use of sleeping medication, and daytime dysfunction (Buysse et al., 1989). The original authors suggest an overall PSQI cut score of 5 to identify individuals at "high risk" of health issues.

WHAT WERE THE MAIN RESULTS AND CONCLUSIONS OF THE REVALIDATION?

See Box 11.1 and refer back to relevant parts of Chapters 8–10 to interpret the statistics, as needed. Empirical methods for each type of evidence are discussed in the sections to follow.

For their intended score-based inferences in the ethnic subsamples, the authors gathered evidence on (1) **norms**, with descriptive statistics on the PSQI

BOX 11.1 Evidence on PSQI Scores in Elderly Black and White Women

I. Internal Consistency Reliability and Subscale Homogeneity

	Cronbach's α total sample	Cronbach's α White women	Cronbach's α Black women
PSQI global scores	0.72	0.72	0.74
Adjusted subscale score to global score correlations			
Subscale 1: Sleep quality	0.62	0.63	0.59
Subscale 2: Sleep latency	0.53	0.53	0.51
Subscale 3: Sleep duration	0.47	0.47	0.51
Subscale 4: Sleep efficiency	0.53	0.53	0.51
Subscale 5: Sleep disturbances	0.38	0.37	0.45
Subscale 6: Sleep medications	0.38	0.28	0.29
Subscale 7: Sleep daytime	0.24	0.23	0.27

II. **Correlations of PSQI's Global Score with External Variables**[a]

	ESS	Daytime inactivity	Total sleep time	Wake after sleep onset	Apnea–hypopnea index	GDS	Mobility
Spearman's r	***.11***	***.05***	–.02	***.14***	.03	***.31***	***.18***
Statistical significance*	*<.001*	*.01*	.34 Not significant	*<.001*	.55 Not significant	*<.001*	*<.001*

*$p < .01$ for statistical significance.

[a]Scales: PSQI, Pittsburgh Sleep Quality Index, higher scores indicate worse sleep quality; ESS, Epworth Sleepiness Scale, higher scores indicate greater sleepiness; GDS, Geriatric Depression Scale, higher scores indicate more depressive symptoms; Mobility, Mobility/Instrumental Activities of Daily Living, higher scores indicate better functioning.

Source: Reprinted with permission from Beaudreau et al. (2012). Copyright © 2012 Elsevier Science & Technology Journals.

scores and other measured health indicators; (2) **internal consistency reliability** of the PSQI total and subscale scores; and (3) the **convergent** and **discriminant validity** of PSQI total scores with a number of external variables. As the first row in Box 11.1 shows, the internal consistency reliability coefficients of the global scores stood just above the minimum acceptability cut point of .70 in the separated subsamples of White versus Black women and the combined sample (Cronbach's α; see Chapter 10). The study reported results on another homogeneity index, the *adjusted subscale-to-total score correlation*, showing that all the subscale scores were correlated in the range of .23 to .63 with the overall PSQI score.

Added convergent and discriminant validity evidence confirmed many of the authors' hypotheses. The so-called actigraph mentioned in their summary below yields measures of a person's measured activity levels (Beaudreau et al., 2012, pp. 39–42):

> Multiple measures were significantly associated with poorer sleep quality, as measured by the PSQI total score, such as greater daytime sleepiness . . . ($r = 0.11$); greater actigraphic wake after sleep onset ($r = 0.14$); and actigraphic daytime inactivity ($r = 0.05$). We also observed associations in the expected directions between the PSQI and non-sleep measures, including greater depressive symptoms (GDS; $r = 0.31$), a known correlate of sleep disturbance. . . .

The normative data from the study are not shown here, but results suggested that using separate norms for the ethnic subsamples might be more appropriate for making comparative score interpretations with the PSQI's scores. The Black participants in the dataset were, on average, slightly younger than their White counterparts, with higher rates of smoking, diabetes, heart and pulmonary disease. When a PSQI cut score of >5 was used, there were higher rates of Black women with poor sleep quality than White women. These differences were statistically significant with less than 1% error.

11.2.4 Devising a Validation Plan for the PSQI Study

What would be the essential parts of a unified validation plan for the PSQI study? See Table 11.1 in conjunction with Box 11.1 now. A first step would be to specify the contextual parameters addressing the assessment use context in detail, as follows (see Section 11.2.2 and Figure 11.1).

The PSQI "Assessment Use" Context: Phase I of the Process Model

- *What?* **Construct:** Subjective perceptions of sleep quality
  - **Score types to validate:** Global PSQI score and subscale scores, PSQI-1 to PSQI-7
  - **Score-based inferences:** Self-perceived sleep-quality levels
- *Why?* **Assessment purposes:**
  - **Specific uses:** Clinical research and screening for poor sleep quality and sleep disorders, and preliminary classifications of "at-risk" versus "not at-risk" individuals
  - **Primary users:** Clinicians, medical staff, and researchers
  - **Stakes tied to score-based uses:** Moderate to high
- *Who?* **Population:** Older women in the United States; specifically, Black and White women age 70 and older living in community dwellings
  - **Population units for making inferences:** Individual women with the above sociodemographic and ecological characteristics

11.2.4.1 Parts of the Validation Plan

Given the context specifications, we can turn to the core parts of a validation plan for the study. See the headings displayed in Table 11.1, which is built retroactively. A complete validation plan should include validation questions, (selected types of) evidence, empirical methods, and a rationale for each question to be investigated. The plan in Chapter 10 incorporated only the questions, evidence, and rationale; Table 11.1 now adds the fourth key part: empirical methods. Reviewing Box 11.1 and Table 11.1 together, now consider each part separately.

VALIDATION QUESTIONS

We find that the authors investigated four main issues in the revalidation effort, with attention to the global scores mainly as the focal construct measures. Although not labeled as "unitarian," the study integrated several different categories of evidence in the two ethnic subpopulations of interest, guided by the validation questions. The excerpted evidence in Box 11.1 suggests that the validation focus was mainly on the global PSQI scores, with some information reported on subscale scores. If used and interpreted, *all* eight score types would need validation.

EMPIRICAL METHODS AND EVIDENCE

To address the empirical components of a validation plan, assessment designers and researchers could draw from a wide array of optional research designs and psychometric procedures. The selected empirical methods could look significantly different for new instrument design efforts, as opposed to a revalidation study. The PSQI study illustrates the use of a preexisting, multivariate dataset from the prior study conducted with a survey research design. Hence, the revalidation represents a "secondary analysis" of that data.

Different empirical methods, as we will see, have their advantages and disadvantages. The choice of appropriate methods, how effectively each is deployed, along with the trustworthiness of the evidence reported on relevant measures, count equally when evaluating the results of a validation study. The evidence produced could be solid and trustworthy in segments, while less compelling in others.

TABLE 11.1. Validation Plan: Investigating the Pittsburgh Sleep Quality Index (PSQI) Scores

Validation questions *To what extent . . .*	Evidence	Empirical methods	Rationale
1. . . . are PSQI global scores correlated with selected external variables?	Convergent and discriminant validity	*Research design:* Survey research—Secondary analysis of a subsample of adults *Psychometric analysis:* Spearman's rank order and Pearson correlations of PSQI global scores with selected variables	To verify construct-relevant hypotheses about the PSQI scores, as consistent with theory
2. . . . are PSQI score distributions similar in Black and White women? Is the combined group's composition suitable for norm-referenced inferences of the PSQI scores?	Norms and normative distributions	*Research design:* As above *Psychometric analysis:* Descriptive data distributions of PSQI scores and selected variables in Black and White subsamples, and combined group	To ensure meaningful comparative interpretations of PSQI scores
3. . . . are PSQI global and subscale scores reliable?	Internal consistency reliability	*Research design:* As above *Psychometric analysis:* Internal consistency estimates of PSQI scores (Cronbach's alpha)	To ensure within-person consistency of PSQI scores in combined sample and subsamples
4. . . . are the PSQI subscale scores correlated, as expected, with the adjusted PSQI global scores in the sample?	Homogeneity of PSQI subscale and global scores	*Research design:* As above. *Psychometric analysis:* Adjusted subscale to PSQI global score correlations	To examine within-person consistency of subscale and total scale scores and domain sampling assumptions

VALIDATION RATIONALE

The contextual specifications and evidence-gathering plan need some rationalization during validation. For executing this step, refer back again to the four criteria discussed in Section 11.2.2. A justification for each type of evidence proposed is desirable.

A main driver for the PSQI revalidation study appears to have been clinical research and health screening uses of the scores in specified subpopulations of women. In such contexts, medical researchers, health care providers, and community professionals are the most likely primary users of the measures. Were the proposed uses of the PSQI scores "high stakes"? Screening older adults for sleep disturbances and sleep-related health problems (especially older women in ethnic minority groups) could carry high stakes with several serious consequences. Less valid inferences, or improper uses of the PSQI results, could lead to errors in screening health needs, or perhaps oversights of other health issues. Applied research, on the other hand, carries far lower stakes. All such matters need due consideration during the rationalization process.

11.2.4.2 Next Steps

Once a validation plan is in place, empirical studies must follow. The validation options generally fall under one or more of the Evidence Clusters I–III, and reliability and utility evidence categories presented earlier in Chapter 10.

QUICK RECAP: Empirical methods are a core component of all validation plans and must be selected with judgment. Unified validation plans integrate pertinent kinds of validity, reliability, and/or utility evidence on the focal construct measures of interest to the primary assessment users. For feasibility, validation studies should focus on the highest user priorities. A number of qualitative and quantitative research designs and psychometric methods could be useful, each with strengths and limitations.

Reflection Break 11.1: Objective 1

Refer to the PSQI revalidation case description to answer these questions.

- What is a *focal construct measure* in a validation effort? Why is it important to identify the focal construct measures prior to validation planning?
- Think of a new instrument that you might design. What would be the major components of your validation plan? Specify the assessment uses and user context first, addressing the four criteria described in Sections 11.2.2 and 11.2.3.
- From a unitarian perspective, list any *strengths* and *limitations* of the PSQI validation plan presented in Table 11.1, such as any omissions or unclear areas. Explain.
- Give an example of a validation scenario where *more than one score type* should be investigated. Explain.
- Give an example of a validation scenario where investigations should be carried out on *more than one population unit*? Explain.

11.3 Evaluating Item Performance

We begin with item analysis methods, introduced under Evidence Cluster I in Chapter 10. This section details quantitative item analysis methods applicable to *three* item types, namely, (1) structured-response items for designing norm-referenced tests (NRTs); (2) structured-response items for designing criterion-referenced tests (CRTs); and (3) rated items and tasks for designing survey-based, performance-based, and other assessments. The methods are illustrated with multiple-choice and self-report items and fall broadly under classical test theory (CTT). All the computations shown can be performed with standard statistical analysis software packages in the social sciences, such as SPSS, SAS, or Systat.

11.3.1 General Procedures for Item Analysis

11.3.1.1 Purposes of Item Analysis

The main purpose of item analysis is to ensure that items function optimally according to the instrument's purposes and design specifications. The methods should be combined with careful evaluative judgments to help diagnose the causes for item malfunctioning, including any early signs of item bias. Qualitative data gathering from respondents *after* item analysis could assist in gaining insights into these causes.

11.3.1.2 When to Do It?

As item analysis falls under Evidence Cluster I, item functioning should be investigated early in the assessment design or selection process. In a best-case scenario, item evaluations would be initiated concurrently with or soon after a preliminary content-validity screening of the initially drafted items. Any item flaws detected should be addressed before the assessment instrument is compiled in final form.

11.3.1.3 The Item Analysis Sample

To begin item analysis, we need to select an appropriate *item analysis sample* of typical respondents. From this sample, two or more comparison groups may be further selected for computing and evaluating specific item statistics. The statistics could be generated separately for each subgroup to be compared, or for the combined group, consistent with the assessment's purposes. The specific procedures and statistics differ depending on the purposes of the assessment.

11.3.1.4 Item Analysis Statistics for Structured-Response Items

For multiple-choice or structured-response items, there are two main statistics: the **item difficulty index** (p_i) and the **item discrimination index** (D). Alongside, we should also perform a **distracter analysis**, involving a review of the response data distributions in the optional answer categories. The descriptive results of all three procedures are evaluated together.

The item difficulty statistic, p_i-value, is the proportion (%) of examinees who select the correct or keyed response option to a multiple-choice item. The p_i-values could range from 0 to 1, corresponding to 0% to 100% of the examinees answering an item correctly. The higher the p_i-value, the easier the item, and vice versa. Item difficulty levels alone provide only a partial picture of item functioning; hence, item discrimination statistics D should be considered in unison.

The D-value shows how well an item is able to distinguish between groups that are *known* to be at different levels on the measured construct. Logically, each item is expected to reveal the differences between individuals documented to be in different subgroups.

A well-designed item should perform *above* or *well above* a "chance level" based on the p_i-value. A chance level is when the examinees' responses are governed largely by random factors rather than systematically learned knowledge or abilities in the tested domains. The chance level would be 25% for a four-option multiple-choice item, 20% for a five-option item, and so forth. For example, a four-option achievement test item with a p_i-value in the neighborhood of .28 (28%) would be performing barely above the chance level. When the item p_i-value is close to the random level, the item is probably too difficult or obscure for most. Such results call for a reexamination of both the items and the characteristics of test-takers. Is the item content, wording, or presentation problematic? Did respondents meet the designer's assumptions with respect to backgrounds and past preparation levels in the domains tested? Are the item's distracters functioning as intended? Did random factors generate the small number of correct responses, or were identifiable variables at play?

Finally, a well-written multiple-choice item should have effective distracters, the incorrect foils (Chapter 5). With well-performing distracters, the correct answer is not an obvious "give-away" to examinees. Rather, the options contribute to an effectively performing item that separates individuals who have a good grasp of the domains tested from those who have partial knowledge, no knowledge, or other confusions. In any tested domain, the weaker examinees should be drawn to the item distracters.

11.3.1.5 Item Analysis Statistics for Rated Items

For rated but structured items, such as Likert-type items, item analysis involves examinations of various **descriptive statistics** of the item-level data and *homogeneity indices*. These statistics could be useful for evaluating all item types, including multiple-choice items.

Homogeneity indices provide insights into the extent to which the data generated by each item or subscale correlate with the data obtained from the remaining items that define a test or scale. As the items are purposefully designed to tap into different dimensions of the same construct (according to domain sampling theory), the correlations should be positive and reasonably strong. The variance in the data obtained from each item or subscale is expected, by design and in theory, to contribute to the variance of the total scores.

There are two main homogeneity indices for evaluating the functioning of items or subscales. The first is the adjusted item-to-total score correlation $r_{\text{i-tot}}$ and, analogously, we could apply an adjusted subscale-to-total score correlation $r_{\text{s-tot}}$. For example, the PSQI study employed the $r_{\text{s-tot}}$ statistic for examining inter-subscale homogeneity (Box 11.1).

In essence, the $r_{\text{i-tot}}$ index is obtained by correlating each item's scores with the total scale score, by adjusting for each item under investigation. (That is, by correlating the data from an item or subscale with the total scores computed *minus* that data.) For items yielding binary (0/1) response data, the correlational statistic is a point biserial coefficient; when items yield ordinal data, a Spearman's rank-order correlation or Kendall's tau is appropriate; and finally, with continuous variables, a Pearson correlation coefficient is applied (Chapter 8).

Another homogeneity index is the *squared multiple correlation* (SMC). Here, we would remove the particular item under investigation and examine how well the other items that define the test, scale, or subscale predict that item's scores. This is performed with a multiple regression procedure, with the item in question serving as the dependent variable. When squared, the multiple correlation coefficient is interpreted as the percent of variance in the item variable explained by the other items.

11.3.2 Item Analysis for NRT Design

Now, let's turn to item analysis procedures for building NRTs. Refer back to Chapter 9 for the general design requirements for NRTs. Suppose we are constructing an NRT with multiple-choice items to measure an achievement domain. To facilitate norm-referenced score interpretations, the objective would be to maximally spread out the test scores of the examinees. To support this basic function, each item should also demonstrate similar properties; that is, individually, well-functioning items should discriminate adequately between individuals at the highest and lowest levels on the overall measures, yielding positive D-values.

11.3.2.1 Steps in Item Analysis

There are five procedural steps for item analysis that apply for both NRT and CRT construction purposes, with qualifications for selecting the comparison groups and interpreting results, as follows:

1. Administer the test to an *item analysis sample* comprising a group of typical test-takers.
2. Select two subgroups from the item analysis sample for comparison. For designing NRTs, these should be the highest- (H) and lowest-performing (L) subgroups based on the total score distribution; usually, we select the top and bottom 25%, 27%, or 33% of the total sample. For CRT design purposes, we select specifically designated examinees belonging in the master and nonmaster, pre- and post-instruction, or expert versus novice categories.
3. Calculate the item p_i-values and D-values.
4. Interpret the item p_i- and D-values.
5. Evaluate the item statistics in conjunction with a distracter analysis.

11.3.2.2 The Item Analysis Sample and Comparison Groups for NRTs

The item analysis sample is obtained by administering the items (or the entire test) to a small group of 30–100 typical examinees from the specified population. A "typical" sample for an item analysis study should meet the basic requirements of the assessment context outlined in Phase I (Figure 1.4). For appropriate sample selection, we should refer back to the purposes, population characteristics, and construct specifications. When measuring achievement, for example, the item statistics would be more meaningful when examinees are reasonably prepared to take the test items; by definition, achievement is a measure of performance after curriculum-based instructional delivery (see Chapters 3 and 5).

For NRTs, the item analysis sample is broken down further into two comparison groups representing the *extreme segments* of the test score distribution to form "high" and "low" subgroups. Traditionally, large-scale NRT projects select the top and bottom 27% of a test score distribution, leaving the middle group out (Allen & Yen, 2002). Makers of many published achievement tests report using the top and bottom 25%, 33%, or 37% of test-takers or even the entire dataset for item analysis (see, e.g., Pearson, 2017). The most relevant information for NRT construction is obtained from the high and low groups; hence, the extreme group selection is deliberate.

A number >30 for the overall item analysis sample is ideal for obtaining adequate variability in the response data and statistics that remain stable across samples. Standardized test designers often conduct item analysis with extremely large samples of respondents (e.g., test developers of the Smarter Balanced Assessment Consortium [SBAC] report $N = 23{,}000$; see CRESST, 2017, 2018). Such large numbers are unnecessary for most assessment projects.

11.3.2.3 Calculating and Interpreting Item p_i and D Statistics for NRTs

See Tables 11.2 and 11.3 next. The formulas for computing the statistics are given at the bottom of the former. For NRTs, the item difficulty p_i is given by $p_i = (P_H + P_L)/N$, where the P_H and P_L terms refer, respectively, to the proportions in the high and low groups selecting the correct answer and N is the total number of participants in the item analysis sample. Item D is given as a difference between P_H and P_L.

Table 11.2 breaks down the response data for an item with five options. The correct answer is Option 4. The high and low comparison groups, each with $N = 10$, represent the top and bottom thirds of the test-taking sample. This item shows desirable properties for an NRT with a p_i of .65 and a D of +.50. The item p_i-value for the high group is .90, indicating 90% answered correctly, compared to a p_i-value of only .40 for the low group. Hence, we have a robust and positive D of +.50. The latter indicates a 50% difference in the estimated

TABLE 11.2. NRT Item Analysis Data for a Five-Option Multiple-Choice Item

				Correct answer (Option 4)		
	Answer Options:					
Item A	→ 1	2	3	4	5	Omit
High group (H)	0	1	0	***9***	0	0
Low group (L)	1	4	1	***4***	0	0
$N_H = 10$						
$N_L = 10$						

Note. Calculation: High group $p_H = 9 \div 10 = .9$
Low group $p_L = 4 \div 10 = .4$
Mean p_i-value $= (p_H + p_L)/2 = (.9 + .4)/2 = 1.30 \div 2 = \mathbf{.65}$
D-value $= p_H - p_L = .9 - .4 = \mathbf{+.50}$

item difficulty in the two groups, consistent with NRT design expectations. Another good sign is that no one omits the item.

The table enables a distracter analysis. Comparing the frequency of responses in each answer category, we find that Option 2 is functioning better as a distracter than the others. Option 5 is ineffective as it draws no respondents. The overall data show that the incorrect answers are generally attracting more examinees from the low group, a desirable pattern.

For item analysis statistics with greater variation, see Table 11.3 next with results on six items of a test. Here, the two extreme subgroups of $N = 25$ were selected of a total of 100. The bottom and top quarters were placed in the low and high groups, respectively. Assuming that the advanced group had greater opportunities to learn, we find the expected differences in the p_i-values for Items 2, 4, and 5.

TABLE 11.3. Item Analysis Results on Six Structured-Response Items

	Item difficulty (p_i)		
Item no.	Low group (beginner students) $n = 25$	High group (advanced students) $n = 25$	Item discrimination (D)
1	*0.64*	*0.26*	*−0.38*
2	***0.35***	***0.88***	+0.53
3	*0.91*	*0.92*	*+0.01*
4	0.48	0.68	+0.20
5	0.43	0.68	+0.25
6	**0.92**	**0.48**	*−0.44*

Note. Total group $N = 100$.

Looking at Item 2 more closely, we find the p_i-value for the advanced group is .88, as compared to only .35 for the beginner group, yielding a strong D of +.53. The p_i of .35 is sufficiently above the .20 chance level for a five-option item, and as expected, the item is much easier for the advanced group. This item meets the logical expectations of NRTs.

On the other hand, Item 3 in Table 11.3 appears too easy for both groups with p_i-values >.90. A D-value of 0.01 further indicates that Item 3 is not differentiating between the high and low groups. Too many items on NRTs with these properties would not meet the design specifications.

Lastly, Items 1 and 6 in Table 11.3 show *negative* D-values, with a reverse distribution of responses in the comparison groups. This result is problematic and points to inherent problems with the items that contradict the logical assumptions of NRTs. Possible causes could be that the item measures an opposing construct that reverses the item information for high and low groups. At other times, a negative D-value points to highly ambiguous items that have no correct answer or where an incorrect answer choice appears correct to large numbers in the high group. Incorrectly scored responses could also produce negative item D-values, such as a miscoding or use of an incorrect answer key. Generally, negative D-values are undesirable.

11.3.2.4 Distracter Analysis for NRT Items

For NRT construction purposes, as mentioned, good item distracters should attract more members in the low group. In Table 11.2, the item has the expected response distribution sorted by distracter, with the exception of Option 5. The difference in the low and high groups is clearly evident in Option 4, the correct answer. Deleting Option 5 would likely retain the item's properties with little loss of information.

Item omission issues could indicate that an item is of a prohibitive difficulty level, outside the domain specifications, too confusing, or placed toward the very end of an overly long or difficult test that many cannot complete. Elsewhere, it could point to limited time allocation for a test overall, or built-in issues of bias, such as an inflammatory bias in the language that causes item avoidance.

11.3.2.5 Actions after Item Analysis

Box 11.2 offers some general "rules of thumb" for interpreting item analysis results for designing NRTs. Good judgment is key to effective application of these guidelines, with thoughtful attention to other relevant information on the test. For example, if the assessment is purported to measure an achievement construct, the data for item analysis should be collected after instruction is delivered. In general, the items included in an NRT should have a near normal distribution of item difficulty levels with a median p_i-value of around .50 and positive D-values.

11.3.3 Item Analysis for CRT Design

Recall that a CRT is purposefully designed to assess domain-referenced competence and sometimes competence in very specific skill areas or subdomains (Chapter 9). CRTs are typically used in educational or training contexts, with the emphasis placed on mastery attainment rather than rank ordering or sorting of candidates. The characteristics of the comparison groups we select for item analysis must therefore change accordingly. Well-functioning items on a CRT must show sensitivity to instruction and to mastery or expertise levels of examinees.

11.3.3.1 Steps in CRT Item Analysis

See Table 11.4 and the five steps given in Section 11.3.2 for NRTs. We would apply the same steps for performing item analysis with CRT items, with an important change in the selection of the item analysis sample and comparison groups. To interpret the results meaningfully for CRT design purposes, groups compared must differ clearly on their mean proficiency levels in the tested domains.

BOX 11.2 Item Analysis Guidelines for Designing Norm-Referenced Tests

Item statistics	Interpretation	Actions
Item p_i-value range: .40 to .75 Median p_i of all items: ~.50 D-value range: ≥ +.10 to +.50 Answer options show expected response distributions.	*Desirable items*	Keep items.
Item p_i-value range: >.75–1.00, with many >.90 Item D-value range: 0.0 to +.10	*Items tending toward easy or too easy*	Keep items. Revise distracters to raise item difficulty levels.
Item p_i-values of ≤.40 Item D-value range: ≥ +.50 Answer options show some unexpected response distributions.	*Items tending toward difficult or too difficult*	Consider item revisions. Drop highly difficult items.
Item p_i-values equal to or close to "chance" levels Item D-values negative or 0 Items omitted by many respondents	*Poor and problematic items*	Drop or reexamine items for issues. Revise items.

11.3.3.2 Group Selection and Research Designs for CRT Item Analysis

A comparative one-group design to evaluate CRT item performance utilizes the same group of participants twice, tested on the items first at a pre-instruction stage, and again at a post-instruction stage. The assumption is that the group would have little or no mastery of the domain prior to instruction, on average, and that level would reverse following instruction.

Alternatively, we could compare item performance in two distinct groups that are *known* to be different, such as experts and novices in a domain (Berk, 1984a). With the two-group design shown in Table 11.4, we could select instructors or graduates of an educational program as the "experts" (masters), with new student enrollees as "novices" (non-masters). The items must be administered to both groups concurrently. Criteria for executing sound experimental designs apply to both one- and two-group item analysis studies. The goal is to isolate the performance of individual items in the selected groups. Hence, the research design should attempt to control for possible confounding effects of various other external variables on item performance (Babbie, 2020; Best & Kahn, 2016) such as practice and previous item exposure.

11.3.3.3 Computing and Interpreting Item Statistics for CRT Design

Other than the differences in group selection and logic for CRT design, the general computation steps for item p_i-values, D-values, and distracter analysis are similar to those discussed for NRT design purposes. For CRTs, the item difficulty p_i is given by $p_i = (P_M + P_{NM})/N$, where the P_M and P_{NM} terms refer, respectively, to the proportions in the master and non-master groups selecting the correct answer and N is the total number of participants in the item analysis sample. Item D is given as a difference between P_M and P_{NM}.

TABLE 11.4. CRT Item Analysis Data for a Five-Option Item

Answer Options: →	1	2	3	4 (Correct answer, Option 4)	5	Omit
Masters group (M)	2	3	2	***30***	3	0
Non-masters group (N-M)	10	6	7	***8***	2	7
$N_M = 40$						
$N_{NM} = 40$						

Note. Calculation:
Masters group $p_M = 30 \div 40 = .75$
Non-masters group $p_{NM} = 8 \div 40 = .20$
Mean p_i-value $= (p_M + p_{NM})/2 = (.75 + .20)/2 = .95 \div 2 = \mathbf{.43}$
D-value $= p_M - p_{NM} = .75 - .20 = \mathbf{+.55}$

Table 11.4 displays the calculations and results of a CRT item analysis with a two-group comparison method, using master (M) and non-master (NM) groups. The item difficulty notations are p_M and p_{NM}. The groups have $N = 40$ in each, with Option 4 being the correct answer. Item $p_{i(NM)} = .20$, Item $p_{i(M)} = .75$, yielding a robust positive $D = +.55$. All the distracters appear to be functioning effectively. A small item omission rate is evident in the NM group only (7/40 = 17.5%); however, this issue is absent in the M group, as expected. It is reasonable for a few individuals in the NM group to omit items that are too difficult. Although the combined group's mean p_i is shown, it is not as relevant for decisions on CRT construction; instead, for assembling the best-functioning items, a clear difference in p_i-values in the M and NM groups is necessary.

11.3.3.4 Actions Based on CRT Item Analysis

Box 11.3 offers some general guidelines for CRT construction. As before, these interpretive criteria should be employed with judgment, accounting for other factors in the assessment context.

CRT items with D-values of 0 are not ideal. Undifferentiated group selection for CRT item analysis purposes could confound the interpretation of D-values. The response distributions on item distracters should also meet the assumptions of CRTs, with larger numbers of the proficient group choosing the correct answer with the nonproficient attracted to the item foils.

Distributions of item p_i statistics obtained from the proficient/master candidates may be negatively skewed, in contrast to the p_i-values of items for NRTs that often distribute normally. Negatively skewed p_i distributions suggest that a majority of the examinees are highly proficient on most of the items. This result is consistent with the design assumptions of CRTs. In educational practice, we expect CRTs to be administered at points when students reach high levels of competence in the domains measured.

BOX 11.3 Guidelines for Criterion-Referenced Tests: Interpreting Item Difficulty and Discrimination Statistics

Item statistics	Interpretation	Actions
Item p_i-value range: ≥ .70 to .99 Item D-value range: ≥ +.30 Expected response pattern differences clearly favoring proficient groups	*Desirable items*	Keep items.
Item p_i-values unexpectedly high (e.g., for non-mastery group, the expected $p_i = .25$, obtained ≥ .70)	*Items tending toward easy or too easy*	Reexamine and revise items. Ensure item performance is dependent on competency level.
Item p_i-values show no difference in groups. Item D-values 0 or lower than expected. Items with negative D-values (e.g., expected $D = +.50$, obtained $D = +.05$, or $D = -.23$)	*Poor or problematic items*	Drop items. Reexamine and revise items. Revise group selection methods for item analysis. Revamp instruction in educational contexts.
Item omissions	*Several possible issues*	Review items. Detect and correct issues.

Negative D-values point to issues and possible item design flaws. The typical defects are testing of very obscure or complex material unmatched to the domain specifications; poor item presentation formats, graphics, supplements, or directions; use of confusing or ambiguous language; and issues of item bias.

11.3.4 Item Analysis Using Item Response Theory Models

Although outside the scope of this book, specific item response theory (IRT) models are helpful in selecting items ordered on a unidimensional continuum based on their estimated difficulty and/or discrimination levels. These procedures impose strict requirements of a selected mathematical model on the item data, allowing determinations of the extent to which the data "fit" that model. When there are adequate levels of fit, we can claim that the ordered items collectively measure a dominant construct scaled along a singular line. Variations of the one-parameter logistic model—-called the Rasch model—are popular in many large-scale test design programs. The Rasch mathematical model, applicable to cognitive and noncognitive assessments, specifies that all the items will increase progressively by their estimated difficulty levels while maintaining similar levels of discrimination (Wright & Masters, 1982; Wright & Stone, 1979).

For a brief example of an application with the Rasch model (after Wyer & Chatterji, 2013), think of designing a competency test to be scaled on a single construct continuum, like a measure of height. After the items are administered to a group of typical examinees, results on the item difficulty estimates and item "fit" statistics are evaluated. The difficulty estimates enable ordering of items on a linear scale, with the item fit statistics showing the degree to which the items meet the statistical criteria of similar discrimination. Items that fail to meet the mathematical criteria set for adequate fit can be flagged, along with items of different difficulty levels not adequately separated from the others. Most Rasch software programs report an item separation reliability statistic, indicating whether their separate locations on the scale continuum are better than chance. Reexaminations, revisions, or deletions of these items then follow.

11.3.5 Item Analysis for Rating Scale Data

Item analysis methods for Likert-type or rating scale items rely on selected descriptive statistics and homogeneity indices with item- and scale-level data described in Section 11.3.1. These item types are typically found in instruments measuring noncognitive, social, health, or behavioral constructs, such as items of the PSQI. Rated items may also be found on constructed response or performance assessments of cognitive or skill-based cognitive domains (Chapters 5–7).

11.3.5.1 Item Analysis Statistics for Likert-Scaled Items

In Table 11.5, we see item level and total scale data from a survey of "attitudes toward vaccinations" of college-going students (Ganguly & Banerji, 2000). One item is shown as an example.

Descriptive statistics on four of the 15-item attitude scale are displayed. The mean of the total scale score is 45.8, with a variance of 34.69. At the item level, the statistics vary. Items 1, 3, and 4 have means ranging from 3.29 to 3.34, with variances from .302 to .369. In comparison, the mean for Item 2 is lower at 2.68, with twice the variance at .608. Such a difference sets Item 2 apart. In the extreme right-hand columns, we see the degree to which each item contributes to the variance of the overall scale score. Removal of Item 2 brings down the total score variance from 34.69 to 29.09, a considerable drop. Given that the item is making the largest contribution to the variability of the total scale score, we would retain such an item.

The adjusted item-to-total score correlation $r_{i\text{-}tot}$ for Item 2 further supports the above decision. It is positive and robust +.47, suggesting that the item is homogeneous with the rest of the items. All four items have satisfactory $r_{i\text{-}tot}$ values ranging from +.37 to +.51. Although not reported, the SMC values for the items corresponded similarly, lying in the range of .42 to .63.

TABLE 11.5. Item Homogeneity Statistics for Four Self-Report Items

An example of an item from the 'attitude toward vaccinations" scale:
*I am willing to take the hepatitis B vaccine.** 1 2 3 4 5
SD—D—U—A—SA

A: Descriptive Statistics on Item-Level and Scale Scores

					Scale score minus item	
Item no.	Item mean	Item variance	Scale score mean	Scale score variance	Adjusted mean	Adjusted variance
1.	3.34	0.336	45.80	34.69	42.46	31.02
2.	2.68	0.608	45.80	34.69	43.12	29.09
3.	3.29	0.369	45.80	34.69	42.52	30.78
4.	3.34	0.302	45.80	34.69	42.46	32.05

B: Homogeneity Index

Item no.	Adjusted item-to-total score correlations *(minus item)*
1.	.51
2.	.47
3.	.50
4.	.37

*SD, Strongly disagree; D, Disagree; U, Uncertain; A, Agree; SA, Strongly agree.

11.3.5.2 Interpreting $r_{i\text{-tot}}$ and SMC Statistics and Suggested Actions

We should aim to retain the smallest number of items that yield sufficiently unique information while adding to the construct validity and reliability of the measures. Items with poor homogeneity statistics should be flagged for reviewing possible issues with the content, wording, response options, or format.

The acceptability cut point for $r_{i\text{-tot}}$ values is usually +.20; ideally, the item values would lie in the range of +.20 to +.70. Very high $r_{i\text{-tot}}$ values for a large number of items—in the region .90 to .99—could suggest item redundancies. Items that fall too far below the +.20 minimum or approach 0 do not adequately "fit" the rest of the items defining the scale. Dropping the latter items may improve the homogeneity levels of the overall scale, simultaneously raising the internal consistency reliability of the scores.

Negative $r_{i\text{-tot}}$ values are undesirable and, like negative *D*-values, indicate questionable item properties. Typically, those items yield information that is opposite to that produced by the others. The exception is an item that is reverse-oriented by design, for example, negatively worded items inserted to control for socially desirable responses. Otherwise, the content, structure, and language of items with negative $r_{i\text{-tot}}$ values should be critically reviewed for revisions or possible deletions.

The SMC for a given item denotes the percent of variance in that item's scores that is explained by the remaining items of the scale. SMCs in the region of 0.30, for instance, would indicate that 30% of the variance in the item's response data is explained by the remaining items. SMCs of 0.30 or higher suggest desirable levels of item homogeneity.

11.3.5.3 Homogeneity Indices, *D* Statistics, and Internal Consistency Reliability

The adjusted item-to-total score correlation is conceptually and empirically a close relative of the item discrimination index *D* and internal consistency reliability indices in Section 11.8. These statistics are all variations of correlation coefficients (Chapter 8).

To obtain the *D*, we establish the high versus low groups based on the total scores and ask: Is this item separating respondents in the same direction as the total score, with the highest scorers tending to answer the item correctly, with low scorers failing to do so? Essentially, with the $r_{i\text{-tot}}$, we ask the same question: Are individuals with the highest total scores also placed at the highest level in the item response distribution, and vice versa? To obtain internal consistency reliability coefficients, such as Küder–Richardson formula 20 (K-R 20) and Cronbach's alpha (α), we would ask: Do the items, taken one at a time, place examinees consistently in the same rank order (from high to low) as the total test scores?

QUICK RECAP: Item analysis procedures assist in selecting items with the desired statistical characteristics, guided by the assessment purposes. The assessment design requirements alter the specific approaches for group selection and comparison for item analysis with CTT methods. Homogeneity indices and descriptive statistics with data from items, subscales, and total scales are useful in evaluating the assumptions of domain sampling theory for either rated and binary-scored items.

Reflection Break 11.2: Objective 2

- Distinguish between the following concepts: *item difficulty*, *item discrimination*, and *distracter analysis*. For which item types and constructs are these applicable? Why is it necessary to interpret the statistics together? How do the procedures differ for NRTs and CRTs?
- Explain the concepts of *item homogeneity*, *subscale homogeneity*, *adjusted item-to-total score correlation*, and *squared multiple correlation*. How are these concepts related to *domain sampling theory*? When would you apply each? Give an example of an item analysis application of each.
- The item analysis results for two multiple-choice items are shown below. Interpret each statistic and evaluate the results. What is the "chance level" of each item? What actions would you take for each item? Explain.
  - Item 1 for constructing an NRT, with three answer options: p_H =. 74, p_L = .33, D = +.41
  - Item 2 for constructing a CRT with five answer options: p_M = .20, p_{NM} =.45, D = –.25

- Item analysis results for two Likert-type items from a psychological scale are given below. Interpret each statistic and evaluate the item. What actions would you take for each? Explain.
  - Item 3: $r_{\text{i-tot}} = .55$, SMC = .37
  - Item 4: $r_{\text{i-tot}} = -.05$, SMC = .04

11.4 Examining Fairness and Measurement Bias

This section presents methods that we could employ to investigate issues of perceived fairness and statistically determined bias in items and overall assessments. It limits the discussion to (1) objective reviews of items and overall instruments for issues of perceived fairness, sensitivity, and bias; and (2) conducting differential item functioning (DIF) studies. Both fall under Evidence Cluster 1; other bias investigations, such as group-specific predictive biases, fall under Evidence Cluster II (Section 11.7; see also Chapter 10).

- **Why investigate perceived fairness, bias, and sensitivity issues?** Investigations of measurement bias and fairness assure stakeholders that eventual inferences and actions taken with the measures are backed by evidence of a *lack* of statistically determined or perceived biases toward specific minority individuals or groups (e.g., minorities in demographic, special needs, or disability groups). Generally, fairness and bias investigations should be carried out for all assessments designed for diverse or global populations, especially when intended for high-stakes decisions. The aim should be in removing or mitigating the observed biases. For example, builders of standardized assessments aiming to test international test-takers should incorporate bias and fairness investigations in their validation plans (AERA et al., 2014).

- **What is bias in measurement?** Different types of **measurement bias** can affect the validity levels of the construct measures. In a widely accepted definition, "bias in tests and testing refers to construct-irrelevant components that result in systematically lower or higher scores for identifiable groups of examinees, who are otherwise of similar levels on the measured construct" (AERA et al., 1999, p. 76; 2014). The sources of measurement bias serve as systematic interferences in measuring the construct. Usually, the issues are linked to oversights in specifying the populations, such as specific sociodemographic and ecological characteristics of minority individuals and special groups that present barriers to these individuals during testing (Chapter 3).

- **What is fairness in assessments?** The literature separates the notion of "fairness" from measurement biases. Fairness is viewed as a social construct. Albeit related to measurement biases, it is without a technical or formal definition in measurement (AERA et al., 1999, p. 74). Regardless, as assessment designers, we must be diligent that respondents, users, and stakeholders do not *perceive* unfairness or bias, especially with high-stakes assessment uses.

11.4.1 Investigating Perceived Sensitivity, Fairness, and Bias Issues

11.4.1.1 Purpose

The goals of perceived fairness, sensitivity, and bias studies are to try to identify (and correct) issues inherent in the language, presentation, or content of the individual items or the overall instrument. The items, tests, and supporting materials should not be perceived as overtly biased toward any individual respondents, specific groups of respondents, or other stakeholders.

11.4.1.2 Methods

To conduct perceived bias and fairness investigations, survey research and interview methods could be employed, as well as group consensus methods (Chapter 4). For example, studies could involve *cognitive interviews* of respondents/test-takers and the primary users probing into any culturally influenced interpretive issues or perceived biases in the assessment's content, language, or formats. Section 11.6 describes cognitive interview methods.

Perceived fairness and bias reviews could also be performed by external experts. As an extension of content validation reviews (described in Section 11.5 next), we could add reviews by cultural experts of sensitivity, bias, and fairness issues. Experts we select to conduct bias reviews must have a trained eye for detecting sensitive sociocultural issues and potential perceptions of unfairness, including inadvertent but real barriers to equitable assessment for specific individuals/groups.

11.4.1.3 Typical Questions

Questions guiding perceived fairness, sensitivity, and bias studies could be the following (see also Chapters 5–7):

- *Materials-related barriers.* Could some individuals or groups be unfairly treated during the assessment procedure compared to the rest, due to limited or no access to required technologies, materials, or support systems?
- *Unequal access and opportunity.* For achievement testing, do the items or overall assessment measure content (knowledge or skills) to which all groups of test-takers *may not* have had equal exposure and opportunity to learn?
- *Inflammatory issues.* Compared to the majority, could any items or parts of the assessment inflame (disrespect, anger, offend, or otherwise upset) some respondents, showing a so-called inflammatory bias? For example, inflammatory issues could be related to self-identified gender, disability, culture, race, or native language.
- *Lack of necessary accommodations.* Could any disabled or diverse subgroups be treated differently during assessment by oversight of, or lack of accommodations of, a physical or language barrier?
- *Appearance of unfairness or bias.* Could any part of the assessment appear unfair or biased toward a minority individual or subgroup? Could some feel less favored, compared to others?

11.4.2 Investigating Differential Item Functioning

11.4.2.1 Purpose

A **differential item functioning (DIF)** analysis is a type of item analysis for statistical detection of biased item performance in selected subgroups of participants. Once detected, thoughtful evaluations should follow to revise or delete the items, considering various background factors. Follow-up interviews with respondents and/or primary users can help in understanding reasons for observed DIF patterns. Refer back to Chapter 3 for a concrete illustration of a DIF analysis, describing how to interpret the results.

In contrast to expert reviews and user-perception surveys, DIF procedures examine the extent to which a given item on an assessment yields significantly different outcomes in two or more groups that are otherwise at the *same level* on a measured construct. For instance, we could ask: Do members of a minority or disadvantaged group have the same chances of succeeding on an item as those in the majority group, given that they are of equal ability levels? Both CTT and IRT methods exist for investigating DIF questions.

11.4.2.2 Methods

The procedure begins by collecting data from a field test of the assessment items and comparing how each item performs in a *focal group* versus a *reference group*. The focal group is suspected of being affected by a systematic barrier to item performance, usually due to the interference of race, gender, language, culture, or a disability condition unrelated to the construct. The reference group comprises respondents or test-takers without the same barriers. Both groups are initially matched to be similar in ability, based on either the total scores or other ability estimates from the assessment. DIF is then investigated for each item separately, by comparing the item statistics in each group. Typically, we look for statistically significant differences in the estimated item difficulty levels for the focal versus reference groups. Several alternative DIF statistics could be employed for this purpose.

For an illustration, an application of the Mantel–Haenszel "D-DIFF" statistic is shown in Table 11.6 (Mantel & Haenszel, 1959). D-DIFF is a modified item discrimination index. This method is employed by many standardized test-makers of achievement tests for investigating DIF in dichotomously scored items (see, e.g., CRESST, 2020). Excerpts of SBAC's reported results for grade 8 items of the mathematics test are shown, where items that exhibited DIF were identified using fixed statistical parameters with the statistic. Specifically, the SBAC group set criteria of <1 for items with negligible bias (A grade items), 1 to 1.5 for items with marginal to moderate levels of bias (B+ or B– grade items), and >1.5 for items showing a moderate to large bias (C+ or C– grade items). Both positive

TABLE 11.6. Graded Items (A–C) Meeting Statistical Criteria of Differential Item Functioning (DIF)

DIF levels	Female (vs. male)	Asian (vs. White)	Black (vs. White)	Native American (vs. White)
Items with negligible DIF levels (A)	968	678	743	37
Items with slight to moderate DIF levels, with positive values (B+)	8	42	17	1
Items with slight to moderate DIF levels with negative values (B–)	17	19	22	1
Items with moderate to large DIF levels with positive and negative values (C+ or C–)	1	15	2	0
(B–) + (C+) + (C–) items	18	34	24	1

Note. DIF levels were estimated with Mantel–Haenszel D-DIFF statistics. Adapted as in original in the public domain from *Technical Manual for Summative Assessments* (2018–19) (Table 3.10), by CRESST (2020), Smarter Balanced Assessment Consortium.

and negative D-DIFF statistics could be obtained, as noted in the table.

Applying these criteria to the comparison between the female (focal) to male (reference) groups, we find that 968 items met the SBAC criteria for an A grade, showing negligible DIF; 25 items showed marginal to moderate levels of DIF (B+ and B–), and 1 showed moderate to large levels of DIF. For the Asian (focal group) to White (reference group) comparison, as many as 61 items were detected with mild to moderate DIF levels, with 15 items flagged with significant DIF.

As with all item evaluations, once items with DIF are flagged, evaluative decisions must follow to revise or delete the items. As indicated, qualitative contextual data are often useful in shedding light on the causes for DIF.

QUICK RECAP: Fairness and bias have different definitions in measurement and are investigated with different methods. For assessments designed for populations that include highly diverse and minority subgroups, we should plan to investigate issues of sensitivity, fairness, and bias. DIF methods are a specialized type of item analysis for detecting bias in structured-response items.

Reflection Break 11.3: Objective 3

- Describe the difference between the concepts of *fairness* and *bias* in measurement.
- Describe methods you would apply for investigating fairness, bias, and sensitivity issues with assessments that you design or select.
- What is DIF? How can DIF analyses be useful for identifying measurement biases? How would you improve the items detected with high DIF statistics? What could be some limitations of quantitative studies of DIF issues? Explain.
- Formulate *validation questions* matched to specific *empirical methods* for investigating specific issues of statistical and perceived bias, sensitivity, and fairness.

11.5 Gathering Evidence of Content-Based Validity

Methods for collecting evidence of **content-based validity** fall under Evidence Cluster I (Chapter 10). The concept has several labels in the literature with essentially the same connotations: *content validity*, *content-oriented validity*, and *evidence based on test content* (AERA et al., 1999, p. 11; AERA et al., 2014; Crocker & Algina, 2006, p. 222). This section abbreviates the terminology to content validity (CV), with discussions of two quantitative indices, the CV-I and CV-S, to refer, respectively, to the content validity levels of items and scales. Recall that CV is distinguished from face validity, with the latter denoting the *appearance of validity* of an assessment to laypersons (Guilford,

1954; Mosier, 1947; Waltz & Bausell, 1981; Chapter 10)

11.5.1 Purpose

Effectively performed, content validation yields data useful for improving the content aspects of an instrument in specific ways prior to its assembly. The procedures involve in-depth and critical reviews performed by the designers themselves, or peers and independently solicited *content experts*. In the main, establishing CV requires evidence of the **content relevance** and **content representativeness** of the domains, indicators, and items that operationalize the constructs against established theory and knowledge, as well as guided by well-researched item-writing or design conventions. Simultaneously, we also examine the clarity and succinctness of the language, presentation, and format of items, including the appearance of bias (Chapters 4–7).

11.5.2 When to Do It

Evidence of CV is most useful when gathered in the developmental stages of instrument building so that items and the overall instrument can be refined using the results before finalization.

11.5.3 Methods

Informally, content validation can be performed using quality review checklists of the kind provided in Chapters 4–7. The procedures were described at length there, embedded in specific cases of instrument design with the Process Model.

Formal content validation studies could be carried out with interview and survey methods, as well as mixed-methods approaches (Creswell & Creswell, 2023). The goals are served best when external reviewers have the necessary levels of expertise in the domains and populations, as well as the requisite measurement knowledge. The four basic components of a formal CV study are as follows.

1. Select the external experts.
2. Obtain objective guided reviews of the content of different parts of the assessment.
3. Summarize the data using statistical and/or qualitative methods.
4. Delete, add to, or revise the domains, items, or overall tool based on the results.

11.5.4 Who Should Review the Items, Scale, and Tool?

As content validation results rely heavily on expertise, criteria for selecting judges should be arrived at with care. For example, judges must be knowledgeable about the theory and related literature on the constructs of interest to primary users, as well as the most appropriate assessment techniques suited to specific professional fields or academic disciplines. Defining the minimal qualifications necessary beforehand, preferably in consultation with other professionals and peers, can be helpful.

11.5.5 What Should Be Reviewed?

Typical CV questions focus on the degree of match of items with domain's indicators and their relevance to the construct theory; consistency of items with established item-writing guidelines; clarity (lack of ambiguity) of item wording, format, graphics, or directions; the (lack of) appearance of item biases; appropriateness of response scales or scoring systems, and overall content representation and coverage by the items. The assessment design specifications could also be subjected to reviews; for example, a *table of test specifications* can be useful in gauging the content representativeness of a test.

11.5.6 How Many Judges?

The literature suggests that we use three to five qualified judges. Use of more than 10 judges could make the studies unwieldy. From a statistical error estimation standpoint, the use of only two experts is discouraged (Lynn, 1986). Sometimes, however, that might be the only feasible option (Polit & Beck, 2006; Polit, Beck, & Owen, 2007; Waltz & Bausell, 1981, p. 71).

11.5.7 Designing CV Tools

For gathering the CV ratings, it is necessary to design a survey or an interview protocol. Like other self-report instruments, CV tools should be designed following the standard guidelines given in Chapter 7. Here are two item examples with accompanying instructions:

CV Survey Directions—*Example 1*

Following a review of the domain, indicators, and items, please indicate the extent to which you agree with these statements with the rating scale provided. Please clarify your selected response in the comments section.

Item 1

The domain of knowledge and skills is *relevant* to the most current practice guidelines and literature in the profession.

1 = Strongly disagree (several major modifications needed)

2 = Disagree (major modifications needed)

3 = Agree (only minor changes needed)

4 = Strongly agree (no modifications needed at all)

Please insert a comment to clarify your response:
[Space provided]

To elicit the maximum information, it is advisable to include both closed-ended and open-ended items that draw the reviewers' attention to specific aspects of the items or the tool, such as relevance, clarity, or conciseness of the presentation. To avoid obtaining data that are unusable or of poor quality, adequate guidance may be necessary for the reviewers to complete the procedure. To clarify the directions, well-designed surveys sometimes add an illustrative completed item. An "unable to evaluate" option allows experts greater freedom to critique the item beyond the criteria offered in a structured set of responses.

11.5.8 Analysis of CV Data

As shown in Tables 11.7–11.8 and Box 11.4, the numeric ratings can be summarized descriptively as a **Content Validity Index (CVI)**. These indices could be obtained for individual items (**CVI-I**) and the full test or scale (**CVI-S**). The CVI-I denotes the absolute percentage of interexpert agreement for each item, across all the participating raters. For example, for Item 1 in

TABLE 11.7. Validation Results on Content Relevance of Items: Expert Agreement Levels

Item no.	Expert A	Expert B	Expert C	Content validity index (CVI-I)
1	No	Yes	Yes	0.66
2	No	No	Yes	0.33
3	Yes	Yes	Yes	1.00
4	Yes	Yes	Yes	1.00
5	No	No	No	0.00
6	Yes	Yes	Yes	1.00

Note. CVI-I index based on agreement percentages, uncorrected for chance. Rating categories: 0 = No, not relevant; 1 = Yes, relevant.

Table 11.7, we find that two of three raters agreed on the content relevance of the item yielding a CVI-I of .67. On Item 5, the CVI-I is 0, making it a clear candidate for deletion.

CV Survey Directions—*Example 2*

Item 1

Review the indicator and matching item given below. Please rate the *relevance* of the item with the rating scale provided. Add comments in the space below, as needed.
[Indicator and item provided]

Item relevance rating scale

1 = Not relevant at all (does not match the indicator)

2 = Somewhat relevant (matches the indicator only partially)

3 = Relevant (matches the indicator well)

4 = Highly relevant (shows a strong match with the indicator and is important to measure)

5 = Unable to evaluate

Please insert a comment to clarify your response.
[Space provided]

By contrast, we find complete agreement among raters on the content relevance of Items 3, 4, and 6 in Table 11.7. Assuming the six items shown define a "scale," we could determine the CVI-S by obtaining the average of the CVI-I values of all the items. The CVI-S is .665 in the case illustrated (Polit et al., 2007).

TABLE 11.8. Adjusting CVI-I Results for Chance: Proportional Interexpert Agreements

Number of Experts	Number of Experts Endorsing Item or Instrument as Content Valid								
	2	3	4	5	6	7	8	9	10
2	1.00								
3	.67	1.00							
4	.50	.75	1.00						
5	.40	60	.80	1.00					
6	.33	.50	.67	.83	1.00				
7	.29	.43	.57	.71	.86	1.00			
8	.25	.38	.50	.63	.75	.88	1.00		
9	.22	.33	.44	.56	.67	.78	.89	1.00	
10	.20	.30	.40	.50	.60	.70	.80	.90	1.00

Note. Reprinted with permission from Lynn (1986). Copyright © 1986 John Wiley & Sons.

In theory, the number of raters could vary from 2 to 10 or more. Hence, the criteria for acceptability of CVI-I values like those above should be adjusted for any agreements obtained by chance. Using the standard error of proportions at the 5% statistical significance level, the criteria adjusted for random errors are given in Table 11.8. The table shows the number of experts crossed with the number of observed endorsements of each item. When these criteria are applied to the CVI-I data based on three raters in Table 11.7, only the items that meet the cut point of 1 are acceptable. That is, the items with CVI-I values of 0, .33, and .67 would all be rejected when corrected for the given *standard error of proportion* estimates (Lynn, 1986).

11.5.9 Correcting for Chance Agreements Using Cohen's κ

In CV study designs where we have two raters and categorical data, Cohen's kappa (κ) provides another measure of interrater agreement corrected for chance. See Box 11.4. The κ coefficient shown is given by the following formula:

$$\kappa = \frac{(P_A - P_C)}{(1 - P_C)}$$

where P_A is the observed relative percent agreement between raters and P_C is the percent agreement expected by chance, given by

$$\left[\frac{(a+b)(a+c)}{N^2}\right] + \left[\frac{(b+d)(c+d)}{N^2}\right]$$

To apply Cohen's κ, several assumptions must be met. (1) The rating must be measured on an ordinal or nominal scale with mutually exclusive categories; (2) the rated data must be based on paired observations of the same set of items; (3) each rating must have the same number of categories yielding a symmetric cross-tabulation, such as a 2 × 2 or 3 × 3, or $n \times n$ table; and finally, (4) the two raters must be independent where one rater's judgment will not influence the other's. There are added versions of κ specifically intended for ordinal variables and multiple raters (Fleiss, 1981), as well as a weighted κ. These are not shown here.

Box 11.4 gives the calculations of κ applied to a dataset with 25 items that were evaluated for CV with satisfactory versus unsatisfactory categories. The binary categories can be derived from multipoint rating scales by collapsing the counts in two consecutive categories together. The *highly relevant* and *relevant* are collapsed in the data shown and compared with the combined data from the *somewhat relevant* and *not relevant* categories (after Polit & Beck, 2006; Polit et al., 2007).

In Box 11.4, the collapsed ratings are presented in a 2 × 2 contingency table, with each cell identified with *a*, *b*, c, and *d*. Chance agreement in each cell is a probability of .25, given that there are four cells. The two

BOX 11.4 Computing Rater Agreement Levels with Cohen's κ

	Ratings from Rater A			
		Satisfactory	Unsatisfactory	
Ratings from Rater B	Satisfactory	a (11)	b (4)	$a + b$
	Unsatisfactory	c (1)	d (9)	$c + d$
		$a + c$	$b + d$	$N = a + b + c + d$

N (items) = 25

P_A = observed relative percent agreement

$= a/N + d/N = 11/25 + 9/25$

$= .80$

P_C = percent agreement expected by chance

$= [(a + b)(a + c)/N^2] + [(b + d)(c + d)/N^2]$

$= [(15)(12)/25^2] + [(13)(10)/25^2]$

$= .50$

$\kappa = (P_A - P_C)/(1 - P_C)$

$= (.80 - .50)/(1 - .50)$

$= .30/.50$

$= .60$

Source: Adapted with permission from Chatterji (2003). Allyn & Bacon. © Madhabi Chatterji.

expert raters disagree on five items. P_C overall is calculated at .50. With respect to CV, we find total agreement that 11 items are satisfactory, with the same agreement level that 9 are unsatisfactory. Based on the formula, κ is calculated to be .60. The κ yields a conservative estimate of rater agreement, as compared to absolute agreement levels, with a value >.60 usually considered acceptable, with estimates of .65 to .80 denoting substantial agreement (Crocker & Algina, 2006). More on κ to follow in the discussion of reliability.

11.5.10 Qualitative Comment Summaries on CV

Alongside the quantitative results, qualitative comments from experts are frequently of greater value from a formative perspective. The open-ended expert feedback specific to items could be used directly for making revisions. For example, here is CV data on an attitudinal item intended to measure political beliefs:

Draft Item: *I am inclined toward political activism.* (SA, A, U, D, SD)

Expert Feedback: *Does "inclined toward" refer to identity, beliefs, or behaviors? If this question is asking about a person's political beliefs, "inclined" is not the best word. "Political activism" is also very broad. . . . More context is necessary for interpreting a political belief. Liberal? Conservative? Giving an example would help.*

Action: Item should be revised to say *I support liberal causes (e.g., equal pay for men and women).*

When the volume of data is large for given items, comments could also be coded and summarized with **content analysis** methods. One useful approach is the *keywords in context* or *key themes in context* method. In this method, the main themes in the running text data are first highlighted and identified in the passage. Next, the number of unique and recurring themes are categorized for taking action (Creswell & Creswell, 2023; Miles & Huberman, 1994).

QUICK RECAP: Content validation is necessary during the instrument design process to improve content-oriented aspects of an assessment. The procedures can be performed informally or formally. Combining quantitative and qualitative methods offers several advantages over using either alone.

Reflection Break 11.4: Objective 2

- Describe two assessment design situations where content validation could be performed (1) *informally* versus (2) *formally*. Create a validation plan for each. What would be the essential steps in the *CV procedure* in each case, and how would these differ? Justify your answers.
- Distinguish between CV-I and CV-S data that may be gathered on an assessment you design. What are three ways by which *qualitative data* enhance the *quantitative* information obtained from a CV study?
- See Table 11.4. Following a CV survey, a researcher organized the expert data on 40 items in a 2×2 table with the following data in each cell: cell $a = 25$; $b = 3$; $c = 2$; and $d = 10$. Calculate and interpret Cohen's kappa (κ) coefficient in this scenario.
- Design a *CV survey* to gather data on an instrument you might adopt. Breakdown the assessment user context (Phase I of the Process Model). Who are your experts? List their qualifications. Which aspects of the instrument will they validate and how?

11.6 Validating Response Processes: The Cognitive Interview

Evidence on the **validity of the response processes** also falls under Evidence Cluster I (Chapter 10). This section will elaborate on one method, called the **cognitive interview** or *cognitive testing* that can be effectively employed to validate responses obtained in a variety of assessment situations.

Cognitive interviewing for validating response processes can be performed in an exploratory or confirmatory mode. Carbone et al. (2002) utilized the method to revise and correct problems in questions on nutrition surveys and cancer prevention messages aimed for lower-income populations. They reported that the procedure helped in defining a lesser known construct and drafting self-report questions.

11.6.1 Purpose

These methods are intended to improve the quality of individual tasks or items by delving into the *information-processing* aspects of intellectual, affective, or behavioral domains, as respondents engage with the constructs and different parts of an instrument. Typically, items intended to measure **process indicators** are examined and probed (Chapter 4). For example, we might want to verify the respondents' use of reasoning processes in mathematics. For little known or unknown constructs, validation of response processes yields evidence to gain insights, and as possible, verify construct theories about the mental processes engaged by respondents during the assessment process.

11.6.2 When to Do It

Validation of response processes also belongs under Evidence Cluster I and should be performed in the early stages of instrument design (Chapter 10).

11.6.3 Timing of the Cognitive Interview

To begin, decide on whether a *concurrent* or *post hoc* cognitive interview would be most useful. In a concurrent interview, we would conduct the interview while the respondent is taking the instrument, with deliberate pauses after each task or segment is completed, to insert the interview questions. The *post hoc* approach is often more practical. It is conducted shortly after the respondent completes an assessment. The time gap should be no more than a week to avoid lapses in memory.

11.6.4 Respondents in a Cognitive Interview

The number of interviewees should be small but strategic to enable in-depth knowledge extraction on the response processes ($N = 2$ to 6, no more than 10). That is, interviewee selection should be purposive. For example, if the goals of a project are to examine response processes tied to issues of gender identity, each known gender identity group should be represented. A somewhat more efficient alternative is cognitive probing in a focus group format (Creswell & Creswell, 2023).

11.6.5 Designing the Cognitive Interview Protocol

A cognitive interview encourages "think-alouds" by participants with reference to specific items, phrases, words, or parts of the assessment, allowing deep interviewing and probes about response processes as follow-ups. For example,

- "How did you approach this question? Why?"
- "What were your thought processes when you saw these words [words inserted] in the question?"
- "Tell me more about what these words or parts of the question mean to you."
- "How did you come up with your answer? Describe your thinking process and steps."

The typical cognitive interview utilizes a six-step procedure (see also Chapter 7): (1) an opening, declaration of purposes, obtaining participant consent, with assurances of anonymity and confidentiality; (2) allocation of time for participants to engage with the instrument, items, or tasks; (3) conducting the interview with specific prompts and probes for the item; (4) repeating the process for the major parts of the instrument, tasks, and items; (5) sharing of the interview notes and recordings with participants to ensure accuracy; (6) concluding with appreciation for interviewee participation.

11.6.6 Analyzing/Synthesizing Interview Data and Taking Actions

As with content validation data, the cognitive interview findings are qualitative in nature and must be coded and analyzed systematically with a suitable analytic method. Findings must lead to some actionable refinements of the domains, items, or instruments. Extracting and organizing the key themes is the most common procedure. Carbone et al. (2002, p. 694), for instance, extracted the following four themes from their content analysis of cognitive interview data:

> Four key themes emerged from the analyses. They were: 1) vague or ineffective instructions, respondents expressed confusion about how to answer survey questions when terms were vague; 2) confusing questions and response options, that is, use of awkward or unfamiliar language in a question or in response options confused respondents; 3) variable interpretation of terms . . . even if words were familiar to participants, it could not be assumed that their meaning was consistent for all respondents and terms or phrases that were not explicitly defined were subject to misunderstanding; and 4) misinterpretation of dietary recommendations.

11.6.7 Benefits and Limitations

Methods for validating response processes are usually time-consuming and resource-dependent. Furthermore, assessment designers must acknowledge their own biases and assumptions before undertaking the procedure with qualitative methods (Creswell & Creswell, 2023).

The benefits of a cognitive interview are the researcher's ability to probe thought processes; clarify the meanings that specific words may carry for respondents; ascertain the most appropriate item and response formats for the desired types of information processing, including the best response categories to use; identify the sources of respondent confusion; and clarify construct definitions through interactive designer–respondent exchanges.

QUICK RECAP: Validation of response processes is necessary for constructs and construct indicators that involve specific theories about how respondents will engage different mental processes to arrive at answers to assessments. Qualitative research methods like the cognitive interview yield useful data on the processual aspects of how respondents interact with items.

Reflection Break 11.5: Objective 2

- What are the similarities and differences in the evidence we obtain from content validation studies versus validation of response processes? Compare the validation questions, methods, and steps in the procedures for each.
- Apart from cognitive interviews, describe other empirical methods that could be useful for procuring evidence on the validity of response processes.
- Design a cognitive interview protocol to gather data on the validity of response processes for an assessment design scenario. Describe the assessment context, the population and purposes of your study.

11.7 Gathering Correlational Evidence of Validity

We could investigate the correlational properties of measures from assessments both internally *or* externally (Chapter 10). The methods discussed next deal with gathering and evaluating evidence on (1) the validity of the internal structure; (2) convergent and discriminant validity; and (3) concurrent and predictive validity, including possible predictive biases.

11.7.1 Purpose

The purposes of these validation studies are to evaluate theory-guided hypotheses about the expected relationships of item- or subscale-level data of an assessment internally, or the expected interrelationships of the overall construct measures with other variables and measures.

11.7.2 When to Do It

These studies fall under Evidence Cluster II. They should be undertaken after the instrument is initially tested and found to be acceptable, usually with some evidence of item quality, content-based validity, and score reliability in hand (Chapter 10).

11.7.3 Commonly Applied Methods

We could employ psychometric procedures from both CTT and IRT for this purpose. In this section, we focus only on selected CTT methods involving estimation and testing of hypotheses about the proposed factor and covariance structures of items and subscales, and correlation–regression procedures for examining relationships of the scores with external variables. To evaluate the results, both the size and direction of the correlations must be evaluated. All the procedures can be performed with standard statistical software like the SPSS, SAS, and Systat packages.

11.7.3.1 Factor Analysis Methods

Two useful methods for validating the internal structure of assessments are **exploratory factor analysis (EFA)** and **confirmatory factor analysis (CFA)**. The basics of EFA and CFA procedures are described in this section with applied examples. Much of the "hard work" in mathematics is delivered by computer software today. Highlights of the main concepts, steps, interpretation of the results, and limitations follow.

For factor analysis purposes, by convention, we refer to the item response vectors in the dataset as the *item variables*. The mathematically derived factors are called the *latent dimensions*, *latent factors*, or simply, *factors*. See the diagram inserted next to start and Figure 11.2.

EXPLORATORY FACTOR ANALYSIS

EFA Purposes. The primary goal of EFA is to validate mathematically derived factors against a theoretical framework, starting with empirically gathered data on the items of an instrument. The EFA procedure is guided by the question: To what extent is the variance in item variables explained by the fewest possible factors that fit the construct theory? Parsimony is a goal—that is, we desire to discard any redundant or weakly performing items that are not explained by the intended factors. When performed in a purely open-ended "discovery" mode, EFA is useful for deriving a smaller number of common factors from a large number of item variables taken from different instruments or multivariate datasets.

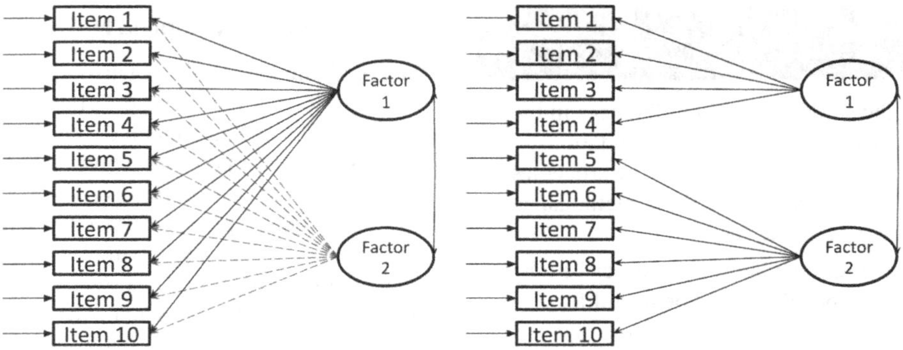

FIGURE 11.2. Examining the internal structure of a 10-item assessment: Alternate models for exploratory factor analysis (EFA; left) and confirmatory factor analysis (CFA; right).

The EFA Model and Logic of the Procedure. The EFA model is a common factor model. It is basically a modified multiple regression model, as shown in the diagram and equations that follow. A common factor is a linear combination of the item variables.

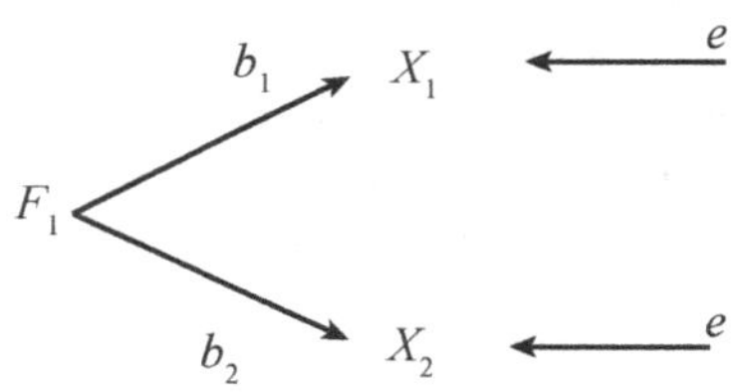

In the diagram shown above, we see two item variables, X_1 and X_1, explained by the common factor F_1 with the directional arrows. Each item is expected to be related to the factor with a loading of b on the factor that shows the size of the shared relationship.

The factor loadings are given as b_1 and b_2, with the e referring to the unique "error" components in the equations. The e affects the variance of the item variables, as shown. But this error variance is separate from the portion explained by the factor F_1:

$$X_1 = a + b_1F_1 + e_1$$
$$X_2 = a + b_2F_1 + e_2$$

Typically, the factor loadings in EFA are standardized regression coefficients (the b_1 and b_2 terms in the equations). They denote the degree to which a unit change in the latent "factor scores" influences a corresponding change in each observed, item variable, both measured as z-scores (Chapter 8).

The a term in the equations is the intercept, or the point of origin of the regression line. The intercept is held constant in the equations of an EFA model. Hence, with $a = 0$, both equations can be restated as follows:

$$X_1 = b_1F_1 + e_1$$
$$X_2 = b_2F_1 + e_2$$

Now, suppose we assume that X_1 and X_2 in the picture are *math ability* items, intended to tap into a common factor F_1. What would be a satisfactory EFA solution from a validity standpoint? The EFA should confirm that F_1 explains *most* of the variance in both the items, yielding large b estimates and small amounts of estimated errors.

For a more realistic EFA model, now see the left-hand side of Figure 11.2 showing a proposed internal structure of a 10-item test. Here, two factors, F_1 and F_2, are hypothesized to explain the variability in 10 items measuring two separate constructs (say, math ability and verbal ability). Items 1–5 (X_1–X_5 in the equations) are intended to measure the first construct, with Items 6–10 (X_6–X_{10} in the equations) measuring the second. The EFA procedure tests *all* of the items together with the two-factor EFA model shown, keeping in mind the substantive differences in the two constructs. Should most of the variance in X_1–X_5, be explained by F_1, with the variances of remaining five items, X_6–X_{10}, explained largely by F_2, we would have confirmation of the hypothesized internal structure. That is, the empirical evidence would validate that the intentionally *different* item variables are explained by two distinguishable latent constructs, verbal and math ability.

To achieve maximum interpretability, the factors need to be rotated following extraction. There are different methods of factor rotation that should be selected rationally. The two main rotation techniques are *orthogonal*, applied when factors are expected to be uncorrelated, and *oblique*, when they are assumed to be related.

In theory, we could extract as many factors as there are item variables in a dataset. The key is to evaluate the merits of each factor against the construct theory and previously set mathematical criteria. The mathematical criteria for identifying the most dominant factors should be preset, and the theoretical meaningfulness of the factors must be supported by pertinent literature. Some commonly used psychometric criteria are the magnitude of the item-to-factor loadings following rotation (the b estimates); the percentage of item-level variance explained by each factor (called the *eigenvalues*); the number of factors that are better than chance; and the fewest factors that cumulatively explain the largest amount of the total variance in items.

An optimal EFA solution has a "simple structure" that is easy to interpret. To claim a simple factor structure, the individual items designated to measure a particular construct should have the largest loadings on only one factor (say, F_1), but not the others.

EFA Sample Size. EFAs require large samples for stable factor solutions. A general rule of thumb is to have 10 people for each item and a minimum of 200 subjects.

EFA Steps. Broadly, EFA methods could use a principal components analysis (PCA), which assumes no error components in the linear equations, and principal axis factor (PAF) extraction techniques, for which the equations include the e components. Both are applicable when factors are expected to be intercorrelated. The general steps are as follows:

1. Start with an inter-item correlation or covariance matrix.
2. Extract the factors using a selected method (e.g., PAF).
3. Identify the fewest factors that explain the maximum amount of the total variance in the items.
4. Rotate the identified factors with an appropriate factor rotation technique to obtain the best solution in terms of factor loadings and a simple structure.
5. Interpret the factors against appropriate construct theory.

An Applied Example. The steps are now illustrated with a validation study (Chatterji & Lin, 2018). In this work, the authors designed and validated a multiconstruct, self-report survey to measure math self-concept (M-SC), math self-efficacy (M-SE), and math anxiety (M-ANX) in elementary school students. Of the 37 items on the initial survey, 10 items were intentionally marked to measure two subdomains of M-SC: *positive affect* and *perceived competence*. The goal was to validate this internal structure, identifying the most meaningful factors with a simple structure. A part of the solution with a rotated factor pattern is shown in Table 11.9.

Beginning with data from 255 students, responses to all 37 items were subjected to an EFA. From an inter-item covariance matrix, factors were initially extracted with a PAF procedure, with the errors modeled in the equations. The first five factors with the largest eigenvalues explained about 40% of the cumulative variance in all items. These factors were determined to be better-than-chance and met the mathematical criterion set of eigenvalues >1. The factors were rotated for further evaluation with a minimum acceptance criterion of >.30 for the item-to-factor loadings. In large part, the items explained by the five dominant factors corresponded with the two subscales of M-SC, two subscales of M-SE, and one scale of M-ANX, as proposed. With a few item exceptions, the *first two* factors showed item loadings that corresponded almost exactly with the two theorized subdomains of M-SC. However, some of the results also pointed to "misfitting" items or ambiguities.

Look closely at Table 11.9 that shows the excerpted results. The five designated M-SC items had loadings that were positive and well above the criterion of >.30 on Factor 1 or 2, suggesting that these were the two "latent" dimensions of M-SC influencing the item variance The loadings of the designated items were relatively high on the identified Factors 1 and 2, but very low toward 0 on the remaining Factors 3 to 5. Statistically, these results pointed to a simple structure.

The table also shows *structure coefficients* in parentheses along with the loadings. The former are correlations of factor-based scores with the individual item variables. These estimates are usually larger than the loadings. The results generally confirmed the explanatory power of the two M-SC factors on the items.

However, one item *did not* meet the loading criterion of >.30 and had to be dropped. See Item 3 on enjoying math games. This is an ambiguous item with double loadings. It shows close to 0 loadings on three factors, and loadings of .24 on Factor 1 (M-SC) and .25 on Factor 5 (M-SE). As M-SC and M-SE are two different constructs according to the literature, such an item would be problematic; it was reevaluated and discarded. In another unexpected result that is not shown, the deliberately reverse-oriented wording on three items of the M-ANX scale caused them to load on the *positive affect* factor of M-SC instead (with rather high loadings >.60). These items were therefore added to the M-SC subscale. There is published research suggesting that negatively worded survey items could sometimes load on a so-called semantic factor unrelated to the intended constructs (DiStefano & Hess, 2005). The final M-SC scale with a validated two-factor structure had 12 items, as (10 – 1) + 3 = 12.

Advantages and Limitations. Usually, poorly conceived items generate more "noise" in the EFA results. We should begin EFA by studying descriptive distributions of item variables, scales, and subscales ensuring that the statistical assumptions of EFA are met. As correlational statistics are sample-dependent, we should seek to replicate the EFA evidence in different samples. A factorable dataset with sufficient respondents will yield a Kaiser's measure of sampling adequacy >.70, a useful statistic to evaluate assumptions of the EFA procedure. Informed analysts start the EFA with a clear construct theory in mind and use judgment for making decisions with the results obtained at each step of the procedure.

CONFIRMATORY FACTOR ANALYSIS

CFA Purposes. See the right-hand side of Figure 11.1 next. The goal of a CFA is to specify an inter-item *covariance structure* beforehand based on theory and then confirm it empirically with a dataset. That is, CFA models impose fixed covariance structures on the item data drawing on theory, whereby prespecified items on

TABLE 11.9. Exploratory Factor Analysis Results: Factor Loadings and Structure Coefficients (in Parentheses)

Construct	Factor 1	Factor 2	Factor 3	Factor 4	Factor 5
Mathematics Self-Concept Items					
1 Is doing math class work fun for you?	**.60*** **(.66)**	.09 (.35)	.07 (.07)	.05 (.27)	.12 (.30)
2 Do you enjoy number work?	**.50*** **(.63)**	.05 (.30)	–.01 (.03)	–.04 (.19)	.03 (.21)
3 Do you enjoy playing math games?	*.26* (.41)	–.04 (.17)	–.07 (–.00)	–.07 (.10)	*.24* (.19)
4 Are you good at math?	.03 (.41)	**.88*** **(.86)**	–.01 (-.33)	.04 (.47)	–.04 (.27)
5 Have you always done well in math?	.06 (.28)	**.60*** **(.62)**	.02 (–.27)	–.13 (.25)	.08 (.25)

Note. Loadings >.30 in **bold font**, after factor rotation. Adapted from Chatterji and Lin (2018).

a scale are linked to particular latent factors by means of a set of linear equations. When applying CFA, in contrast to the EFA, only specific items are allowed to load on particular factors, as shown. Restrictions could also be imposed on predicted relationships among various factors in a model.

Once specified, the entire CFA model is subjected to empirical testing with a sample of item-level data gathered from the defined populations. Should the prespecified covariance structure in the sample data demonstrate a close match (based on statistical fit criteria) with an estimated population covariance matrix, we have evidence verifying the proposed internal structure. As a method to procure another form of validity evidence on internal structure, CFA models are restrictive analytic tools (DiStefano & Hess, 2005; Harrington, 2009; Kline, 2023).

CFA Model Specification and Procedures. In general terms, the CFA procedure begins with an item-level covariance or correlation matrix from which the latent factors are then estimated. First, a CFA model is specified, as shown on the right in Figure 11.2. The expected inter-item, item-to-factor, or interfactor relationships are all prespecified by the arrows in the CFA model. To draw conclusions on the validity of internal structure, we ask: How closely did the sample covariance matrix "fit" the estimated population covariance matrix, in statistical terms? Is there adequate evidence that the observed relationships among factors and items are consistent with the theoretically specified domain structure? Satisfactory "fit" for CFA models can be evaluated using a number of statistical indices. Popular software packages for performing CFA are LISREL, EQS, AMOS, and Mplus.

CFA Sample Size. To support the estimation procedures, CFAs require large datasets with at least 200–300 subjects.

An Applied Example. For a CFA illustration, we return to the earlier study on validating survey-based measures of M-SC, M-SE, and M-ANX (Chatterji & Lin, 2018). Recall that the best-performing 25 items of the original pool of 37 were retained following the EFA from the first iteration. These 25 items were validated with a restrictive five-factor CFA model in a new dataset. Testing competing CFA models adds rigor to the procedure; thus, the authors compared the fit statistics of a one-factor CFA that went against the theorized structure, to a five-factor structure consistent with theory. Detailed results appear in the published article.

The fit statistics for the five-factor CFA model met the statistical criteria set on several indices but, as expected, were below par with the one-factor competing model. For the two M-SC dimensions, *perceived affect* and *perceived competence*, the item-to-factor loadings were reasonably high at .40 to .88. The expected inter-correlations of items with factors and interfactor correlations, as modeled, were all confirmed with a reasonable and consistent pattern of results on all statistics (Chatterji & Lin, 2018).

Advantages and Limitations. CFA is best applied in the latter stages of assessment development, with EFA applied during the early, exploratory stages. Employing EFA to start with in an exploratory dataset, followed by a CFA in an independent dataset to confirm the obtained structure, as described, is the recommended approach. Performing both EFA and CFA with the same dataset is inadvisable and compromises scientific standards. Note that CFA is a conceptually and statistically different analytic approach. A benefit is that CFA enables the removal of the modeled error variance when obtaining estimates of factor loadings and correlations. While useful for confirming prespecified covariance structures, designers could run into problems if the CFA model is specified incorrectly or is atheoretical and ill-conceived.

11.7.3.2 Convergent and Discriminant Validity

PURPOSE

This type of evidence helps confirm or disconfirm hypotheses about the innate nature of the focal construct measures based on their correlations with selected external variables. The external measures could be of similar or markedly different constructs. While convergent validity investigates correlations of the focal measures with measures of the same or highly similar constructs, discriminant validity examines correlations with measures known to be distinctly different (Chapter 10).

METHODS

Convergent or discriminant validity evidence is typically reported as empirical correlation coefficients at the appropriate units of analysis. Pearson's *r* is applied when measures are continuous, interval-scaled variables (Chapter 8). Interfactor correlations obtained through CFA or EFA could also be used to evaluate convergent or discriminant validity. Selection of appropriate construct measures is the key to proper implementation of these procedures.

Empirically, two measures may be related to some degree simply because they utilize the same assessment method (e.g., a self-report modality). Campbell and Fiske (1959), therefore, recommended that we control for *method variance* when analyzing convergent and discriminant validity. To rule out the effects of the assessment methods from the overlapping variance in two construct measures, they proposed the use of a multitrait–multimethod matrix (MTMM) of correlations. An empirical MTMM application with a 3 × 3 matrix involving medical education assessments is available from Baig et al. (2010) with clinical competency constructs. MTMM correlations can also be estimated with CFA procedures accounting for errors in items and latent factors (see, e.g., Henseler, Ringle, & Sarstedt, 2015).

AN MTMM ILLUSTRATION

Table 11.10 provides an illustration of MTMM with a hypothetical matrix of bivariate correlations of different construct measures. Assume we are measuring two different constructs focusing on mathematics versus language arts skills, *A* and *B*. Each construct is measured in three assessment modalities: Method 1 (multiple-choice tests); Method 2 (interview-based assessments); and Method 3 (essay tests). To begin the procedure, a selected sample of examinees is administered the assessments in all three modes on both constructs, with the correlational results displayed in an MTMM table as shown.

The diagonal of the MTMM table presents *test–retest reliability coefficients.* These denote correlations of the *same construct measure*, administered twice to the same examinees, with the *same assessment method.* If reliable, we would expect the scores from Test A_1 (math skills, multiple-choice test) to yield high correlations showing acceptable reliability (>.70 and approaching .90–.99). All the underscored corre-

TABLE 11.10. Illustration of a Multitrait–Multimethod Matrix

		Method 1: Multiple-choice			Method 2: Interview-based assessment		Method 3: Written open-ended tasks	
Domains	*Test*	A_1	A_{11}	B_1	A_2	B_2	A_3	B_3
Math	A_1	<u>.90</u>						
	A_{11}	.81	<u>.89</u>					
Language arts	B_1	.50	.45	<u>.88</u>				
Math	A_2	.75	.71		<u>.85</u>			
Language arts	B_2	.44	.48	.60	.65	<u>.82</u>		
Math	A_3	.52	.59	.62	.70		<u>.78</u>	
Language arts	B_3	.26	.30	.63	.41	.68	.56	<u>.85</u>

Note.
.81 = Convergent validity with same methods
.75 = Convergent validity with different methods
.65 = Discriminant validity with same methods
.41 = Discriminant validity with different methods
<u>.89</u> = Reliability coefficient (all reliability coefficients <u>underlined</u>)

Adapted with permission from Chatterji (2003). Allyn & Bacon/Pearson. © Madhabi Chatterji.

lations in the diagonal represent test–retest reliability coefficients.

Similarly, we would expect convergence in the form of positive and strong correlations of test scores measuring the *same trait* (math skills) but with two different instruments that use the *same method* (multiple-choice tests). The correlation of .81 of Test A_1 with Test A_{11} shows this strong overlap in the construct domain and common methods. Convergent validity evidence under conditions where we have *different methods* (multiple-choice vs. interview-based assessment) for the *same trait* (math skills) is illustrated in the .75 correlation coefficient. Because the correlation drops in magnitude from .81 to .75, we are able to see the influence of the assessment methods.

In a similar vein, to be able to confirm discriminant validity, we would expect scores from Test A_1 to have much lower correlations with the language arts skills test (Test B_t), a qualitatively different trait even when the same method is used (e.g., multiple-choice test). Discriminant validity is evident in the drop in size of the correlation coefficients (e.g., r_{B1A1} = .50, suggesting only 25% overlapping variance). When assessment methods and traits *both vary*, we would expect the lowest correlations confirming the discriminant validity. In the matrix, we see the correlation between A_2 and B_3, $r_{A,B3}$ = .41 (with only about 16% overlapping variance). In sum, the general pattern of correlations supports the conclusion that the math and language arts measures have sufficient convergent and discriminant validity levels, even after accounting for the "assessment methods."

AN EMPIRICAL EXAMPLE

Readers may refer back to the results of the PSQI validation study in Box 11.1 for a real-world example, to be discussed again at the end of the chapter.

Returning to investigating the properties of the M-SC, M-SE, and M-ANX measures, Chatterji and Lin (2018) presented interfactor correlations from the CFA as evidence of convergent and discriminant validity. Given the literature at the student level, they expected negative correlations of the two M-SC factors with the M-ANX factor as these yield opposite kinds of information. To confirm convergent validity, on the other hand, they expected moderate to strong positive correlations between M-SC factors with each other and with the validated M-SE factor. The interfactor correlations, controlling for the error factors in CFA models, yielded results consistent with these hypotheses, as follows:

Discriminant validity evidence

Factor 1 (M-SC, *positive affect*) and Factor 3 (M-ANX, *negative affect*): –.11

Factor 2 (M-SC, *perceived competence*) and Factor 3 (M-ANX): –.53

Convergent validity evidence (same construct)

Factors 1 and 2 (M-SC, *postive affect*, and M-SC, *perceived competence*), different dimensions of math self-concept, correlated at +.72.

Convergent validity evidence (different constructs)

Factors 1 and 2 (M-SC, *positive affect*, and M-SC, *perceived competence*) correlated with the M-SE factor, a separate construct at +.39, and +.63, respectively

ADVANTAGES AND LIMITATIONS

Convergent and discriminant validity studies are relatively easy to implement even with small-scale field tests of instruments with <100 respondents; hence, such evidence should be procured when possible. Careful sample selection matters as correlation coefficients are affected by the variability of measures and the sample size. Reliability of all the measures should be estimated *before* computing the validity coefficients (see Section 11.8); correlation coefficients are known to be attenuated by unreliability. Attention must also be given to the units of analysis when designing correlational studies. To generalize the results from the samples to the population, statistical significance tests should accompany the descriptive correlations.

11.7.3.3 Predictive and Concurrent Validity Evidence

PURPOSE

The purpose of predictive validity evidence is to confirm that an assessment's scores are able to predict an expected, future "criterion" behavior in examinees to a sufficient degree. Evidence of concurrent validity is usually sought when the aim is to substitute a preexisting measure with a new one. Both classes of evidence, described throughout, are traditionally placed under *criterion-related validity* (Chapter 10).

METHODS

Methodologically, concurrent validity overlaps exactly with convergent validity in terms of using a concurrent data-collection design. Both rely on correlational statistics of the focal measure with a chosen criterion in a given sample.

For predictive validity studies, the validation involves a longitudinal data-collection design followed by correlation–regression analyses. Scatterplots, correlation coefficients (usually Pearson's r), and the r^2-values (coefficients of determination) provide evidence of the predictive power of the predictor. Results can also be obtained as *expectancy tables*, which present the calculated probabilities of a criterion score, given a predictor score range. Confidence bands around predicted scores on the criterion measure allow users to take into account the standard errors of measurement (SEMs) during decision making, as elucidated in Section 11.8.

AVOIDING PREDICTION ISSUES

Chapter 3 discussed a scenario with different predictive validity coefficients in males and females for an admissions test, where the cut score set on the combined group's distribution of scores could lead to a prediction bias. The effectiveness of prediction using an assessment's scores depends on the cut scores set by users on the predictor and criterion score distributions and the strength of the observed, bivariate relationship. Users should be alerted to two kinds of prediction errors when using assessments designed for prediction: *false positive* errors, where we select unqualified candidates by mistake, and *false negative* errors, where we fail to select qualified candidates. When the predictive validity coefficient varies significantly in different subgroups of the population, these decision-making errors are more likely. In the typical case, uninformed decision-makers rely on the combined group's predictive validity results.

The Taylor–Russell tables (Taylor & Russell, 1939) continue to be useful for taking into account the interdependencies among predictive validity coefficients, the selection ratio, and the proportion that would be successfully selected in the absence of the "predictor" assessment.

In high-stakes candidate-selection scenarios, according to Taylor and Russell (1939), we should consider three statistics: the selection ratio, the base rate, and the success ratio. The selection ratio is the proportion of candidates that would be selected based on their scores only on the predictor (i.e., those who meet the cut point set by decision-makers on the predictor). The base rate is the proportion that would be selected based on their scores only on the criterion (i.e., those who meet the cut on the criterion). The success ratio is the proportion that is actually selected.

Weaker predictive validity coefficients yield greater statistical errors in prediction. These issues are compounded by unreliability levels around cut scores in the predictor and criterion measures. On top of this, when the predictive validity coefficients vary significantly in diverse subgroups of test-takers, in practice, the success ratios for one or the other groups can have greater numbers of false positive or false negative errors. More on error rates in tests used for classification follows in our discussion of reliability.

EMPIRICAL STUDY EXAMPLES

In a recent concurrent validation study, Famodu et al. (2018) validated a shortened version of the PSQI in young adults. The authors rationalized the work claiming that the length of the original PSQI compromised its utility in clinical contexts. As concurrent validity evidence, they reported very high and statistically significant correlations between the global scores of the original PSQI and the shorter versions, with a Spearman's rho (ρ) of .94. Furthermore, they found high levels of agreement in classifying good and poor sleepers ($\kappa = .83$) using the long and short versions of the tool, supporting the substitution of one with the other.

A very recent predictive validity study was performed on the SAT by a university-led task force of researchers at the University of California (2020, pp. 21–22). The study was prompted by a need to review institutional admissions policies and questions as to whether the SAT scores predicted similar outcomes for diverse subsets of students entering the university. The study presented prediction models disaggregated by various demographic groups of undergraduate students, such as family income and race. To evaluate predictive validity, the regression models combined SAT scores with high school GPA as the predictors, using subsequently gathered university grades as a criterion measure. Regardless of ethnic group membership, just 14–22% of the variance in grades was explained by the two combined predictors, with only 18–20% explained for students at all income levels. The authors acknowledged that this was not a large amount of shared variance, albeit consistent with prior research evidence on the properties of SAT scores.

ADVANTAGES AND LIMITATIONS

Like all types of correlational evidence, interpretations of concurrent and predictive validity evidence should be situated in information about the constructs, the caliber of measures on external variables, and the population characteristics. If the goal of prediction studies is to support accurate decision making in high-stakes applications, we should adhere to rigorous technical standards. All the interpretive guidelines and cautionary caveats for correlations would apply to predictive and concurrent validity data.

QUICK RECAP: Correlational evidence speaks most directly to the construct validity and interpretability of measures. The methods range from simple to more complex, and allow examinations of the items, subscales, and assessments both internally and externally. We should plan to procure the necessary types for most assessment design or adoption situations.

Reflection Break 11.6: Objectives 1 and 2

- Clarify the distinctions between *convergent validity, discriminant validity*, and *concurrent validity* evidence.
- Which statistic is most important in a *predictive validity* study for making selection and placement decisions: (1) predictive validity coefficient; (2) coefficient of determination; (3) r^2; (4) classification error rates; or (5) other? Explain your answer.
- Why are *units of analysis* important when you gather *correlational evidence* of validity?
- Why is consulting the literature important when evaluating *correlational evidence* of validity?
- Compare the application of *EFA with CFA methods* for validating the internal structure of assessments on the following: (1) when to use each, (2) assumptions and models, (3) main steps, and (4) interpreting the results.
- Draw a *graphic* for (1) an EFA model and (2) a CFA model for validating the internal structure of an assessment you might design or adopt.
- Is factor analysis better used as a technique for *discovery, data reduction*, or *validation*?

11.8 Empirical Estimation of Reliability

The estimation of random or unspecified errors in the assessment results and the differentiation of these "errors" from the "true scores" are the central problems of reliability. Reliability of the measures is essential, but it cannot substitute for evidence of validity. Four reliability coefficients treated in this section are **internal consistency reliability, test–retest reliability, parallel forms reliability**, and **interrater reliability**. Some discussion is provided on domain score reliability and classification consistency, useful for testing situations that rely on cut scores.

Under the CTT framework, specific types of reliability coefficients are estimated tied to different sources of random error. Different data-collection designs and computational procedures apply to each. See Table 11.11 as we proceed.

11.8.1 Which Reliability Coefficient to Use?

To identify the reliability coefficient(s) most appropriate for a given assessment situation, assessment designers, adopters, and users must identify the potential sources of random error, such as domain sampling, parallel forms, raters, or occasions (Table 11.11). Focusing on item data, internal consistency reliability is a standard requirement for *all* assessments designed

TABLE 11.11. Procedures for Reliability Estimation

Question: *To what extent . . .*	Reliability coefficient	Empirical methods
1. . . . do the construct measures remain stable over short time periods?	Test–retest reliability coefficient	Correlate the measures from given assessments in the same group of individuals, gathered on two occasions with a time gap of 10–15 days. *Interpretation: Consistency of measures over time*
2. . . . do the construct measures remain consistent on two parallel and equivalent forms of the assessment?	Parallel forms reliability coefficient	Correlate the measures in the same group of individuals gathered concurrently on two or more forms of the same assessment. *Interpretation: Consistency of measures in parallel forms*
3. . . . do the responses to different items, subparts, and overall assessment consistently measure the same domains in given persons?	Internal consistency reliability coefficients	Administer the assessment to a group of individuals on one occasion. Split the assessment data randomly by item and subparts, and intercorrelate the measures from each component to evaluate homogeneity levels. Common indices: split-half reliability, KR-20 and Cronbach's α. *Interpretation: Within-person consistency of measures*
4. . . . do the measures remain consistent, regardless of observer or rater?	Interrater reliability coefficients	Administer the assessment to a group of individuals on one occasion, with observations and ratings made by two or more raters; correlate the ratings obtained from different raters. *Interpretation: Interrater consistency in measures*

using a domain sampling approach. Test–retest reliability is also necessary to claim stability of item-level data or total scores obtained from tests and subtests over short durations of time. For single-item measures, like stand-alone survey items, test–retest reliability may be the *only* type of reliability information we can feasibly gather. With parallel forms and interrater reliability concerns, the investigations are more situation-specific.

11.8.2 Internal Consistency Reliability

11.8.2.1 Purpose

Internal consistency reliability estimates yield within-person consistency levels in the responses to items defining a scale or test. These statistics are closely related to item homogeneity indices (see Item Analysis in Chapter 11; see also Chapter 10). Essentially, the assumption is that responses to randomly sampled items or item sets on an assessment would be closely and positively correlated with scores built from the remaining items. To be acceptable, internal consistency reliability estimates should be at least .70 and tending toward >.90.

11.8.2.2 Methods

Methods for gauging internal consistency reliability require a single administration of the assessment and hence are easier to implement logistically. Although the formulas and procedures differ somewhat, the three major methods detailed next are conceptually and mathematically equivalent: split-half, KR-20, and Cronbach's α.

STEPS FOR SPLIT-HALF RELIABILITY ESTIMATION

See Box 11.5 next. A split-half reliability coefficient can be computed by hand and is easy for practitioners to use. Once data are collected and organized, the steps in computation are as follows:

1. Split the test or assessment in two halves randomly, for example, by using the odd-numbered (A) and even-numbered items (B).

2. Obtain total scores for the two half-forms, *A* and *B*.
3. Calculate a Pearson's correlation of the scores from half-forms *A* and *B*.
4. Apply the *Spearman–Brown prophecy formula* given in Box 11.5 to statistically adjust for the initial estimate from halved test forms to obtain a final estimate.

In shortening of the test's length when halved, the reliability is at first underestimated. We use the Spearman–Brown prophecy formula to correct for this issue in the final step to obtain the reliability of .45. The approach assumes that the two forms are "strictly parallel" (Chapter 10).

In the data shown, the corrected reliability is only .45, even after the Spearman–Brown adjustment, well below par. The reasons may be due to the lack of consistent agreement in the paired scores we see for individual examinees. The data suggest that items on the half-forms, *A* and *B*, are yielding inconsistent response patterns for individual examinees. This could possibly be due to nonhomogeneous content or other intrinsic flaws that violate the statistical assumptions of strictly

BOX 11.5 Computing Split-Half Reliability with the Spearman–Brown Correction

Corrected Split-Half Reliability

	Split-half reliability examination						Scores	
	Items						Odd items	Even items
Examinee	*1*	*2*	*3*	*4*	*5*	*6*	Form *A*	Form *B*
A	0	1	0	1	0	1	0	3
B	1	0	1	1	1	0	3	1
C	1	1	1	1	1	1	3	3
D	1	1	1	1	0	0	2	2
E	0	1	1	1	1	1	2	3
F	0	1	1	1	1	1	2	3
G	0	0	0	0	0	0	0	0
H	4	1	1	1	1	0	3	2

$N = 8$

$\Sigma X_A = 15$ $\quad \Sigma X_B = 17$

$\bar{X}_A = 1.88$ $\quad X_B = 2.13$

$s_A = 1.905$ $\quad s_B = 1.052$

$$r_{AB} = \frac{\Sigma z_A z_B}{N} = \frac{2.31}{8} = .29 \checkmark\checkmark$$

Spearman–Brown prophecy formula applied to half-tests:

$$r_{XX'} = \frac{2r_{AB}}{1 + r_{AB}}$$

Corrected Split-half Reliability

$$r_{XX'} = \frac{2(.29)}{1 + .29} = \frac{.58}{1.29} = .45 \checkmark\checkmark$$

Source: Reprinted with permission from Chatterji (2003). Allyn & Bacon/Pearson. © Madhabi Chatterji.

parallel tests (e.g., equal means and equal variances of scores on half-forms for the group). In addition, notice that the test in the example has only six items. The small number of items may also contribute to unreliable scores. Such issues must be deliberated following analysis.

KR-20 RELIABILITY

The KR-20 applies to tests with items yielding dichotomous (0, 1) responses, such as a knowledge test. It is computed using the following formula:

$$\text{KR}_{20} = \frac{k}{k-1}\left(1 - \frac{\Sigma pq}{s_x^2}\right)$$

The mathematical procedure is shown in Box 11.6 with a five-item test comparing the sum of the item score variances on k items, Σpq, with the variance of the summated total scores of the tool, s_X^2. Results yield a Σpq of 1.15, with a total score variance of 4. The calculated internal consistency reliability is .89, which lies above the acceptable minimum of .70.

CRONBACH'S α

The Cronbach's α coefficient developed by Cronbach and his colleagues in 1951, is a more general form of the KR-20. The α coefficient is commonly applied to rated item data (e.g., a Likert scale), or partial credit scales with two or more response categories. It has a computational formula like the KR-20:

$$\alpha = \frac{k}{k-1}\left(1 - \frac{\Sigma\sigma_i^2}{\sigma_X^2}\right)$$

The α coefficient is obtained with the computational steps shown in Box 11.7. Here, the obtained α reliability, also with a five-item scale, is .72 and just above the acceptability cut point of .70.

BOX 11.6 Internal Consistency Reliability with the Küder–Richardson Formula 20

Computing KR-20 Reliability

Item	p	q	pq
1	.30	.70	.21
2	.60	.40	.24
3	.70	.30	.21
4	.60	.40	.24
5	.50	.50	.25
$\bar{X} = 3.0$			$\Sigma pq = 1.15$
$s_X = 2.0$			
$s_X^2 = 4.0$			

$$\text{KR}_{20} = \frac{k}{k-1}\left(1 - \frac{\Sigma pq}{s_X^2}\right)$$

$$\text{KR}_{20} = \frac{5}{4}\left(1 - \frac{1.15}{4.00}\right)$$

$$= \frac{5}{4}(1 - .29)$$

$$= 1.25(.71)$$

$$\text{KR}_{20} = .89 \checkmark\checkmark$$

Note. The formula using population estimates appears as follows:

$$\text{KR}_{20} = \frac{k}{k-1}\left(1 - \frac{\Sigma pq}{\sigma_X^2}\right)$$

Source: Reprinted with permission from Chatterji (2003). Allyn & Bacon/Pearson. © Madhabi Chatterji.

11.8.3 Test–Retest Reliability

11.8.3.1 Purpose

A test–retest reliability coefficient denotes how consistent scores remain in a given group of examinees on *two* occasions of testing with a short time gap (10–15 days), holding everything else constant.

BOX 11.7 Internal Consistency Reliability with Cronbach's α Coefficient

Item	Item variance s_i^2
1	8
2	5
3	10
4	7.2
5	12.5
	$\Sigma s_i^2 = 42.7$

$$\alpha = \frac{k}{k-1}\left(1 - \frac{\Sigma s_i^2}{s_x^2}\right)$$

$s_X = 10.0$

$s_X^2 = 100.0$

$$\alpha = \frac{5}{4}\left(1 - \frac{42.7}{100}\right)$$

$$\alpha = \frac{5}{4}(.573)$$

$$\alpha = 1.25(.71)$$

$$\alpha = .72 ✓✓$$

Note. The formula using population estimates appears as follows:

$$\alpha = \frac{k}{k-1}\left(1 - \frac{\Sigma \sigma_i^2}{\sigma_x^2}\right)$$

Source: Reprinted with permission from Chatterji (2003). Allyn & Bacon/Pearson. © Madhabi Chatterji.

11.8.3.2 Method

Table 11.11 shows a guiding question for a test–retest study with a longitudinal data-collection design. A 2-week time delay is the standard gap that helps manage possible interferences of practice effects or other confounders. A test–retest reliability is usually estimated with a Pearson correlation coefficient $r_{XX'}$ using the paired scores from individuals on the two different testing occasions, Time 1 and Time 2. Because of repeated testing with the same items and examinees, test–retest coefficients tend to be very high. The cutoff for acceptability is therefore set higher at 0.90.

When the assumptions are reasonably met in field settings, the resulting $r_{XX'}$ indicates the extent to which the scores are free of random factors associated with occasions of testing. When the time gap is too long, systematic interferences may be difficult to control between Time 1 and Time 2. Common obstacles in interpreting results are the maturation of examinees from Time 1 to Time 2 and unforeseen interventions altering the examinees' standing on the measured construct, or other environmental interferences.

11.8.4 Parallel Forms Reliability Coefficient

11.8.4.1 Purpose

Also called the *alternate forms reliability coefficient* and symbolically represented as r_{AB} for a test with two parallel Forms *A* and *B*, this reliability coefficient indicates the extent to which users can be confident that multiple parallel forms sampled from the same domain will yield interchangeable scores for the same persons. This form of reliability evidence is only necessary for assessments designed with parallel forms.

11.8.4.2 Methods

Table 11.11 shows that the design of a parallel forms study requires concurrent administration of all the test forms under similar controlled conditions to the same group of examinees. A parallel forms reliability coefficient is also computed using a Pearson correlation coefficient of paired scores of the same persons on the forms. The size of a parallel forms coefficient depends on how effectively assessment designers are able to construct *strictly parallel*, or equivalent test forms from the same domain. The acceptability cut point of the parallel forms reliability coefficient is around 0.80.

11.8.5 Interrater Reliability Coefficients

11.8.5.1 Purpose

As Table 11.11 shows, interrater reliability evidence denotes the degree to which scores remain consistent regardless of random variations of different judges, raters, or observers. This form of evidence is required for constructed-response and performance assessments. These are multifaceted assessment systems where raters serve as a major facet through which the scores are produced (Chapter 6). The evidence confirms that ratings are not unduly influenced by random rater-related factors and are thus essentially interchangeable.

11.8.5.2 Methods

Interrater reliability data are usually collected concurrently from all raters involved and evaluated through correlational statistics, as shown in Box 11.4 with the κ. As Chapters 5 and 6 emphasized, raters may need formal orientation or training to implement rubrics in a valid and consistent manner in high-stakes situations. Multifaceted measurement designs and studies of rater behaviors could involve interrater comparisons, or comparison of trained raters with a "gold standard" rater (Mor et al., 2003).

In a more commonly applied interrater study, we gather data from two independent raters on the same group of respondents with the assessment and then examine the agreement levels in ratings. Agreement levels may be evaluated in absolute terms, using indices like the κ coefficient (see the κ formula and demonstrations in presented earlier in Section 11.5.9 on computing CVIs under content validity). Correlation coefficients of rank-ordered or interval-scaled data from two raters could also be useful, such as Kendall's tau (τ) coefficients or Sommer's d for ordinal data, or Pearson's r for interval-scaled variables (Chapter 8).

11.8.6 Applying the Standard Error of Measurement

Recollect from reliability theory that the observed score X for a person on a given assessment is the sum total of a true score (T) and a random error (E) component. These measurement errors cause the X to be normally distributed over multiple measurements. The **standard error of measurement (SEM)** describes the extent of random variability of the scores. There is an inverse relationship between the reliability coefficient and SEM that enables the derivation of the SEM, as given by the formula below (Chapter 10):

$$\text{SEM} = s_X\sqrt{1 - r_{XX'}}$$

SEM = the standard error of measurement

s_X = the standard deviation of the observed scores

$r_{XX'}$ = the reliability coefficient

11.8.6.1 Confidence Intervals with SEM

Once the reliability of scores is estimated for a given assessment, it is possible to derive the SEM and create *confidence intervals* (CIs) around an individual's scores or a group's mean scores using the SEM. The use of CIs provides users with greater confidence that those results will be replicable within given margins of error.

11.8.6.2 Applying Confidence Intervals

For an illustration, we will use reliability information reported for the grade 3 mathematics battery developed by the PARCC (Pearson, 2017, pp. 78–79). Based on try-outs of various test forms and modalities, the developers reported an average reliability of .93 on the test with very large samples of students ($N > 99{,}000$). The SEM reported for both raw scores and IRT-based scale scores of the computer-based test for individual students as 3.46 and 9.03, respectively.

Suppose we wish to create a 95% CI around a hypothetical student's raw score. Based on the normal curve, we know that the probability (percent area) defined by +/–1.96 σ-units is 95%. The 1.96 is usually rounded to +/–2 σ-units in practice. To build a 95% CI, we would simply substitute the σ-units in the standard normal curve with the SEM units. For a student in grade 3 receiving a raw score of 80 on the computer-based mathematics battery, the following CI is obtained:

$$X = 80$$

$$\text{SEM} = 3.46$$

$$X + (2 * \text{SEM}) = 80 + 2\,(3.46) = 80 + 6.92 = \mathit{86.92}$$

[*Upper limit of CI*]

$$X - (2 * \text{SEM}) = 80 - 2\,(3.46) = 80 - 6.92 = \mathit{73.08}$$

[*Lower limit of CI*]

As shown, the SEM reported is 3.46 for the raw scores of the computer-based test. For building a 95% CI, we simply add and subtract two SEM units to that observed score of 80, yielding 73.08 to 86.92 as the upper and lower limits of the band, respectively. We can now conclude that 95% of the time that examinee's true score would lie somewhere in the range of 73.08 to 86.92 on repeated testing, given the reported SEM estimates.

Applying the CI procedure is a useful practice for high-stakes, test-based decisions, particularly when using cut score points. CIs aid in making the decisions more defensible, providing classification consistency ranges when taking the following types of actions:

- Determining pass versus fail classifications of individuals using a performance standard or cut score
- Making clinical diagnoses or treatment classifications of individuals with a cut score
- Grading individuals or organizations with aggregated scores (e.g., score means)
- Conducting performance reviews using multi-indicator composite scores for individuals or organizations

11.8.6.3 Methods for Assuring Reliability of Domain Scores in CRTs

The reliability coefficients described so far all assume high variability in the item response distributions and total scores. Assessments designed for criterion-referenced score interpretations in instructional contexts *may not* yield sufficient variability in the score distributions, especially at the end of a course of study when most students are likely to approach mastery levels. Two reliability concerns arise with CRT scores. First, how well does the individual's raw score approximate their *domain score*? Second, how consistently can we place a person in a mastery category using the cut score?

11.8.6.4 Classification Consistency Rates

In CRT applications, decision consistency concerns the extent to which a categorical classification of an examinee as a master versus a non-master is replicable. Four types of decisions can result after measurement involving a cut score, already touched on under issues with predictive validity and candidate selections. We could make (1) correct decisions when a master is classified as a master (a true positive); (2) a non-master is repeatedly classified as such (a true negative); (3) a false positive classification, an error where we classify a non-master as a master; and (4) a false negative classification, another error in which we mistakenly place a master in the non-master category.

The estimation of error rates is possible starting with 2 × 2 quadrants to evaluate how consistently the cut score permits accurate master versus non-master classifications. For example, see Box 11.8, showing quadrants for obtaining a κ coefficient. We could examine classification consistency over two administrations of the same test on a group of examinees, as shown, yielding a *test–retest classification consistency rate*. Performed on two forms of a test, the procedure yields a *parallel forms classification consistency rate*.

In Box 11.8, the agreement levels in classifications are given by the total descriptive counts and percentages of examinees in the diagonal. The data in the diagonal quadrants yield the classification consistency rate, as shown. The counts and percentages in off-diagonal quadrants yield the false positive and false negative error rates. A κ coefficient is calculated here, yielding a summary statistic corrected for chance. Here, the estimate is .68, a substantial agreement level.

We could similarly apply regression procedures to predict the probabilities of the categorical classifications of examinees over two assessment occasions or test forms. The latter would utilize appropriate correlation coefficients. Added details are available in more advanced psychometric books for interested readers (e.g., Bandalos, 2018; Crocker & Algina, 2006).

BOX 11.8 Classification Consistency Rate across Two Testing Occasions

		Time 1	
		Non-masters	Masters
Time 2	Non-masters	***a*** **10**	*b* 3
	Masters	*c* 1	***d*** ***12***

Note. $N = 26$.

Observed relative agreement percentage: (Cell $a + d$)/N = 22/26 (84.6%)

False-positive error rate: Cell b/N = 3/26 (11.5%)

False-negative error rate: Cell c/N = 1/26 (3.8%)

$\kappa = [(P_A - P_C)/1 - P_C] =$ **.68**

11.8.7 Examining Reliability with Generalizability Theory

11.8.7.1 Reliability of the Domain Score Estimate

Reliability theory on domain score estimates is drawn from a specialized area called generalizability theory (GT). A generalizability coefficient is related to Cronbach's α and addresses the extent to which we can generalize from the observed score to the "true" domain score. A higher generalizability coefficient indicates more precise and reliable domain scores. The generalizability coefficient is a perfect 1 when every examinee's observed score is equal to that individual's true domain score. A full treatment of GT lies outside the scope of this book, but the concept of generalizability of the domain score is briefly described. The key question is still: How much of the observed score variance is due to the person's true domain scores?

11.8.7.2 GT Methods

A generalizability coefficient is calculated by partitioning different components of the observed variance in total scores. Multifaceted designs assist in the partitioning and estimations by separating the variance components attributable to different sources, such as persons, items, raters, or unexplained error (Chapter 6). The statistical analysis uses mixed-model ANOVA designs (analysis of variance) to obtain the variance estimates. Once estimated, ratios of selected variance components yield the generalizability coefficients for the facets of interest to users and analysts. Results of the procedure are affected by the test length, variability of the domain scores, as well as the accuracy of the variance estimates (Crocker & Algina, 2006).

11.8.7.3 Advantages and Limitations of GT

GT tends to be mathematically inaccessible to many practitioners, with CTT methods taking precedence in applied settings. Shavelson et al. (1989), however, noted GT provides a flexible framework for examining the dependability of measures in several ways. They stated:

> GT extends classical theory by (a) estimating the magnitude of multiple sources of measurement error, (b) modeling the use of a measurement for both norm-referenced and domain-referenced decisions, (c) providing reliability (*generalizability*) coefficients tailored to the proposed uses of the measurement, and (d) isolating major sources of error so that a cost-efficient measurement design can be built. (p. 922)

QUICK RECAP: Reliability studies should be tailored to the proposed uses of the measures. Under the CTT framework, there are four main reliability coefficients, each interpreted differently. Confidence intervals constructed around individual scores and cut score points aid in defending classification decisions. For CRTs, classification consistency could be evaluated with κ coefficients or more advanced methods drawn from generalizability theory.

Reflection Break 11.7: Objectives 1 and 4

- Define each different reliability coefficient below. What source of error does each address?: (1) *internal consistency reliability*, (2) *test–retest reliability*, (3) *parallel forms reliability*, and (4) *interrater reliability*. Interpret a calculated $r_{xx} = .75$ for each type of reliability coefficient.
- What kind(s) of reliability evidence would you gather for your own assessment design project? Formulate the questions and methods with a justification for each, with a brief description of the specific context of assessment use.
- An estimated SEM of 2 in raw score units is reported in the technical manual for a test. Calculate and interpret the *99% confidence interval* for a person obtaining a raw score of 50 on the test.
- Which kinds of *reliability evidence* would you require for a CRT used for classification of examinees as competent versus incompetent? Explain.

11.9 Methods to Examine Utility

Evidence of assessment utility falls under both Evidence Clusters I and III (Chapter 10). The concept of utility, as this book defines it, lies at the crux of a user-centered assessment design process. It centers around investigating (1) the *usefulness* and (2) the *usability* of the assessment and its different components for its intended functions (Chapters 1 and 10).

11.9.1 Purpose

The purpose of utility studies is to ensure that the assessment (or overall assessment system) is both useful and usable for the primary assessment users, including respondents and other stakeholders. These studies are essentially user-centered *product evaluations*. The specific purposes should be crafted differently for formal and less formal assessment design projects.

Questions guiding early utility studies could focus on the assessment's physical structure and form, accessibility, administration, scoring and reporting procedures, or supporting materials. Later studies could focus on short- and long-term benefits and consequences of assessment uses. More complex questions should be investigated for large-scale and high-stakes assessment programs that could impact large numbers of respondents, examinees, or stakeholders.

11.9.2 When to Do It

Consistent with user-centered design principles, usability studies should be initiated during the earliest stages of the design process and embedded throughout (Norman, 2013). Utility studies are formatively oriented, with findings informing specific improvements to the assessments, assessment-related products, or large-scale assessment programs. Design–testing–redesign cycles occur in an ongoing manner. Consequential validity studies require some lag time after assessments are in use in final form.

11.9.3 Methods

Empirical evidence on assessment usability and usefulness are commonly gathered via interviews, focus groups, and small- or large-scale surveys of the major user groups. The data could also be gathered from *action research* projects to inform different aspects of the design process.

Consequential validity questions on complex assessment programs could be studied with longitudinal designs guided by causal path diagrams (*logic models*). Both the expected positive impacts, and any unforeseen negative consequences of assessment uses, should be evaluated comprehensively. Combining experiments or quasi-experiments for evaluating long-term impacts of tests or testing programs, with contextual data-gathering methods, may add insights into the causes for any unexpected issues (see Chatterji, 2004; Henry et al., 2019).

11.9.4 An Empirical Example: Studying the Usefulness of CRT Reports

This study, titled *Use of the Georgia Eighth Grade Criterion-Referenced Tests: Reports by Ninth Grade Teachers*, was performed by H. Suarez DeCasper (Jaeger, 1997, pp. 339–387). It involved a large-scale survey of over 900 ninth-grade teachers, the major user group, at schools under the Georgia State Department of Education's jurisdiction. The researcher initiated the study to comply with a policy mandate requiring an evaluation of the state's criterion-referenced testing program aligned to the curricula then in operation. The policy required that the test-based information has high levels of utility for classroom instructors and school leaders, with the following language in legislative documents (as given in Jaeger, 1997, p. 343): "The program should provide the teachers and administrators in every school basic information for assessing the effectiveness of the principal phases of instruction, both for individual students and for groups of students."

While the primary users included both teachers and administrators, teachers in the eighth and ninth grades were expected to use the information from assessment reports to improve their instruction on a day-to-day basis so that, eventually, students' pass rates on the tests would improve. Hence, the student score reports were intentionally designed to be teacher-friendly and skill-referenced, with timely dissemination to support classroom decisions on student grouping, remediation, or acceleration. The survey results were reported as summaries of the quantitative and qualitative teacher responses. In all, 572 ninth-grade teachers responded (~67% response rate).

A small excerpt of the results on user-perceived "usefulness" of the CRT reports is shown in Box 11.9, where teachers reacted to the "scale scores," "cut

BOX 11.9 User Survey Results: Teacher-Perceived Usefulness of Criterion-Referenced Test Reports of a Statewide Assessment Program

	Usefulness	
Reported information	Frequency	%
Scale scores	390	68.2
Cutoff scores for objective mastery	394	68.9
Listing of each objective	450	78.7
No. of items answered correctly	427	74.7
No. of items needed to pass	436	76.2
Whether students achieved the objective	463	80.9
Listing of areas of additional instruction	441	77.1

Two teacher comments

It might be helpful to know in which areas the student has excelled. The survey mentions acceleration, but little seems to be done about it.

Overall, the reports are outstanding; we teachers need help in using the results.

Note. Counts and percentages of "Yes" responses.

Source: Adapted with permission from Jaeger (1997). Copyright © 1997 American Educational Research Association.

scores," and other information on student mastery levels on the curriculum's objectives. As seen, about 70–80% of the responding teachers indicated that the CRT reports were "useful" on a number of items. Elsewhere, however, 30–50% indicated that they had inadequate access to the different reports, and a vast majority indicated they needed further assistance in interpreting the results, especially on how to use the reports to meet their instructional needs. To determine overall utility levels of the CRT program and take the next steps, the information was evaluated against the goals of the state's policy.

QUICK RECAP: Evidence gathering on the usability and usefulness of assessments can be conducted with various research methods. Formative and informal data should be gathered in an ongoing and cyclic manner to fine-tune the utility of various aspects of the tools, with examinations of consequential validity undertaken more strategically at a later point.

Reflection Break 11.8: Objectives 5 and 6

- Identify research methods and actions you would take to gather information on and ensure high levels of (1) usefulness and (2) usability of an instrument and construct measures you plan to design or adopt. Identify the primary users and suggest how you would tailor the instrument for meeting their needs.
- Formulate two utility questions to include in your validation plan.

11.10 Evaluating the Evidence: The PSQI Case Revisited

Evidence evaluation prior to using an assessment falls under Phase V of the Process Model (Figure 11.1). Assessment tools like the PSQI, to which we return again to close this chapter, are widely adopted and used by other researchers and practitioners who were not necessarily involved in the original design process. Given that reality, how would a prospective adopter conduct a comprehensive and user-centered review of the evidence available on the validity, reliability, and utility of PSQI measures? Let us reexamine Box 11.1 with a focus on Phase V and Figure 11.1, specifically. The Standards advises us: "Ultimately, the validity of an intended interpretation of test scores relies on all the available evidence relevant to the technical quality of a testing system. This includes evidence of careful test construction, adequate score reliability, appropriate test administration and scoring, accurate score scaling, equating, and standard-setting, and careful attention to fairness for all examinees. . . ." (AERA et al., 1999, p. 13; 2014).

Taking the above perspective, we could begin a review of the PSQI instrument and study with some guiding questions like these:

- Do the data on the background characteristics and life circumstances of the sample match those of the groups we plan to assess? Could we make norm-referenced score interpretations using the descriptive evidence reported, or should we collect new data for making comparisons?
- Does the convergent and discriminant validity evidence help in interpreting PSQI global and subscale scores accurately? What added evidence might we need?
- Is there adequate reliability information on the PSQI scores that we plan to use? To better classify individuals into "good" and "poor" sleep quality categories, what added reliability data would we need?
- There is no utility evidence reported. Will we need to gather these data?
- What other kinds of evidence would shed greater light, and help defend, the interpretations and uses of the PSQI scores that we plan?

- **Positive observations.** Bearing in mind that the primary uses of the PSQI were to conduct clinical evaluations of sleep quality in specific groups of women, there were several positive aspects to the PSQI revalidation. First, the researchers attempted to address evidence gaps on the PSQI with respect to elderly Black and White women and were able to fill in several with systematic analysis of data from both these demographic groups. Second, they integrated more than one type of evidence to examine the overall construct validity levels of PSQI scores, consistent with a unitarian view. Finally, they supplied important background data on the samples to support better interpretation of the validity and reliability coefficients. As correlational evidence is sample-dependent, the work made a contribution to support future applications of the tool in the focal demographic groups situated in community dwellings. As with most studies, however, there are some limitations.

- **Did the reliability evidence look adequate for the proposed uses?** On reliability, the study reported satisfactory internal consistency estimates of the PSQI global scores. The estimates hold in all the sample breakdowns, just meeting the minimum acceptability cut of .70 for Cronbach's α estimates. Furthermore, subscale and total scores were internally homogeneous in various subgroups and overall, showing the reasonable and expected overlaps with each other.

- **Are the normative data useful?** As the validation study was constrained by the fact that it was a secondary analysis of a preexisting dataset, the norms are limited. While the authors had a large dataset, the case selection procedure may have yielded unbalanced racial-ethnic groups. The normative data reported are no longer *recent*, with the original data dated from the 1980s–1990s. The descriptive evidence on the background variables in the sample is also no longer likely to be *representative* of current Black and White women in the nation today. Extrapolating all three of the "recent, relevant, and representative" criteria for evaluating norms (Chapter 9), however, we find the study may meet the "relevance" criterion adequately, given that it was informed by clinical research on sleep disorders of adults, particularly Black and White elderly women. For current uses of the PSQI, we might seek to gather fresh data and compare the background characteristics of the new sample against the latest information available nationally, with a specific focus on subpopulations of interest to users.

- **Did the validity evidence add insights into what the PSQI scores convey?** To interpret the convergent and discriminant validity evidence meaningfully, we need to be informed about prior theory and research on sleep disorders in these demographic groups and adult populations overall. For instance, some correlations appear to be very low or close to zero with the selected external variables. We see, for example, the $r = +.11$ value with another sleep measure (ESS) and the $r = .05$ with actigraph data, both statistically significant results. These low-magnitude r values may raise concerns at first glance. In fact, however, these are reasonable correlations when compared to relevant literature on the same or related measures (Landry, Best, & Liu-Ambrose, 2015). Although the shared variance ranges are very small, the low correlations of PSQI scores and the selection of external variables therefore suggest that PSQI may measure a *different* aspect of sleep quality than the other instruments. The report may, subject to further verification, offer evidence of discriminant validity.

- **Could other validity and reliability questions have been examined?** With the large dataset, validity of the internal structure of the PSQI could have been investigated. It would also have been useful to have validity and reliability evidence on the categorizations of "good" and "poor" sleepers with the PSQI cut score (e.g., Did the categories with the PSQI correlate with classifications with other measures of sleep quality? What were the errors in classification rates?)

- **Was utility evidence overlooked?** Utility studies usually require current and "in the moment" data collection from direct users and respondents of a tool. As the authors conducted a secondary analysis of a preexisting dataset, these issues could not be investigated. This may be viewed as an omission and an added component of future studies.

QUICK RECAP: Evidence evaluation is a necessary part of instrument design and construct validation efforts and should be undertaken before a newly designed or adopted instrument is applied. Critical reviews of the technical evidence of validity, reliability, and utility of the measures should be situated in given user contexts and conducted in a unified manner. As necessary, evidence gaps should be addressed before instruments and measures are put to use.

Reflection Break 11.9: Objectives 5 and 6

- In which areas do you *agree* or *disagree* with the evaluation of the PSQI revalidation study given here? Expand the review, with an explanation of your approach.
- Think of an existing instrument you would adopt. Prepare a list of "to-do's" for gathering and evaluating empirical evidence. In what ways can the Process Model help in evaluating the measures with a unitarian and user-centered perspective?

11.11 Summary

Validation should be a planned evidence-gathering and evaluation exercise (Section 11.2). This chapter endorsed the unitarian perspective on construct validation, discussing a range of research methods and evidence-gathering approaches with numerous examples of applied studies. The timing of specific empirical studies should be appropriate; some evidence is more useful *during* the assessment design phases, while other evidence is better collected *after* the assessments have been field-tested or applied on a larger scale (Sections 11.3–11.9).

User-centered design principles call for ongoing data collection to optimize the user experience with assessments, measures, and related products. The Process Model as a framework can guide the execution of required validation studies in an iterative manner, situated in the specified user contexts.

By itself, validation cannot correct any design flaws or issues detected with instruments or measures. These evaluative studies should be followed by deliberate corrective actions or further evidence gathering to improve and maximize performance of the measures in the intended user contexts. Instrument adoption requires systematic reviews of the existing evidence on given instruments and construct measures. When major evidence gaps are evident for the user-intended interpretations and uses of existing tools, a redesign and revalidation effort could become necessary.

CHAPTER 12

User-Centered Assessment Design

Revisiting the Principles, Comparisons, and Conclusions

12.1 Chapter Overview

12.1.1 Introduction

This closing chapter presents a final word on how to incorporate user-centered principles guided by the Process Model, through the medium of two instrument design projects in medical education. It revisits an extended application of the Process Model for an overall curriculum design project in health information technology (Chapter 6). The chapter compares and contrasts the present version of the Process Model for Assessment Design, Validation, and Use® (Figure 12.1) with prevailing models of test/instrument development promulgated or endorsed by other authors, groups, or organizations in the social and behavioral sciences, and with the earlier version of the model. The chapter ends by reiterating the connections of the Process Model with current Standards (AERA et al., 2014). There are two Reflection Breaks in the chapter, given its shorter length.

12.1.2 Chapter Objectives

After reading this chapter and completing the accompanying exercises, the reader should be able to:

1. Implement the key principles of the user-centered Process Model during assessment design–validation–use.
2. Extend applications of the Process Model from assessment design to added product development endeavors.
3. Distinguish between the former and present version of the Process Model.
4. Compare and contrast the Process Model with other approaches and models of assessment design.
5. Identify connections of the Process Model with the latest *Standards for Educational and Psychological Testing.*

12.2 Principles Undergirding the Process Model: A Quick Revisit

> The design of everyday objects is not always intuitive and at times it leaves the user frustrated and unable to complete a simple task. . . . Do we have to put up with designs like these?
>
> —Chadia Abras, Diane Maloney-Krichmar, and J. Preece (2004, p. 445)

Designing instruments that function optimally in user-specific contexts calls for thoughtful designs and

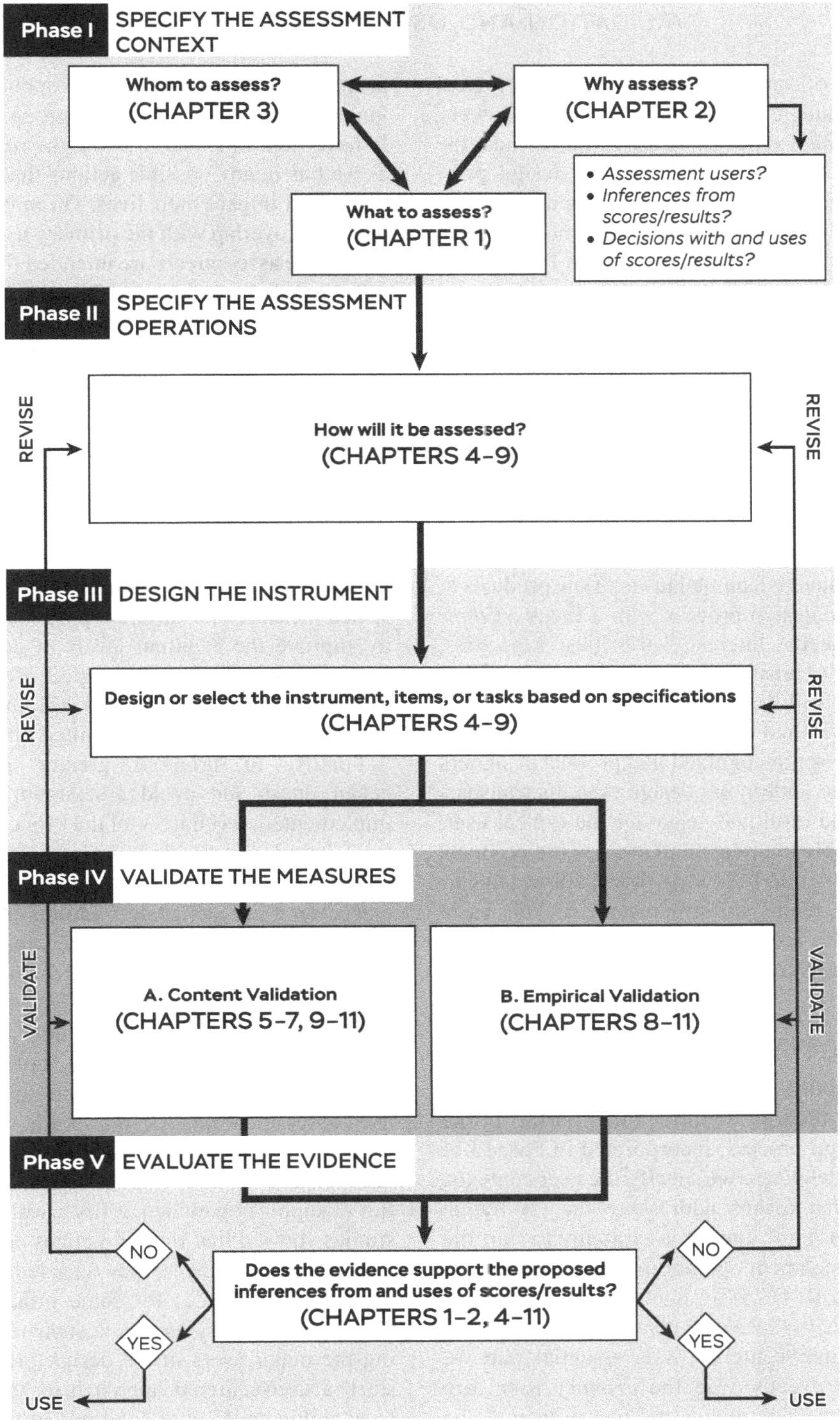

FIGURE 12.1. Connecting Chapter 12 to the Process Model and the rest of the book.

implementation of sometimes complex methodological procedures. Strategic decisions are required at every phase of the design process. To serve these ends, the Process Model combines user-centered design principles with foundational knowledge and technical procedures drawn from the measurement-evaluation sciences. The framework, shown again in Figure 12.1, is applicable for measuring an array of constructs in individuals, groups, or entities, who may be situated in diverse and multidisciplinary settings. To close, this chapter asks: How could designers conduct the design process in a deliberately user-centered way? The main principles and themes on which the Process Model is built are now reviewed.

Recollect that a fundamental principle of user-centered design (UCD), borrowed from the fields of technology, engineering, and the computer sciences, is to place the prospective human users of the products at the center of the design process with a focus on *their* backgrounds, needs, interests, priorities, capacities, and limitations (Abras et al., 2004; Giacomin, 2014; Norman, 2013; Still & Crane, 2017). Norman (2013), the author of a seminal book on UCD, *The Psychology of Everyday Things*, recognized that product designers need to make the underlying design systems transparent, obvious, and intuitively easy for the typical user. Users must be able to understand and use the products just as intended while following their natural tendencies, situated in their own circumstances. This basic principle is useful for the design of tests, assessments, and construct measures of all types as well.

12.2.1 Foundational Principles: Chapters 1–3

Chapter 1 introduced the main principle of user-centered design through the three main portals of the assessment design process, incorporated in Phase I of the Process Model where we specify the user contexts. In operation, that means addressing the (1) *What?* (2) *Why?* and (3) *Who?* questions explicitly to start the process. The assessment operations, crafted afterward in Phases II and III (*How?*), should be guided by and closely aligned with those user contexts.

To be truly user-centered, it is essential that we recognize early exactly who the *primary users* are likely to be, as the instrument and measures must be designed or adapted to function optimally for meeting their information needs, in the circumstances that they prioritize. The test-takers and respondents (*Who?*) belong among these primary user groups, as they typically have high interests in using the results themselves, as well as in any possible actions that others may take that could impact their lives. On many occasions, the designers overlap with the primary users. In other situations, the assessments are intended for applications by *other* researchers, professionals, decision-makers, and sometimes, the lay public. Regardless, attention to the primary users assists in creating tools and measures that perform best for their intended needs, bearing in mind their backgrounds, capacities, and situations.

Chapter 1 also emphasized the *convergence principle*, recommending a merging of qualitative and quantitative methods of inquiry to gain greater understandings of the constructs and attributes we wish to measure. This principle helps in the choice of appropriate operations and procedures to create appropriately scaled measures for different purposes and is expected to improve the eventual levels of construct validity. Convergence of methods is especially useful when the constructs to be measured are still novel, hypothetical ideas about which we have limited knowledge.

Finally, to promote greater levels of user-centeredness and avoid assessment misuses during implementation (Phase V of the Process Model), Chapter 1 broadened the concept of assessment utility to include usefulness and usability. Redefined, utility is placed on a par alongside traditionally valued criteria of validity and reliability for evaluating the overall quality of instruments and construct measures.

Chapter 2, dealing with the *Why?* portal of the Process Model, stressed the connections between validity, appropriate and inappropriate uses of assessments, and the potential consequences of actions that rely on misused assessment results. While it is common practice to use any given assessment or measure for more than one purpose without a mind to its necessary properties or supporting evidence, historical and current case studies showed that these practices could be problematic. In some instances, they have led to adverse, long-lasting consequences for some groups of test-takers and related primary users and stakeholders. By involving the major users in the design processes from the start, a user-centered approach to assessment design or adoption could offer solutions in this area. Specifically, such steps could build greater awareness among users—who are typically not technically trained, of both the intended *benefits* and *limitations* of the instruments/measures. Likewise, engaging users as participants or co-designers could help structure procedures that are more *user-friendly* and *usable*, reducing the chances for unexpected issues and barriers.

To assist assessment designers and adopters in distinguishing between the interests and action-taking priorities of different user groups, Chapter 2 identified the eight user paths informed by a literature review.

1. Science, research and development
2. Professional certification and credentialing
3. Clinical screening, diagnosis, treatment placements, and/or monitoring
4. Candidate selection for admissions, scholarships, and awards in education
5. Personnel evaluations in the workplace, including recruitment, selection, recognition, and promotion
6. Program or organizational evaluations, accreditation, and accountability
7. Classroom teaching and learning
8. Guidance and counseling

Bearing in mind that specific uses of assessments are not always bound by these fixed user paths, we should stand ready to undertake renewed validation efforts, or a redesigning and adaptation of the assessments. Here, too, the Process Model could serve as a guide to optimize the performance of measures in the altered user contexts.

Chapter 3 focused on *Who?* and emphasized the interdependencies between the *Who* and *How* portals of the design process. The dependencies between user-centeredness and construct validity were underscored again, this time with respect to systematic errors that might interfere with construct measurement. Measurement biases and other operational barriers may be introduced by oversight of specific background characteristics or ecological circumstances of subgroups of respondents, usually minorities. Here, following the fundamental principle of user-centered design, the designers could *include* both minority and majority test-takers/respondents (also primary users) in relevant aspects of the design and validation processes. Given the chance to engage directly with the assessment items, tasks, technologies, reports, and other operational interfaces while these are still being designed could not only improve the final products but also enhance the eventual user experience. Depending on user contexts, each of the optional assessment modalities in Chapter 3 may be better or less suited for measuring different constructs and populations.

12.2.2 Design Principles: Chapters 4–7

Chapter 4 focused on procedures for specifying construct domains and subdomains guided by the principles from *domain sampling theory* (Phases I and II, *What* and *How* portals). The chapter recommended that we draw on existing research, theoretical literature, or practice-based knowledge, and group consensus methods to specify the construct indicators, followed by content validation efforts (Phases I, II, and IV, A). As appropriate to the assessment contexts, again, involving potential respondents and primary user groups in these aspects of the design process could help tailor the domains, indicators, and initial items/tasks to their circumstances and profiles.

Chapters 5–7 detailed specific item-writing methods and guidelines for designing performance tasks and multistep exercises of different formats and modalities (Phases I–III). For each different assessment method treated, the demonstration cases applied user-centered design principles in different ways and to different degrees.

Adopting a user-centered approach, in theory, would again involve the relevant user groups in executing these various steps. Conversely, leaving key users out altogether (or keeping them at too great a distance) could lead to problems during instrument administration, scoring, communication of results, score interpretation, or subsequent points of assessment use. In incorporating user-centered ideas, the objective should be to promote overall construct validity of the measures within the limits set, anticipating where and how the tool would likely be applied subsequently.

12.2.3 Validation and Use Principles: Chapters 8–11

Chapter 8 laid the statistical groundwork for an array of psychometric and research methods that were demonstrated and treated in greater depth in the chapters that followed. *Chapter 9* dealt with the theory and technical derivation procedures for various types of statistically transformed scores and scales, most generated from raw scores (Phase III of the Process Model, *How*). Several of these score transformations require complicated steps and advanced statistical procedures. The designer's motivation is generally to improve the inferences and usefulness of the assessment results for the uses prioritized by users (Phase I, *Why*). However, the various transformed score types have their own built-in limitations, and many are *not* transparent to the typical user. To make the scores "user-friendly" and prevent unforeseen misinterpretations or misuses of results, we should bear in mind the quality criteria of usefulness, transparency, and ease of interpretation for both the test-takers/respondents and decision-makers (Phase I, *Why?* and *Who?*).

Consistent with the latest Standards, *Chapters 10 and 11* endorsed the unitarian principles of construct validation (Phase IV, A and B, guided by Phase I in Figure 12.1), discussing relevant measurement theory and research methods useful for construct validation. Wide-ranging types of evidence were clustered under validity, reliability, and utility and illustrated through cases, demonstrations, and applied examples. For making determinations of overall construct validity in a user-centered manner, the *evidence* we gather must be integrated and evaluated together and referred back to the projected *assessment uses* and *user contexts* (Phase I). Based on the evidence obtained, not all aspects of the instruments/measures may be validated with evidentiary support. When technical limitations are detected, users may need to alter how the measures can be interpreted and used in a defensible manner, or modify the instruments significantly.

As designers, we may need to consciously manage the *user interfaces* during Phases IV and V of the instrument design or adoption processes. These phases are generally conducted by trained researchers and measurement-evaluation specialists. To the extent necessary and at strategic points of the process, therefore, assessment designers should involve, orient, and educate the key users and stakeholders who are technically untrained. That may mean learning about the primary users' needs, limitations, and capacities at the points where they are most likely to interact directly with the items/tasks, directions, scores, reports, or other aspects of the assessments. Such steps could avert untoward consequences, especially with high-stakes assessment applications.

12.3 A User-Centered Design Process: Comparing the Old with the New

12.3.1 Five Features

The Process Model has evolved over time. Compare Figure 12.1 to Figure 12.2, the older version (Chatterji, 2003). The updated version is characterized by five main features; namely, it is user-centered, systematic, iterative, generalizable, and integrative.

1. **The Process Model is user-centered.** Essentially, and as indicated in the opening section, the process works best when guided by the primary users' purposes, capacities, and prioritized assessment contexts. Depending on the user contexts and/or user paths, the methodology could lend itself to either: (1) designing new assessment tools, (2) selecting preexisting instruments in intact form, or (3) excerpting and adapting parts of preexisting instruments. Validation needs could change, as indicated, depending on whether the users desire to adopt and use existing tools for the originally specified assessment contexts, or for entirely *different* purposes, populations, and situations. Regardless, the users' interests should guide the specific actions we take during assessment development/adoption and validation.

2. **The Process Model is systematic.** In an ideal application, the process is specifications-driven and disciplined, guided by the assessment context specifications (Phases I and II in Figure 12.1). If we start with thoughtful planning and actions tied to the context, the next tasks—that is, specifying domains, building the assessment tasks, and overall tool, validation, and evidence evaluation—should flow automatically (Phases III–V in Figure 12.1). In this sense, the recommended process is systematic.

3. **The Process Model is iterative.** The cyclic framework is grounded in selected literature on product design, product evaluation, improvement science, and unitary validation theory (elaborated in Chapters 1, 10, and 11). The feedback loops in Figure 12.1 show

that we would continue the instrument design, validation, and revision cycles until we obtain the levels of quality necessary for the predesignated contexts of use. To keep the process manageable and efficient, however, we must continually refer back to the primary users' needs and ask: Are the construct measures sufficiently meaningful and precise in the population units of interest to the users? Is there sufficient evidence of validity, reliability, and utility to support those targeted uses? Are the expected benefits likely to be achieved, without any unforeseen adverse consequences, when the assessment tool and measures are applied as designed? Depending on the answers, the process can be concluded at an appropriate point. It should not, and need not, be unending.

4. The Process Model is generalizable. The process is broadly applicable, as suggested in Chapter 1 and throughout, across disciplines and fields of practice, and in diverse global settings. We could employ the framework to design or select assessments tied to *any* user's needs, to measure *any* constructs in any profession or field of study, to engage in assessment development endeavors at any scale (small or large, from very formal to relatively informal) and in *any* assessment modality (from surveys and multiple-choice tests to modern technology-enhanced assessments). The basic process would entail only minor variations that are situation-specific.

Importantly, the framework allows the implementation of a variety of research methods, psychometric models, or statistical procedures—both quantitative and qualitative—during the design, validation inquiry, and evidence evaluation phases (Chapters 9–11). Similarly, it can accommodate more specialized models of assessment design, such as cognitively based item design approaches, within the larger process.

5. The Process Model is integrative. Lastly, it is important that the phases in the framework are interconnected during implementation; we must think of *design–validation–use* as integrated processes that are responsive to user profiles and contexts. Such integrative links, in theory, would promote better assessment practices by helping designers and users coordinate their thinking and actions throughout. The interlinking of the assessment use and user context with actions we take during the assessment design and validation phases is intended to optimize the overall construct validity of the tools/measures we design.

12.3.2 The Process Model Version 2.0: What's Different and Why?

What's new or different in Figure 12.1 (current) compared to Figure 12.2 (old) shown next? The specific changes, and the rationale for the same, are the following:

1. The current model has *five* integrated phases instead of four, intended to guide user-centered actions by assessment designers, validators, and users. In Phase I, the Assessment Context specifications box in the updated Process Model is broadened to include information on the users, specifics of the populations, and the assessment context. Phase V, the evidence evaluation phase, is added and linked back to Phase I.

2. The Assessment Purposes boxes in Phase I (*Why?*) require more explicit specification *assessment users* with a separation of the *inferences* and *uses* of the measures. We know that the two words "inferences" and "uses" have distinct connotations with respect to construct measures and measurement. Their separation is to ensure the terms are not conflated during the design process, or when the instruments are applied.

3. Likewise, the delineation of *population characteristics, socio-ecological contexts,* and *population units* separately for inference-making purposes of the updated model is a new addition (*Who?* in Phase I). This change was imperative, given the globalization of assessment applications in a multitude of professional and research settings today. Furthermore, we saw via actual case studies that multilevel inferences and uses of measures designed originally for individual-level applications, are far too common. This observation gave the impetus for identifying the *population units* for inference making when the process begins; that is, we need to specify the units as individuals, groups, or organizations for the measures and score types we design.

4. Finally, the model integrates the *design–validation–use* phases. Phase V has been added to

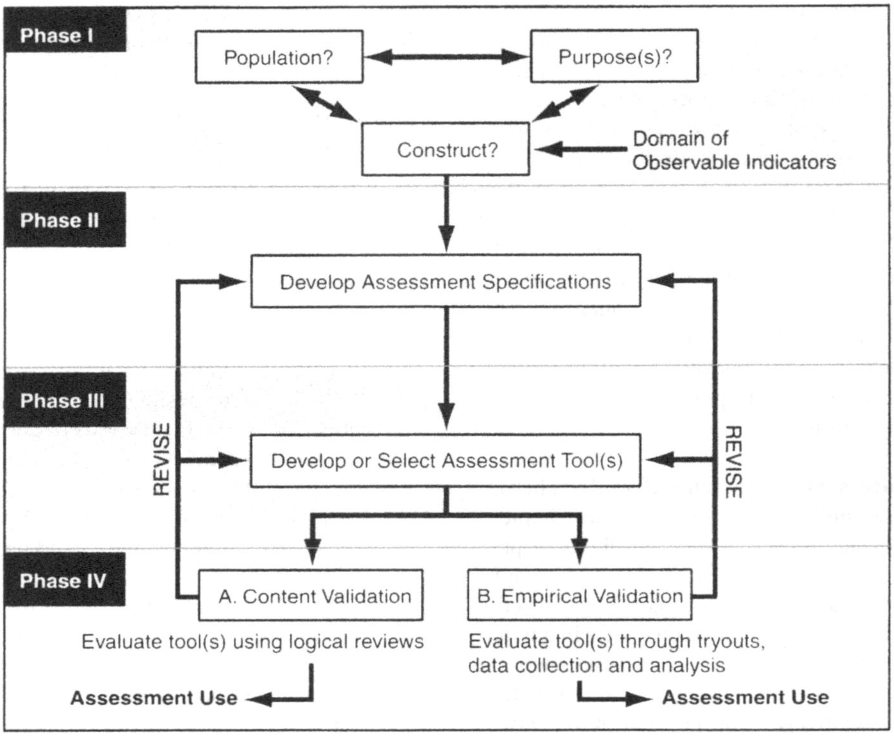

FIGURE 12.2. Earlier version of the Process Model. Reprinted with permission from Chatterji (2003). © Madhabi Chatterji.

emphasize the need for a comprehensive, unified, and user-centered evaluation of the evidence on given instruments and construct measures as a part of the overall process. It should occur with reference to Phase I, allowing returns to Phases II–IV for redesigning or revisions, if necessary, prior to applications.

As an aside, the earlier Process Model was associated with a more limited taxonomy of six user paths instead of eight that were generally applicable to educational assessment contexts (Chatterji, 2003). The revised taxonomy with two added user paths is more consistent with the multidisciplinary focus of the present book and has been updated based on the literature review presented in Chapter 2.

12.4 Extended Applications with the Process Model

The general framework of the Process Model lends itself to designing assessments, as well as curriculum-related products and service interventions. Three recent projects are described next, where the principles of user-centeredness and iterative improvement cycles afforded several advantages.

12.4.1 Assessment Design to Evaluate the Effects of Video-Based Learning Modules

Lee et al. (2018, 2019a, 2019b, 2023) recently developed a multiple-choice item pool to build parallel test forms using the Process Model. Their aim was to support research, product development, and instruction with a "serious video game" that they also designed called EmergenCSim^{TM}.

EmergenCSim is a three-dimensional screen-based digital simulation training tool. The lead authors designed the serious game for teaching novice resident physicians participating in their initial clinical rotation in anesthesiology to perform general anesthesia for emergency Cesarean delivery. The video game replicates the context of an operating room and uses a first-person perspective, with actions occurring from the viewpoint of the trainee (player). The player interacts with avatars representing the patient, attending anesthesiologist, obstetrician, and a nurse.

The researchers were interested in measuring the learning outcomes of the trainees after providing exposure to experiences with EmergenCSim. The particular assessment design effort detailed here was undertaken as part of a randomized experiment investigating the effects of EmergenCSim. Respectively, the parallel test forms yielded the pre- and postintervention outcome measures on the trainee participants.

12.4.1.1 What Were the Main User Path and Assessment Context?

In the immediate term, the primary user path for this multiyear project led by Lee and colleagues, based on the eight categories identified in Chapter 2, was (1) *science, research and development*. Projected long term, the user path also included (7) *teaching and learning* at university medical centers. Other than the researchers themselves, the primary users of the module and accompanying assessments were other medical educators and researchers in anesthesiology located in similar university settings in the United States, alongside the resident physicians who were undergoing training in these programs. Broken down, the details of the assessment context were as follows. See Phase I in Figure 12.1.

- *Assessment purposes.* Research and development
  - *Primary users.* Medical educators and researchers in anesthesiology, and resident physicians undergoing training
  - *Measure-based inferences.* Effectiveness of the video intervention based on the average test performance of resident trainees
  - *Specific uses of the results.* The parallel form scores combined with other outcome measures, were used for ascertaining the effects of the simulated video module on trainees' developmental outcomes
- *Construct?* Curriculum-based knowledge and skills in an obstetric anesthesiology domain
- *Population?* Resident physicians in training in specified anesthesiology programs
  - *Population units for making inferences.* Training outcomes as individual, trainee-level scores, and average "group scores"
  - *Population characteristics.* Sociodemographic profiles and ecological backgrounds of typical cohorts of resident physicians in the selected medical institutions

To elaborate, the experiment was designed to evaluate the comparative effects of EmergenCSim combined with two different debriefing components in two cohorts of resident physicians at the authors' university. For this purpose, the lead authors designed two separate parallel test forms tied to the objectives of the same curricular domain that would help mitigate any possible "practice effects" due to resident exposure to the same test items twice. They field-tested the items in similar participants from three outside medical institutions.

12.4.1.2 How Was the Process Model Implemented?

The authors built on an earlier assessment design–validation effort also using the Process Model (Lee et al., 2018). To develop and validate the test forms for the present experiment, the authors implemented all five phases of the Process Model with roughly three iterations embedded, as follows: (1) specifying the assessment purposes and context (Phase I, see above); (2) specifying the content domains and writing/selecting/revising items (Phases II and III, Iteration 1); (3) content-validating matched-item pairs linked to specific topics and cognitive levels with external expert reviewer involvement (Phase IV, A, Iteration 2); (4) field-testing and empirically validating a refined 52-item pool with examinee-participants from three medical institutions (Phase IV, B, Iteration 3); and (5) evaluating the compiled evidence to determine the overall quality of the parallel test forms and measures for the specified uses (Phase V, cycling back to Phase I).

12.4.1.3 What Were the Evidence and Results?

Specifically, the researchers gathered evidence with content validity indices at the domain and item levels (CVIs); item *p* and *D* indices to examine statistical properties of items for making criterion-referenced score interpretations in instructional contexts; comparative analysis of group scores of expert versus novice participants, to see if the test forms were sensitive to differences in their proficiency levels; internal consistency reliability of test scores; parallel test forms reliability of the test scores; and a participant-user survey to gauge the general utility of the video game–based module and assessment experiences. Refer back to Chapters 10 and 11 for details of these procedures, as needed.

All in all, the collective evidence indicated that the instruments and measures (total test scores) were sufficiently robust for supporting formative applications in instructional contexts with beginning anesthesiology residents, as well as the research goals of the experimental stages of product design. Once the item and test form prototypes were compiled, the designer-researchers invited external faculty experts and practicing anesthesiologists to perform a formal content validation. This process yielded more refined items that were distributed over the four main subdomains of the curriculum. Paired multiple-choice items matched to the test design specifications were then allocated to each test form comprising 26 items.

The online field test involved 49 participants, including novice and more experienced residents, fellows, and supervising anesthesiologists from the three selected institutions. The results validated a vast majority of the authors' hypotheses about the properties of the total scores from the parallel test forms. For example, the parallel forms reliability estimate was .87, indicating that the scores from the two forms were adequately correlated in the field-tested sample of examinees. Each parallel test form further yielded scores with near normal distributions, with highly similar means, medians, ranges, and standard deviations in the field-test sample. Readers may examine the original articles for further details on the evidence.

12.4.1.4 How Were User-Centered Design Principles Implemented?

All along, other medical educators and researchers in anesthesiology, education, and measurement were directly involved in the various design phases, such as the domain specification, test form and item development, content validation, and field testing. Anesthesiology residents from three typical university settings served as a major part of the field-test sample. A "user survey" accompanying the parallel test form try-outs yielded added valuable data on the functionality of both the video-simulation game and the accompanying assessments with typical participant groups.

12.4.2 Gender-Equity in Anesthesiology Education: A Survey-Based Tool for Research and Program Evaluation Purposes

In contrast to the above project, Hastie (2019) and Hastie et al. (2024) were interested in designing survey-based measures of noncognitive constructs for conducting research on gender bias issues in the workplace. In academic medicine and anesthesiology departments in university-affiliated hospitals, Hastie noticed that women tended to encounter disproportionately greater barriers in progressing to leadership positions as compared to men. But she was unable to locate well-designed survey instruments that drew on relevant literature in academic medicine, educational leadership, business administration, and gender equity issues in the workplace.

To fill the observed gap, Hastie et al. (2024) undertook a project guided by the Process Model. Specifically, their aim was to design and validate construct measures of the perceived facilitators, barriers, and challenges to career progress for men and women who taught at medical schools, and more specifically, in anesthesiology education settings at university hospitals.

12.4.2.1 What Were the Main User Path and the Assessment Context?

Hastie (2019) was initially interested in designing the survey to support research on gender equity issues in academic medicine contexts, with a focus on women in anesthesiology only. The primary user path was, therefore, (1) *science, research and development*. The projected users of the assessment tool (and the survey's results) were other men and women doctors in anesthesiology, along with medical educators and researchers in medicine located at similar university/hospital settings. However, once designed, Hastie et al. (2024) recognized that the instrument could also be employed in User Path 6, *program evaluations, accreditation, and accountability*. The details of the assessment context (Phase I) for these two potential applications follow:

- *Assessment purposes.* Science, research and development

  Primary users of the survey and measures. Doctors, medical educators, and researchers in anesthesiology education, and academic medicine settings generally

  - *Measure-based inferences.* Individual perceptions of leadership facilitators and barriers
  - *Specific uses of survey results.* Adding to the knowledge base on gender equity in academic medicine settings (User Path 1); once validated, possible future uses for formative evaluations of equity issues in similar programs/organizations (User Path 6)
- *Constructs?* Perceived leadership facilitators and barriers for women and men
- *Population?* Doctors (women and men) in academic medicine and anesthesiology
  - *Population units for making inferences.* Program-level outcomes as averages or aggregated "group scores" on the survey measures for comparing perceived conditions for men and women
  - *Population characteristics.* Sociodemographic profiles and ecological backgrounds of typical doctors in academic medicine settings in anesthesiology and general medicine

12.4.2.2 How Was the Process Model Implemented?

The authors (Hastie, 2019; Hastie et al., 2024) applied the five phases with several iterations. These were (1) specifying the assessment context (see above) and developing a conceptual framework for the survey instrument; (2) specifying three main construct domains with subdomains based on relevant literature review and an exploratory case study (Iteration 1); (3) designing a pool of survey items to represent the domains and subdomains; (4) content validation and refining of the survey items by outside content experts in anesthesiology education and other fields (Iteration 2); and (5) field testing, empirical validation, and evidence evaluation to arrive at a final version of the survey instrument (Iteration 3).

12.4.2.3 What Was the Evidence on the Construct Measures?

Hastie utilized a literature-based framework to conceptualize three survey-based scales to measure the main constructs, namely, environmental, structural, and motivational factors that facilitated or posed barriers to leadership. She measured a fourth construct, situational factors, with item-level data on demographic characteristics, marital status, the presence of dependent care, and relative contributions to the household income of the doctors surveyed.

With case study research in her own institution, Hastie (2019) was able to validate the domain's indicators and items in early iterations; she then used CVI agreement levels of outside experts to select 38 items that were most content-relevant. The survey items were rated for clarity and concept inclusiveness by experts selected from academic leadership, anesthesiology, psychometrics and measurement, and business administration in four institutions.

The field-test results were based on data from 91 respondents in anesthesiology settings and validated several of the authors' hypotheses (Hastie et al., 2024). Although the initial reliability levels of some scales and subscales were subpar, by deleting the malfunctioning items (with low or negative adjusted item-to-total score correlations), the researchers improved reliability levels to meet or exceed the established minimum of .70.

The convergent and discriminant validity evidence of the scale scores confirmed most of their theoretical hypotheses as well, showing the expected male versus female differences on several scale scores based on past research. Women were found to be significantly more motivated to take on leadership roles than men, and there were statistically significant differences suggesting perceived biases against women on some major environmental factors, as predicted by the literature.

12.4.2.4 How Were User-Centered Design Principles Implemented?

Here, too, Hastie (2019) engaged the main user groups in various phases of the instrument design process. Doctors and medical educators in anesthesiology and other appropriate fields were involved in domain and item development, while men and women doctors from typical university-hospital settings were included in the field-test sample. The final version of the survey resulted from multiple quality reviews and iterations with direct user involvement.

12.4.3 Designing Curriculum-Instruction-Assessment Modules in Health Information Technology

Lastly, Chapter 6 described a nationally funded project in health information technology demonstrating how the Process Model could be useful in designing and validating curriculum-based instructional modules paired with classroom assessments. That particular project was designed for community college instructors, in-service trainers, and workers/trainees in regional health care systems. It utilized multiple *design-quality review-feedback* cycles to improve on the prototype versions of the products (Chatterji et al., 2017).

The project was guided by User Path 7, *assessment for teaching and learning*, and involved several of the major user groups and stakeholders in the design work, namely, community college instructors and trainee-students, university-based researchers and health educators in different state education systems, health department professionals and hospital workers in different regions, and national-level health policymakers. Although the project period ended before field tests could be carried out on a large scale with trainee populations, one of the collaboratively designed "products" was a *systems-based logic model*. The logic model, also called a program theory model in the evaluation literature, is a causal path diagram to help evaluate the consequential validity and expected long-term benefits of using the curricular products at various levels of health care systems and community colleges (Chatterji et al., 2017; Rogers, Petrosino, Huebner, & Hacsi, 2000).

QUICK RECAP: The updated version of the Process Model is a user-centered, pragmatic framework based on established measurement-evaluation theory. To design assessments that function optimally in the desired user contexts, we need to combine user-centered design and measurement-evaluation principles during the design process. The Process Model is adaptable for designing curricular products along with assessments.

Reflection Break 12.1: Objectives 1–3

- Summarize the main principles of user-centered design (UCD) that you see in the recommended assessment design process in Figure 12.1.
- What could be the consequences of *not* being user-centered during assessment development?
- Review the demonstration cases described in this chapter again. For each, identify two advantages that the user-centered Process Model offered to the designers and users. Explain.
- Define "construct validity" from a unitarian standpoint. In an assessment context of your choice, explain how UCD could improve the construct validity of the inferences and uses of your measures.

12.5 The Process Model Compared to Existing Models of Assessment Design

Over time, various models of instrument/test development have been proposed or recommended by different researchers, scholarly groups, and professional organizations. In what ways is the updated Process Model similar to, or different from, these models? While this chapter does not provide an exhaustive review of the topic, the predominant trends in assessment design are described next to enable comparisons with the Process Model.

12.5.1 Models for Designing Standardized Tests

12.5.1.1 Developing Standardized Achievement Tests

The relatively recent and updated edition of the *Handbook of Test Development* (Lane et al., 2016a) provides a comprehensive guide to procedures for designing standardized educational tests intended for large-scale dissemination and applications, incorporating up-to-date developments in the field. The audience identified for the guide is chiefly test developers and psychometricians (including graduate students under training for these roles), along with policymakers and administrators at state and national education systems who typically adopt the tests.

The first chapter of the handbook describes the recommended process of test development as "a systematic approach to ensure the validity of test score interpretations and uses based on those interpretations" (Lane et al., 2016b, p. 3). The 12 interactive components are presented as a framework aligned with the 2014 Standards (AERA et al., 2014). The components are (Table 12.1):

- Starting with an overall, detailed plan for the test development project
- Domain definition and preparing a claims statement, indicating the claims to be made about knowledge, skills, and abilities of test-takers from the test scores
- Content specifications, indicating the item and test design specifications with respect to the content to be tested
- Item development with try-outs and evidence on item-level validity
- Test design and assembly, including the creation of test forms, scoring, scaling, and equating of test forms
- Test production, including printing or presentation of the test forms on computer interfaces
- Test administration, or developing policies and standardization procedures that avoid "threats to validity" during administration
- Scoring, with associated quality control procedures
- Cut score setting according to the overall plan
- Test score reporting, with materials that are accessible and understandable to the audiences
- Test security, or setting up policies and procedures to keep items secure during administration and scoring
- Test documentation, involving preparation of reports with evidence supporting the "validity, fairness and technical adequacy of the test"

The authors recommend that validity evidence be accumulated at various junctures of this process. To execute specific parts of the recommended process, the chapters present the advancements in technology and psychometrics that could be incorporated.

Generally, all the parts of the process and recommendations of Lane et al. (2016b) are consistent with traditional guidelines for developing standardized achievement tests for large-scale applications in grades K–12 and higher education settings (Brennan, 2006; Linn, 1989). Notably, this handbook chapter emphasizes the 2014 Standards on equity, fairness, and the consequences of achievement test uses (AERA et al., 2014). Based on the discussions of the "claims statement," the implicit focus of the test development process is the validity of interpretations of *individual student's* test scores.

12.5.1.2 Developing Standardized Psychological Tests

Along similarly traditional lines, Kline (2015) describes a psychometric approach for designing a "good" psychological test in the *Handbook of Test Construction*. Kline's approach embraces several elements of an empirically guided psychometric approach to instrument design. As discussed in Chapter 4, empirical methods differ conceptually and in implementation from the domain sampling approach presented in this book, with primacy given to the empirical data and psychometric methods applied for analysis.

The major parts of Kline's design process are predicated on the characteristics of a good test, defined as follows. A good test "should be at least an interval scale, be further reliable, valid, and discriminating, and either have good norms or fit a Rasch or similar model with precision, or be expertly tailored to its subjects" (2015, p. 1). Three separate chapters in this guide describe the different approaches to item writing and item content for intelligence and ability tests, personality assessments, projective tests, attitude scales, and other psychological instruments. The emphasis is placed on the statistical and psychometric properties of the individual-level scores determined based on reliability, item trials, validity and discriminating power, standardization and norms, and scaling (in chapter order).

12.5.2 Models for Measuring Noncognitive and Social-Behavioral Constructs

12.5.2.1 A Four-Phase Model with Strong Validation Components

The development of the Children's Test Anxiety Scale (CTAS) followed an iterative four-phase model of instrument development and validation offered by Benson and Clark (1982). Starting with a 50-item scale, they produced a revised and refined scale with 30 items following an item analysis and reliability study. The authors of CTAS, Wren and Benson (2004), applied the model as follows:

- A planning phase, which involved specifying the "target group for which the instrument was intended and defining the theoretical and empirical domains of the construct"
- A construction phase, involving "the creation of the initial item pool, review of the items, preliminary item tryouts, and final editing of the items"
- Quantitative evaluation phase, involving three parts, estimating the internal consistency of the new scale and subscale scores (evidence of reliability); an initial examination of the three-factor structure proposed (evidence of internal structure); and investigating the relationship among the factors (evidence of convergent validity). (pp. 227–230)

Benson (2005) distinguished between strong and weak validation, emphasizing the role of theory and nomological networks in the instrument development process. A "strong" validation research program would have three progressive validation stages (p. 14): a substantive stage, involving theory-guided and science-based approaches to defining and establishing content-based validity of the construct domains, items, and overall instruments; a structural stage, involving theory-guided, exploratory, and confirmatory evaluations of the *internal* structure and dimensionality of measures; and an external stage, involving validation of theorized relationships with *external variables*.

12.5.2.2 A 15-Step Process for Designing Attitude Scales

Speaking specifically to instrument development in the affective domain, Gable and Wolf (1993) also offered an iterative 15-step process. This process was consistent with the then current Standards, offering guidelines for appropriate score interpretations.

The authors delineated the 15 steps as follows: (1) developing conceptual definitions of constructs; (2) developing operational definitions of constructs; (3) selecting a scaling technique; (4) conducting a content validation of instruments through judgment-based reviews; (5) selecting a response format; (6) developing directions for respondents; (7) drafting and pilot testing the instrument; (8) preparing the final instrument; (9–10) gathering and analyzing final pilot-test data with exploratory factor analyses, item analyses, and reliability analyses; (11–12) revising the instrument and conducting a final pilot test; (13) producing the final instrument; (14) conducting added validity and reliability studies; (15) preparing a manual documenting key aspects of the theory and evidence from validation studies, and guiding scoring and score interpretation guidelines.

12.5.3 Cognitively Based Assessment Design: Inferences about Learning

12.5.3.1 A Cognitively Based Assessment Triangle for Item Design

A 2001 National Research Council report *Knowing What Students Know* (Pellegrino et al., 2001; see also Pellegrino, 2020) argued that the design of assessments for teaching and student learning purposes should start with an explicit and well-conceptualized cognitive model of learning. The NRC committee viewed assessment in teaching and learning contexts as "a tool designed to observe students' behavior and produce data that can be used to draw reasonable inferences about what students know" (pp. 42–43). In theory, the chain of reasoned inferences starts from the cognitive model and links directly to the observed data we gather from assessment items and tasks. Such evidence from assessment items, the authors argue, would give teachers a window into the learners' minds when they are engaged in learning new material.

The committee used the notion of *reasoning from evidence,* credited to Mislevy (1994, 1996), to refer to the process of collecting evidence to support the types of inferences that educators would want to make about student learning. All modes of assessment, including internal tests, externally administered standardized assessments, a constructed-response or multiple-choice items, and other item forms, lend themselves to the recommended approach. These assessments could include, for example, teacher-made classroom quizzes, a school district's adopted standardized tests, computerized assessments embedded in instructional modules, or interview-based assessments implemented during a science experiment.

The committee's model depicted the process of reasoning from evidence as an *assessment triangle*. See Figure 12.3. The triangle has three key elements that should underpin the design of assessment tasks for making learning-related inferences.

- *Cognition.* A theory or model of student *cognition and learning* in the domain.
- *Observations (data).* A set of beliefs about the kinds of *observations* that will provide evidence of students' competence in the domain.
- *Interpretation.* A model of an inference-making process that is tied to specific statistical procedures and measurement models that are expected to add meaning to the data or evidence we collect. As data are error-prone, various measurement and statistical approaches (many of which are discussed in the book), along with new developments with Bayesian models, may be useful in enhancing interpretations of learning from the evidence.

The NRC report provides several task and item examples to help readers grasp these concepts.

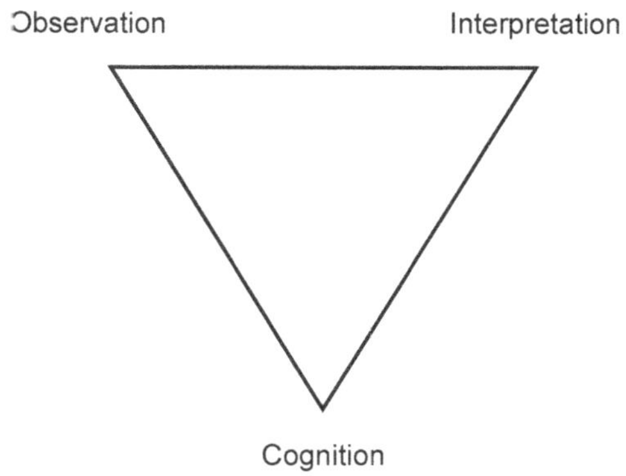

FIGURE 12.3. A cognitively based model of assessment of learning: The assessment triangle. Reprinted with permission from Pellegrino, Chudowsky, and Glaser (2001). Copyright © 2001 The National Academies Press.

12.5.3.2 Evidence-Centered Design: Learning Inferences from Large-Scale Educational Assessment Tasks

Evidence-centered assessment design (ECD), from which the notion of "evidence" is borrowed in the assessment triangle just discussed, is a technically sophisticated and complex approach for constructing educational assessments based on evidentiary arguments (Mislevy, Almond, & Lukas, 2004; Riconscente, Mislevy, & Corrigan, 2015). The approach focuses on assessment design as part of a large-scale assessment delivery system, using probability-based reasoning for making inferences about student learning from evidence obtained from students' response data. All assessments and task try-outs with students would generate data—this is referred to as *evidence* in ECD nomenclature.

In the Educational Testing Service (ETS) report mentioned above (Mislevy et al., 2004), the approach is portrayed with a conceptual assessment framework and a four-process delivery architecture for assessment delivery systems. The authors rely on probability-based reasoning tied to the evidence obtained from students' task performances, as given by the underlying beliefs about the unobservable knowledge, skills, and/or abilities measured. They apply graphical approaches, showing how models could fit with such educational and psychological assessment applications. More recently, Riconscente et al. (2015) described ECD principles and processes with reference to expert systems, software design, and legal argumentation.

The ECD model focuses on understanding, modeling, and refining the evidence-to-interpretation links pertinent to learning, as captured through responses to items and tasks from standardized educational assessments implemented on a large scale. It does so by employing probability-based mathematical models, reasoning akin to legal argumentation, and graphical display methods.

12.5.4 What Are the Similarities and Differences?: Existing Models versus the Process Model

The Process Model shares several characteristics with the Wren and Benson (2004), Benson (1998), and Gable and Wolf (1993) models, such as specifying the population and the constructs at the start, employing an iterative approach to the design, validating measure-based inferences based on construct theory, and unifying multiple kinds of evidence to make claims about what the measures mean. In a general sense, the phases of the Process Model also overlap with the specifications-driven, systematic procedure including validation that is recommended by Lane et al. (2016b).

The Process Model differs from all three approaches in taking an intentionally user-centered approach with broader applicability for multidisciplinary designers, users, and settings. Its phases are purposefully interlinked to promote the integration of the components and activities tied to various user contexts. It is built on the premise that keeping users at the forefront will help optimize construct validity levels and functionality of the assessments and measures in the end.

Depending on the specified assessment use context, likewise, the Process Model could incorporate all of the psychometric components recommended in Kline's (2015) approach, such as item construction for different psychological constructs, reliability, interval scaling, and validity investigations. In contrast, when applying the Process Model, we would be guided by user-specific contexts to make the *choices* of particular assessment operations and validation procedures, including issues like interval scaling. The logic of the design-related decisions, flow of activities, and cycles of the design–validation–use would change according to user contexts and information needs.

Where would evidence-centered item or task design fit within the Process Model's framework? Broadly, both ECD and the assessment triangle could be viewed as frameworks compatible with Figure 12.1. Depending on the designer's objectives, the Process Model allows flexible inclusion and assimilation of parts of, or the entire approach to cognitively based assessment or task design that are recommended by these groups.

For example, the assessment triangle is one that the Process Model could potentially accommodate in Phases II and III as a cognitively based model for designing items that enable inferences about learning. However, we would start by identifying the learners, educators, and other learning facilitators as the primary users of the information in those given learning settings first. The triangle, once situated within the Process Model and User Path 7, *teaching and learning*, could then facilitate the design and validation of the items, tasks, and scoring rubrics that function best in those environments for those user contexts. Validation would entail linking of the evidence from the item response data with reasoned inferences about learning as defined by a theoretically grounded cognitive model. Similarly, the Process Model is a broad enough framework to accommodate the logical arguments, expert systems, mathematical models, and other procedures of ECD as a component of building a larger assessment design and delivery system.

12.6 Connecting the Process Model with the 2014 Standards

To conclude, this section summarizes specific overlaps of the Process Model with selected Standards (AERA et al., 2014), with the rationale for any departures. See Table 12.1 again. The Standards, both current and past, have been referenced throughout this book because they represent a consensus-based summary of updated measurement knowledge and theory that can guide instrument designers. These are useful guidelines for any assessment design endeavor, bearing in mind that they were written for standardized and commercial test developers and adopters/users of large-scale assessment programs.

12.6.1 Alignments of Each Phase with the Standards

In Table 12.1, we see each phase of the Process Model connected with the different Standards identified by number. The Standards' descriptions are abbreviated. Interested readers should look up the details under specific Standards.

For example, Standard 1.0 dealing with validity targets assessment designer audiences, and states: "Clear articulation of each intended test score interpretation for a specified use should be set forth, and validity evidence for each intended interpretation should be provided" (AERA et al., 2014, p. 23). Below it, Standard 1.1 further elaborates on this statement, saying: "The test developer should set forth clearly how the test scores should be interpreted and subsequently used. The population(s) for which a test is intended should be delimited clearly, and the construct or constructs that the test is intended to assess should be described clearly" (AERA et al., 2014, p. 23).

In contrast, Standard 1.4 addresses prospective test adopters and users, stating: "If a test score is interpreted for a given use in a way that has not been validated, it is incumbent on the user to justify the new interpretation for that use, providing a rationale and collecting new evidence, if needed" (AERA et al., 2014, p. 24).

12.6.1.1 Phase I

Validity theory as pertinent to assessment uses, and the consequences of those uses, was a major driving focus of the Process Model. Many of the validity Standards in the old and newer versions of the Standards influenced Phase I.

Table 12.1 lists the main Standards under validity (1.0) and testing applications (10.0, 11.0, 12.0, and 13.0) that served as guides, the latter having to do with assessment uses and user contexts. Together, the validity Standards speak to criteria for specifying the planned interpretations and uses of the construct measures, laying the construct foundations and construct-related theories, and populations. Under the testing applications section, the Standards recognize four broad application contexts for tests: psychological uses of tests; workplace uses of tests, mainly for credentialing; educational uses of tests; and uses of tests for program evaluation, policy studies, and accountability.

WHAT ARE THE DEPARTURES OR ADDITIONS?

The Process Model adds the details on specifying the assessment context with assessment users and population units, settings, and social ecologies. Assessment uses are tied to eight separate user paths, allowing crossovers for multiple uses of given instruments.

12.6.1.2 Phases II and III

Phases II and III drew on Standards 4.0–6.0 under test development; administration and scoring; and (derived) scores, scales, linking, and cut scores. These Standards provide quality criteria for the assessment design specifications and operations, including development of domains, items, scoring, assessment administration conditions, and derived scores and scales. Issues of accessibility and fairness are treated under Standard 3.0.

WHAT ARE THE DEPARTURES OR ADDITIONS?

The Process Model adds user-centered principles and design criteria for usability and usefulness. The model and book have adopted the spirit of the Standards for a variety of formal and informal assessment design projects in eight broad user paths.

12.6.1.3 Phases IVA and B

The Standards for validity, reliability, and fairness set the parameters for undertaking comprehensive validation efforts. The evidence gathered should be well rationalized, according to the Standards, given the proposed interpretations and uses of the measures. These criteria influenced the Process Model and accompanying recommendations.

WHAT ARE THE DEPARTURES OR ADDITIONS?

The Process Model broadens the Standards, allowing validation of multiple score types with a range of qualitative and quantitative methods and psychometric and analytic approaches in both formal and informal assessment contexts.

The organization of the evidence clusters, reliability, and utility evidence categories in the book differs somewhat from those in the 2014 Standards, to align with the logical flow of the phases of the Process Model. The additions incorporate user-centered design

TABLE 12.1. Alignment of the Process Model with the 2014 Standards

Process model	Match with 2014 Standards	Focus
Phase I: Specify the Assessment Context *What?* Constructs and attributes *Why?* Assessment purposes— Assessment users? Inferences? Uses? *Who?* Populations— Population characteristics? Population units? Population settings and ecologies?	Standard 1.0 Standard 10.0 Standard 11.0 Standard 12.0 Standard 13.0	• Validity • Testing applications
Phase II: Specify the Assessment Operations	Standard 4.0 Standard 3.0 Standard 5.0 Standard 6.0	• Test development • Interlinkages of components of the test development process with uses • Administration and scoring • (Derived) scores, scales, linking, and cut scores • Fairness, accessibility, and accommodations
Phase III: Design the Assessment, Items, Tasks, and Supporting Materials to Match the Specifications	Standard 4.0 Standard 3.0 Standard 5.0 Standard 6.0	As above
Phase IV: Validate the Measures	Standard 1.0 Standard 2.0 Standard 3.0 Standard 4.0	• Validity • Reliability • Fairness, accessibility, and accommodations • Interlinkages of components of the test development process with uses
Phase V: Evaluate the Evidence and Use	Standard 1.0 Standard 2.0 Standard 3.0 Standard 4.0 Standard 10.0 Standard 11.0 Standard 12.0 Standard 13.0	• Validity • Reliability • Fairness, accessibility, and accommodations • Interlinkages of components of the test development process with uses • Testing applications

Note. Testing applications include uses of psychological tests; uses of workplace tests for credentialing; uses of educational tests; uses of tests for program evaluation, policy studies, and accountability.

principles, with suggested methods for collecting usability and usefulness data.

12.6.1.4 Phase V

Selected Standards for validity, reliability, and fairness set parameters for evaluating evidence to support specific inferences and uses of measures. These, again, influenced the Process Model and accompanying recommendations with adaptations. The test applications Standards come into play here again, as evidence evaluation and use are reciprocal activities in Phase V.

WHAT ARE THE DEPARTURES OR ADDITIONS?

The Process Model adds the user-centered principles to the evidence evaluation criteria for usability and usefulness and adapts the Standards for a broader array of construct measures in a variety of assessment use contexts.

12.6.1.5 Phases I–V

Finally, Standard 4.0 is listed under Phases II–V in Table 12.1. It recommends that we should aim for tighter interlinkages between various aspects of assessment development procedures and subsequent uses of tests and test scores. It states: "Tests and testing programs should be designed and developed in a way that supports the validity of the interpretations of test scores for the intended uses. Test developers should document steps taken during the design and development process to provide evidence of fairness, reliability, and validity (of results) for the intended uses for individuals in the intended examinee populations" (AERA et al., 2014, p. 85).

The Process Model attempts to underscore these interconnections and keep the design-validation actions closely tied to the intended interpretations and uses of measures. Despite the recommendations, this aspect needs continuing attention in assessment-use environments. As Case Studies in Chapter 2 and elsewhere in this book show, we see far too many disconnects in assessment practice.

12.6.2 Conclusions, Limitations of the Process Model, and Looking to the Future

To end, we must remember that all frameworks are limited in some ways. Their efficacy depends on the extent to which they are implemented as intended. As we have seen, assessment development is a complex process. The usefulness of the recommended process will depend on the capacities of the assessment designers and the resources available in given assessment situations. When executing the different phases and parts of the process, we must be prepared to make informed choices with actions taken judiciously. Outside of involving appropriate users and stakeholders, depending on the occasion, we may need to call on technically trained consultants to facilitate complex aspects of the process.

Many have noted recently that opposition to standardized testing and large-scale uses of assessments is growing in the United States (see, e.g., Bennett, 2023). The cases and literature in Chapters 2 and 3 indicated that when users are overlooked, distanced from the instrument design process, or uninformed, validity issues could arise. Here, this book argues that implementing a user-centered process could assist in improving transparency and user education levels, thereby promoting better assessment practices. For example:

- Users could be educated to *not* develop a blind trust in assessment results, with a belief that all tests and assessments yield "scientific" and "objective" data, regardless of their technical shortcomings or lack of evidence in given contexts.
- Users could be better oriented to read and/or interpret the scores, measures, and assessment information accurately.
- Greater user involvement in the design processes could build better understandings of appropriate ways to use given tests and assessments (e.g., for the appropriate populations and purposes).

One answer to thwarting potential issues, therefore, is to grant users a place in the assessment design process.

However, we must remember that the Process Model cannot solve the documented problems in assessment practices or policies at large, such as the issues of test-based inequities. Subject to empirical verification, some of these *may* be exacerbated by misinterpretations and misuses of the results of tests and assessments by users; other issues may be design-related. Hence, a coordinated approach involving designers and users together may provide solutions.

The cases of instrument design with the Process Model demonstrated how different groups of designers (including this author) were able to apply the approach to design assessments for a number of practice settings in education, health, and psychology, as well as for research, program evaluation and accreditation purposes in medical education and grade K–12 systems. Assessment tools and measures are imperfect instruments, no matter the procedures we follow; hence, the book has argued that the goal should be to achieve optimal functioning levels of the measures for the desired application contexts. Each such project will have its own strengths and limitations. Looking to the future, the hope is that the book and model together will continue to serve instrumentation needs in a wide variety of situations while building greater assessment capacities of designers, researchers and other users.

QUICK RECAP: A number of existing models of assessment development have similarities with the Process Model. The general framework can accommodate specialized models and methods within it and is aligned with many of the 2014 Standards. What sets the Process Model apart is that it is user-centered, valuing evidence on the usefulness and usability of the instruments and multiple types of measures measures, alongside validity and reliability.

Reflection Break 12.2: Objectives 3-5

- List three similarities and three differences of the Process Model with the *other* approaches to test and assessment development presented in Chapter 12. Which would you prefer for your own project? Explain.
- What is *evidence-centered design* in assessment? Where would you apply the approach? How is the assessment triangle offered by Pellegrino et al. (2014) related to evidence-centered design?
- See Table 12.1. How would you apply Standards 1.0–4.0 in your own instrument design project? Describe the steps you would take and the model of assessment design you would follow. In what ways could the Process Model facilitate your activities? (For reference, the complete 2014 Standards are available online.)

12.7 Summary

The Process Model stands on the theoretical ideas of validity with respect to test and assessment uses. The earlier version was a more general framework. Albeit similar and also guided by the then current Standards, the updated version incorporates user-centered design principles more purposefully. The model presents the design–validation–use as integrated and reciprocal processes. The broad foundational literature for the model was discussed in the first chapter and throughout the book.

The summary by section reviewed the main themes highlighted in the book's chapters. It suggested specific actions that designers could take to improve and tighten each phase of the instrument design process.

Iterative assessment design–validation models are not new in measurement. But user-centered design, validation, and evidence–evaluation processes guided by well-specified contexts of assessment use are a new direction that the Process Model offers. The model's defining features are that it is user-centered, systematic, iterative, generalizable, and integrative. The approach concurs with several recommendations of the 2014 Standards and is broad enough to accommodate specialized methods, models, and psychometric approaches for validation, as applicable to different score types and measures. Together, the book and model are aimed at promoting better assessment practices and outcomes in a variety of situations.

GLOSSARY

Glossary

Achievement Test, Scholastic Achievement Test Educational assessments that are designed to measure what students are expected to have learned following the delivery of a formal curriculum. *See* Domain, Educational Objectives, Learning Outcomes.

Acquiescence Bias In designing self-report assessments, the tendency of respondents to readily agree, rather than disagree, with attitudinal items.

Alternative Assessments Assessments that offer items with alternative response modalities as compared to a traditional, multiple-choice, or structured-response test item (e.g., performance assessment tasks).

Analytic Scoring Rubrics Domain-referenced criteria to rate/score *different parts* of answers to constructed-response tasks. Useful for formative assessment uses, diagnosis, or feedback.

Answer Key The pre-identified correct answers to structured-response test items allowing objective scoring by machine or human examiners.

Aptitude A cognitive construct describing one's potential to succeed in given domains in the future.

Assessment Systematic procedures, compiled in the form of an instrument or measurement system to serve user-specified needs, that yield quantified information on selected characteristics of persons, objects, or entitites in given populations.

Synonyms: Instrument, Test, Assessment Tool, Assessment Instrument, Measuring Tool, Tool, Assessment System, Multilevel Assessment System

Plural: Assessments

Assessment Context In assessment design, the prespecified context in which the assessment is intended to be used, and the construct measures interpreted; defined by designers based on the *What?*, *Why?*, and *Who?* boxes of the Process Model. *See* User-Centered Assessment Design, Process Model.

Assessment (or Test) Design Specifications Parameters and requirements set by assessment designers to build an assessment tool, such as the design parameters for domains, indicators, items, facets, scoring protocols, and the like.

Assessment Methods Six broad categories of assessment devices based on different response modalities: (1) written structured-response assessments; (2) written constructed-response assessments;

(3) product- and portfolio-based assessments; (4) behavior-based assessments; (5) survey-based assessments; and (6) interview-based assessments.

Assessment Operations Specific procedures that designers create or select to build an assessment, such as the task/item modality, scoring methods, measurement scales, and score types. *See* Operational Definition.

Assessment Purposes, Assessment Uses The intended uses of an assessment and the information it generates in given contexts, as specified by the designers and primary users of a tool.

Assessment Users *See* Primary Users.

Assessments for Accountability Assessments designed to support specific uses of the results to hold persons, programs, services, and entities accountable for their performance by external government authorities, stakeholders, or other constituents. *See* User Paths.

Assessments for Awards, Scholarships, or Recognitions Assessments designed to support specific uses of the results for granting awards, recognitions, or opportunities selectively to individuals, usually based on cut score points on the scale. *See* User Paths, Cut Scores.

Assessments for College Entrance Assessments designed to support specific uses of the results for making admission decisions for students entering higher or professional education, usually based on cut score points on the scale. *See* User Paths, Cut Scores.

Assessments for Educational Evaluation Assessments designed to support specific uses of the results for improving or evaluating the performance, quality, or overall effectiveness of educational programs, institutions, curricula, policies, interventions, and services. *See* User Paths.

Assessments for Identifying Mild Handicaps or Learning Disabilities Assessments designed to support specific uses of the results for the diagnosis of mild handicaps or learning disabilities and placement of individual students in special education or treatment programs. *See* User Paths.

Assessments for Job Selection and Recruitment Assessments designed to support specific uses of the results in the workplace for hiring, promotion, or performance evaluations of individual workers and groups. *See* User Paths.

Assessments for Professional Certification Assessments designed to support specific uses of the results for certifying professional competence of individuals in different fields. *See* User Paths.

Assessments for Screening, Diagnosis, and Placement Assessments designed to support specific uses of the results for screening or identifying specific health conditions, disorders, learning disabilities, or special education needs, and/or placement of persons in patient care, rehabilitation, treatment, or intervention settings. *See* User Paths, Cut Scores.

Attributes Characteristics of individuals/entities that are the focus of assessment design or selection efforts.

Synonyms: Constructs, Concepts, Traits, Latent Traits

Authentic Assessments Assessments that incorporate real-life tasks and expectations of performance, usually requiring demonstrations of higher-order skills in actual school, workplace, or community contexts.

Antonyms: Simulated or Semi-Simulated Assessments, Structured-Response Tests

Basic Skills Test Assessments designed to measure concept knowledge or skill areas at a very rudimentary level, associated with low-performance standards set for passing. Also called *minimum competency tests* in math, reading, and language.

Behavior Dimension In assessment design, an essential component of the indicators defining a construct domain. *See* Domain Specification.

Behavior-Based Assessments A type of performance assessment requiring individuals to demonstrate or exhibit behaviors relevant to the construct under natural or "live" conditions. Measured via direct observations.

Behavioral Sample In domain sampling theory, a sample of the responses to the items and tasks intended to measure a construct, as obtained from individual test-takers/respondents. *See* Construct Domain.

Behaviorist View, Constructivist View Two alternative views from educational psychology that have influenced assessment design traditions. (1) *Behaviorist view:* Human behavior and learning occur largely by human reflexes or via stimulus-response chains triggered by external rewards or punishments. (2) *Constructivist view:* Human learning and knowledge of the world are constructed through experiences in social and cultural contexts.

Bimodal Distribution In descriptive statistics, a distribution of test scores/measures with two modes.

Bipolar Rating Scale In designing self-report assessment items, multipoint response scales anchored at two points reflecting extreme views/positions—for example, Strongly agree, Strongly disagree, Very good, Very bad. *See* Likert Scale.

Bivariate Correlation A statistical relationship between two variables. *See* Correlation Coefficient.

Case Study Methods *See* Case Study Research.

Case Study Research In-depth studies of single/selected cases useful for construct specification and content validation phases of assessment design. Cases could focus on individuals, groups, or organizations.

Census A large-scale data-gathering effort using questionnaires focused on counting every member of a population.

Central Tendency, Measures of Central Tendency In descriptive statistics, refers to the mean, median, and mode—the average of the measures in a distribution.

Checklist In assessment design, a binary scoring method where boxes are checked for each item observed, such as "Yes/No."

Class Interval In a grouped frequency arrangement of test scores/measures, a score interval that includes two or more consecutive scale units.

Classical Test Theory (CTT) The traditional branch of measurement theory based on the true score–observed score model for each individual, given by X (Observed score) = T (True score) + E (Error).

Classroom Assessments Formal or informal assessments, usually designed by classroom teachers and instructional personnel, to support teaching and learning needs in education/training settings.

Closed-Ended Item In designing self-report assessments, attitudinal statements or items requiring a highly structured response, such as selecting only one response of several.

Cloze Exercise A variation of the completion-item format that uses paragraphs of text, with words removed at regular intervals. Useful for measuring reading comprehension.

Cluster Analysis In assessment design, mathematical methods used to study patterns in numerically coded data obtained from assessments, useful for validating proposed internal structures and scaling properties of constructs.

Coefficient of Determination The squared correlation coefficient r^2, denoting the percent of shared variance between two or more correlated variables.

Cognitions In the cognitive sciences, organized knowledge structures (stored knowledge) in the human brain.

Cognitive Interviewing, Cognitive Interviews In assessment design, a qualitative research method that engages participants in guided metacognitive and reflective exercises with probing interview techniques; useful for validating response processes and item quality.

GLOSSARY

Completion Item, Fill-in-the-Blank Item A structured-response item format where the examinees supply a one-word or very brief answer to complete an incomplete statement or respond to question prompt. Useful for measuring cognitive constructs.

Composite Score A type of derived score, obtained by summing the scores from different subtests of given assessments, or the calculation of a single, multi-indicator index, often with weights and complex statistics.

Computer Adaptive Testing (CAT) A computer-delivered or Web-based test that relies on mathematical algorithms to present questions adapted to the measured capacities of examinees/respondents using their responses to prior questions.

Concept Mapping In assessment design, a diagramming method used for sorting and interrelating themes, useful during the domain specification and content validation with qualitative research methods.

Concepts *See* Constructs, Attributes.

Concurrent Validity A kind of correlational validity evidence gathered to evaluate properties of the measures, with the intent of substituting one assessment with another (e.g., replacing a longer version of a test with a shorter version). *See* Validation, Validity, Construct Validity.

Condition Dimension In assessment design, a component of indicators specifying the conditions under which a performance would be observed or demonstrated. Necessary for some constructs, for example, achievement, workplace learning. *See* Domain Specification.

Confirmatory Factor Analysis (CFA) Specific factor analysis methods conducted in a confirmatory mode starting with a proposed model specifying the internal structure of a construct. *See* Factor Analysis.

Consequential Validity, Consequences of Test Use Specific kind of validity evidence gathered to verify the extent to which the use of assessments in the specified contexts yields the intended positive impacts on the test-takers/respondents and other stakeholders, with minimal unintended or adverse effects. *See* Construct Validity, Usefulness, Utility.

Construct Domain In assessment design, a defined set of observable indicators representing a hypothesized construct, supported by theory, the literature, or some established knowledge base(s). *See* Domain, Indicators.

Construct Invariance Extent to which the construct definition and score meanings remain constant, even when the measured individuals or groups change.

Construct Validity An integrated body of evidence that together supports the validity, reliability, and utility of the construct measures for the inferences and uses that the primary users of the tool desire in given contexts. *See* Unitarian View of Validity, Process Model.

Construct-Irrelevant Variance Systematic variability found in the measures/scores that is *not* attributable to the construct being measured (i.e., variance due to outside factors).

Constructed-Response Tasks A question or task prompt with an open-ended response format where the examinee must compose and supply a response. Includes short-answer or essay formats for measuring cognitive constructs.

Constructs Hypothetical concepts, usually unobservable, that are the focus of assessment design or selection efforts.

Synonyms: Concepts, Attributes, Characteristics, Traits, Latent Traits

Content Analysis In qualitative research, methods for coding and analyzing running text data, useful for domain specification and content validation phases of the assessment design process.

Content Dimension In assessment design, an essential component of the indicators defining a construct domain. *See* Domain Specification.

Content Relevance In assessment design, evidence verifying that the content of the domains, indicators, and items/tasks is relevant to the theory or knowledge bases on which the constructs rest; confirms content-based validity. *See* Validation, Construct Validity.

Content Representativeness In assessment design, evidence verifying that the content of the domains, indicators, and items/tasks is adequately representative of the theory or knowledge bases on which the constructs rest; confirms content-based validity. *See* Validation, Construct Validity.

Content Standards In standards-based education reforms, the expected student learning outcomes in different subject areas, usually tested at strategic points of schooling.

Content Validation In assessment design, a procedure for critically evaluating the content of the domains, items, tasks, and overall instrument, usually performed via self-reviews, peer reviews, or expert reviews. *See* Validation, Construct Validity, Content Relevance, Content Representativeness.

Content Validity Index (CV-I, CV-S) In assessment design, a quantitative index of the content-based validity levels of individual items (CVI-I) or a full test or scale (CVI-S) based on interexpert agreement.

Content-Based Validity, Content Validity, Content-Oriented Validity Specific type of validity evidence confirming that the items and assessment reflect the content, behaviors, and mental processes matched to the constructs to be measured. *See* Content Relevance, Content Representativeness, Content Validation, Construct Validity.

Convergent Validity A type of correlational validity evidence, concurrently gathered on two or more instruments to confirm whether the measures of the *same or similar* constructs overlap to the degree expected.

Correlation In assessment design, statistical procedures for describing the degree and direction of the relationships between different construct measures, either taken in pairs (bivariate correlation) or in a group (multiple correlation).

Correlation Coefficients Quantitative indices denoting the degree to which variables are related, such as Pearson's r for interval scaled variables or kappa (κ) coefficient, for nominally scaled variables.

Criterion Measure The measured behavior/outcome in evaluating predictive validity levels of construct measures designed for prediction. *See* Predictive Validity, Predictor Measure.

Criterion-Referenced Scores, Criterion-Referenced Score Interpretations Score categories in a tested domain, obtained by setting a performance standard or cut score on the score continuum for interpretation purposes. *See* Cut Score, Domain-Referenced Test, Performance Standard, Domain-Referenced Score Interpretation.

Criterion-Referenced Test (CRT) Assessments designed to enable interpretations of performance with reference to specified standards and domains of indicators, with preset cut scores for placing examinees/respondents in categories (e.g., proficiency levels). *See* Domain-Referenced Assessment, Criterion-Referenced Score Interpretations.

Critical Incident Techniques In assessment design, live recording methods for critical episodes or defining behaviors of individuals or groups, useful for specifying and validating construct domains.

Culminating Learning Outcomes The expected end products of learning when building expertise in a domain; useful for measuring learning and development constructs. *See* Domain Specification.

Cut Score A point set on a scaled construct measure (e.g., a test score of 50) that separates subgroups of respondents/examinees, usually for determining eligibility for programs, treatments, or selective opportunities. *See* Performance Standard, Performance Criterion, Criterion-Referenced Test.

Delphi Method In assessment design, a facilitated, consensus-seeking process, useful for domain specification and content validation with expert groups.

Derived Scores Mathematically transformed measures from the "raw scores" produced originally by an assessment tool.

Descriptive Statistics Statistics that describe the distributions and properties of measured constructs/ variables in given populations.

Developmental Assessments Assessments designed to map the developmental changes over time on measured constructs in the individuals, groups, or entities assessed.

Difference Score, Gain Score In measurements of change, the calculated difference between a pretreatment and posttreatment measures on given constructs on the individuals or groups assessed.

Differential Item Functioning (DIF) A type of measurement bias for an item showing statistically that two groups of the same ability have significantly different response distributions. *See* Measurement Bias, Construct Validity, Systematic Errors of Measurement.

Direct Observation In assessment design, methods for recording observations of live behaviors of individuals or groups with behavior-based assessments, useful for domain specification and content validation phases.

Discriminant Validity A type of correlational validity evidence, concurrently gathered on two or more instruments to confirm whether the measures of *dissimilar* constructs are uncorrelated or negatively correlated to the degree expected.

Distracter Analysis In multiple-choice test design, evaluating the item response distributions to each answer choice of an item against the expected distributions.

Domain In assessment design, a defined set of observable indicators of hypothetical construct(s), as supported by theory, the literature, or some established knowledge base in a field. *See* Construct Domain, Indicators.

Domain Sampling Theory In assessment design, the theoretical perspective that an assessment represents a sample of all possible items, tasks, or exercises taken from an infinite universe, for given construct(s) being measured.

Domain Specification, Domain Specification Procedures In assessment design, the systematic methods and steps for identifying and stating the visible indicators of unobservable constructs explicitly. *See* Construct Domain, Indicators, Operational Definition.

Domain Specificity, Domain Generality Alternative theoretical views from the cognitive/developmental sciences useful for assessing cognitive constructs. (1) *Domain specificity:* Specific regions of the brain control human learning in specialized domains. (2) *Domain generality:* Human brain development occurs broadly across domains with transferable knowledge.

Domain-Referenced In assessment design, the linkages of the assessment items to the specified domains and indicators of given constructs. Directly influences measure-based inferences from responses to tasks and items.

Domain-Referenced Assessment *See* Domain-Referenced, Criterion-Referenced Test, Criterion-Referenced Score Interpretations.

Educational Evaluation Studies or data-gathering efforts focused on judging the performance, merit, and worthwhileness of education programs, institutions, curricula, interventions or policies. *See* Evaluation, Evaluation Research.

Educational Objectives, Learning Objectives In educational curricula, the expected learning outcomes for students, as the stated indicators of what students should know and be able to do following the delivery of a curriculum. *See* Domain, Operational Definition of Constructs.

Synonyms: Indicators, Learning Outcomes, Learning Targets, Domains

Emotions In the cognitive sciences, learned structures (stored knowledge) in the human brain governing our mindsets, habits, behavioral tendencies, and feelings in specific domains.

Empirical Validation In assessment design, the field testing and research conducted to investigate/evaluate the validity, reliability, utility of the items, assessment parts, or overall instrument for the specified user contexts. Performed before finalizing assessments.

Essay Question A constructed-response item format requiring the examinee to supply a lengthy open-ended response to a question prompt, but within some structured parameters and time limits.

Eugenics A discredited early-20th-century scientific movement holding that human societies could be built through selective breeding of inherited traits (like intelligence).

Evaluation Judgments on the merit, value, worth, standing, or quality of an individual or an entity for a specified purpose (usually with assessments and other relevant information).

Evaluation Research Systematic data-gathering efforts, including formal research studies, aimed at ascertaining the quality, value, worth, merit, or effectiveness of social service programs, policies, or interventions for the participants and stakeholders.

Exploratory Factor Analysis (EFA) Specific factor analysis methods conducted in an open-ended and exploratory mode to investigate the internal structure of constructs. *See* Factor Analysis.

Face Validity Evidence of credibility of the surface features of items or an instrument as judged by lay audiences, test-takers, and other lay assessment users.

Factor Analysis In assessment design, a family of mathematical techniques for studying patterns in the item response data, employed to validate the proposed internal structures of the constructs. *See* Construct Validity, Validation, Evidence of Internal Structure.

Fairness In assessment, perceptions of equal access, equal opportunity, or equal treatment of all persons and groups of participants. *Note:* Social, ethical, and legal definitions can vary.

Focus Group Interviews In assessment design, a facilitated interview procedure with small groups, useful during domain specification and content-validation phases.

Formative Assessment(s) Assessments designed for identifying/diagnosing needs; giving feedback; improving or supporting the development of individuals in an area; or for planning, designing, improving, and developing products, programs, interventions, or services in organizations.

Synonyms/Related Concepts: Formative Uses, Formative Decisions, Formative Assessment Uses, Formative Evaluations

Formative Use *See* Formative Assessment(s).

Frequency (*f*) In descriptive statistics, the number of times a given score/measure appears in a distribution.

Frequency Polygon In descriptive statistics, a graphical display of a frequency distribution with a line graph.

Generalizability Theory, G-Theory A theory of reliability where the reliability estimates can be obtained for each facet of a multifaceted assessment, called *generalizability coefficients*; useful for performance assessment measures.

Global Scoring *See* Holistic Scoring Rubric.

Grouped Frequency Distribution In descriptive statistics, a frequency distribution built with class intervals of the scores/measures.

Growth Curve Models Complex statistical approaches for evaluating change in individuals or groups over time on given construct measures.

Halo Effect In scoring performance assessments and essays, a favorable subjective bias of examiners/judges toward given examinees, unrelated to the constructs.

High-Stakes Assessments Assessments for which the results are used specifically for actions that may have significant, irreversible, or lasting consequences on the individuals/entities assessed or other stakeholders.

Histogram In descriptive statistics, a graphical display of a frequency distribution with a vertical bar graph.

Holistic Scoring Rubrics Domain-referenced criteria to rate/score answers *as a whole* to constructed-response tasks. Useful for summative assessment uses in classroom or large-scale testing settings.

Horizontal Linking, Horizontal Scaling A statistical procedure for placing scores from several tests on a common metric, with examinees at the same level (e.g., linking scores from two different math tests in grade 12 students).

Human Intelligence A cognitive construct with many different theoretical and operational definitions; commonly refers to a range of mental abilities and capacities.

Inclusive Range An index of the variability of scores/measures in a distribution, given by $R = X_{max} - X_{min} + 1$.

Indicators In assessment design, statements describing the visible signals of constructs, as words, actions, behaviors, symptoms, or physical appearance signs, that are manifested in the individuals/entities being assessed. *See* Domain, Domain Specification.

Individual Differences The observed differences on a measured characteristic in individuals of a given population. *See* Variable.

Inferences In assessment design, the construct meanings deduced from the scores/measures produced by an assessment tool.

Synonyms: Measure-Based Inferences, Measure-Based Interpretations, Test Score Interpretations, Interpretations of Assessment Results

Inflammatory Bias A systematic difference in an assessment's results found between groups or individuals at the same level on the overall construct domains, attributable to use of offensive language or culture-related material on the test; a type of measurement bias and validity issue.

Internal Consistency Reliability A specific type of reliability estimate denoting within-person consistency levels of the responses to items in a defined domain/subdomain.

International Large-Scale Assessments (ILSA), ILSA Studies A series of global assessment programs designed to facilitate comparative studies in education and/or monitoring of the quality of education systems.

Interrater Reliability A statistical reliability estimate, denoting the degree to which individual raters, observers, or examiners behave consistently.

Interval Scale A type of linear measurement scale that starts with an arbitrary zero point and has equal-sized units. *See* Levels of Measurement.

Synonym: Equal-Interval Scale

Item In assessment design, a formally crafted question, task, or prompt that requires a response from the respondent or examinee.

Item Analysis Statistical methods for conducting empirical evaluations of item performance against the assessment design specifications.

Item Difficulty Index A calculated item statistic based on the proportions (%) of examinees who select the correct answer to a multiple-choice item. *See* Item Analysis.

Item Discrimination Index A calculated item statistic based on the *difference in proportions* (%) of examinees in two preselected groups who select the correct answer to a multiple-choice item. *See* Item Analysis.

Item Homogeneity A calculated item statistic indicating individuals' consistency levels when responding to items measuring the same construct domain or subdomain (e.g., item-to-adjusted score correlation).

Item Probes In interview-based assessments, follow-up items to a main question, intended to obtain deeper or added levels of information on the topic. *See* Probing Questions.

Item Response Theory (IRT), IRT Models A modern branch of measurement theory that utilizes mathematical models, called IRT models, to represent the expected functional relationship between an item's responses, the item's statistical properties, and the respondent's standing on the construct measure in given groups of individuals. Useful for unidimensional scaling of constructs.

Job Competency A cognitive construct describing the requisite knowledge, skills, and proficiency levels for success at given jobs in the workplace.

Kappa (κ) Coefficient A specific type of correlation coefficient suited to nominally scaled data, useful in reliability and validity studies.

Key Facet, Facet In performance assessment design, the specific dimensions of the assessment that are intended to contribute to the variance of the measures/scores.

Kurtosis An index of the flatness or peaked-ness of a frequency distribution of scores/measures.

Large-Scale Tests, Large-Scale Testing Assessments designed for administration to very large groups of test-takers or respondents on a regulated schedule, such as annual testing of all students in an education system.

Latent Trait The underlying construct intended to be measured by a set of items on an assessment tool. *See* Construct, Trait.

Learning and Development A cognitive construct describing learning progress over time in specified domains on a developmental continuum. *See* Domain Specification.

Learning Outcomes, Learning Targets *See* Educational Objectives.

Learning Processes, Learning Process Indicators Indicators describing *how* learners build expertise in a domain, including errors made, steps taken, attempts, and pathways to success; useful for designing assessments of learning and development constructs. *See* Domain Specification.

Learning Progressions, Learning Pathways Indicators describing steps and pathways learners take when building expertise in a domain; useful for measuring learning and development constructs. *See* Domain Specification.

Levels of Measurement Four scale types, hierarchically arranged, based on Stevens's 1946 taxonomy: nominal (lowest level), ordinal, interval, and ratio (highest level).

Likert Scale In assessment design, a 5-point, Agree–Disagree response scale accompanying self-report items, first proposed by Likert to measure attitudes.

Low-Stakes Assessments Uses of an assessment's results that typically carry little or no serious lasting consequences for the respondents and other stakeholders, or any harm.

Many-Faceted Assessment Systems Assessments built with identifiable but separate dimensions (the facets), each adding to the variance of the measures/scores (e.g., a three-faceted system with tasks, raters, examinees).

Many-Faceted Rasch Measurement, Rasch Measurement In item response theory, an approach to scaling assessment data using a one-parameter mathematical model; many-faceted Rasch models incorporate different facets of a performance assessment.

Matching Items, Matching Exercise A set of structured-response items where the items and answers are presented in two columns that must be matched correctly in pairs by examinees. Useful for measuring cognitive constructs.

Mean (M) A statistical index of central tendency, based on the sum of the scores divided by the number of scores in a distribution.

Measure of Relative Position A descriptive measure indicating the distance or location of a given test score/measure in relation to the average score or mean in a distribution.

Measurement In assessment design, the operations and procedures used by designers to generate numeric construct measures.

Measurement Bias A statistically determined, systematic difference found between specific groups or individuals on an assessment's results, which are otherwise at the same level on the measured constructs; a validity issue.

Measurement Scale In assessment design, the specific, built-in operations that yield the numeric construct measures. *See* Levels of Measurement, Scaling, Scaling Methods.

Synonyms: Metric, Scaling Operations, Scale

Measures, Construct Measures The quantified information produced by an assessment describing the properties of the measured construct(s) in given persons/entities.

Synonyms: Scores, Test Scores, Assessment Results, Score Types, Data

Median (Mdn) A statistical index of central tendency, given by the 50th percentile in a distribution of scores/measures.

Meta-Analysis Statistical methods for summarizing the quantitative results of multiple studies into a single index; used in reliability generalization or validity generalization studies for given instruments/instrument types.

Metacognition From the cognitive sciences, capacities and skills of learners to reflect on and evaluate their own learning on given tasks and domains.

Minimum Competency Standard *See* Cut Scores, Basic Skills Test.

Minimum Competency Tests Assessments designed to measure concept knowledge or skills at a very basic level with low-performance standards set for passing. *See* Basic Skills Tests.

Mode (Mo) A statistical index of central tendency, given by the most frequent score in a distribution.

Multi-Item Scale In designing self-reported assessments, several interrelated items intended to measure a single construct, yielding a scale score.

Multimodal In descriptive statistics, a distribution of test scores/measures with more than two modes.

Multiple Correlation A statistical index describing the extent to which multiple, selected variables are related. *See* Correlation Coefficient.

Multiple-Choice (MC) Item A structured response item format designed with a stem and several answer options of which only one is correct. Useful for measuring cognitive constructs. *See* Multiple-Choice Test.

Multiple-Choice Test Test built with highly structured response items where the respondents must select one correct response from several answer choices given, usually five.

Multipurposed Assessments Assessments used for more than one purpose (or in more than one user path), typically without meeting the design/validation requirements. *See* User Paths, User-Centered Assessment Design.

Multivariate In statistics, analyses or analytic results involving multiple variables.

GLOSSARY

Nominal, Ordinal, Interval, and Ratio *See* Measurement Scales, Levels of Measurement.

Nominal Group Techniques In assessment design, a facilitated group process for naming and clustering themes in qualitative data, useful for domain specification and content validation with expert groups.

Nominal Scale A type of categorical measurement scale where numerals represent qualitatively different classes of the population units. *See* Levels of Measurement, Measurement Scales.

Nomological Network When validating construct meanings, a hypothetically proposed set of associations of new construct measures with a group of other variables.

Noncognitive Construct Broadly, psychological constructs dealing with attitudes and dispositions, social behaviors/tendencies, personality characteristics, interests, and other social-emotional attributes of individuals.

Norm-Referenced Scores A class of mathematically transformed scores derived from the individual raw scores of examinees/respondents on given assessments, for enabling comparative score interpretations with reference to a selected norm group. *See* Norming, Norms Tables, Percentile Rank, Norm Group.

Norm-Referenced Test (NRT) An assessment designed to generate specific types of norm-referenced scores for enabling comparative score interpretations among examinees/respondents. *See* Norming, Norms Tables, Norm-Referenced Scores.

Normal Distribution, Standard Normal Distribution A bilaterally symmetrical, bell-shaped curve based on a mathematical probability function describing the expected distribution of a continuous, random normal variable.

Normalize, Normalized Distributions, Normalization In assessment design, a statistical procedure of transforming the raw score distribution to take on the shape of the standard normal distribution.

Normalized Percentile Ranks Percentile ranks derived mathematically for given scores/measures obtained from an empirical distribution that is normalized to take the shape of a standard normal distribution.

Norming In assessment design, systematic methods for gathering data on a given test/assessment from a selected group of individuals for enabling comparative score interpretations. *See* Norms Tables, Norm-Referenced Scores, Norm-Referenced Score Interpretations, Standardization, Standardization Sample, Standardized Test.

Norms In norm-referenced test design, data collected on an assessment from a carefully selected comparison group. *See* Norm-Referenced Test.

Norms Tables Tables of norm-referenced scores derived from the raw scores in a selected group of test-takers or respondents serving as the "norm group" for enabling comparative score interpretations. *See* Raw Scores, Norming, Norm-Referenced Scores, Norm Group.

Objective-Type Tests Assessments built with highly structured response items and "objective" scoring procedures using answer keys, which do not involve subjective opinions of human examiners.

Objectives-Based Evaluation An approach to educational program evaluation started by Ralph Tyler, whereby instructional programs are evaluated based on their stated goals and objectives.

Objectives-Based Tests In education, tests and assessments built to measure the expected learning outcomes of students of a curriculum, or the objectives.

Observational Assessments *See* Behavior-Based Assessments.

Ogive In descriptive statistics, a graphical display of a frequency distribution that is based on cumulative frequencies and percentages of each score/measure at each interval.

Open-Ended Survey Item In designing self-report assessments, items allowing a response to be supplied by respondents, usually a short response.

Operational Definition The definition of a construct based on the specific operations that the assessment designers choose or craft when building the instrument. *See* Assessment Operations.

Opportunity-to-Learn Bias A statistically confirmed, systematic difference in measured achievement found between groups/individuals at the same level on the overall construct, attributable to a lack of similar instruction, educational resources, or opportunities to learn; a type of measurement bias and validity issue.

Order Effects In performance assessments and essay scoring, the changing behaviors of examiners/judges, unrelated to the constructs measured, due to the order in which the papers are read or observations made.

Ordinal Scale A type of ordered measurement scale with increasing unequal-sized units enabling "greater than" or "lesser than" inferences. *See* Levels of Measurement.

Paper-and-Pencil Format Assessments designed with items that require a written response using paper and pencil. Useful for measuring cognitive constructs.

Parallel Forms Reliability In classical test theory, an empirically obtained reliability coefficient on given persons using the measures/scores from two parallel test forms, holding all else constant.

Parallel Test Forms In classical test theory, multiple test forms created by sampling items from the same construct domains, yielding scores that have the same statistical properties and distributions in given groups. *See* Strictly Parallel Test Forms.

Percent Score The proportion of correct answers on an assessment/test out of a maximum possible score, expressed as the percentage of correct answers.

Percentile Rank The location of a person's test score/measure in a comparison group's distribution, indicating its rank based on the percent of test-takers or respondents it surpasses; a type of norm-referenced score. *See* Percentile, Norm-Referenced Scores.

Percentile Ranks (PRs) In measurement theory, the ranked score corresponding to a specific percentile point in a frequency distribution, below which certain percentages of the examinees/respondents fall. For example, a PR = 50 corresponds to a raw score at the 50th percentile.

Percentiles In descriptive statistics, specific points in a frequency distribution below which certain percentages of the examinees/respondents fall. The *median* is a point in a distribution below which 50% of the group lies.

Performance Carryover Effect In scoring performance assessments and essays, biases of examiners/judges carrying over from one examinee to the next, unrelated to the constructs.

Performance Criterion Dimension In assessment design, a component of the indicators defining a standard or criterion for acceptable performance. Necessary for making criterion-referenced score interpretations in some construct domains. *See* Domain Specification, Criterion-Referenced Test.

Performance Gaps, Achievement Gaps Average measured gaps on standardized achievement or ability tests found in different social groups of test-takers, such as gender, racial/ethnic, or socioeconomic groups

Performance Standards Cut scores set on tests/scales to determine proficiency levels in education or the workplace. *See* Cut Score, Criterion-Referenced Test.

Population In assessment design, the predefined group(s) of persons and/or entities with some shared characteristics that are to be assessed.

Population Unit In assessment design, each member of the defined population to be assessed.

Portfolio-Based Assessments A type of collective performance assessment based on multiple observation records, work samples, and/or tangible products created by examinees/respondents, as relevant to one or more constructs being measured.

Practical Significance Evaluating the implications of the results of a statistical significance test for applied actions, practice, or theory.

Predictive Validity A type of correlational validity evidence confirming that the construct measures predict performance on a desired future outcome measure in given groups/individuals, as logically/theoretically expected. *See* Construct Validity, Validation.

Predictive Validity Coefficient In classical test theory, an empirical correlation coefficient denoting the predictive validity levels of a given construct measure. *See* Predictive Validity, Predictor Measure, Criterion Measure.

Predictor Measure The measure expected to predict a future outcome in examinees/respondents, employed for evaluating predictive validity of construct measures. *See* Predictive Validity, Criterion Measure.

Primary Users, Assessment Users In given assessment scenarios, the individuals with a direct interest in using an assessment tool for a specified need, and in interpreting the assessment's results in given action-taking contexts. *See* User-Centered Assessment Design, Process Model.

Probing Question A type of cognitively based item or item series designed to delve into existing knowledge structures of individuals, as stored in the brain.

Process Model; Process Model for Assessment Design, Validation, and Use® A five-phase iterative and interlinked model for assessment design, validation, and use, guided by specified user contexts and information needs of the primary assessment users. *See* User-Centered Assessment Design.

Product-Based Assessments A type of performance assessment requiring individuals to create tangible products relevant to the construct, usually under flexibly timed conditions.

Product–Moment Correlation, Pearson's Product–Moment Correlation A specific correlation coefficient, Pearson's *r*, indicating the degree and direction of the correlation between two interval- or ratio-scaled variables.

Progressive Education An education movement in the early-20th-century United States that has persisted in modern times, promoting democratic, society-centered values and learning-by-doing experiences.

Psychological Assessment *Several definitions:* In typical psychological testing scenarios, a broad evaluation process for understanding a person's mental health needs and problems based on the information from one or more assessments.

Psychological Scale Development *See* Scale Construction (in Psychology).

Psychological Test *Several definitions:* In typical psychological testing scenarios, a formal means for obtaining an objective sample of human behavior tied to given psychological construct(s), gathered under controlled conditions.

Purposive Sampling A nonprobability sampling technique used widely in social research, where the researchers rely on informed judgments to select the subjects or entities to be studied.

Qualitative In assessment design, the substantive, underlying qualities of the constructs.

Quantitative In assessment design, the numeric measures or numeric data on the construct produced on a quantified scale.

Random Measurement Error Chance fluctuations in test scores or construct measures that lead to poor reliability levels.

Range (R) In descriptive statistics, the calculated distance between the maximum and minimum score in a distribution, given by $R = X_{max} - X_{min}$.

GLOSSARY

Rank-Ordered Distribution In descriptive statistics, a high to low arrangement of the scores/measures in a given distribution.

Rating Scale In assessment design, a multipoint scoring scale for items, for example, 4-point rating scale: Poor (0), Fair (1), Good (2), Very good (3).

Ratio Scale The most advanced type of linear measurement scale with a true zero and equal-sized units. *See* Levels of Measurement, Measurement Scales.

Raw Score In assessment design, the original score, measures, or data produced directly by an assessment tool in unmodified form.

Readability Bias In assessment design, high reading or vocabulary levels unrelated to the construct that exclude some respondents from being able to respond fully to the assessment.

Regression In measurement and statistics, a method that describes the relationship of one or more independent variables (the predictor measures) with a dependent variable (the criterion measure) in given groups.

Reliability The degree to which the construct measures are free from random errors of measurement, consistent and replicable in the same individuals under different conditions. A desired quality of construct measures produced by an assessment.

Reliability Coefficient In classical measurement, empirical evidence denoting the consistency levels of given construct measures, with estimable errors of measurement from different sources. Reported in the form of a correlation coefficient ranging from 0 to 1. *See* Parallel Forms Reliability, Test–Retest Reliability, Internal Consistency Reliability, Interrater Reliability.

Reliability Generalization Evidence synthesis studies that summarize the reliability statistics for given instruments taken from a number of studies.

Response Sets The human tendency to mark a particular response repeatedly on self-report items without considering the item content.

Sample A selected subset of members from a given population.

Scale Construction (in Psychology) Methods and formal models for building measurement scales for psychological constructs, as proposed by different researchers/scientists.

Synonym: Scaling

Scaling The scoring and quantification steps that designers employ when building an instrument.

Synonym: Scaling Methods

Scatterplot In descriptive statistics, a graphical display of the correlation between two or more variables.

Score Interval In a simple or ungrouped frequency distribution of test scores/measures, an interval that includes one scale unit defined by an upper and lower limit.

Scoring Key *See* Answer Key.

Scoring Rubric *See* Analytic Scoring Rubric, Holistic Scoring Rubric.

Selection, Selection Decisions *See* User Paths.

Selection Biases With assessment data, refers to imbalanced composition of test-takers in a population, leading to biased intergroup comparisons.

Self-Report Assessments Assessments that, by design, rely on voluntarily offered opinions and responses of respondents.

Semantic Differential Scale A self-report assessment technique using 7-point bipolar items to measure the meanings that individuals attribute to various social concepts, developed by Osgood.

Short-Response Task A constructed-response item format requiring the examinee to supply a short response to a question, usually no more than half a page.

Short-Term Learning Outcomes, Interim Learning Indicators Periodic learning status indicators reached as expertise grows in a domain; useful for measuring learning and development constructs. *See* Domain Specification.

Simple Domain Structure In assessment design, a construct domain specified with *no* discernible substrata, with all the indicators homogeneous and interchangeable in terms of content and behaviors to be assessed.

Synonyms: Nonstratified Domain, Construct Domain

Simple Frequency Distribution, Ungrouped Frequency Distribution In descriptive statistics, a frequency distribution built with single score intervals.

Simulated Performance, Simulated Assessment Aspects of constructs demonstrable by examinees/respondents in artificially created situations, not actual settings.

Situation Specificity In assessment design, specific contexts in which behaviors are observed/measured on examinees or respondents, and in which the evidence of validity, reliability, and/or utility would apply (cannot be generalized beyond).

Situation-Specific Performance, Situational Testing Aspects of constructs that are demonstrable by examinees/respondents in specific situations only, usually natural (real-world) settings.

Skewness A measure of non-normality of a data distribution, calculated as the difference between the mean and mode in standard deviation units.

Social Desirability Bias (SD) On self-report assessments, the tendency of individuals to say or endorse items that are known to have broad social approval.

Social Index A group of items on a questionnaire that are intended to measure a social construct (e.g., socioeconomic status).

Social Realist, Social Realism A philosophy of science positing that aspects of the social world can be studied using the same methods of science applied to study nature and natural systems. Combines qualitative and quantitative inquiry methods.

Socioecological Context *See* Socioecological Factors.

Socioecological Factors In assessment design, the social, demographic, and situational (ecological) characteristics of the population units to be assessed; context factors that influence construct definitions and understandings.

Synonym: Socioecological Setting

Stakeholders Individuals with vested interests in an assessment's results and any associated evaluative actions; includes the primary users of an assessment tool.

Standard Deviation An index of variability of scores/measures of a distribution, calculated as the positive square root of the mean-squared deviations of the scores from the mean of the distribution.

Standard Error of Measurement (SEM) In classical measurement, an estimate of reliability that is the mathematical inverse of the reliability coefficient for the scores/measures.

Standard Normal Distribution *See* Normal Distribution.

Standard of Excellence *See* Cut Scores, Performance Standard.

Standard Score, *z*-Score In descriptive statistics, expressing the location of a raw score in a distribution in terms of its distance from the mean in standard deviation units.

Standardization In assessment design, methods for ensuring controlled and uniform assessment operations and score meanings for all test-takers/respondents. *See* Standardized Test, Norming.

Standardization Studies *See* Norming.

Standardized Tests Instruments that, by design, are crafted and scored under uniform and controlled conditions, and administered with the same strict protocols for all test-takers or respondents.

Standards-Based Reforms (in Education) A successive series of education reform initiatives implemented in the United States that are intended to raise academic standards in grades K–12.

Statistically Significant The results of a statistical hypothesis test showing a very low probability (usually <1–5%) that the observations in a controlled research study occurred due to sampling error or by chance.

Stratified Domain Structure In assessment design, a construct domain specified with clearly discernible strata (the subdomains), with indicators organized in heterogeneous subsets in terms of content and behaviors to be assessed.

Synonym: Subdomain

Structured-Response Test A test built with items that offer only highly structured response options to examinees, like fill-in-the blank or multiple-choice items.

Subdomain In assessment design, a discernible substratum of indicators within a specified construct domain that defines a subscale or subtest.

Subscale In assessment design, a subset of items on an instrument tied to a subdomain that yields a separate score/measure.

Synonym: Subtest

Summative Assessments Uses of assessment results for making final, summary judgments about individuals/entities.

Synonyms: Summative Decisions, Summative Evaluations, Summative Uses of Assessments

Summative Use *See* Summative Assessments.

Survey Research, Sample Survey Research A social research method utilizing self-report instruments with selected samples/cases for making generalizations to the population.

Systematic Errors of Measurement In assessment design, the observed variance in the test scores/measures that is *not* systematically related to the constructs being measured, lowering validity levels. *See* Construct-Irrelevant Variance.

Systematic Variance In assessment design, the observed variance in the construct measures that is systematically related to the construct(s) intended to be measured; determines validity levels. *See* Construct Validity.

Table of Specifications, Table of Test Specifications In assessment design, the specified domain presented in the form of a table. *See* Domain Specification.

Task Carryover Effects In scoring performance assessments and essays, biases of examiners/judges carrying over from one task to the next, unrelated to the constructs.

Technology-Mediated Assessments Assessments with items delivered using various forms of technology or media, such as video, iPads, or tablets.

Test Equating Methods for statistically adjusting scores from parallel test forms of given domains that yield different scores for the same people.

Test-Based Accountability Models (in Education) High-stakes, summative uses of standardized test scores of students for holding teachers, leaders, and educational entities accountable for their performance.

Test–Retest Reliability An empirically obtained reliability coefficient from the measures/scores on given persons taken on two different occasions with a 2-week time delay, holding all else constant.

Test-Wise A construct describing an examinee's capacity to successfully take a test without having the necessary knowledge/skills in the tested domains.

Theoretical Definitions of Constructs In assessment design, the definition of a construct based on established literature, practice-based knowledge, a theory, or proposed conceptual framework, as given by the designers and/or primary users. *See* Operational Definition

Trait A hypothetical construct (from psychology).

Synonyms: Construct, Concept, Latent Trait, Trait

Tree diagram For construct domain specification in assessment design, a method for organizing/diagramming the indicators with a main central trunk and branches and subbranches beneath. *See* Domain Specification.

True–False (T/F) Item A structured-response item format designed with a propositional statement or question stem followed by two answer options, of which only one is correct—True–False, Yes–No, Correct–Incorrect. Useful for measuring cognitive constructs.

Unidimensional, Unidimensional Scale A continuous linear scale for a construct measure with equal interval or ratio units.

Unified Validation In given contexts, gathering and evaluating a collective body of evidence on validity, reliability, and utility that is necessary to justify the proposed inferences and uses of the construct measures. *See* User-Centered Assessment Design, Process Model.

Unitarian View of Validity The current and dominant conception of validity positing that evidence gathered must collectively justify the proposed inferences and uses of the construct measures of a tool.

Synonym: Unified Validation

Usability The ease of use, accessibility, practicality, transparency, and overall suitability of an assessment and the construct measures for the primary assessment users in given contexts; an aspect of *utility* and desired quality of assessments and construct measures. *See* User-Centered Assessment Design.

Usefulness The expected benefits of using an assessment tool and its construct measures for the specific uses that primary users and stakeholders desire; an aspect of *utility* and desired quality of assessments and construct measures. *See* User-Centered Assessment Design.

User Paths Eight categories of assessment uses, each associated with specialized groups of users: (1) science, research, and development; (2) professional certification and credentialing; (3) clinical screening, diagnosis, treatment placement, and monitoring; (4) candidate selection for admissions in education, or grade-level promotions and other recognitions; (5) personnel evaluations in the workplace, including recruitment, selection, recognitions, and promotions; (6) program/organizational evaluations, accreditation, and accountability; (7) classroom teaching and learning; (8) guidance and counseling.

User-Centered Assessment Design An approach to assessment design, founded on the principles of human-centered design, that aims to optimize the functionality of a tool and the construct measures in given user contexts. *See* Process Model.

Uses In assessment design, specific decisions or actions that the primary users of an assessment intend to take with the construct measures in designated user contexts. *See* Assessment Purposes, Assessment Uses.

Utility The overall functionality of an assessment and the construct measures it yields for the designated uses and user contexts; a desired quality of assessments and measures combining the criteria of *usefulness* and *usability*. *See* User-Centered Assessment Design.

Validation, Construct Validation Evidence-gathering and evidence-evaluation efforts undertaken as a part of the assessment design process to determine validity, reliability, and utility levels of measures for the inferences and uses that the primary users desire. *See* Unitarian View of Validity, Unified Validation, Construct Validity, User-Centered Assessment Design, Process Model.

Validation Plan In assessment design, a plan for collecting and evaluating a unified body of evidence to investigate the quality of an assessment and the construct measures it yields. *See* Validation, Construct Validity.

Validity Broadly, the degree to which the measures are meaningful with respect to the intended constructs and free from outside interferences, showing the expected variability in the designated population units. *See* Construct Validity, Systematic Variance, Validation.

Validity Evidence *See* Construct Validity, Validation.

Validity Generalization Evidence synthesis studies that summarize the validity evidence taken from a number of studies for given instruments.

Validity of the Response Processes Specific type of validity evidence confirming that the items require the examinees/respondents to engage in the relevant cognitive processes when responding. *See* Construct Validity, Validation.

Variability, Measures of Variability In descriptive statistics, a measure of the spread of the scores/measures in a distribution, such as the variance, standard deviation, and range.

Variable A measured construct that distributes with different values in members/units of given populations.

Variance An index of variability of scores/measures of a distribution, calculated as the mean-squared deviation of the scores from the mean of the distribution

Vertical Linking, Vertical Scaling A statistical procedure for placing scores of several tests at increasing grade levels on a common numeric scale, regardless of differences in construct definitions—for example, linking math test scores in grade 3–12 students.

Workplace Learning A cognitive construct describing the learning progressions over time for acquiring the requisite knowledge/skills for given jobs in the workplace. *See* Domain Specification, Learning and Development.

References

Abras, C., Maloney-Krichmar, D., & Preece, J. (2004). User-centered design. In W. Bainbridge (Ed.), *Encyclopedia of human–computer interaction* (Vol. 2, pp. 445–456). Berkshire.

Aikin, W. M. (1942). *The story of the eight-year study.* Harper & Brothers.

Allen, M. J., & Yen, W. M. (2002). *Introduction to measurement theory.* Waveland Press.

Alrqiq, H. (2020). *Use of an animated video for child oral health education as a brief online intervention designed for parent-child dyads: Predictors of parental self-efficacy to engage in recommended behaviors.* PhD dissertation, Teachers College, Columbia University. https://academiccommons.columbia.edu/doi/10.7916/d8-4a7f-sp80.

American Educational Research Association. (2015). Statement on use of value-added models (VAM) for the evaluation of educators and educator preparation programs. *Educational Researcher, 44*(8), 448–452.

American Educational Research Association, American Psychological Association, & National Council on Measurement in Education. (1999). *Standards for educational and psychological testing.* Author.

American Educational Research Association, American Psychological Association, & National Council on Measurement in Education. (2014). *Standards for educational and psychological testing.* Author.

American Evaluation Association. (2018). *Guiding principles for evaluators.* www.eval.org/About/Guiding-Principles.

American Psychiatric Association. (2022). *Diagnostic and statistical manual of mental disorders* (5th ed., text rev.). Author.

American Psychological Association. (2007). *Report of the APA Task Force on Socioeconomic Status.* www.apa.org/pi/ses/resources/class/measuring-status.

American Psychological Association. (2011). *Assessment tools.* www.apa.org/pi/about/publications/caregivers/practice-settings/assessment/tools.

American Psychological Association, American Educational Research Association, National Council on Measurement in Education, & American Educational Research Association. Committee on Test Standards. (1966). *Standards for educational and psychological tests and manuals.* American Psychological Association.

Andrich, D. (1978). Relationships between the Thurstone and Rasch approaches to item scaling. *Applied Psychological Measurement, 2*(3), 451–462.

Angoff, W. H. (1971). Scales, norms, and equivalent scores. In R. L. Thorndike (Ed.), *Educational measurement* (2nd ed., pp. 508–600). American Council on Education.

Angoff, W. H. (1988). Validity: An evolving concept. In

H. Wainer & H. I. Braun (Eds.), *Test validity* (pp. 19–32). Erlbaum.

Arbuthnot, K. (2020). Reimagining assessments in the postpandemic era: Creating a blueprint for the future. *Educational Measurement, Issues and Practice, 39*(3), 97–99.

Aron, A., & Elliott, J. (2012). *Statistics for social and behavioral sciences* (6th ed.). Amazon.

Astin, A. W. (2012). *Assessment for excellence: The philosophy and practice of assessment and evaluation in higher education.* Rowman & Littlefield.

Atwell, C. R. (1937). Relationship of scores and errors on the Army Alpha test. *Journal of Applied Psychology, 21*(4), 451–455.

Babbie, E. R. (1998). *Survey research methods* (2nd ed.). Wadsworth.

Babbie, E. R. (2015). *The practice of social reserach* (14th ed.). Cengage.

Babbie, E. R. (2020). *The practice of social research* (15th ed.). Cengage.

Backhoff, E. (2013). Validity issues in international large scale assessment (ILSA) programs: Thoughts for developing countries. In M. Chatterji (Ed.), *Validity and test use: An international dialogue on educational assessment, accountability and equity* (pp. 233–249). Emerald Group.

Baig, L., Violato, C., & Crutcher, R. (2010). A construct validity study of clinical competence: A multitrait multimethod matrix approach. *Journal of Continuing Education in the Health Professions, 20*(1), 19–25.

Baker, E. L. (2013). The chimera of validity. *Teachers College Record, 115*(9), 1–26.

Bandalos, D. L. (2018). *Measurement theory and applications for the social sciences.* Guilford Press.

Banerji, M. (1999). Validation of scores/measures from a K–2 developmental assessment in mathematics. *Educational and Psychological Measurement, 59*(4), 694–715.

Banerji, M., Anderson, R. H., & Kerstyn, C. (2000). Designing assessment systems for nongraded environments: Pedagogical foundations and classroom applications. *National Forum of Teacher Education Journal, 10*(2), 19–39.

Banerji, M., & Ferron, J. (1998). Construct validity of a developmental assessment made up of mathematical patterns tasks. *Educational and Psychological Measurement, 58*(4), 634–660.

Barret, L. F. (2017, December). *You aren't at the mercy of your emotions—your brain creates them* [Video]. TED Talks. www.ted.com/talks/lisa_feldman_barrett_you_aren_t_at_the_mercy_of_your_emotions_your_brain_creates_them?utm_campaign=tedspread&utm_medium=referral&utm_source=tedcomshare.

Bass, B. M., Burger, P. C., Doktor, R., & Barrett, G. V. (1979). *Assessment of managers: An international comparison.* Free Press.

Beaudreau, S. A., Spira, A. P., Stewart, A., Kezirian, E. J., Lui, L. Y., Ensrud, K., . . . Study of Osteoporotic Fractures. (2012). Validation of the Pittsburgh Sleep Quality Index and the Epworth Sleepiness Scale in older Black and White women. *Sleep Medicine, 13*(1), 36–42.

Becker, B. J., & Gözütok, A. S. (2022). Measurement issues in synthesizing survey-item responses. In H. K. T. Ng & D. F. Heitjan (Eds.), *Recent advances on sampling methods and educational statistics* (pp. 119–140). Springer.

Belarmino, B., Jr. (2003). A performance assessment for measuring competence in physical therapy in cardiac care units. Submitted in partial fulfillment of course requirements for ORL 5523, Teachers College, Columbia University. See under "Process Model Applications" at www.columbia.edu/~mb1434/EdAssess.htm.

Benjamin, L. T., Jr. (2009). The birth of American intelligence testing. *APA Monitor, 40*(1), 20.

Bennett, R. E. (2010). Cognitively based assessment of, for, and as learning (CBAL): A preliminary theory of action for summative and formative assessment. *Measurement: Interdisciplinary Research and Perspectives, 8*(2–3), 70–91.

Bennett, R. E. (2016). *Opt out: An examination of issues.* ETS Research Report Series. Educational Testing Services. https://doi.org/10.1002/ets2.12101.

Bennett, R. E. (2023). Toward a theory of socioculturally responsive assessment. *Educational Assessment, 28*(2), 83–104.

Benson, J. (2005). Developing a strong program of construct validation: A test anxiety example. *Educational Measurement: Issues and Practice, 17*(1), 10–17.

Benson, J., & Clark, F. (1982). A guide for instrument development and validation. *American Journal of Occupational Therapy, 36*(12), 789–800.

Berk, L. E. (1986). Relationship of elementary school children's private speech to behavioral accompaniment to task, attention, and task performance. *Developmental Psychology, 22*(5), 671–680.

Berk, R. A. (Ed.). (1982). *Handbook of methods for detecting test bias.* Johns Hopkins University Press.

Berk, R. A. (1984a). Conducting the item analysis. In R. A. Berk (Ed.), *A guide to criterion-referenced test construction* (pp. 97–143). Johns Hopkins Press.

Berk, R. A. (Ed.). (1984b). *A guide to criterion-referenced test construction.* Johns Hopkins Press.

Best, J. W., & Kahn, J. V. (2016). *Research in education* (10th ed.). Pearson.

Beveridge, W. I. B. (1950). *The art of scientific investigation.* Norton.

Binet, A. (1909). *Les idées modernes sur les enfants.* Flammarion.

Black, P., Harrison, C., Lee, C., Marshall, B., & Wiliam, D. (2007). *Assessment for learning.* McGraw-Hill International (UK).

Black, P., & Wiliam, D. (1998). Assessment and classroom learning. *Assessment in education: Principles, Policy & Practice, 5*(1), 7–74.

Bloom, B. S. (1956). *Taxonomy of educational objectives: The classification of educational goals* (1st ed.). Longman Group.

Bloom, B. S., Englehart, M. D., Furst, E. J., Hill, W. H., & Krathwohl, D. R. (1956). *Taxonomy of educational objectives: The classification of educational goals: Handbook 1. Cognitive domain.* Longman.

Blum, R. H., Muret-Wagstaff, S. L., Boulet, J. R., Cooper, J. B., & Petrusa, E. R. (2018). Simulation-based assessment to reliably identify key resident performance attributes. *Anesthesiology, 128*(4), 821–831.

Bogart, J. A. (2003). Subjective perceptions of unhealthy intimate relationships. Unpublished manuscript, Teachers College, Columbia University.

Borsboom, D., & Mellenbergh, G. J. (2007). Test validity in cognitive assessment. In J. P. Leighton & M. J. Gierl (Eds.), *Cognitive diagnostic assessment for education: Theory and applications* (pp. 85–115). Cambridge University Press.

Borsboom, D., Mellenbergh, G. J., & van Heerden, J. (2004). The concept of validity. *Psychological Review, 111*(4), 1061–1071.

Brennan, R. L. (1984). Estimating the dependability of scores. In R. A. Berk (Ed.), *A guide to criterion-referenced test construction.* Johns Hopkins Press.

Brennan, R. L. (2006). Perspectives on the evolution and future on educational measurement. In R. L. Brennan (Ed.), *Educational measurement* (4th ed., pp. 1–14). American Council of Education/Praeger.

Briggs, S. R., & Cheek, J. M. (1986). The role of factor analysis in the development and evaluation of personality scales. *Journal of Personality, 54*(1), 106–148.

Brookhart, S. M., & Chen, F. (2014). The quality and effectiveness of descriptive rubrics. *Educational Review, 67*(3), 343–368.

Buehl, M. M., Alexander, P. A., & Murphy, P. K. (2002). Beliefs about schooled knowledge: Domain specific or domain general? *Contemporary Educational Psychology, 27*(3), 415–449.

Burge S. K. (1998). How do you define abuse? *Family Medicine*, 7(1), 31–32.

Butler, P. (Ed.). (1997). *Issues in alternative assessment: The Japanese perspective.* Kwansei Gaikuin University, Nishinomiya. Language Center.

Buysse, D. J., Reynolds, C. F., Monk, T. H., Berman, S. R., & Kupfer, D. J. (1989). The Pittsburgh Sleep Quality Index: A new instrument for psychiatric practice and research. *Psychiatry Research, 28*(2), 193–213.

Byers, H. (1994). *General meteorology.* McGraw-Hill.

Cacioppo, J. T., Petty, R. E., & Feng Kao, C. (1984). The efficient assessment of need for cognition. *Journal of Personality Assessment, 48*(3), 306–307.

Campbell, D. T., & Fiske, D. W. (1959). Convergent and discriminant validation by the multitrait–multimethod matrix. *Psychological Bulletin, 56*(2), 81.

Cannell, J. J. (1988). The Lake Wobegon effect revisited. *Educational Measurement: Issues and Practice, 7*(4), 12–15.

Carbone, E. T., Campbell, M. K., & Honess-Morreale, L. (2002). Use of cognitive interview techniques in the development of nutrition surveys and interactive nutrition messages for low-income populations. *Journal of the American Dietetic Association, 102*(5), 690–696.

Carroll, L. (1865/2011). *Alice's adventures in wonderland* (2nd ed.). Broadview Press.

Carson, J. (1993). Army alpha, army brass, and the search for army intelligence. *Isis, 84*(2), 278–309.

Carter, R., & New, C. (Eds.) (2004). *Making realism work: Realist social theory and empirical research.* Routledge.

Chatterji, M. (2003). *Designing and using tools for educational assessment.* Allyn & Bacon/Pearson.

Chatterji, M. (2004). Evidence on "what works": An argument for extended-term mixed method (ETMM) evaluation designs. *Educational Researcher, 33*(9), 3–13.

Chatterji, M. (2012). Development and validation of indicators of teacher proficiency in diagnostic classroom assessment. *International Journal of Educational and Psychological Assessment, 9*(2), 4–25.

Chatterji, M. (Ed.). (2013a). *Validity and test use: An international dialogue on educational assessment, accountability, and equity.* Emerald Group.

Chatterji, M. (2013b). Bad tests or bad test use? A case of SAT use to examine why we need stakeholder conversations on validity. *Teachers College Record, 115*(9), 1–10.

Chatterji, M. (2014, March 11). Validity counts: Let's mend, not end, educational testing. *Education Week*. www.edweek.org/policy-politics/opinion-lets-mend-not-end-educational-testing/2014/03.

Chatterji, M. (2019). *A consumer's guide to testing under the Every Student Succeeds Act (ESSA): What can the common core and other ESSA assessments tell us?* National Educational Policy Center. https://nepc.colorado.edu/publication/rd-assessment-guide.

Chatterji, M., & Freda, P. (2003). Designing and using tools for educational assessment: A computer module. http://www.columbia.edu/~mb1434/EdAssess.htm.

Chatterji, M., Graham, M. J., & Wyer, P. C. (2009a). Mapping cognitive overlaps between practice-based learning and improvement and evidence-based medicine: An operational definition for assessing resident physician competence. *Journal of Graduate Medical Education, 1*(2), 287–298.

Chatterji, M., Koh, N., Choi, L., & Iyengar, R. (2009b) Closing learner gaps proximally with teacher-mediated diagnostic assessment. *Research in the Schools, 16*(2), 60–77.

Chatterji, M., & Lin, M. (2018). Designing non-cognitive construct measures that improve mathematics achievement in grade 5–6 learners. A user-centered approach. *Quality Assurance in Education, 26*(1), 70–100.

Chatterji, M., Tripken, J., Johnson, S., Koh, N., Sabain, S., Allegrante, J. P., & Kukafka, R. (2017). Development and validation of a health information technology curriculum: Toward more meaningful use of electronic health records. *Pedagogy in Health Promotion, 3*(3). 154–166.

Cizek, G. J. (1997). Learning, achievement, and assessment: Constructs at a cross-roads. In G. D. Phye (Ed.), *Handbook of classroom assessment: Learning, adjustment, and achievement* (pp. 1–32). Academic Press.

Cizek, G. J. (2012). Defining and distinguishing validity: Interpretations of score meaning and justifications of test use. *Psychological Methods, 17*(1), 31.

Cizek, G. J. (2013). Conjectures on the rise and call of standard setting: An introduction to context and practice. In *Setting performance standards* (pp. 17–32). Routledge.

Cohen, R. J., & Swerdlik, M. E. (2010). *Psychological testing and assessment: An introduction to tests and measurement*. McGraw-Hill.

Cohen R. J., Tobin, R. M., & Schneider W. J. (2022). *Psychological testing and assessment: An introduction to tests and measurement* (10th ed.). McGraw Hill.

Cole, N. S. (1981). Bias in testing. *American Psychologist, 36*(10), 1067.

Comrey, A. L. (1988). Factor-analytic methods of scale development in personality and clinical psychology. *Journal of Consulting and Clinical Psychology, 56*(5), 754–761.

Conley, D. T. (1987). Critical attributes of effective evaluation systems. *Educational Leadership, 44*(7), 60–64.

Copple, C., Jerlean, D., & Tomlinson, H. B. (2007). Revisiting the NAEYC position statement on developmentally appropriate practice. *YC Young Children, 62*(4), 74.

Cremin, L. A. (1961). *The transformation of the school: Progressivism in American education, 1876–1957*. Knopf.

Creswell, J. W., & Creswell, J. D. (2023). *Research design: Qualitative quantitative and mixed methods approaches* (6th ed.). SAGE.

Crocker, L., & Algina, J. (2006). *Introduction to classical and modern test theory*. CBS College Publishing.

Cronbach, L. J. (1971). Test validation. In R. L. Thorndike (Ed.), *Educational measurement* (2nd ed., pp. 443–507). American Council on Education.

Cronbach, L. J. (1988). Five perspectives on validity argument. In H. Wainer & H. L. Braun (Eds.), *Test validity* (pp. 3–17). Erlbaum.

Cronbach, L. J., Gleser, G. C., Nanda, H., & Rajaratnam, N. (1972). *The dependability of behavioral measurements: Theory of generalizability for scores and profiles*. Wiley.

Cronbach, L. J., & Meehl, P. (1955). Construct validity in psychological tests. *Psychological Bulletin, 52*(4), 281–302.

Cureton, E. E. (1951). Validity. In E. F. Lindquist (Ed.), *Educational measurement* (pp. 621–694). ACE.

Curran, P. G. (2016). Methods for the detection of carelessly invalid responses in survey data. *Journal of Experimental Social Psychology, 66*, 4–19.

Dalkey, N., & Helmer, O. (1963). An experimental application of the Delphi method to the use of experts. *Management Science, 9*(3), 458–467.

Dang, K. V., Rerolle, F., Ackley, S. F., Irish, A. M., Mehta, K. M., Bailey, I., . . . Morris, M. D. (2021). A randomized study to assess the effect of including the Graduate Record Examinations (GRE) results on reviewers scores for underrepresented minorities. *American Journal of Epidemiology, 190*(9), 1744–1750.

Davis, K., Christodoulou, J., Seider, S., & Gardner, H. (2011). The theory of multiple intelligences. In R. J.

Sternberg & S. B. Kaufman (Eds.), *Cambridge handbook of intelligence* (pp. 485–503). Cambridge University Press.

de Onis, M., Onyango, A. W., Borghi, E., Siyam, A., Nishida, C., & Siekmann, J. (2007). Development of a WHO growth reference for school-aged children and adolescents. *Bulletin of the World Health Organization, 85*, 660–667.

de Wilde, J. A., van Dommelen, P., van Buuren, S., & Middelkoop, B. J. C. (2014). Height of South Asian children in the Netherlands aged 0–20 years: Secular trends and comparisons with current Asian Indian, Dutch and WHO references. *Annals of Human Biology, 42*(1), 38–44.

Deary, I. J. (2001). *Intelligence: A very short introduction*. Oxford University Press.

Delbecq, A. L., & Van de Ven, A. H. (1971). A group process model for problem identification and program planning. *Journal of Applied Behavioral Science, 7*, 466–491.

Dewey, J. (1897). My pedagogic creed. *School Journal, 54*(1), 77–80.

Dewey, J. (1902). The school as social center. *The Elementary School Teacher, 3*(2), 73–86.

Dick, W., Carey, L., & Carey, J. O. (2022). *The systematic design of instruction* (9th ed.). Pearson.

Dillman, D. A. (2011). *Mail and internet surveys: The tailored design method—2007 update with new internet, visual, and mixed-mode guide*. Wiley.

Dillman, D. A., Smyth, J. D., & Christian, L. M. (2014). *Internet, phone, mail, and mixed mode surveys: The tailored design method* (4th ed.). Wiley.

DiStefano, C., & Hess, B. (2005). Using confirmatory factor analysis for construct validation: An empirical review. *Journal of Psychoeducational Assessment, 23*, 225–241.

DiStefano, C., & Motl, R. W. (2006). Further investigating method effects associated with negatively worded items on self-report surveys. *Structural Equation Modeling: A Multidisciplinary Journal, 13*(3), 440–464.

Dodou, D., & de Winter, J. C. (2014). Social desirability is the same in offline, online, and paper surveys: A meta-analysis. *Computers in Human Behavior, 36*, 487–495.

Dorans, N. J., Pommerich, M., & Holland, P. W. (2007). *Linking and aligning scores and scales*. Springer.

Du Bois, P. H. (1970). *A history of psychological testing*. Allyn & Bacon.

Eagly, A. H., & Chaiken, S. (1998). Attitude, structure and function. In D. T. Gilbert, S. T. Fisk & G. Lindsey (Eds.) *Handbook of social psychology* (pp. 269–322). McGowan-Hill.

Eaton, J. S. (2015, November). *An overview of US accreditation*. Council for Higher Education Accreditation.

Ebel, R. L. (1961). Must all tests be valid? *American Psychologist, 16*, 640–647.

Ebel, R. L., & Frisbie, D. A. (1972). *Essentials of educational measurement* (2nd ed.). Prentice Hall.

Eisenstat, B. D. (1999). Examples of abusive behavior. *New England Journal of Medicine, 341*(12), 886–892.

Ercikan, K., & Oliveri, M. E. (2013). Is fairness research doing justice? A modest proposal for an alternative validation approach in differential item functioning (DIF) investigations. In M. Chatterji (Ed.), *Validity and test use: An international dialogue on educational assessment, accountability and equity* (pp. 69–86). Emerald Group.

Famodu, O. A., Barr, M. L., Holásková, I., Zhou, W., Morrell, J. S., Colby, S. E., & Olfert, M. D. (2018). Shortening of the Pittsburgh Sleep Quality Index survey using factor analysis. *Sleep Disorders, 2018*, 9643937.

Feuer, M. (2013). Validity issues in international large-scale assessments: "Truth" and "Consequences." In M. Chatterji (Ed.), *Validity and test use: An international dialogue on educational assessment, accountability and equity* (pp. 197–215). Emerald Group.

Feuerstein, R., Rand, Y., & Hoffman, M. (1979). *The dynamic assessment of retarded performers: The learning assessment potential device, theory, instruments and techniques*. University Park Press.

Fink, A. (1995). *How to ask survey questions*. SAGE.

Fischer, D. G., & Fick, C. (1993). Measuring social desirability: Short forms of the Marlowe–Crowne social desirability scale. *Educational and Psychological Measurement, 53*(2), 417–424.

Fitzpatrick, J. L., Sanders, J. L., & Worthen, B. R. (2003). *Program evaluation: Alternative approaches and practical guidelines* (3rd ed.). Pearson.

Fleiss, J. (1981). *Statistical methods for rates and proportions* (2nd ed.). Wiley.

Freeman, R. (2010). *Strategic management: A stakeholder approach*. Cambridge University Press.

Friedlander Moore, A., McCallum, R., & Bracken, B. (2017). *The Universal Nonverbal Intelligence Test: Second Edition*. PRO-ED.

Gable, R. K., & Wolf, M. B. (1993). *Instrument development in the affective domain: Measuring attitudes and values in corporate and school settings*. Springer Netherlands.

Gagné, R. M. (1965). *The conditions of learning.* Holt, Rinehart & Winston.

Ganguly, R., & Banerji, M. (2000). Hepatitis B virus infection and vaccine acceptance among university students. *American Journal of Health Behavior, 24*(2), 96–107.

Gardner, W. L., & Martinko, M. J. (1996). Using the Myers-Briggs Type Indicator to study managers: A literature review and research agenda. *Journal of Management, 22*(1), 45–83.

Gauvain, M. (2005). Sociocultural contexts of learning. In A. E. Maynard & M. I. Martini (Eds.), *Learning in cultural context* (pp. 11–40). Springer.

Gershon, R. C. (2005). Computer adaptive testing. *Journal of Applied Measurement, 6*(1), 109–127

Gewertz, C. (2017, February 15). Which states are using PARCC or smarter balanced? *Education Week.* www.edweek.org/ew/section/multimedia/states-using-parcc-or-smarter-balanced.html.

Ghiselli, E. E., Campbell, J. P., & Zedeck, S. (1981). *Measurement theory for the behavioral sciences.* Freeman.

Giacomin, J. (2014). What is human centered design? *The Design Journal, 17*(4), 606–623.

Gitomer, D. H., Phelps, G., Weren, B. H., Howell, H., & Croft, A. J. (2014). Evidence on the validity of content knowledge for teaching assessments. In T. Kane, K. Kerr, & R. Pianta (Eds.), *Designing teacher evaluation systems: New guidance from the Measures of Effective Teaching Project* (pp. 493–528). Jossey-Bass.

Gitomer, D. H., & Zisk, R. C. (2015). Knowing what teachers know. *Review of Research in Education, 39,* 1–53.

Glaser, R. (1984). Education and thinking: The role of knowledge. *American Psychologist, 39*(2), 93.

Glaser, R. (1994). Criterion-referenced tests: I. Origins. *Educational Measurement: Issues and Practice, 13,* 9–11.

Glickman, T. S. (2000). *Meteorology glossary* (2nd ed.). American Meteorological Society.

Goldman, A. W., & Kane, M. (2014). Concept mapping and network analysis: An analytic approach to measure ties among constructs. *Evaluation and Program Planning, 47,* 9–17.

Good, C. V. (Ed.). (1973). *Dictionary of education* (3rd ed.). McGraw-Hill.

Goodlad, J. I., & Anderson, R. H. (1987). *The nongraded elementary school.* Teachers College Press.

Gordon, E. W., & Bridglall, B. L. (2007). *Affirmative development: Cultivating academic ability.* Rowman & Littlefield.

Gordon, E. W., McGill, M. V., Sands, D. I., Kalinich, K., Pellegrino, J. W, & Chatterji, M. (2014). Bringing formative assessment to schools and making it count. *Quality Assurance in Education, 22*(4), 336–350.

Gorsuch, R. L. (2014). *Factor analysis: Classic edition.* Routledge.

Gould, S. J. (1981). *The mismeasure of man.* Norton.

Gould, S. J. (1996). *The mismeasure of man* (rev. ed.). Norton.

Graham, M. J., Naqvi, Z., Encandela, J., Harding, K. J., & Chatterji, M. (2009). Systems-based practice defined: Taxonomy development and role identification for competency assessment of residents. *Journal of Graduate Medical Education, 1*(1), 49–60.

Gravetter, F. J., & Forzano, L. B. (2012). *Research methods for the behavioral sciences* (4th ed.). Wadsworth.

Gray, E. (2015, June 11). Find out if your personality fits your job. *Time.* https://time.com/3915807/personality-fits-job.

Greenacre, Z. A. (2016). The importance of selection bias in internet surveys. *Open Journal of Statistics, 6*(3), 397.

Greenbaum, T. (2000). *Moderating focus groups.* SAGE.

Greeno, J. G., Moore, J. L., & Smith, D. R. (1993). Transfer of situated learning. In D. K. Detterman & R. J. Sternberg (Eds.), *Transfer on trial: Intelligence, cognition, and instruction* (pp. 99–167). Ablex.

Gregorich, S. E. (2006). Do self-report instruments allow meaningful comparisons across diverse population groups?: Testing measurement invariance using the confirmatory factor analysis framework. *Medical Care, 44*(11, Suppl. 3), s78–s94.

Gronlund, N. E. (1981). *Measurement and evaluation in teaching* (5th ed.). Macmillan.

Guilford, J. P. (1954). *Psychometric methods.* McGraw-Hill.

Gulliksen, H. (1950). *Theory of mental tests.* Wiley.

Guttman. L. (1941). The quantification of class attributes: A theory and method of scale construction. In P. Horst et al. (Eds.), *The prediction of personal adjustment* (pp. 321–348). Social Science Research Council.

Guyatt, G., Rennie, D., Meade, M., & Cook, D. (Eds.). (2002). *Users' guides to the medical literature: A manual for evidence-based clinical practice* (Vol. 20). AMA Press.

Hafferty, F. W., O'Brien, B. C., & Tilburt, J. C. (2020). Beyond high-stakes testing: Learner trust, educational commodification, and the loss of medical school professionalism. *Academic Medicine, 95*(6), 833–837.

Haladyna, T. M. (2015). *Developing and validating multiple-choice test items.* Routledge.

Hambleton, R. K., & Pitoniak, M. J. (2006). Setting performance standards. In R. L. Brennan (Ed.), *Educational measurement* (4th ed., pp. 433–470). American Council on Education/Praeger.

Harmon, L. W. (1989). Counseling. In R. L. Linn (Ed.), *Educational measurement* (pp. 13–103). American Council on Education.

Harrington, D. (2009). *Confirmatory factor analysis*. Oxford University Press.

Harvey, A., Rosenbaum, P., Graham, H. K., & Palisano, R. J., (2009). Current and future uses of the gross motor function classification system. *Developmental Medicine & Child Neurology, 51*(4), 328–329.

Hastie, M. J. (2019). *Perceptions of leadership among women in academic medicine: A case study comparing the perspectives of full-time faculty with and without institutionally defined leadership titles*. Doctoral dissertation, Teachers College, Columbia University. Available from ProQuest.

Hastie, M. J., Kim, M., Lin, M., & Chatterji, M. (2024). Survey validation for measuring perceptions of work-related factors that influence career paths of men and women in academic anesthesiology. *Anesthesia & Analgesia, 138*(1), 187–197.

Hattie, J., & Timperley, H. (2007). The power of feedback. *Review of Educational Research, 77*(1), 81–112.

Henry G. T. (1998). *Practical sampling*. SAGE.

Henry, G. T., Lipsey, M. W., & Rossi, P. H. (2019). *Evaluation: A systematic approach*. SAGE.

Henseler, J., Ringle, C. M., & Sarstedt, M. (2015). A new criterion for assessing discriminant validity in variance-based structural equation modeling. *Journal of the Academy of Marketing Science, 43*(1), 115–135.

Herman, J. L., Aschbacher, P. R., & Winters, L. (1992). *A practical guide to alternative assessment*. Association for Supervision and Curriculum Development.

Hidecker, M. J. C., Paneth, N., Rosenbaum, P. L., Kent, R. D., Lillie, J., Eulenberg, J. B., . . . Taylor, K. (2011). Developing and validating the Communication Function Classification System for individuals with cerebral palsy. *Developmental Medicine and Child Neurology*, 53, 704–710.

Hilts, V. L. (1978). *Aliis exterendum*, or the origins of the Statistical Society of London. *Journal of the American Statistical Association, 69*(1), 21–43.

Holden, R. B. (2010). Face validity. In I. Weiner, B. Craighead, & W. Edward (Eds.). *The Corsini encyclopedia of psychology* (4th ed., pp. 637–638). Wiley.

Holland, J. G., & Skinner, B. F. (1961). *The analysis of behavior: A program for self-instruction*. McGraw-Hill.

Hopkins, K. D. (1998). *Educational and psychological measurement and evaluation* (8th ed.). Allyn & Bacon.

Horowitz, M. E. (2022). The vaccine-hesitant moment: Letters to the editor. *New England Journal of Medicine, 387*, 1050–1051.

Hovland, C. I., & Rosenberg, M. J. (Eds.). (1960). *Attitude organization and change*. Yale University Press.

Hughes, G. (2017). *Ipsative assessment and personal learning gain*. Palgrave Macmillan.

Isitan, S. (2021). Psychometric properties of the Self-Description Questionnaire for preschoolers in a sample of 3- to 5-year-old Turkish children. *International Journal of Progressive Education, 17*(1), 86–96.

Jackson, D. (2014). Business graduate performance in oral communication skills and strategies for improvement. *International Journal of Management Education, 12*(1), 22–34.

Jaeger, R. M. (1997). *Complementary methods for research in education* (2nd ed.). American Educational Research Association.

Jaeger, R. M., & Tittle, C. K. (Eds.) (1980). *Minimum competency testing: Motives, models, measures, and consequences*. McCutchen.

Jethwa, A., Mink, J., MacArthur, C., Knights, S., Fehlings, T., & Fehlings, D. (2010). Development of the Hypertonia Assessment Tool (HAT): A discriminative tool for hypertonia in children. *Developmental Medicine and Child Neurology, 52*, 82–87.

Jick, T. (1979). Mixing qualitative and quantitative methods: Triangulation in action. *Administrative Science Quarterly, 24*(4), 602–611.

Johanningmeier, E. V., & Richardson, T. (2008). *Educational research, the national agenda, and educational reform: A history*. Information Age.

John-Steiner, V., & Mahn, H. (1996). Sociocultural approaches to learning and development: A Vygotskian framework. *Educational Psychologist, 31*(3–4), 191–206.

Johnson, C. C., Sondergeld, T. A., & Walton, J. B. (2019). A study of the implementation of formative assessment in three large urban districts. *American Educational Research Journal, 56*(6), 2408–2438.

Kane, M. (2006). Validation. In R. L. Brennan (Ed.), *Educational measurement* (4th ed., pp. 17–64). Praeger.

Kane, M. (2013a). Validity and fairness in the testing of individuals. In M. Chatterji (Ed.), *Validity and test use: An international dialogue on educational assessment, accountability, and equity* (pp. 17–55). Emerald Group.

Kane, M. T. (2013b). Validation as a pragmatic, scientific

activity. *Journal of Educational Measurement, 50*(1), 115–122.

Katz, D. (1960). The functional approach to the study of attitudes. *Public Opinion Quarterly, 24*(2), 163.

Kerr, C. C., Mistry, D., Stuart, R. M., Rosenfeld, K., Hart, G. R., Núñez, R. C., . . . Klein, D. J. (2021). Controlling COVID-19 via test-trace-quarantine. *Nature Communications, 12*(1), 2993.

Klenowski, V., Askew, S., & Carnell, E. (2006). Portfolios for leaning, assessment and professional development in higher education. *Assessment and Evaluation in Higher Education, 31*(3), 267–286.

Kliebard, H. M. (1992). *Forging the American curriculum: Essays in curriculum history and theory*. Routledge.

Kliebard, H. M. (2004). *The struggle for the American curriculum, 1893–1958*. Psychology Press.

Kline, P. (2015). *A handbook of test construction (psychology revivals): Introduction to psychometric design*. Routledge.

Kline, R. B. (2023). *Principles and practice of structural equation modeling* (5th ed.). Guilford Press.

Kok, G., Gottlieb, N. H., Commers, M., & Smerecnik, C. (2008). The ecological approach in health promotion programs: A decade later. *American Journal of Health Promotion, 22*, 437–442.

Kolen, M. J., & Brennan, R. L. (2013). *Test equating scaling and linking: Methods and practices* (3rd ed.). Springer Science & Business Media.

Kolen, M. J., & Brennan, R. L. (2014). *Linking*. Springer.

Kolen, M. J., & Hendrickson, A. B. (2013). Scaling, norming, and equating. In K. F. Geisinger, B. A. Bracken, J. F. Carlson, J.-I. C. Hansen, N. R. Kuncel, S. P. Reise, & M. C. Rodriguez (Eds.), *APA handbook of testing and assessment in psychology: Vol. 1. Test theory and testing and assessment in industrial and organizational psychology* (pp. 201–222). American Psychological Association.

Krathwohl, D. R., Bloom, B. S., & Masia, B. B. (1964). *Taxonomy of educational objectives: Handbook II. Affective domain*. David McKay.

Krumpal, I. (2013). Determinants of social desirability bias in sensitive surveys: A literature review. *Quality & Quantity, 47*(4), 2025–2047.

Landry, G. J., Best, J. R., & Liu-Ambrose, T. (2015). Measuring sleep quality in older adults: A comparison using subjective and objective methods. *Frontiers in Aging Neuroscience, 7*, 166.

Lane, C. (2013, May 4). The NIMH withdraws support for DSM-5. *Psychology Today*. www.psychologytoday.com/intl/blog/side-effects/201305/the-nimh-withdraws-support-dsm-5.

Lane, S., Raymond, M. R., & Haladyna, T. M. (Eds.). (2016a). *Handbook of test development*. Routledge.

Lane, S., Raymond, M. R., Haladyna, T. M., & Downing, S. M. (2016b). Test development process. In S. Lane, M. R. Raymond, & T. M. Haladyna (Eds.), *Handbook of test development* (pp. 3–18). Routledge.

Larson, H. J., Gakidou, E., & Murray, C. J. (2022). The vaccine-hesitant moment. *New England Journal of Medicine, 387*(1), 58–65.

Larson, R., & Farber, E. (2004). Elementary statistics: Picturing the world. www.stat.tamu.edu/~lzhou/stat302/standardnormaltable.pdf.

Laster Pirtle, W. N. (2020). Racial capitalism: A fundamental cause of novel coronavirus (COVID-19) pandemic inequities in the United States. *Health Education & Behavior, 47*(4), 504–508

Lau, Y. L., Wong, W., Hattangdi-Haridas, S. R., & Chow, C. B. (2020). Evaluating impact of school outreach vaccination programme in Hong Kong influenza season 2018–2019. *Human Vaccines & Immunotherapeutics, 16*(4), 823–826.

Laurie, R. (2013). Applying Feuer's validation framework in a Canadian context: A look at international large scale assessment programs. In M. Chatterji (Ed.), *Validity and test use: An international dialogue on educational assessment, accountability and equity* (pp. 263–271). Emerald Group.

Lee, A., Chen, C., Landau, R., & Chatterji, M. (2019, January). *Learning outcomes of a serious video game for anesthesia residents: A battle of the sexes*. Paper presented at the 20th International Meeting on Simulation in Healthcare (IMSH 2019), San Diego, CA.

Lee, A. J., Goodman, S. R., Banks, S. E., Lin, M., & Landau, R. (2018). Development of a multiple-choice test for novice anesthesia residents to evaluate knowledge related to management of general anesthesia for urgent cesarean delivery. *Journal of Education in Perioperative Medicine, 20*(2), 1–11.

Lee, A. J., Goodman, S., Corradini, B., Chen, C, M., Chatterji, M., & Landau, R. (2019). *Learning outcomes of a serious video game-based experiment: A battle of the sexes*. Paper presented at the Society for Obstetric Anesthesia and Perinatology 51st Annual Meeting, Phoenix, AZ.

Lee, A. J., Goodman, S., Corradini, B., Chen, C. M., Chatterji, M., & Landau, R. (2023). A serious video game—

EmergenCSim™—for novice anesthesia trainees to learn how to perform general anesthesia for emergency Cesarean delivery: A randomized controlled trial. *Anesthesiology and Perioperative Science, 1*(14), 1–10.

Lee, J. (2002). Racial and ethnic achievement gap trends: Reversing the progress toward equity? *Educational Researcher, 31*(1), 3–12.

Lee, J. (2006). *Tracking achievement gaps and assessing the impact of NCLB on the gaps: An in-depth look into national and state reading and math outcome trends.* The Civil Rights Project at Harvard University.

LeMahieu, P. G., Bryk, A. S., Grunow, A., & Gomez, L. M. (2017). Working to improve: Seven approaches to improvement science in education. *Quality Assurance in Education, 25*(1), 2–4

Li, D., Christ, S. E., & Cowan, N. (2014). Domain-general and domain-specific functional networks in working memory. *NeuroImage, 102*(2), 646–656.

Likert, R. (1932). A technique for the measurement of attitudes. *Archives of Psychology, 22*(140), 1–55.

Lin, M. (2018). *Examining the influence of yutori education in Japan on opportunity to learn (OTL) and student achievement on the TIMSS: A multiple cohort analysis* (Publication No. 586742). PhD dissertation, Teachers College, Columbia University. Available from ProQuest.

Linacre, J. M. (2006). *Facets-Rasch measurement computer program.* Winsteps.

Linacre, J. M., & Wright, B. D. (2002). Construction of measures from many-facet data. *Journal of Applied Measurement, 3*(4), 486–512.

Linn, R. L. (Ed.). (1989). *Education measurement.* American Council of Education.

Lockwood, J. R., McCaffrey, D. F., Hamilton, L. S., Stecher, B., Le, V. N., & Martinez, J. F. (2007). The sensitivity of value-added teacher effect estimates to different mathematics achievement measures. *Journal of Educational Measurement, 44*(1), 47–67.

Lombardo, P. A. (2011). *A century of eugenics in America: From the Indiana experiment to the human genome era.* Indiana University Press.

Lord, F. M. (1953). On the statistical treatment of football numbers. *American Psychologist, 8*, 750–751.

Lord, F. M. (2009). *Applications of item response theory to practical testing problems.* Routledge.

Lorge, I. (1951). The fundamental nature of measurement. In E. F. Lindquist (Ed.), *Educational measurement* (pp. 533–559). American Council of Education.

Lowdermilk, T. (2013). *User centered design: A developer's guide to designing user-friendly applications.* O'Reilly Media.

Lynn, M. R. (1986). Determination and quantification of content validity. *Nursing Research, 35*(6), 382–386.

Madni, A., Baker, E. L., Chow, K. A., Delacruz, G. C., & Griffin, N. C. (2015). Assessment of teachers from a social psychological perspective. *Review of Research in Education, 39*(1), 54–86.

Maitland, A., & Presser, S. (2016). How accurately do different evaluation methods predict the reliability of survey questions? *Journal of Survey Statistics and Methodology, 4*(3), 362–381.

Mantel, N., & Haenszel, W. (1959). Statistical aspects of the analysis of data from retrospective studies of disease. *Journal of the National Cancer Institute, 22*(4), 719–748.

Marini, J. P., Westrick, P. A., Young, L., Ng, H., Shmueli, D., & Shaw, E. J. (2019). *Differential validity and prediction of the SAT®: Examining first-year grades and retention to the second year.* College Board.

Martiñez-Arboleda, A. (2021). Ipsative assessment: Measuring personal improvement. In T. Beaven & F. Rosell-Aguilar (Eds.), *Innovative language pedagogy report* (pp. 77–82). Research-publishing.net.

Marzano, R. J., Pickering, D., & McTighe, J. (1994). *Assessing student outcomes: Performance assessment using the dimension of learning model.* Association for Supervision and Curriculum Development.

Mayher, J. S. (1990). *Uncommon sense: Theoretical practice in language education.* Boynton/Cook-Heinemann.

Mazzeo, J., Lazer, S., & Zieky, M. J. (2006). Monitoring educational progress with group-score assessments. In R. L. Brennan (Ed.), *Educational measurement* (4th ed., pp. 17–64). Praeger.

McCallum, R. S. (Ed.). (2003). *Handbook of nonverbal assessment.* Kluwer Academic/Plenum.

McCallum, R. S., & Bracken, B. A. (2018). The universal nonverbal intelligence test: A multidimensional nonverbal alternative for cognitive assessment. In D. P. Flanagan & E. M. McDonough (Eds.), *Contemporary intellectual assessment: Theories, tests, and issues* (pp. 567–583). Guilford Press.

McDermott, P. A., Fantuzzo, J. W., Glutting, J. J., Watkins, M. W., & Baggaley, A. R. (1992). Illusions of meaning in the ipsative assessment of children's ability. *Journal of Special Education*, 25(4), 504–526.

McMullan, M., Endacott, R., Gray, M. A., Jasper, M., Miller, C. M., Scholes, J., & Webb, C. (2003). Portfolios and assessment of competence: A review of the literature. *Journal of Advanced Nursing, 41*(3), 283–294.

McReynolds, P., Rosen, J. C., & Chelune, G. J. (Eds.). (2012). *Advances in psychological assessment* (Vol. 7). Springer Science & Business Media.

Mendoza-Denton, R. (2014). A social psychological perspective on the achievement gap in standardized test performance between White and minority students: Implications for assessment. *Journal of Negro Education, 83*(4), 465–484.

Meredith, W. (1993). Measurement invariance, factor analysis, and factorial invariance. *Pyschometrika*, 58, 525–543.

Mertens, D. M. (2020). *Research and evaluation in education and psychology: Integrating diversity with quantitative qualitative and mixed methods* (5th ed.). SAGE.

Mertler, C. A. (2002). *Using standardized test data to guide instruction and intervention.* ERIC Clearinghouse on Assessment and Evaluation.

Messick, S. (1989). Validity. In R. L. Linn (Ed.), *Educational measurement* (pp.13–103). American Council on Education.

Miles, M. B., & Huberman, A. M. (1994). *Qualitative data analysis: An expanded sourcebook.* SAGE.

Miller, G. D. (1990). The assessment of clinical skills/competence/performance. *Academic Medicine, 65*(9) 63–67.

Miller, M. D., Linn, R. L., & Gronlund, N. (2013). *Measurement and assessment in teaching* (11th ed.). Pearson Education South Asia.

Mislevy, R. J. (1994). Evidence and inference in educational assessment. *Psychometrika, 59*(4), 439–483.

Mislevy, R. J. (1996). Test theory reconceived. *Journal of Educational Measurement, 33*(4), 379–416.

Mislevy, R. J. (2006). Cognitive psychology and educational assessment. *Educational Measurement, 4*, 257–305.

Mislevy, R. J. (2019). Advances in measurement and cognition. *Annals of the American Academy of Political and Social Science, 683*(1), 164–182.

Mislevy, R. J., Almond, R. G., & Lukas, J. F. (2004). *A brief introduction to evidence-centered design.* National Center for Research on Evaluation, Standards, and Student Testing (CRESST), Center for the Study of Evaluation (CSE), University of California. https://files.eric.ed.gov/fulltext/ED483399.pdf.

Montana Office of Public Instruction. (2018). *Montana American Indian student achievement data report fall 2018.* https://files.eric.ed.gov/fulltext/ED520721.pdf.

Montenegro, E., & Jankowski, N. A. (2017, January). *Equity and assessment: Moving towards culturally responsive assessment* (Occasional Paper No. 29). National Institute for Learning Outcomes Assessment.

Montenegro, E., & Jankowski, N. A. (2020, January). *A new decade for assessment: Embedding equity into assessment praxis* (Occasional Paper No. 42). National Institute for Learning Outcomes Assessment

Moore, A. F., McCallum, R. S., & Bracken, B. A. (2017). The universal nonverbal intelligence test. In R. S. McCallum (Ed.), *Handbook of nonverbal assessment* (2nd ed., pp. 105–125). Springer International/Springer Nature.

Mor, V., Angelelli, J., Jones, R., Roy, J., Moore, T., & Morris, J. (2003). Inter-rater reliability of nursing home quality indicators in the U.S. *BMC Health Services Research, 3*(1), 20.

Morgan, J. L. (2016). *The impact of summer intervention on reading regression as measured by student normal curve equivalent scores when grouped by grade level and socioeconomic status for 2013, 2014 and 2015.* Doctoral dissertation, Baker University. www.bakeru.edu/images/pdf/SOE/EdD_Theses/MorganJessica.pdf.

Mosier, C. I. (1947). A critical examination of the concepts of face validity. *Education and Psychological Measurement, 7*, 191–205.

Mukherjee, S. (2010). *The emperor of all maladies: A biography of cancer.* Scribner/Simon & Schuster.

Naliboff, B. D., & Mayer, E. A. (2006). Brain imaging in IBS: Drawing the line between cognitive and noncognitive processes. *Gastroenterology, 130*(1), 267–270.

National Assessment of Educational Progress. (2013). *An overview of NAEP: Brochure.* National Center for Education Statistics.

National Assessment of Educational Progress. (2015). *School composition and the Black-White achievement gap.* National Center for Education Statistics.

National Assessment of Educational Progress. (2017). *NAEP 4th- and 8th-grade mathematics and reading report card for the nation and the states.* National Center for Education Statistics.

National Center for Research on Evaluation, Standards, and Student Testing. (2017). *Smarter Balanced Assessment Consortium: Formative technical report.* CRESST.

National Center for Research on Evaluation, Standards, and Student Testing. (2018). *Smarter Balanced Assessment Consortium: Summative technical report.* CRESST.

National Center for Research on Evaluation, Standards, and Student Testing. (2020). *Smarter Balanced Assessment Consortium: Technical Manual for Summative Assessments.* CRESST.

National Commission for Excellence in Education (1983). *A nation at risk: The imperative for education reform.* Government Printing Office.

National Research Council. (2012). *A framework for K–12 science education: Practices, crosscutting concepts, and core ideas.* National Academies Press.

National Research Council. (2013). *Education for life and work: Developing transferable knowledge and skills in the 21st century.* National Academies Press.

New Hampshire Department of Education. (2018). *Consolidated state plan. The Elementary and Secondary Education Act of 1965, as amended by Every Student Succeeds Act.* https://oese.ed.gov/offices/office-of-formula-grants/school-support-and-accountability/essa-consolidated-state-plans.

Newman, C. W., Weinstein, B. E., Jacobson, G. P., & Hug, G. A. (1990). The Hearing Handicap Inventory for Adults: Psychometric adequacy and audiometric correlates. *Ear and Hearing, 11*(6), 430–433.

Nichols, P., Mittelholtz, D., Adams, J., & van Deusen, R. (2008, March). *User-centered assessment design.* Paper presented at the Annual Conference of the American Educational Research Association, New York, NY.

Norman, D. (2013). *The design of everyday things* (Rev. ed.). Basic Books.

Northouse, P. G. (2018). *Leadership: Theory and practice.* SAGE.

Nunnally, J. C., & Bernstein, I. H. (1994). *Psychometric theory* (3rd ed.). McGraw-Hill.

Olver, J. M., & Mooradian, T. A. (2003). Personality traits and personal values: A conceptual and empirical integration. *Personality and Individual Differences, 35*(1), 109–125.

Organisation for Economic Co-operation and Development. (2010). *PISA 2009 results: Overcoming social background: Equity in learning opportunities and outcomes* (Vol. II). Author.

Ortiz, C. (2016). *Racism and inequity are products of design. They can be redesigned.* Medium. https://medium.com/equity-design/racism-and-inequity-are-products-of-design-they-can-be-redesigned-12188363cc6a.

Osgood, C. E. (1964). Semantic differential technique in the comparative study of cultures. *American Anthropologist, 66*(3), 171–200.

Palmer, E. (2014). *Teaching the core skills of listening and speaking.* ASCD.

Patton, M. Q., & Campbell-Patton, C. E. (2022). *Utilization-focused evaluation* (5th ed.). SAGE.

Paulhus, D. L. (1991). Measurement and control of response bias. In J. P. Robinson, P. Shaver, & L. S. Wrightsman (Eds.), *Measures of personality and social psychological attitudes* (pp. 17–34). Academic Press.

Pawson, R. (1989). *A measure for measures: A manifesto for empirical sociology.* Routledge.

Pawson, R., & Tilley, N. (1997). *Realistic evaluation.* SAGE.

Pearson. (2017). *Partnership for assessment of readiness for college and careers: Final technical report for 2016 administration.* https://parcc-assessment.org/wp-content/uploads/2018/02/PARCC-2016-Tech-Report.pdf.

Pellegrino, J. W. (2002). Knowing what students know. *Issues in Science and Technology, 19*(2), 48–52.

Pellegrino, J. W. (2020). Important considerations for assessment to function in the service of education. *Educational Measurement: Issues and Practice, 39*(3), 81–85.

Pellegrino, J. W., Chudowsky, N., & Glaser, R. (2001). *Knowing what students know: The science and design of educational assessment.* National Academies Press.

Pellegrino, J. W., Wilson, M. R., Koenig, J. A., & Beatty, A. S. (2014). *Developing assessments for the next generation science standards.* National Academies Press.

Penn, P. R., & Wells, I. G. (2018). Making assessment promote effective learning practices: An example of ipsative assessment from the school of psychology at UEL. *Psychology Teaching Review, 24*(2), 70–74.

Phelps, R. P. (2017). The "teaching to the test" family of fallacies. *Revista Iberoamericana de Evaluación Educativa, 10*(1).

Pittenger, D. J. (2005). Cautionary comments regarding the Myers-Briggs type indicator. *Consulting Psychology Journal: Practice and Research, 57*(3), 2010.

Pizmony-Levy, O., Harvey, J., Schmidt, W., Noonan, R., Engel, L., Feuer, M. J., . . . Chatterji, M. (2014). On the merits of, and myths about, international assessments. *Quality Assurance in Education, 22*(4), 316–335.

Plisko, V. (2013). Validity and international large scale assessment programs: A reaction to Feuer's "truth" and "consequence." In M. Chatterji (Ed.), *Validity and test use: An international dialogue on educational assessment, accountability and equity* (pp. 251–261). Emerald Group.

Polit, D. F., & Beck, C. T. (2006). The Content Validity Index: Are you sure you know what's being reported?

Critique and recommendations. *Research in Nursing & Health, 29*, 489–497.

Polit, D. F., Beck, C. T., & Owen, S. V. (2007). Is the CVI an acceptable indicator of content validity? Appraisal and recommendations. *Research in Nursing & Health, 30*(4), 459–467.

Popham, W. J. (2014). The right test for the wrong reason. *Phi Delta Kappan, 96*(1), 46–52.

Porter, A., McMaken, J., Hwang, J., & Yang, R. (2011). Common core standards: The new US intended curriculum. *Educational Researcher, 40*(3), 103–116.

Price, L. R. (2018). *Psychometric methods: Theory into practice*. Guilford Press.

Rabiee, F. (2004). Focus-group interview and data analysis. *Proceedings of the Nutrition Society, 63*(4), 655–660.

Raudenbush, S., & Jean, M. (2012). *How should educators interpret value-added scores?* Carnegie Knowledge Network. www.carnegieknowledgenetwork.org/briefs/value-added/interpreting-value-added.

Ravitch, D. (2016). *The death and life of the great American school system: How testing and choice are undermining education*. Basic Books.

Reardon, S. F. (2016). *School district socioeconomic status, race, and academic achievement*. Stanford University.

Rees, C. J., & Metcalfe, B. (2003). The faking of personality questionnaire results: Who's kidding whom? *Journal of Managerial Psychology, 18*(2), 156–165.

Reiser, R. A., Reiser, R. A., & Dempsey, J. V. (2011). *Trends and issues in instructional design and technology*. Pearson.

Reynolds, C. R., & Suzuki, L. A. (2012). Bias in psychological assessment: An empirical review and recommendations. In J. R. Graham, J. A. Naglieri, & I. B. Weiner (Eds.), *Handbook of psychology: Assessment psychology* (2nd ed., pp. 82–113). Wiley.

Reynolds, W. M. (2004). The Reynolds Adolescent Depression Scale—Second Edition (RADS-2). In M. J. Hilsenroth & D. L. Segal (Eds.), *Comprehensive handbook of psychological assessment* (Vol. 2, pp. 224–236). Wiley.

Rice, J. M. (1893). *The public-school system of the United States*. Century.

Rice, J. M. (1898). *The rational spelling book*. American Book Company.

Rice, J. M. (1913). *Scientific management in education*. Publishers Printing Company.

Riconscente, M. M., Mislevy, R. J., & Corrigan, S. (2015). Evidence-centered design. In S. Lane, M. R. Raymond, & T. M. Haladyna (Eds.), *Handbook of test development* (pp. 40–63). Routledge.

Robson, C. (2024). *Real world research*. Wiley.

Robson, C., & McCartan, K. (2016). *Real world research* (4th ed.). Wiley.

Rogers, P. J., Petrosino, A., Huebner, T. A., & Hacsi, T. A. (2000). Program theory evaluation: Practice, promise, and problems. *New Directions for Evaluation, 2000*(87), 5–13.

Roid, G. H. (2003). *Stanford–Binet Intelligence Scales* (5th ed.). Riverside.

Rollnick, S., Miller, W. R., & Butler, C. C. (2008). *Motivational interviewing in health care: Helping patients change behavior*. Guilford Press.

Roozenburg, N. F., & Eekels, J. (1995). *Product design: fundamentals and methods* (Vol. 2). Wiley.

Rosas, S. R., & Kane, M. (2012). Quality and rigor of the concept mapping methodology: A pooled study analysis. *Evaluation and Program Planning, 35*(2), 236–245.

Rossi, P. H., Lipsey, M. W., & Henry, G. T. (2018). *Evaluation: A systematic approach* (8th ed.). SAGE.

Rotberg, R. I. (2014). Good governance means performance and results. *Governance, 27*(3), 511–518.

Russ-Eft, D., & Preskill, H. (2009). *Evaluation in organizations: A systematic approach to enhancing learning, performance, and change*. Basic Books.

Russell, E. W. (2010). The "obsolescence" of assessment procedures. *Applied Neuropsychology, 17*(1), 60–67.

Ryan, K., & Cousins, J. B. (Eds.). (2009). *The SAGE international handbook of educational evaluation*. SAGE.

Santos, M. (1997). Portfolio-based assessment. In P. Butler. (Ed.), *Issues in alternative assessment: The Japanese perspective* (pp. 23–49). Kwansei Gaikun University, Nishinomiya. Language Center.

Sarafian, A. J. (2020). *Development and validation of an observational tool to evaluate upper extremity functioning or hand-object interaction for children diagnosed with bilateral cerebral palsy GMFCS III, IV, and V.* Unpublished doctoral dissertation, Teachers College, Columbia University.

Sattler, J. M. (1988). *Assessment of children*. Author.

Scavone, B. M., Toledo, P., Higgins, N., Wojciechowski, K., & McCarthy, R. J. (2010). A randomized controlled trial of the impact of simulation-based training on resident performance during a simulated obstetric anesthesia emergency. *Simulation in Healthcare, 5*(6), 320–324.

Schmeiser, C. B., & Welch, C. J. (2006). Test development. In R. L. Brennan (Ed.), *Educational measurement* (4th ed., 307–353). American Council on Education.

Schmidt, F. L., & Hunter, J. E. (1977). Development of a general solution to the problem of validity generalization. *Journal of Applied Psychology, 62*(5), 529.

Schölmerich, V. L., & Kawachi, I. (2016). Translating the socio-ecological perspective into multilevel interventions: Gaps between theory and practice. *Health Education & Behavior, 43*(1), 17–20.

Scriven, M. (1991). *Evaluation thesaurus* (4th ed.). SAGE.

Sedera, D., & Gable, G. G. (2010). Knowledge management competence for enterprise system success. *Journal of Strategic Information Systems, 19*(4), 296–306.

Shavelson, R. J., Webb, N. M., & Rowley, G. L. (1989). Generalizability theory. *American Psychologist, 44*(6), 922.

Shaw, E. J., & McKenzie, E. (2010). *The National SAT Validity Study: Sharing results from recent college success results.* College Board.

Shea, S. C. (2017). *Psychiatric interviewing: The art of understanding* (3rd ed.). Elsevier.

Shepard, L. A. (1989). Identification of mild handicaps. In R. L. Linn (Ed.), *Educational measurement* (pp. 13–103). American Council on Education.

Shepard, L. A. (2000). *The role of assessment in teaching and learning.* CRESST/CREDE, University of California, Los Angeles.

Shepard, L. A. (2006). Classroom assessment. In R. L. Brennan (Ed.), *Educational measurement* (4th ed., pp. 623–646). ACE/Praeger.

Shepard, L. A. (2013). Validity for what purpose? *Teachers College Record, 115*(9), 1–12.

Siegler, R. S. (2021). *Children's thinking.* Pearson.

Sireci, S. G. (2021). NCME presidential address 2020: Valuing educational measurement. *Educational Measurement: Issues and Practice, 40*(1), 7–16.

Sireci, S. G., & Faulkner-Bond, M. (2015). Promoting validity in the assessment of English learners. *Review of Research in Education, 39*(1), 215–252.

Sireci, S. G., Wells, C. S., & Keller, L. A. (2016). *Why we should abandon student growth percentiles* (Research Brief 16-1). Center for Educational Assessment, University of Massachusetts Amherst. www.umass.edu/remp/pdf/CEAResearchBrief-16-1_WhyWeShouldAbandonSGPs.pdf.

Sirin, S. R. (2005). Socioeconomic status and academic achievement: A meta-analytic review of research. *Review of Educational Research, 75*(3), 417–453.

Sloutsky, V. M. (2010). Mechanisms of cognitive development: Domain-general learning or domain-specific constraints? *Cognitive Science, 34*(7), 1125–1130.

Smarter Balanced Assessment Consortium. (2018). *Sample questions.* www.smarterbalanced.org/assessments/sample-questions.

Smedley, B. D., Stith, A. Y., & Nelson, A. R. (Eds.). (2003). *Unequal treatment: Confronting racial and ethnic disparities in health care.* National Academies Press.

Smith, E. R., & Tyler, R. W. (1942). *Appraising and recording student progress.* Harper.

Smith, G. (2005). Communication skills are critical for internal auditors. *Managerial Auditing Journal, 20*(5), 513–519.

Spies, R. A., & Plake, B. S. (2003). *The sixteenth mental measurements yearbook.* Buros Center, University of Nebraska, Lincoln.

Stake, R. E. (2015). *Multiple case study analysis.* Guilford Press.

Stanley, J. C. (1971). Reliability. In R. L. Thorndike (Ed.), *Educational measurement* (2nd ed., pp. 359–442). American Council on Education.

Steele, J. L., Hamilton, L. S., & Stecher, B. M. (2010). *Incorporating student performance measures into teacher evaluation systems.* RAND Corporation.

Sternberg, R. J. (2003). What is an "expert student?" *Educational Researcher, 32*(8), 5–9.

Sternberg, R. J. (2018). The triarchic theory of successful intelligence. In D. P. Flanagan & E. M. McDonough (Eds.), *Contemporary intellectual assessment: Theories, tests, and issues* (pp. 174–194). Guilford Press.

Sterne, J. A., White, I. R., Carlin, J. B., Spratt, M., Royston, P., Kenward, M. G., . . . Carpenter, J. R. (2009). Multiple imputation for missing data in epidemiological and clinical research: Potential and pitfalls. *British Medical Journal, 338*, 2393.

Stevens, S. S. (1946). On the theory of scales of measurement. *Science, 103*, 677–680.

Stevens, S. S. (1951). Mathematics, measurement, and psychophysics. In S. S. Stevens (Ed.), *Handbook of experimental psychology* (pp. 1–49). Wiley.

Stevens, S. S. (1968). Measurement, statistics and the schemapiric view. *Science, 161*, 849–856.

Stiggins, R. J. (2002). Assessment crisis: The absence of assessment for learning. *Phi Delta Kappan, 83*(10), 758–765.

Still, B., & Crane, K. (2017). *Fundamentals of user-centered design: A practical approach.* CRC Press.

Strachan, T., Cho, U. H., Kim, K. Y., Willse, J. T., Chen, S. H., Ip, E. H., . . . Weeks, J. P. (2020). Using a projection IRT method for vertical scaling when construct shift is present. *Journal of Educational Measurement, 58*(2), 211–235.

Student, S. R. (2022). Vertical scales, deceleration, and empirical benchmarks for growth. *Educational Researcher, 51*(8), 536–543.

Taylor, H. C., & Russell, J. T. (1939). The relationship of validity coefficients to the practical effectiveness of tests in selection: Discussion and tables. *Journal of Applied Psychology, 23*(5), 565.

Taylor, W. L. (1953). Cloze procedure: A new tool for measuring readability. *Journalism Quarterly, 30*, 415–433.

Teachers College, Columbia University. (2021, May 13). *Rebuilding assessment to help students learn.* www.tc.columbia.edu/articles/2021/may/rebuilding-assessment-to-help-students-learn.

Thissen-Roe, A., Hunt, E., & Minstrell, J. (2004). Combining assessment and learning. *Behavior Research Methods, Instruments, & Computers, 36*(2), 234–240.

Thomson Reuters. (2018, September 8). *Thomson Reuters D&I Index ranks the 2018 Top 100 most diverse and inclusive organizations globally.* www.thomsonreuters.com/en/press-releases/2018.

Thorndike, E. L. (1918). The nature, purposes and general methods of measurement of educational products. *The seventeenth yearbook of the National Society for the Study of Education.* Public School Publishing Company.

Thorndike, R. L. (1971). Educational measurement for the seventies. In R. L. Thorndike (Ed.), *Educational measurement* (2nd ed., pp. 3–14). American Council on Education.

Thorndike, R. M. (1990). Origins of intelligence and its measurement. *Journal of Psychoeducational Assessment, 8*(3), 223–230.

Thorndike, R. M. (1997). *Measurement and evaluation in education and psychology* (6th ed.). Merrill.

Thornton, G. C., & Byham, W. C. (1982). *Assessment centers and managerial performance*. Academic Press.

Thurstone, L. L. (1930). A scale for measuring attitude toward the movies. *Journal of Educational Research, 22*(2), 89–94.

Thurstone, L. L. (1959). *The measurement of values.* University of Chicago Press.

Thurstone, L. L., & Chave, E. J. (1929). *The measurement of attitude*. University of Chicago Press.

Tryon, R. C. (1957). Reliability and behavior domain validity: Reformulation and historical critique. *Psychological Bulletin, 54*(3), 229.

Twain, M. (1876/1996). *The adventures of Tom Sawyer and Huckleberry Finn.* Thomas Nelson.

Tyack, D. B. (1974). *The one best system: A history of American urban education* (Vol. 95). Harvard University Press.

Tyler, R. W. (1949). *Basic principles of curriculum and instruction*. University of Chicago Press.

Tyler, R. W. (1951). The function of measurement in improving instruction. In E. F. Lindquist (Ed.), *Educational measurement.* ACE.

University of California. (2020, January). *Report of the UC Academic Council Standardized Testing Task Force (STTF).* UC, Systemwide Academic Senate. https://senate.universityofcalifornia.edu/committees/sttf/reports.html.

U.S. Department of Education. (2015). *Every Student Succeeds Act.* www.ed.gov/essa?src=rn.

U.S. Department of Education. (2017). *Every Student Succeeds Act—Accountability, state plans and data reporting: Summary of final regulations.* www2.ed.gov/policy/elsec/leg/essa/essafactsheet170103.pdf.

Vacha-Haase, T. (1998). Reliability generalization: Exploring variance in measurement error affecting score reliability across studies. *Educational and Psychological Measurement, 58*(1), 6–20.

Valentino, R. A., & Reardon, S. F. (2015). Effectiveness of four instructional programs designed to serve English learners: Variation by ethnicity and initial English proficiency. *Educational Evaluation and Policy Analysis, 37*(4), 612–637.

VandenBos, G. R. (2007). *APA dictionary of psychology.* American Psychological Association.

Von Davier, A. (2013). Standardized assessments and implications for improving test and sampling design: Applying Kane's principles for validation. In M. Chatterji (Ed.), *Validity and test use: An international dialogue on educational assessment, accountability and equity* (pp. 55–67). Emerald Group.

Wagemaker, H. (2013), International large scale assessment (ILSA) programs and the challenges of consequential validity. In M. Chatterji (Ed.), *Validity and test use: An international dialogue on educational assessment, accountability and equity* (pp. 217–231). Emerald Group.

Walsh, B. W., & Betz, N. E. (2001). *Tests and assessment* (4th ed.). Prentice Hall.

Waltz, C. F., & Bausell, R. B. (1981). *Nursing research: Design, statistics, and computer analysis*. F.A. Davis.

Ward, A., Stoker, H. W., & Murray-Ward, M. (1996). *Educational measurement: Theories and applications* (Vol. 2). University Press of America.

Wechsler, D. (1989). *Wechsler Preschool and Primary Scale of Intelligence—Revised.* Psychological Corporation.

Wiersma, J. D., Cleveland, H. H., Herrera, V., & Fischer, J. L. (2010). Intimate partner violence in young adult dating, cohabitating, and married drinking partnerships. *Journal of Marriage and Family, 72*(2), 360–374.

Wiggins, G. (1989). Teaching to the (authentic) test. *Educational Leadership, 46*(1), 41–47.

Wiggins, G. (2011). A true test: Toward more authentic and equitable assessment. *Phi Delta Kappan, 92*(7), 81–93.

Wiliam, D., & Thompson, M. (2007). Integrating assessment with instruction: What will it take to make it work? In C. A. Dwyer (Ed.), *The future of assessment: Shaping teaching and learning* (pp. 53–82). Erlbaum.

Willcox, W. F. (1934). Note on the chronology of statistical societies. *Journal of the American Statistical Association, 29*, 418–420.

Wren, D. G., & Benson, J. (2004). Measuring test anxiety in children: Scale development and internal construct validation. *Anxiety, Stress, and Coping, 17*(3), 227–240.

Wright, B. D., & Masters, G. N. (1982). *Rating scale analysis*. MESA Press.

Wright, B. D., & Stone, M. H. (1979). *Best test design*. Rasch Measurement.

Wundt, W. (1873/1948). Principles of physiological psychology. In W. Dennis (Ed.), *Readings in the history of psychology* (pp. 248–250). Appleton-Century-Crofts.

Wyer, P. W., & Chatterji, M. (2013). Designing outcome measures for the accreditation of medical education programs as an iterative process combining classical test theory and Rasch measurement. *International Journal of Educational and Psychological Assessment, 13*(2), 35–61.

Yarbrough, D. B., Caruthers, F. A., Shulha, L. M., & Hopson, R. K. (2011). *The program evaluation standards: A guide for evaluators and evaluation users* (3rd ed.). SAGE.

Yen, W. M., & Fitzpatrick, A. R. (2006). Item response theory. In R. L. Brennan (Ed.), *Educational measurement* (pp. 111–153). American Council of Education.

Author Index

B

C

D

E

F

G

H

I

J

K

L

M

T

V

W

Y

Z

Subject Index

Note. *b*, *f*, or *t* following a page number indicates a box, figure, or table

B

C

T

U

W

X

Z

About the Author

Madhabi Chatterji, PhD, is Professor Emerita of Measurement, Evaluation, and Education at Teachers College, Columbia University, where she founded the Assessment and Evaluation Research Initiative (AERI). AERI is dedicated to promoting meaningful use of assessment and evaluation information to improve equity and the quality of practices and policies in education, psychology, and the health professions. An award-winning, internationally recognized methodologist and educationist, Dr. Chatterji has taught and mentored numerous doctoral students and postdoctoral researchers over her 30-plus-year career. She is author or editor of more than 100 publications and is a Fellow of the National Education Policy Center. A public intellectual, Dr. Chatterji has spoken out frequently on the limitations of large-scale tests and the adverse social consequences of misused high-stakes educational assessments. Her longstanding scholarly interests lie in instrument design, validation, validity, and test use issues; improving program and policy evaluation designs to support evidence-based practices; and closing learning gaps with proximal diagnostic assessments.